Age has been identified as the strongest risk factor for Alzheimer's disease, and is also strongly associated with the cerebrovascular risk factors for vascular dementia. When a disorder is so strikingly age dependent, it is appropriate to examine its relationship to normal aging, and this book is based on the premise that the challenge of dementia lies in establishing its true relationship with normal aging.

The traditional disease model which regards dementia as categorically distinct from the normal aging process may have obscured important clues about the underlying causes of dementia, its frequency, course, management and social consequences. With contributions from leading neurobiologists, psychologists, clinicians and epidemiologists, this book makes an important contribution to the understanding of these and other aspects of dementia by reappraising the latest research in the light of the continuity model, which proposes that dementia lies along a continuum with normal aging. In examining the evidence for and against the continuum and disease models of dementia, most of the discussion concentrates on the relationship between Alzheimer's disease and normal aging, with other subtypes of dementia also being considered. Ranging from molecular genetics and fundamental neuro-biology to issues of diagnosis and the provision of services, this is a challenging work in its breadth and in the level of its argument, which has far-reaching implications for the study of dementia and, indeed, of the mind itself.

As a review of current thinking and research, it will serve as an essential text for clinicians and scientific investigators, and it will also stimulate further enquiry and debate in areas as diverse as research strategy, treatment and prevention, social attitudes and health policy.

Dementia and normal aging

Dementia and normal aging

EDITED BY

Felicia A. Huppert

Lecturer in the Psychology of Aging, Department of Psychiatry, University of Cambridge, UK

Carol Brayne

Lecturer in Epidemiology and Honorary Consultant in Public Health Medicine, Department of Community Medicine, University of Cambridge, UK

Daniel W. O'Connor

Professor of Psychogeriatrics, Department of Psychological Medicine, Monash University, Melbourne, Australia

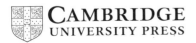

CAMBRIDGE
UNIVERSITY PRESS

Published by the Press Syndicate of the University of Cambridge
The Pitt Building, Trumpington Street, Cambridge CB2 1RP
40 West 20th Street, New York, NY 10011-4211, USA
10 Stamford Road, Oakleigh, Melbourne 3166, Australia

First published 1994

Printed in Great Britain at
the University Press, Cambridge

A catalogue record for this book is available from the British Library

Library of Congress cataloguing in publication data

Dementia and normal aging / edited by Felicia A. Huppert, Carol
    Brayne, Daniel W. O'Connor.
        p. cm.
    Includes index.
    ISBN 0-521-41393-1(hc)
    1. Senile dementia.   2. Brain – Aging.   3. Alzheimer's disease.
4. Dementia.   I. Huppert, Felicia A.   II. Brayne, Carol.
III. O'Connor, D. W. (Daniel W.)
    [DNLM: 1. Dementia.   2. Age Factors.   3. Aging.   4. Dementia,
Senile.   WT 150 D3755 1994]
RC523.D46   1994
616.89'83 – dc20
DNLM/DLC
for Library of Congress 93-745 CIP

ISBN 0 521 41393 1 hardback

RO

Contents

List of contributors   x

Foreword   E. S. Paykel   xiv

Preface   F. A. Huppert   xv

Acknowledgement   xvi

PART I   Introduction

1   What is the relationship between dementia and normal
aging?   3
F. A. Huppert and C. Brayne

PART II   The development of contemporary views of dementia

2   Dementia and aging since the nineteenth century   15
G. E. Berrios
3   The history of research into dementia and its
relationship to current concepts   41
W. A. Lishman
4   The relationship between dementia and normal aging
of the brain   57
Sir Martin Roth

PART III   The diagnosis of dementia today

5   International criteria and differential diagnosis   79
A. S. Henderson and N. Sartorius

6   Mild dementia: a clinical perspective   91
     D. W. O'Connor
7   Neurological aspects of dementia and normal aging   118
     J. R. Hodges
8   Imaging and dementia   130
     C. E. L. Freer

PART IV   Research methodology and population studies

9   How common are cognitive impairment and dementia?
     An epidemiological viewpoint   167
     C. Brayne
10   What are the risk factors for dementia?   208
     J. A. Mortimer
11   How do risk factors for dementia relate to current
     theories on mechanisms of aging?   230
     T. B. L. Kirkwood
12   A method for measuring dementia as a continuum in
     community surveys   244
     A. F. Jorm

PART V   Behaviour and cognition in dementia and normal aging

13   The meaning of dementia to those involved as carers   257
     P. A. Pollitt
14   Personality and behaviour in dementia and normal
     aging   272
     T. Hope
15   Memory function in dementia and normal aging –
     dimension or dichotomy?   291
     F. A. Huppert
16   Language in dementia and normal aging   331
     D. Kempler and E. M. Zelinski
17   Visuospatial dysfunction in dementia and normal aging   366
     J. V. Filoteo, D. C. Delis, P. J. Massman and N. Butters

PART VI   Neurobiology of dementia and normal aging

18   Dementia and normal aging: neuropathology   385
     M. Esiri
19   Cholinergic component of dementia and aging   437
     E. K. Perry, J. A. Court, M. A. Piggott and R. H. Perry
20   Molecular characterization of the neurodegenerative
     changes which distinguish normal aging from
     Alzheimer's disease   470
     C. Wischik, C. Harrington and E. B. Mukaetova-Ladinska
21   Genetic linkage in Alzheimer's disease   492
     S.-J. Richards and C. van Broeckhoven

PART VII   Health care and social policy issues

22   Health-care policy and planning for dementia: an
     international perspective   519
     B. Cooper
23   Public health implications of a continuum model of
     dementia   552
     K.-T. Khaw

     Index   561

Contributors

GERMAN E. BERRIOS
Department of Psychiatry, Box 189, Addenbrooke's Hospital, Hills Road, Cambridge CB2 2QQ, UK

CAROL BRAYNE
Department of Community Medicine, Institute of Public Health, Forvie Site, Robinson Way, Cambridge CB2 2SR, UK

NELSON BUTTERS
Psychology Service (116B), Department of Veterans Affairs Medical Center, 3350 La Jolla Village Drive, San Diego,CA 92161, USA

BRIAN COOPER
Department of Old Age Psychiatry, Institute of Psychiatry, De Crespigny Park, Denmark Hill, London SE5 8AF, UK

JENNIFER A. COURT
MRC Neurochemical Pathology Unit, Newcastle General Hospital, Westgate Road, Newcastle upon Tyne NE4 6BE, UK

DEAN C. DELIS
University of California, San Diego, School of Medicine, Psychology Service (116B), Department of Veterans Affairs Medical Center, 3350 La Jolla Village Drive, San Diego, CA 92161, USA

MARGARET M. ESIRI
Departments of Clinical Neurology and Neuropathology, Radcliffe Infirmary, Oxford OX2 6HE, UK

J. VINCENT FILOTEO
University of California, San Diego, School of Medicine, Psychology Service (116B), Department of Veterans Affairs Medical Center, 3350 La Jolla Village Drive, San Diego, CA 92161, USA

CHARLES E. L. FREER
Department of Radiology and MRIS Unit, Box 219, Addenbrooke's Hospital, Hills Road, Cambridge CB2 2QQ, UK

CHARLES R. HARRINGTON
Cambridge Brain Bank Laboratory, Department of Psychiatry, University of Cambridge, MRC Centre, Hills Road, Cambridge CB2 2QH, UK

A. S. HENDERSON
National Health and Medical Research Council Social Psychiatry Research Unit, The Australian National University, Canberra ACT 0200, Australia

JOHN R. HODGES
Neurology Department, Box 165, Addenbrooke's Hospital, Hills Road, Cambridge CB2 2QQ, UK

TONY HOPE
Department of Psychiatry, University of Oxford, Warneford Hospital, Oxford OX3 7JX, UK

FELICIA A. HUPPERT
Department of Psychiatry, Box 189, Addenbrooke's Hospital, Hills Road, Cambridge CB2 2QQ, UK

ANTHONY F. JORM
National Health and Medical Research Council Social Psychiatry Research Unit, The Australian National University, Canberra ACT 0200, Australia

DANIEL KEMPLER
Department of Otolaryngology, Director, Speech Pathology, (OPD-2P52), 1175 N. Cummings Street, Los Angeles, CA 90033, USA

KAY-TEE KHAW
Clinical Gerontology Unit, University of Cambridge, Level 2, Addenbrooke's Hospital, Hills Road, Cambridge CB2 2QQ, UK

THOMAS B. L. KIRKWOOD
Department of Geriatric Medicine and School of Biological Sciences, University of Manchester, Stopford Building, Oxford Road, Manchester M13 9PT, UK

WILLIAM ALWYN LISHMAN
Institute of Psychiatry, De Crespigny Park, Denmark Hill, London SE5 8AF, UK

PAUL J. MASSMAN
Department of Psychology, University of Houston, 4800 Calhoun Drive, Houston, TX 77204, USA

JAMES A. MORTIMER
Geriatric Research, Education and Clinical Center (11G), Veteran's
Affairs Medical Center, Minneapolis, MN 55417, USA

ELIZABETA B. MUKAETOVA-LADINSKA
Cambridge Brain Bank Laboratory, Department of Psychiatry,
University of Cambridge, MRC Centre, Hills Road, Cambridge
CB2 2QH, UK

DANIEL W. O'CONNOR
Department of Psychological Medicine, Heatherton Hospital,
Kingston Road, Heatherton, Victoria 3202, Australia

ELAINE K. PERRY
MRC Neurochemical Pathology Unit, Newcastle General Hospital,
Westgate Road, Newcastle upon Tyne NE4 6BE, UK

ROBERT H. PERRY
Department of Neuropathology, Newcastle General Hospital,
Westgate Road, Newcastle upon Tyne NE4 6BE, UK

MARGARET A. PIGGOTT
MRC Neurochemical Pathology Unit, Newcastle General Hospital,
Westgate Road, Newcastle upon Tyne NE4 6BE, UK

PENELOPE A. POLLITT
National Health and Medical Research Council Social Psychiatry
Research Unit, The Australian National University, Canberra, ACT
0200, Australia

SARAH-JANE RICHARDS
Department of Medicine, Box 157, Addenbrooke's Hospital, Hills
Road, Cambridge CB2 2QQ, UK

SIR MARTIN ROTH
Trinity College, Cambridge CB2 1TQ, UK

NORMAN SARTORIUS
Department of Psychiatry, University of Geneva, Centre
Psychosocial, Boulevard St Georges, 16–18 Geneva, Switzerland

CHRISTINE VAN BROECKHOVEN
Neurogenetics Laboratory, Department of Biochemistry, University
of Antwerp, Universitetsplein 1, B-2610 Antwerp, Belgium

CLAUDE M. WISCHIK
Cambridge Brain Bank Laboratory, Department of Psychiatry,
University of Cambridge, MRC Centre, Hills Road, Cambridge
CB2 2QH, UK

ELIZABETH M. ZELINSKI
The Leonard Davis School of Gerontology, University of South California, University Park, Los Angeles, California 90089-0191, USA

Foreword

This is a time of awareness of aging. Never before has such a large proportion of the population, at least in developed countries, survived to middle age and beyond. Becoming elderly is now a long-term expectation for an adult.

It is usual to undergo some impairment of memory as we become older. Most of us notice occasional difficulty in remembering names of people, by middle age. Memory loss is expected in old age, as the vignettes from carers by Pollitt in this volume attest.

Dementia, with severe impairment of intellectual and other functions, also becomes increasingly common in old age. Prevalence rates double approximately every five years, over the age of 60. Some forms of dementia are due to rare specific diseases, and considerably more is a result of cerebral atherosclerosis, but the largest proportion is due to Alzheimer's disease. But is dementia, and particularly Alzheimer's disease, really a specific disease or is it an extension of the normal phenomena of aging, perhaps even an inevitable consequence if we were to survive even longer? This question bears in a fundamental way on the nature of the disorder, its causes, possible treatments and the best approaches to its prevention.

This is the problem which this book sets out to examine, but it does so in the context of a much broader discussion of dementia and cognitive and other aspects of normal aging. All editors have undertaken major population studies of dementia in Cambridge, where two are currently University Lecturers and the third was formerly a Research Fellow. They have assembled an eminent team of authors who have comprehensively examined recent developments in the field. I commend this excellent volume to all those whose research interests or therapeutic and caring endeavours lie in cognitive impairments in the elderly.

Eugene Paykel
Professor of Psychiatry
University of Cambridge
Addenbrooke's Hospital
Cambridge CB2 2QQ, UK

Preface

This book is based on the premise that the challenge of dementia lies in establishing the true relationship between dementia and normal aging. The medical model assumes that elderly people are either demented or cognitively normal, while recognising that the distinction is not always easy to make. While this approach has been valuable for promoting research and providing services, it may have obscured important clues about the underlying causes of dementia, and about its frequency, course, management and social implications.

The continuity model is based on the observation that most of the variables associated with dementia fall along a continuum with normal aging. The continuum includes cognitive functioning, neuropathology and neurochemistry, including changes which are the hallmarks of Alzheimer's disease. We believe the understanding of dementia will be advanced by reappraisal of the latest research in the light of the continuity model.

The book includes contributions from a wide range of disciplines. Most authors focus on the relationship between normal aging and dementia of the Alzheimer's type (DAT), since this is the area in which research has been most abundant. However, consideration is also given to the relationship between normal aging and vascular forms of dementia, frontal dementia, dementia of the Lewy body type and other forms of dementia.

By understanding the fundamental relationship of aging and dementia, we will also come closer to elucidating the causes and implications of decline in the population. This understanding has far-reaching implications, including the possibility of prevention or reduction of cognitive decline. By applying preventive measures to the whole population, not only may we stop dementia from occurring in small groups of individuals, but we may improve functioning in the whole aging community.

F.A.H.

Acknowledgement

We are most grateful to Mrs Julie Aston for her role in collating, proofreading and correcting the manuscript, which she undertook with patience and good humour.

PART I

Introduction

1

What is the relationship between dementia and normal aging?

FELICIA A. HUPPERT AND CAROL BRAYNE

Dementia is predominantly a disorder of later life, with its prevalence and incidence rising sharply with advancing age. Age has been identified as the strongest risk factor for Alzheimer's disease, the most prevalent form of dementia in most studies. Age is also associated strongly with the cerebrovascular risk factors for vascular dementia. When a disorder is so strikingly age-dependent, it is appropriate to examine its relationship to normal aging.

There are numerous biopathological and cognitive–behavioural changes which are associated with normal aging, and many of these are the same as changes attributed to the dementias. This observation can lend itself to two opposing interpretations. One is that researchers have not yet identified those changes which are unique to the dementias, because the changes observed are confounded with age-related changes. The other is that normal aging and dementia form a continuum, the changes differing in degree but not in kind.

Two conclusions would follow if there was a continuity between normal aging and dementia. One is that the diagnosis of dementia, at least in the mild or early stage, would be particularly difficult to make among individuals who have reached advanced old age. Certainly it is the case that both doctors and lay people are likely to 'excuse away' the memory loss and other cognitive changes of individuals aged 90 years and above. Indeed, the widely accepted NINCDS–ADRDA criteria for the diagnosis of Alzheimer's disease (McKhann et al., 1984) state specifically that onset must be between age 40 years and 90 years. This can be regarded as a tacit recognition that the changes seen in advanced old age merge with dementia.

It should also follow from the continuum hypothesis that everyone who lives long enough will develop dementia. This conclusion is more

Dementia and Normal Aging, eds. F. A. Huppert, C. Brayne & D. W. O'Connor. © Cambridge University Press 1994.

difficult to verify, partly because the relevant age has not been specified. However, if one extrapolates the age-specific prevalence figures
provided by Katzman & Saitoh (1991), everyone should have Alzheimer's disease by 100 years of age (Figure 1.1). However, we know
that many centenarians do not have dementia and a linear extrapolation along these axes may not be appropriate (Dewey, 1991).

The issue of whether dementia should be regarded as a disease
distinct from the normal aging process, or whether it is part of the
normal aging process, is not merely of academic interest. It has implications for research strategy, for treatment and prevention, and for

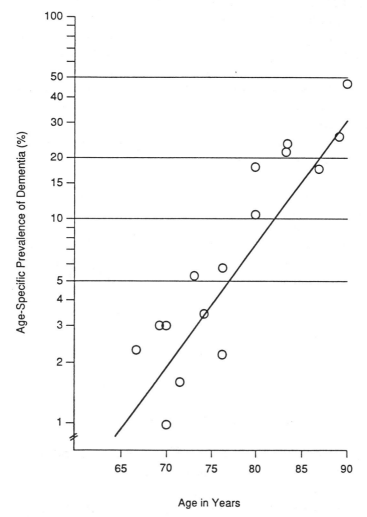

Figure 1.1. Age-specific prevalence of dementia. (From Katzman & Saitoh, 1991.)

social attitudes and social policy. If dementia and normal aging lie along a continuum, then research strategies which seek to understand the nature or aetiology of dementia are bound to fail if they do not also examine representative samples of elderly people. Furthermore, if dementia is virtually universal among the increasing numbers of the very old, treatment of the entire aged population would presumably be impractical and the need to search for preventive factors would become more urgent.

In recognition of the importance of examining this theoretical issue, we have invited researchers from a wide variety of disciplines to review their area of expertise in the context of whether the data best fit the conventional view that dementia is a disease categorically distinct from normal aging, or whether dementia and normal aging fall along a continuum. Since most information is available about dementia of the Alzheimer's type (DAT), most of the discussion concentrates on the relationship between DAT and normal aging, but other subtypes of dementia and their relationship to normal aging are considered in several of the chapters.

The debate about whether there is continuity or discontinuity between normal aging and dementia has a long history. Berrios (Chapter 2) places the debate firmly in its historical context, citing opposing views going back to classical times. More recently, it appears that Alzheimer (1907) supported a continuity view while Kraepelin (1919) supported discontinuity, and it was the latter whose view prevailed for much of this century. However, as Berrios points out, the debate could only be settled once there was a scientific framework to carry out the pertinent tests and stipulations to decide what evidence is to be taken as valid.

In this chapter, we draw together the latest research findings and methodological advances to judge whether a continuity model or a discontinuity model best describes the relationship between normal aging and dementia.

Evidence favouring the continuum model

A continuum model suggests that dementia is at one extreme of a distribution of normal aging. It is based on the observation that advancing age is associated with increasing functional impairment and disability (Chapters 13 to 17) and decline in physiological, pathological and neurochemical measures (Chapter 11 and Chapters 18 to 20). As

Kirkwood points out (Chapter 11), this process is 'normal' and yet by its very nature involves the production of abnormality. The continuum hypothesis suggests that a small amount of functional change in life is related to a small degree of pathology, and larger amounts of functional change are related to larger degrees of pathology.

Increasing age is also associated with increasing diversity, including an increasing range of performance on cognitive tests (Chapter 15), and an increasing heterogeneity in physiological function and a gradual broadening of cell phenotypes (Chapter 11). This increase in diversity is an additional reason why the distinctions between normality and abnormality become harder to make with advancing age. This creates difficulties for the establishment of diagnostic criteria (Chapter 5) and for the practising clinician (Chapters 6 and 8).

The fact that all aged individuals show decline is not to deny that some show very little, while others deteriorate to a marked extent. When changes along a continuum reach the point where the help of a clinician is sought, it may be 'linguistically convenient' (Storandt et al., 1988, p. 232) to speak of the individual as diseased, but, as Storandt and her colleagues point out, such categories tend to take on a life of their own. They suggest that any distinction between normal aging and dementia is arbitrary, because it is based on a cutoff along a continuum which could be placed at many different points. Jorm (Chapter 12) proposes a method for deciding when to apply the label 'dementia', by using regression analysis to calculate the expected cognitive score for an individual, based on their premorbid ability and diagnostically relevant variables, such as symptoms of depression and delirium. Departures of the deserved cognitive score from the expected score are regarded as a measure of dementia.

Consistent with the continuum hypothesis is the lack of any evidence of qualitative differences between individuals with mild dementia and the normal elderly in terms of cognitive performance (Chapters 15 to 17) or neurobiological measures (Chapters 18 to 20). Where dramatic quantitative differences are seen this appears to be due to problems in sample selection, where well-established cases (i.e. with moderate or severe dementia) are compared with selected controls, rather than with a representative elderly sample (e.g. Chapters 16, 18 and 20).

The situation is more complicated if we consider the changes in behaviour which are seen in dementia. While many aspects of personality and behavioural change in dementia may be exaggerations of changes seen in the normal elderly population, some appear to be restricted to dementia (e.g. wandering, aggressiveness not consistent with premorbid personality). However, Hope (Chapter 14) concludes that behaviour which appears to be phenomenologically different from what is seen in normal aging, does not provide evidence against the continuum hypothesis. For example, a person might wander off and get lost only when spatial ability falls below a particular level of functioning; that is, behaviour may change suddenly (qualitatively) but as a result of continuous changes in both the pathology and cognitive function. Similar considerations may apply to some neurological signs which seem to be restricted to dementia, such as myoclonus or epilepsy (Chapter 7). These are clearly abnormal, but may result from continuous changes in the underlying pathology.

Evidence favouring a disease model

The discontinuity or disease/normality model suggests that the dementias are discrete disorders, clearly distinguishable from normality. Fundamental to the ability to examine this hypothesis is the identification of valid and reliable markers for each disease process. Such markers would be associated with qualitative differences between each subtype of dementia and the normal aging process, or at the very least with large quantitative differences; a bimodality of distribution of the relevant variables should be observed in large enough community samples. The search for functional or pathological markers has not yet produced any such measures for DAT, which can be applied to the community, still less for other types of dementia. No definite qualitative differences have yet been found (see above), and all potential markers which have been investigated to date in living patients reveal overlap with age- and sex-matched controls. The post-mortem studies which reveal extreme differences in pathology and chemistry for groups of demented patients and controls are based on highly selected case series and are therefore biased. Indeed, it would be surprising if such differences were not seen with such selected samples, even if the variables were known to be continuous.

Other evidence which has been advanced in favour of the disease model for DAT is that the neurobiological changes are specific and localized and that dementia appears almost invariably once pathology has exceeded a threshold (Chapter 4); also that DAT can affect individuals in middle age, when age-associated decline has not yet had the opportunity to express itself (Chapters 4 and 18). The specificity and localization of DAT changes has been well established but the data at present suggest that the same specificity and localization apply to the normal aging process (Chapters 18 and 19). The observation of threshold effects in dementia (e.g. Blessed et al., 1968) is not incompatible with the notion of an underlying continuum, since pathology is associated with disability on a probabilistic basis. Not everyone with a given amount of pathology shows the clinical syndrome of dementia, and not everyone with dementia appears to have a given amount of pathology.

Mortimer's elegant model (Chapter 10) links the concepts of a continuum and a disease threshold by employing the hypothetical construct of reserve capacity. The threshold corresponds to an amount of brain tissue below which normal function cannot be sustained. Brain reserve capacity is hypothesized to decrease steadily with age, so that among elderly people only a small change is required to tip them over the threshold of dementia. In addition, variation in the age of onset of dementia is explained in terms of individual differences in reserve capacity which may be present from birth (as in Down's syndrome) or altered by environmental influences (e.g. head trauma). Onset of Alzheimer's disease in middle age is attributed to reduced reserve capacity resulting from familial/genetic factors which may be evident at birth, and/or to an increased susceptibility to environmentally produced decreases in brain reserve. Thus, according to this model, the existence of pre-senile Alzheimer's disease does not necessarily constitute evidence in support of the disease model.

Although attractive as the idea of reserve capacity is, it remains a hypothetical entity, for which we do not have direct evidence at present. What appears to be irrefutable, however, is that in a few families where a mutation can be confirmed as causative of Alzheimer's disease (see Richards & van Broeckhoven, Chapter 21), the disorder is distinct from normal aging. But even in this case, the fact that the disorder takes a minimum of 35–40 years to become manifest, leaves open the possibility of complex interactions with environmental variables, head trauma, etc. Moreover, Richards & van Broeckhoven discuss the increasing evidence for heterogeneous aetiology in DAT and the likelihood that abnormal cellular processing may be influenced by a range of age-related events.

Although there is little data at the present time to support the dichotomous disease/normality model for the majority of cases of DAT, we can ask whether the same is true for other age-related forms of dementia. In many case series, vascular dementia is the second most common form of dementia after DAT. Vascular dementia may have an abrupt onset, following a stroke. A stroke is clearly a discrete event which can be regarded as changing the individual from a healthy to a diseased state. Thus, vascular dementia appears to be a good candidate for the disease model. However as Brayne (Chapter 9) and Freer (Chapter 8) point out, a clinically significant stroke may be on a continuum with the micro-infarcts or leucoariosis seen commonly in the normal elderly, and these changes are correlated with cognitive impairment (Chapter 8).

Khaw (Chapter 23) discusses the well-known relationship between blood pressure, which exhibits a normal distribution in the population, and stroke. She draws attention to the evidence that the incidence of stroke is related to the level of blood pressure in the population. The higher the blood pressure levels, the greater the incidence of stroke. This is a clear example where a disease which appears to be either clinically present or absent, such as stroke, is related to an underlying continuum of risk, such as blood pressure. Other examples include coronary heart disease, blood cholesterol level and saturated fat intake, as well as lung cancer and level of cigarette smoking in the population. In all these cases the 'disease' appears following the progressive accumulation of adverse biological changes. Thus vascular dementia, like DAT and other medical conditions, is perhaps best thought of as a useful label to apply once a certain threshold of disability or pathological change has been passed. Ongoing population studies will establish the extent to which the clinical and neurobiological variables characterizing vascular dementia fall along a continuum.

Even less is known about other forms of dementia such as Lewy body dementia or Pick's disease. Perry et al. (Chapter 19) reports that the pathological changes characteristic of Lewy body dementia overlap with normal aging, but the definitive population studies have yet to be done. The selective lobar atrophy characteristic of Pick's disease is an unlikely candidate to lie on a continuum with normal aging. However, Freer (Chapter 8) suggests that an individual with relatively prominent frontal lobe sulci early in life may appear to atrophy selectively in frontal lobes 40 to 50 years later, confounding the diagnostic techniques and leading to a diagnosis of frontal lobe dementia, despite have a typical DAT.

Freer's example raises the possibility that the concept of reserve capacity may apply to local, as well as global, brain areas. One of the pitfalls of searching for subtypes of dementia among clinical cases is that researchers may be misled by failing to take account of pre-existing individual differences in structure or function.

In his historical review of research into dementia, Lishman (Chapter

3) concludes that we may have seized too quickly on the medical model for Alzheimer's disease, partly by analogy with other dementias with known causes, such as Huntington's disease and Creutzfeldt–Jakob disease. This conclusion may apply with equal force to the other forms of age-associated dementia.

Conclusion

The issue of whether dementia is a discrete disease (or group of diseases) distinct from the normal processes of aging, or whether it is part of the normal aging process cannot be decided for certain until cognitive–behavioural and neurobiological data are available from representative population samples. If the markers for dementing diseases had been established unequivocally and showed a bimodal distribution for dementia and normal aging in population studies, then a different explanation would have to be found for the cognitive decline seen in normal elderly people. It seems likely that the causes of both cognitive decline and dementia will prove to be multi-factorial. The current tendency to label each new clinicopathological presentation as a new disease subtype, may bring with it the danger of reifying changes which are really part of a complex, age-related syndrome.

The bulk of the evidence presented in this book is consistent with a continuum model of age-associated decline, where chronological age, intrinsic variables and environmental factors combine to determine when disability becomes manifested. It is a convenience to apply a diagnostic label when a threshold of disability has been reached. Indeed Cooper (Chapter 22) suggests that such labelling is unavoidable when issues of service provision and health-care planning are considered.

Some would argue that the evidence supporting a continuity model paints a grim picture of the aging process, and it is true that we have been focusing on the pathological end of the continuum. However, demonstrating a continuity between normal aging and dementia does not preclude the possibility of preventing the changes associated with cognitive decline and dementia, nor the arrest or reversal of such changes once they have occurred. An important corollary of the continuity notion is that service provision, treatment and prevention should be targeted not only at one extreme of the continuum but also at the bulk of the distribution where individuals are showing milder forms of cognitive impairment. We should take the lead from the public health approaches to the prevention of stroke and heart disease: by attempting to shift the whole distribution away from the pathological end of the continuum (Khaw, Chapter 23), we may be able to reduce the incidence of cognitive decline and dementia. This requires the identification of risk factors for cognitive decline and dementia, and the identification of protective factors for 'successful aging' (to use the terminology of Rowe & Kahn, 1987).

Richards & van Broeckhoven (Chapter 21) advocate that governments should spend more in research programmes aimed at identifying ways of protecting brains from the cellular degeneration that occurs in Alzheimer's disease. How much more poignant is their appeal if the same degeneration occurs in most people as they age?

References

Alzheimer, A. (1907). Über eine eigenartige Erkrankung der Hirnrinde. *Allgemeine Zeitschrift für Psychiatrie und Psychisch-Gerichtlich Medizine*, **64**, 146–8.

Blessed, G., Tomlinson, B. E. & Roth, M. (1968). The association between quantitative measures of dementia and of senile change in the cerebral grey matter of elderly subjects. *British Journal of Psychiatry*, **114**, 797–811.

Dewey, M. E. (1991). How should prevalence be modelled? *Acta Psychiatrica Scandinavica*, **84**, 246–9.

Katzman, R. & Saitoh, T. (1991). Advances in Alzheimer's Disease. *FASEB Journal*, **5**, 278–86.

Kraepelin, E. (1919). *Dementia Praecox and Paraphrenia*. (Translation by R. M. Barclay.) Livingstone, Edinburgh.

McKhann, G., Drachman, D., Folstein, M., Katzman, R., Price, D. & Stadlan, E. M. (1984). Clinical diagnosis of Alzheimer's Disease: report of the NINCDS–ADRDA Work Group under the auspices of Department of Health and Human Services task force on Alzheimer's Disease. *Neurology*, **34**, 939–44.

Rowe, J. W. & Kahn, R. L. (1987). Human aging: usual and successful. *Science*, **237**, 143–9.

Storandt, M., Aufdembrinke, B., Backman, L., Baltes, M. M., Blass, J. P., Braak, H., Gutzmann, H., Hauw, J-J., Hoyer, S., Jorm, A. F., Kauss, J., Kliegl, R. & Mountjoy, C. Q. (1988). Group report: relationship of normal aging and dementing diseases in later life. In A. S. Henderson & J. H. Henderson (eds.) *Etiology of Dementia of Alzheimer's Type*. Life Sciences Research Report 43: Report of the Dahlem Workshop, Berlin 1987, 231–9. John Wiley & Sons, Chichester.

PART II

The development of contemporary views of dementia

2

Dementia and aging since the nineteenth century

G. E. BERRIOS

Behavioural states related to what is now called 'dementia' have existed – and been named differently – since classical times, and it is safe to assume that psychosocial incompetence has been the only feature they all had in common. Beyond this, each historical period has emphasized different symptoms and explanations. Although loss of memory and judgment were included in a number of classical accounts of fatuitas and distraction (Berrios, 1987a), the view that cognitive failure is the 'essence' of dementia originated only during the late nineteenth century (Berrios, 1990a). Since the previous century, a persistent question was whether the cognitive and behavioural changes of dementia were just part of growing older or whether, in fact, a veritable 'disease'. To deal with this issue we must also explore the history of the concepts of aging.

To prevent projecting onto the past perspectives that belong to the present, good method recommends that the history of aging and dementia distinguish between the history of the word and that of the concepts and behaviours associated with it. This chapter will concentrate on the nineteenth century, since it is during this period that the current notion of dementia was constructed. Some concepts will, however, be briefly followed backwards or forwards. The historical hypotheses to be propounded here are that normal aging and dementia have been distinguished, at least since the beginning of the nineteenth century, and that this became clearer after the 1860s, when the clinical scope of 'dementia' became reduced greatly. This process culminated in the early 1900s with the consolidation of the 'cognitive paradigm' i.e. the view that dementia consisted in an irreversible disorder of intellectual functions (Berrios, 1989, 1990a).

Dementia and Normal Aging, eds. F. A. Huppert, C. Brayne & D. W. O'Connor.
© Cambridge University Press 1994.

The study of aging before the nineteenth century

Like most other aspects of human life, aging has always been portrayed in terms of metaphors. Classical views were couched in terms of the nature–nurture controversy, i.e. aging was seen as the result of internal instructions or of external factors (Grmek, 1958; Grant, 1963). The latter, or 'wear and tear' view, became popular during the early nineteenth century, but even then it was just a repetition of the ageless observation that all natural objects, whether animate or not, are subject to the ravages of time. This fatalistic view did not always generate, however, a positive or understanding attitude. In fact, across times and cultures great ambiguity seems to have existed about what to do with the elderly. In some cases there was great fatalism and hostility; in others, great play was made of the wisdom and value of the elderly; but even then protection and respect were not afforded to all aging subjects but only to those in positions of power and influence (Cicero, 1923; Kastenbaum & Ross, 1975). A common thread, however, is the view that aging was undesirable and that life was worth prolonging; to do so, the factors that accelerate wearing and tearing had to be identified (Legrand, 1911; Gruman, 1966)

A second ambiguity can be detected in regard to the extent to which aging necessarily involved the human mind. Whilst it was an objective and palpable fact that the body decayed, not everyone felt that the same process affected the soul or mind. Whilst everyday observation must have dictated that it often did (for there are plenty of stereotyped descriptions of the psychological changes of old age) theory and religion suggested persistently that the spirit ought to escape wear and tear and that, by accumulating experience and knowledge, it should grow ever wiser. This view is likely to have been particularly relevant to those societies that allowed themselves to be governed by intellectual and/or socio-political gerontocracies (Minois, 1987). From the point of view of the relationship between aging and dementia, it is important to know to what extent these pre-conceived ideas were undermined by the appearance of states of chronic cognitive failure amongst the elderly in positions of power (Huber & Gourin, 1987). Historical evidence suggests that dementia and mental illness (occurring at any age) were perceived to be equally disruptive and perturbing. When either was diagnosed, legal devices were enacted to cope with the social upheaval created.

The ideas on aging that the nineteenth century inherited had been reshaped during the previous century by Buffon, Darwin and Goethe.

Buffon ((1774) p. 108; my translation) wrote: 'All changes and dies in Nature. As soon as it reaches its point of perfection it begins to decay. At first this is subtle and it takes years for one to realize that major changes have in fact taken place'. Buffon put this down to 'ossification', a process similar to that affecting trees: 'this cause of death is general and common to animals and vegetables. Oak trees die because their core hardens with age and they can no longer feed. Their trapped humidity eventually makes them rot away' (Buffon (1774), p. 111; my translation).

Erasmus Darwin's views are interesting, for they result from the application of yet another metaphor, namely that of the effects on the brain of silence and isolation (resulting from a loss of communication between man and his environment) (Darwin, 1794–96). Darwin suggested that this may lead to a decline in the power of irritability (a property of nerve fibres) and a decreased response to sensation:

> It seems our bodies by long habit cease to obey the stimulus of the aliment, which support us . . . three causes may conspire to render our nerves less excitable: (1) if a stimulus be greater than natural, it produces too great an exertion of the stimulated organ, and in consequence exhausts the spirit of animation; and the moving organ ceases to act, even though the stimulus is continued, (2) if excitations weaker than natural be applied, so as not to excite the organ into action, they may be gradually increased, without exciting the organ into action, which will thus acquire a habit of disobedience to the stimulus, and (3) when irritative motions continue to be produced in consequence of stimulus, but are not succeeded by sensation.
>
> *(Darwin, 1794–96, p. 365)*

The study of aging during the nineteenth century

At the beginning of the nineteenth century, Sir John Sinclair (1807) published a major work on aging and longevity including references to most pre-nineteenth century views on the subject. It was, in a way, the last grand glance to the past. Soon after the work started of those who, like Léon Rostan, were to base their claims on empirical findings. Rostan, one of the most original members of the Paris school published the first edition of his *Recherches sur le Ramollissement du Cerveau* in 1819 (Rostan, 1823); therein he suggested that vascular disorders might be as important as parenchymal changes to explain the process of cerebral aging. Even more important was his uncompromising anti-vitalistic position, accompanied by the claim that all diseases were related to pathological changes in specific organs (Rostan, 1833; Chereau, 1877).

During the 1850s, another great specialist in this field, Reveillé-Parise, saw his task as writing on 'the history of ageing, that is, mapping the imprint of time on the human body, whether on its organs or on its spiritual essence' (Reveillé-Parise (1853), p. v; my translation). With regard to aging itself he wrote: 'the cause of ageing is a gradual increase in the work of decomposition . . . but how does it happen? What are the laws that control the degradation that affects the organization and mind of man?' (Reveillé-Parise (1853), p. 13; my translation). Reveillé-Parise dismissed the toxic view defended by the Italian writer Michel Lévy (1850) according to which there was a gradual accumulation of calcium phosphates that led to petrification, i.e. to an 'anticipation of the grave'. This view, he stated, had no empirical foundation and was based on a generalization from localized findings. The second hypothesis, which he supported, suggested that aging resulted from a negative balance between composition and elimination. This gradual loss affected equally the cardiovascular, respiratory and reproductive organs. During the 1880s, the defective 'blood supply' view was propounded strongly by Démange (1886) but by then Charcot's views had already taken shape (Charcot, 1881). (For an account of the historical debate during this period see Gimeno, 1910.)

In 1868, J. M. Charcot offered at la Salpêtrière a series of 24 lectures on the diseases affecting the elderly. Charcot's first lecture was dedicated to the 'general characters of senile pathology'. He stated that all books on geriatrics up to his century had 'a particularly literary or philosophical turn [and had been] more or less ingenious paraphrases of the famous treatise *De Senectute*' (Charcot, 1881, p. 25). He praised Rostan for his views on brain softening, and predictably mentioned Cruveilhier, Hourman and Dechambre, Durand-Fardel and Prus. He critized Canstatt and other German theoreticians in whose work 'imagination holds an immense place at the expense of impartial and positive observation' (Charcot, 1881, p. 26). Charcot's own contribution was the general principle that: 'changes of texture impressed on the organism by old age sometimes become so marked, that the physiological and pathological states seem to merge into one another by insensible transitions, and cannot be clearly distinguished' (Charcot, 1881, p. 26).

The relationship between aging and dementia

Throughout history there has been ambiguity on the nature of the relationship between aging and dementia. This was expressed in two views which, since classical times, have vied for supremacy. One, which will be called here the 'discontinuity' view, was expressed by Cicero (1923, pp. 44–5): 'Just as waywardness and lust are more often found in young men than in the old, yet not in all who are young, but only in those naturally base; so that senile debility, usually called 'dotage' [senilis stultitia] is a characteristic, not of all men, but only of those who are weak in mind and will' The Latin text suggests that Cicero saw dementia (senilis stultitia) as a separate state that developed only in elderly people who also were 'naturally base', i.e. tainted by another factor.

The second, or 'continuity' view, according to which dementia is no different from aging, was put forward by Cicero's contemporary Lucretius, who wrote (1975, p. 223):

> Beside, we feel that the mind is begotten along with the body, and grows up with it, and with it grows old. For as toddling children have a body infirm and tender, so a weak intelligence goes with it. Next, when their age has grown up into robust strength, the understanding too and the power of the mind is enlarged. Afterwards, when the body is now wrecked with the mighty strength of time, and the frame has succumbed with blunted strength, the intellect limps, the tongue babbles, the intelligence totters, all is wanting and fails at the same time.

These opposing views remained unchanged until the nineteenth century. It is difficult to imagine how it could have been otherwise. To decide on their merits demands not only a scientific framework to carry out the pertinent empirical tests but also stipulations to decide what evidence is to be taken as valid. It can even be suggested that the continuity view has flourished in times of therapeutic pessimism. This seems to be the case with late eighteenth century writers who felt that dementia could not be cured, and that the solution was to delay aging by means of hygienic measures: Hufeland's concept of *Makrobiotik*, or the 'art of prolonging the individual length of life' is a good example of this (Hufeland, 1797). During this period both German (von Kondratowitz, 1991) and French physicians seem to have supported a continuity view. For example Marcé, whose contribution to the neuropathology of dementia has been sadly neglected (Marcé, 1863), wrote: 'Age as such facilitates the development of dementia even when there is no other complicating factor' (Marcé (1862), p. 396; my translation).

The development of neuropathology during the nineteenth century seemed to provide evidence in favour of the discontinuity view. A good illustration of this position is the work of Reveillé-Parise (1853, p. 232; my translation): 'Many elderly are not ill although their age makes them susceptible to it. Old age is not, by itself, a disease, it only offers a predisposition to illness'. Charcot (1881) lent the weight of his authority to this view (see above). Moreover, based on new physiological ideas, he was able to offer a more refined explanation. Thus, he believed that anatomical continuity was compatible with physiological discontinuity: 'senile changes are not peculiar to man but also met with in aging animals . . . beyond a degree [these changes] upset the physiological state, and are capable of producing functional troubles which may be extremely grave'. (Charcot, 1881, p. 30).

By the end of the nineteenth century the debate flared up again, this time between two great scientists of the period. Elié Metchnikoff (1904, pp. 240–1) believed that 'macrophages play a very important part in bringing about senile decay . . . in the brains of old persons and animals, for instance, it is known that a number of nervous cells are surrounded and devoured by macrophages'. Georges Marinesco disagreed, and in a classical paper wrote: (1900, p. 1137; my translation and italics):

> For Metchnikov, senile atrophy results from a fight between two tissues in which macrophages are victorious . . . this view led me to investigate the death of nervous cells in the spinal cord of individuals between 60 and 110; I am convinced that in the nervous cells senescence causes both a diminution of the cellular body and internal changes . . . which I have given the name *senile chromatolysis* . . . I have never found macrophages destroying nerve cells.

Marinesco went as far as sending some of his slides to Metchnikoff (1904, p. 242) who dismissed the evidence: 'I freely admit the absence of phagocytosis in M. Marinesco's preparations, but these were derived from the cells of spinal marrow, which is much less subject to the ravages of senile decay than is the brain'.

It was against this context that both Alzheimer and Kraepelin developed their ideas. Whilst the former seems to have favoured a continuity view, and hence did not see much that was new (except age of onset) in the case he reported in 1907 (for a full history of these important events see below), Kraepelin – who was keen for such cases to be a new disease – supported a discontinuity view (see Berrios, 1990b). Age of onset had already been discussed before Alzheimer's case: for example, Cullere wrote: (1890, p. 399; my translation) 'senile dementia indicates that this condition pertains to old age. It hardly develops before 60 or 65, except in those individuals who show premature senility, when it may appear before 50'. Fox (1989) has also remarked that age of onset seems to have been the main criterion in the differentiation of Alzheimer's disease.

However, the authority of Kraepelin was so great that, up to the 1950s, great writers in the field of aging still can be found supporting the discontinuity view: 'It used to be believed that senile dementia, the mental weakness of old age, was the final state of brain degeneration in the aged. It is now known that this view was mistaken, for anatomical changes in the brain are not necessarily accompanied by changes in the mental functions. In this respect, the case reported by Professor Kuczynski is instructive: it concerned a man of 109 whose brain showed changes even worse than those seen in senile dementia but who had shown no mental deterioration whatsoever until his death' (Woltereck (1956), p. 114; my translation). Kral's notion of 'benign senescent forgetfulness' can be considered to be another version of the discontinuity view this time expressed in terms of a phenomenological description of the memory disorder itself (Kral, 1962). Also a version of the discontinuity view is the elegant model of aging put forward by Ursula Lehr (1977). But these works are bringing us dangerously close to the present and we must not forget that our brief is the modest one of setting out the history of these events. Let us, therefore, deal now with the history of dementia itself.

Views on dementia before the nineteenth century

The word 'dementia' first appeared in the vernacular in Blancard's popular *Physical Dictionary* as an equivalent of 'anoea' or 'extinction of the imagination and judgment' (Blancard, 1726, p. 21). The earliest adjectival usage ('demented') has been dated by the *Oxford English Dictionary* (OED) to 1644. The OED also dates the earliest substantive usage to Davis's translation of Pinel's (1806) *Treatise of Insanity*. Sobrino's Spanish–French dictionary offers the following definition:

'*demencia* = *démence, folie, extravagance, egarement, alienation d'esprit*' (Sobrino (1791), p. 300; my italics). It would seem, therefore, that the Latin stem 'demens' (without mind) was incorporated into the European vernacular sometime between the seventeenth and eighteenth centuries, and that, after the 1760s, it acquired a medical connotation. Further evidence for this usage can be found in the *French Encyclopaedia* (Diderot & d'Alembert, 1754), where both medical and legal definitions of dementia are stated clearly and show that the basic concepts had already formed during the 1760s. In this encyclopaedia, dementia is distinguished from mania (a term which, at the time, described any state of acute excitement be it schizophrenic, hypomanic or organic) and from delirium (which referred, more or less, to what goes on nowadays under the same name). Dementia was reversible and affected individuals of any age. Reference to many aetiologies suggests that a 'syndromal' view of dementia had developed.

Cullen and 'amentia'

During the eighteenth century, some forms of dementia were also called 'amentia' (for example by W. Cullen, the Edinburgh physician who coined the term 'neuroses'). Cullen (1827; first published in 1777) defined amentia as a loss of intellectual functions and memory, whether congenital or acquired, the latter resulting from infections, vascular disorders, sexual excesses, poisons, and trauma. Cullen distinguished states of idiocy (mental handicap) from acquired brain damage and senile dementia.

Pinel and the end of the eighteenth century

Pinel was, by ideology and temperament, the last great nosologist of the eighteenth century. In the *Nosographie* (1818; first published in 1798), he dealt with cognitive impairment under amentia and morosis, explaining it as a failure in the association of ideas leading to disordered activity, extravagant behaviour, superficial emotions, memory loss, difficulty in the perception of objects, obliteration of judgment, aimless activity, automatic existence, and forgetting of words or signs to convey ideas. He also referred to *démence senile* (paragraph 116) thus disproving Cohen's point (1983, p. 30) that 'the term senile dementia was first used by Esquirol'. Pinel (1818) did not emphasize the difference between congenital and acquired dementia.

Dementia during the nineteenth century

There is a major difference between Pinel's concept of dementia and what was to go under the same name 80 years later. Dementia by then referred to states of cognitive impairment mostly affecting the elderly, and almost always irreversible. The word 'amentia' had changed meaning and named a 'psychosis, with sudden onset following severe, often acute physical illness or trauma' (Meynert, 1890). This section will explore these momentous changes.

French views on dementia

Esquirol   It has been claimed that Esquirol's views on dementia were more advanced than Pinel's (Tomlinson & Corsellis, 1984); this is not borne out by an analysis of the primary sources. Esquirol's notion of dementia changed, in fact, between 1805 and 1838 (Esquirol, 1805, 1814, 1838). In 1805, he used the word (as in *démence accidental*, *démence melancolique*, etc.) to refer to loss of reason; by 1814, however, he was beginning to distinguish between acute, chronic and senile dementia, and to suggest 'composite' types which may have included defect states following melancholia, mania, epilepsy, convulsions, scurvy and paralysis. Acute dementia was short lived, reversible, and followed fever, haemorrhage, and metastasis; chronic dementia was irreversible and caused by masturbation, melancholia, mania, hypochondria, epilepsy, paralysis, and apoplexy; senile dementia resulted from aging, and consisted in a loss of the faculties of understanding.

Esquirol's (1838) final thoughts on dementia were influenced by his controversy with Bayle (1822) who had described *chronic arachnoiditis*. This young Frenchman entertained an anatomical ('organic') view of the insanities and had scorned Pinel's views (Bayle, 1826). Esquirol, together with his student Georget (see below), supported the latter's 'descriptivist' approach. His 1838 chapter on dementia included new terms, clinical vignettes, and post-mortem descriptions. He reported 15 cases of dementia (7 males and 8 females) with a mean age of 34 years (standard deviation = 10.9); 7 being, in fact, cases of general paralysis of the insane with grandiosity, disinhibition, motor symptoms, dysarthria and terminal cognitive failure. There also was a 20-year-old girl with a catatonic syndrome (in modern terms), and a 40-year-old woman with pica, cognitive impairment, and space-occupying lesions in her left hemisphere and cerebellum. The type of patient reported illustrates well Esquirol's concept of dementia. For example, no cases of senile dementia are included and – although this may reflect the type of patient admitted to the Charenton Hospital – it is more likely that age was not a relevant variable for him. Indeed, 'senile dementia' appears in early nineteenth century classifications as an afterthought only. The same holds true for the 'irreversibility' criterion which was mentioned only in cases of severe brain damage: as to the rest, improvement was expected.

Georget   Trained under Rostan, Falret, and Calmeil, Georget had become interested in brain softening and its relationship to intellectual impairment (Ball & Chambard, 1881; see Postel, 1972). He also contributed to the creation of the concept of stupidity or stupor, called 'acute dementia' by Esquirol (Esquirol, 1814; Postel, 1972; Berrios, 1981). Georget (1820, p. 36) believed that 'The brain is the site of madness and gives origin to its symptoms' and recognized five 'genres' of *folie*: idiocy, mania, monomania, stupidity and dementia. He disagreed with Esquirol's view that cognitive impairment in dementia was due to attentional deficit only. He suggested that both idiocy and dementia were irreversible, for both resulted from an abolition of thought, the former from a 'vice' in the organization of the brain, the latter from weakening, old age or intercurrent diseases.

Calmeil   Aware of the importance of clinical description, Calmeil wrote (1835, p. 71; my translation): 'it is not easy to describe dementia, its varieties, and nuances; because its complications are numerous . . . it is difficult to choose its distinctive symptoms'. Dementia followed chronic insanity and brain disease, and was partial or general. Calmeil was less convinced than Georget that all dementias were associated with alterations in the brain. In regard to senile dementia, he remarked (Calmeil, 1835, p. 71): 'there is a constant involvement of the senses, elderly people can be deaf, and show disorders of taste, smell and touch; external stimuli are therefore less clear to them, they have little memory of recent events, live in the past, and repeat the same tale; their affect gradually wanes away'. Although a keen neuropathologist, Calmeil concluded that there was insufficient information on the nature and range of anomalies found in the skull or brain to decide on the cause of dementia.

Guislain   Guislain (1852, p. 10; my translation) defined dementia thus:

> All intellectual functions show a reduction in energy, external stimuli cause only minor impression on the intellect, imagination is weak and uncreative, memory absent, and reasoning pathological . . . There are two varieties of dementia . . . one affecting the elderly (senile dementia as per Cullen) the other (affecting) younger people. Although confused with dementia, idiocy must be considered as a separate group.

Guislain included 'vesanic dementias' amongst the 'acquired' forms (1852, p. 19; my translation): 'there is nothing sadder than seeing a patient progress from mania or monomania to dementia'. In his 'Lectures', Guislain also offered an operational definition for 'cognitive failure' (1852, p. 311; my translation):

> The patient has no memory, or at least is unable to retain anything . . . impressions evaporate from his mind. He may remember names of people but cannot say whether he has seen them before. He does not know what time or day of the week it is, cannot tell morning from evening, or say what two and two add to . . . he has lost the instinct of preservation, cannot avoid fire or water, and is unable to recognize dangers; has also lost spontaneity, is incontinent of urine and faeces, and does not ask for anything, he cannot even recognize his wife or children.

Marc   Marc contributed to the legal concept of dementia (1840, p. 261; my translation): 'From the legal viewpoint, dementia is considered as equivalent to insanity in general; medically, however, it only names one of its forms'. Marc also commented upon the notion of dementia enshrined in article 64 of the French Penal Code (where it is defined as a weakness of the understanding, will, memory, and judgment) and found it wanting in clinical situations when dementia was mild (i.e. some mental faculties were well preserved), or onset was sudden (i.e. no prodromal features were present), or when it was accompanied by 'lucid intervals', hallucinations or delusions, or in cases of malingering. So, he believed that 'black and white' diagnoses were not possible, and that the expert witness ought to offer statements of probability about a subject having dementia.

Morel   Criticizing older taxonomies, Morel (1860, p. 2) wrote that in the past the mentally ill: 'had been categorized only in terms of a [putative] impairment of their mental faculties'. He endeavoured to develop a 'causal' taxonomy, i.e. one based on separating *occasionelle* (e.g. social precipitants) from *determinante* (e.g. genetic factors and brain changes) causes. Six groups were thus identified: hereditary, toxic, associated with the neuroses, idiopathic, sympathetic, and dementia. Morel believed that (1860, pp. 837–8; my translation and italics):

> if we examine dementia (amentia, progressive weakening of the faculties) we must accept that it constitutes a terminal state. There will, of course, be exceptional insane individuals who, until the end, preserve their intellectual faculties; the majority, however, are subject to the law of decline. This results from a loss of vitality in the brain . . . Comparison of brain weights in the various forms of insanity shows that the heavier weights are found in cases of recent onset. Chronic cases show more often a general impairment of intelligence (dementia). Loss in brain weight – a constant feature of dementia – is also present in aging, and is an expression of decadence in the human species.

> [There are] natural dementia and that dementia resulting from a pathological state of the brain . . . some forms of insanity are more prone to end up in dementia (idiopathic) than others . . . it could be argued that because dementia is a terminal state it *should not be classified as a sixth form of mental illness* . . . I must confess I sympathise with this view, and it is one of the reasons why I have not described the dementias in any detail . . . on the other hand from the legal and pathological viewpoints, dementia warrants separate treatment.

Morel's view that the dementias are a terminal state was in keeping with his 'degenerationist' hypothesis (on this see Pick, 1989). Consequently, he dealt with dementia in most chapters of his treatise (Morel, 1860). His view was based on the assumption that insanity always pre-dated dementia; he soon realized that this was nonsense, and explained the frequent exceptions by aging or degeneration. The 'terminal state' hypothesis dissuaded Morel from believing that there were specific brain alterations in dementia.

The fragmentation of the dementia concept

By 1900, senile, arteriosclerotic, and 'subcortical' forms of dementia had been recognized (Berrios & Freeman, 1991). Many clinical forms, however, found no place in this tripartite classification; some had been known for a long time, such as general paralysis of the insane, dementia praecox, and melancholia attonita; others had been described recently, such as the dementias related to alcoholism, epilepsy, brain damage, myxoedema, hysteria and lead poisoning. Their presence created clinical ambiguity, and this was resolved in various ways: some were considered to be independent conditions (e.g. Korsakoff's syndrome and myxoedema), others were hidden under a different name (e.g. dementia praecox became schizophrenia and melancholia attonita became stupor); yet others were explained away as 'pseudo-dementias' (e.g. hysteria). The history of some of these states, however, must be picked up ab initio.

General paralysis of the insane

Bayle (1822) described under the name *arachnitis chronique* cases of what later was to be called 'general paralysis of the insane'. Whether this 'new phenomenon' resulted from 'a mutation in the syphilitic virus towards the end of the eighteenth century' is unclear (Bayle, 1822, p. 623; Hare, 1959). Equally dubious is the claim that its discovery reinforced the belief of alienists in the anatomoclinical view of mental disease (Zilboorg, 1941). In fact, it took more than 30 years for general paralysis to gain acceptance as a 'separate' disease. Bayle's 'discovery' was more important in other ways, because it challenged the 'cross sectional' view of disease; in the words of Bercherie (1980, p. 75): 'for the first time in the history of psychiatry there was a morbid entity which presented itself as a sequential process unfolding itself into successive clinical syndromes'.

By the 1850s, no agreement had yet been reached as to how symptoms were caused by the *periencephalite chronique diffuse* (as general paralysis was known at the time). Three clinical types were recognized and were manic-ambitious, melancholic-hypochondriac and pertaining to dementia; according to the 'unitary view', all three constituted stages of a single disease, the order of their appearance depending on the progress of the cerebral lesions. Baillarger, however, sponsored a 'dualist' view (1883, p. 37; my translation): 'paralytic insanity and paralytic dementia are different conditions'. It is clear that the debate had less to do with the nature of the brain lesions than with how mental symptoms and their contents were produced in general: how could the 'typical' content of paralytic delusions (grandiosity) be explained? Since the same mental symptoms could be seen in all manner of conditions, Baillarger (1883 p. 389) believed that chronic periencephalitis could account for the motor signs only – mental symptoms 'therefore, having a different origin'. The absence of a link between lesion and symptom also explained why some patients recovered.

The view that general paralysis might be related to syphilis (put forward by Fournier, 1875) was resisted. Indeed, the term 'pseudo-general paralysis' was coined to refer to cases of infections causing psychotic symptoms (Baillarger, 1889). In general, there is little evidence that alienists considered general paralysis to be 'paradigm disease', i.e. a model for all other mental diseases. It can even be said that that the new 'disease' created more problems than it solved (for a discussion of this issue see Berrios, 1985).

'Dementia praecox' becomes schizophrenia

Morel (1852) coined the term *démence précoce* to refer to a state of dementia occurring during adolescence or soon after. Many years later, Kraepelin (1919; first published in 1910) borrowed it to name a composite 'disease', soon after to be renamed 'schizophrenia' by Bleuler (1911). In the 1940s, Kurt Schneider (1959; first published in 1946) suggested 'empirical' criteria for its diagnosis.

The term 'dementia' was used to name the same clinical states that Georget had called 'stupidity' – states whose common denominator was a major reduction and/or disorganization of behaviour. Morel (1852) reported the case of a young man who, after a period of religious fanaticism, developed delusions, hallucinations, excitement, and generalized muscular contractions. Six months of stupor followed, during which he maintained awkward bodily positions, would not answer questions, and was incontinent of urine; he remained lacking in initiative and with some automatic behaviour. It is tempting to rediagnose this case as catatonic schizophrenia. Kraepelin believed that these states, and those of dementia paranoides, simplex, and hebephrenia, shared the same course, bad prognosis and unknown cause, and hence constituted the same disease (Berrios & Hauser, 1988). Soon after, dementia praecox was effectively 'psychologized' by Bleuler – under Jung's influence – (Berrios, 1987b), and to many alienists the new disease (schizophrenia) stopped being part of the history of the organic dementias. In practice, fortunately, this has not been so, and the issue of a real 'cognitive defect' has remained alive ever since (Johnstone et al., 1978).

Pseudo-dementia and vesanic dementia

The mechanism and/or concept of 'pseudo-dementia' was created during the 1880s to deal with cases of 'dementia' that recovered eventually; its most common name at the time being *démence melancolique* (Berrios, 1985). Before then, these cases had been considered to be 'vesanic', i.e. dementias caused by a functional psychosis (Berrios, 1987c). Mairet (1883) challenged this compromise by showing that melancholic patients with cognitive impairment may show alterations in the temporal lobe; this led him to hypothesize that these sites were related to feelings, and that nihilistic delusions appeared only when the lesion spread to the cortex. Mairet's cases (some of which would now be called 'Cotard's syndrome' (Cotard, 1882)) showed psycho-motor retardation, refused food, and died in stupor. Another contributor to the understanding of cognitive impairment in the affective disorders was Georges Dumas (1894, p. 64; my translation) who suggested that it was 'mental fatigue that explained the psychological poverty and monotony of melancholic depressions' and that the problem was not 'an absence but a stagnation of ideas'; i.e. he was, therefore, the first to explain the disorder as a failure in performance.

The word 'pseudo-dementia', in turn, originated in a different clinical tradition, and was first used by Carl Wernicke (see Lanczik, 1988) to refer to 'a chronic hysterical state mimicking mental weakness' (quoted in Bulbena & Berrios, 1986). It was used infrequently until the 1950s, when it was given a new lease of life (e.g. Madden et al., 1952; Anderson et al., 1959; Kiloh, 1961). Current usage is ambiguous, for it refers to, at least, three different clinical situations: a real (albeit reversible) cognitive impairment accompanying some psychoses; a parody of such impairment; and the cognitive deficit of delirium (Bulbena & Berrios, 1986).

The term 'vesanic dementia' began to be used after the 1840s to refer to the clinical states of cognitive disorganization following insanity; its meaning, has changed pari passu with psychiatric theory. According to the unitary insanity notion, vesanic dementia was a terminal stage (after mania and melancholia); according to degeneration theory, it was the final expression of a corrupted pedigree; and, according to post-1880s nosology, a final common pathway to some insanities. Vesanic dementias were reversible, and could occur at any age; risk factors such as old age, lack of education, low social class, bad nutrition, etc. accelerated the progression of the dementia or impeded recovery (Ball & Chambard, 1881). By the 1900s, the vesanic dementias became 'pseudo-dementias'.

Brain changes and aging

Since the beginning of the nineteenth century, cases had been described of brain 'softening' followed by cognitive failure. Rostan (1823) reported 98 subjects thus affected, thought to be scorbutic in origin, and divided them into simple, abnormal and complicated (the latter two groups being accompanied by psychiatric changes). Mental symptoms might occur before, during and after the softening itself; thus, senile dementia and insanity might precede the brain changes. Rostan (1823, pp. 214–5; my translation) reported that stroke might be accompanied by cognitive failure and attacks of insanity, and suggested that these symptoms were 'a general feature . . . not a positive sign of localization'. Durand-Fardel (1843) provided an account of the relationship between softening and insanity, warning that softening was used to refer both to a *disease* (stroke) and to a *state* of the brain. Psychiatric complications were acute and long term, the former including confusion, depression, irritability, acute insanity, and loss of mental faculties; the latter had gradual onset, and exhibited an impairment of memory, poverty of thinking, and a regression to infantile forms of behaviour, features which led to 'true dementia' (see Durand-Fardel, 1843, pp. 327–8).

Years later, J. H. Jackson (1875, p. 335) reviewed the problem: 'softening . . . as a category for a rude clinical grouping was to be deprecated'; nonetheless, he followed Durand-Fardel's classification, and suggested that, after a stroke, mental symptoms might be immediate or might follow after a few hours or months; he recognized that major cognitive failure may ensue, and saw this as an instance of 'dissolution': emotional symptoms being release phenomena (for an analysis of this concept see Berrios, 1991a). He believed that anxiety, stress and irritability might be harbingers of stroke.

The concept of arteriosclerotic dementia

Old age was considered to be an important factor in the development of arteriosclerosis (Berrios, 1993) and a risk factor in diseases such as melancholia (Berrios, 1991b). By 1910, there was a trend to include all dementias under 'mental disorders of cerebral arteriosclerosis' (Barrett, 1913). Arteriosclerosis, might be generalized or cerebral, inherited or acquired, and caused by syphilis, alcohol, nicotine, high blood pressure, and aging. In those predisposed genetically, cerebral arteries were considered to be thinner and less elastic. Arteriosclerosis caused mental changes by narrowing of arteries and/or reactive inflammation. The view that arteriosclerotic dementia resulted from a gradual strangulation of blood supply to the brain was also formed during this period; consequently, emphasis was given to prodromal symptoms, and strokes were but the culmination of a process started years before. Some opposed this view from the beginning. For example, Marie (1906, p. 358; my translation) claimed that such explanation was a vicious circle, since alienists claimed both that: 'ageing was caused by arteriosclerosis and the latter by ageing', and Walton (1912) expressed serious doubts from the histopathological point of view. The frequent presence in postmortem of such changes also concerned pathologists who worried that they could not 'safely exclude cerebral arteriosclerosis of greater or less degree in any single case' of senile dementia (Southard, 1910, p. 677). Based on a review of these arguments, Olah (1910) concluded that there was no such thing as 'arteriosclerotic psychoses'. But the 'chronic global ischaemia' hypothesis won the day, and it was to continue well into the second half of the twentieth century. For some it became a general explanation; for example, North & Bostock (1925) reported a series of 568 general psychiatric cases in which around 40% suffered from 'arterial disease', which – according to the authors – was responsible even for schizophrenia. The old idea of an apoplectic form of dementia, however, never disappeared.

Apoplectic dementia

'Apoplectic dementia' achieved its clearest enunciation in the work of Benjamin Ball (Ball & Chambard, 1881). 'Organic apoplexy' resulted from bleeding, softening or tumour and might be 'followed by a notable decline in cognition, and by a state of dementia which was progressive and incurable . . . of the three, localized softening [*ramol-lissement en foyer*] caused the more severe states of cognitive impairment' (Ball & Chambard, (1881), p. 581; my translation). Ball believed that prodromal lapses of cognition (e.g. episodes of somnolence and confusion with automatic behaviour, for which there was no memory after the event) and sensory symptoms were caused by atheromatous lesions. Visual hallucinations, occasionally of a pleasant nature, were also common. After the stroke, persistent cognitive impairment was frequent. Post-mortem studies showed in these cases softening of 'ideational' areas of cortex and white matter.

Ball also suggested a laterality effect in that 'right hemisphere strokes led more often to dementia whereas left hemisphere ones caused perplexity, apathy, unresponsiveness, and a tendency to talk to oneself' (Ball & Chambard (1881), p. 583; my translation). Following Luys, he believed that some of these symptoms resulted from damage to corpora striata, insular sulci and temporal lobes. During Ball's time, attention also shifted from white to red softening. Charcot (1881, p. 267) wrote the following about cerebral haemorrhage (the new name for red softening): 'having eliminated all these cases, we find ourselves in the presence of a homogeneous group corresponding to the commonest form of cerebral haemorrhage. This is, *par excellence*, sanguineous apoplexy . . . as it attacks a great number of old people, I might call it senile haemorrhage' [my italics].

Alzheimer and his disease

Alzheimer (1907) reported the case of a 51-year-old woman, with cognitive impairment, delusions, hallucinations, focal symptoms, and whose brain showed plaques, tangles, and *arteriosclerotic* changes. The existence of neurofibrils had been known for some time (Barrett, 1911; DeFelipe & Jones, 1988); for example, that in senile dementia 'the destruction of the neuro-fibrillae appears to be more extensive than in the brain of a paralytic subject' (Bianchi, 1906, p. 846). Fuller (1907) had remarked in June 1906 (i.e. *five months before* Alzheimer's report) on the presence of neurofibrillar bundles in senile dementia. Likewise, the association of plaques with dementia was not a novelty: Beljahow (1889) had reported them in 1887, and so had Redlich & Leri a few years later (See Simchowicz, 1924); in Prague, Fischer (1907) gave an important paper in June 1907 pointing out that miliary necrosis could be considered to be a marker of senile dementia. Nor was it a new syndrome that was described by Alzheimer: states of persistent cognitive impairment affecting the elderly, accompanied by delusions and hallucinations were well known (Marcé, 1863; Krafft-Ebing, 1873; Crichton-Browne, 1874; Marie, 1906). As a leading neuropathologist, Alzheimer was aware of this work. Did he then mean to describe a new disease? The answer is that it is most unlikely that he did, his only intention having been to point out that such a syndrome could occur in younger people (Alzheimer, 1911). This is confirmed by commentaries from those who worked for him: Perusini (1911, p. 193; my translation) wrote that for Alzheimer 'these morbid forms do not represent anything but atypical forms of senile dementia'.

The naming of the disease

Kraepelin (1910) coined the term in the eighth edition of his *Handbook*: at end of the section on 'senile dementia' he wrote (my italics):

> the autopsy reveals, according to Alzheimer's description, changes that represent the most serious form of senile dementia . . . the "*Drusen*" were numerous and almost one third of the cortical cells had died off. In their place instead we found peculiar deeply stained fibrillary bundles that were closely packed to one another, and seemed to be remnants of degenerated cell bodies . . . The clinical interpretation of *this Alzheimer's disease* is still confused. Whilst the anatomical findings suggest that we are dealing with a particularly serious form of senile dementia, the fact that this disease sometimes starts already around the age of 40 does not allow this supposition. In such cases we should at least assume a "senium praecox" if not perhaps a more or less age-independent *unique disease process*.

The reception of the new disease

Alzheimer (1911) showed surprise at Kraepelin's interpretation, and always referred to his 'disease' as '*Erkrankungen*' (in the medical language of the 1900s a term softer than '*Krankheit*', which was used by Kraepelin). Others also expressed doubts. Fuller (1912, p. 26), whose contribution to this field has been sadly neglected, asked 'why [there was] a special clinical designation – Alzheimer's disease – since, after all, they are but part of a general disorder'. Hakkéboutsch &

Geier (1913), in Russia, saw the disease as a variety of the involution psychosis. Simchowicz (1911) considered 'Alzheimer's disease' to be just a severe form of senile dementia. Ziehen (1911) does not mention the disease in his major review of senile dementia. In a meeting of the New York Neurological Society, Ramsay Hunt (Lambert, 1916) told Lambert, the presenter of a case of 'Alzheimer's disease', that 'he would like to understand clearly whether he made any distinction between the so-called Alzheimer's disease and senile dementia other than . . . in degree and point of age'. Lambert suggested that, as far as he was concerned, the underlying pathological mechanisms were the same (Lambert, 1916). Lugaro wrote (1916, p. 378; my translation): 'For a while it was believed that a certain agglutinative disorder of the neurofibril could be considered as the main "marker" [*contrassegno*] of a pre-senile form [of senile dementia], which was "*hurriedly baptized*" [*fretta battezzate*] as "Alzheimer's disease"'. He went on to say that this state is only a variety of senile dementia. Simchowicz who had worked with Alzheimer, wrote (1924, p. 221; my translation and italics): 'Alzheimer and Perusini did not know at the time that the plaques were typical of senile dementia [in general] and believed that they *might have discovered* a new disease'. These views, from men who lived in Alzheimer's and Kraepelin's time, must be taken seriously (for a detailed discussion of these issues see Berrios (1990b)).

Final commentary

Since the eighteenth century, the concepts of dementia and aging have been found to be interlinked closely. The perfect historical method to unravel this relationship has not yet been devised. What we know is that the history of the words 'dementia' and 'aging' must not be confused with that of the concepts or behaviours involved. During the eighteenth century, the 'wear and tear' and 'internal control' theories of aging are found fully fledged as are the clinical and legal definitions of dementia as a form of insanity and a complete (and often irreversible) state of psychosocial incompetence, respectively. In addition to cognitive impairment, the clinical definition included symptoms such as delusions and hallucinations; irreversibility and old age were not features of the condition. In general, dementia was considered to be a terminal state for most mental, neurological and even physical conditions. It was also asked whether aging per se was the main cause of dementia; but the main argument against this claim was the fact that this condition was often diagnosed in young people, for example the brain damaged.

The adoption of the anatomoclinical model by nineteenth century alienists changed this. Questions were asked about the neuropathological basis of dementia and this, in turn, led to readjustments in its clinical description. The history of dementia during the nineteenth century is, therefore, the history of its gradual attrition. Stuporous states (then called acute dementia), vesanic dementias, and localized memory impairments were gradually reclassified and, by 1900, the cognitive paradigm, i.e. the view that the essential feature of dementia was intellectual impairment, became established. From then on, efforts were made to explain other symptoms such as hallucinations, delusions, mood and behavioural disorders as being epiphenomena which were unrelated to whatever the central mechanism of dementia was.

There has also been a fluctuating acceptance of the parenchymal and vascular hypotheses, the latter leading to the description of arteriosclerotic dementia. The separation of the vesanic dementias (i.e. those following severe functional psychoses) and of the amnestic syndromes (i.e. states with specific impairment of memory) led to the realization that age and aging mechanisms were important after all, and by 1900 a narrow version of the 'senile dementia' concept had become the prototype of the dementias. This chapter does not deal with the history of the 'localized' dementias (e.g. Pick's disease) or the large group of the 'acquired' ones, since they are studied elsewhere in this book.

References

Alzheimer, A. (1907). Über eine eigenartige Erkrankung der Hirnrinde. *Allgemeine Zeitschrift für Psychiatrie und Psychisch-Gerichtlich Medizine*, **64**, 146–8.

Alzheimer, A. (1911). Über eigenartige Krankheitsfälle des späteren Alters. *Zeitschrift für die gesamte Neurologie und Psychiatrie*, **4**, 356–85 (see also translation by Förstl H. and Levy R. (1991) in *History of Psychiatry*, **2**, 71–101).

Anderson, E. W., Threthowan, W. H. & Kenna, J. C. (1959). An experimental investigation of simulation and pseudodementia. *Acta Psychiatrica et Neurologica Scandinavica*, **34**, (supplement 132).

Baillarger, J. (1883). Sur la théorie de la paralysie générale. *Annales Médico-Psychologiques*, **35**, 18–52; 191–218.

Baillarger, J. (1889). Doit-on dans la classification des maladies mentales assigner une place à part aux pseudo-paralysies générales? *Annales Médico-Psychologiques*, **41**, 521–5.

Ball, B. & Chambard, E. (1881). Démence. In Dechambre, A. & Lereboullet, L. (eds.) *Dictionnaire Encyclopédique des Sciences Médicales*, pp. 559–605. Masson, Paris.

Barrett, A. M. (1911). Degenerations of intracellular neurofibrils with miliary gliosis in psychoses of the senile period. *American Journal of Insanity*, **62**, 503–16.

Barrett, A. M. (1913). Presenile, arteriosclerotic and senile disorders of the brain and cord. In W. A. White & S. E. Jelliffe (eds.) *The Modern Treatment of Nervous and Mental Diseases*, pp. 675–709. Kimpton, London.

Bayle, A. L. J. (1822). *Recherches sur les Maladies Mentales*. Thèse de Médecine, Paris.

Bayle, L. J. (1826). *Traité des Maladies du Cerveau*. Gabon et Compagnie, Paris.

Beljahow, S. (1889). Pathological changes in the brain in dementia senilis. *Journal of Mental Science*, **35**, 261–2.

Bercherie, P. (1980). *Les Fondaments de la clinique*. La Bibliothèque d'Ornicar, Paris.

Berrios, G. E. (1981). Stupor: a conceptual history. *Psychological Medicine*, **11**, 677–88.

Berrios, G. E. (1985). 'Depressive pseudodementia' or 'melancholic dementia': a nineteenth century view. *Journal of Neurology, Neurosurgery and Psychiatry*, **48**, 393–400.

Berrios, G. E. (1987a). Dementia during the seventeenth and eighteenth centuries: a conceptual history. *Psychological Medicine*, **17**, 829–37.

Berrios, G. E. (1987b). Introduction to 'the fundamental symptoms of schizophrenia'. In C. Thompson (ed.) *The Origins of Modern Psychiatry*, pp. 200–9. Wiley, Chichester.

Berrios, G. E. (1987c). History of the functional psychoses. *British Medical Bulletin*, **43**, 484–98.

Berrios, G. E. (1989). Non-cognitive symptoms and the diagnosis of dementia. Historical and clinical aspects. *British Journal of Psychiatry*, **154**, (supplement 4), 11–16.

Berrios, G. E. (1990a). Memory and the cognitive paradigm of dementia during the nineteenth century: a conceptual history. In R. Murray & T. Turner (eds.) *Lectures on the History of Psychiatry*, pp. 194–211. Gaskell, London.

Berrios, G. E. (1990b). Alzheimer's disease: a conceptual history. *International Journal of Geriatric Psychiatry*, **5**, 355–65.

Berrios, G. E. (1991a). Positive and negative signals: a conceptual history. In A. Marneros, N. C. Andreasen & M. T. Tsuang (eds.) *Negative versus positive schizophrenia*, pp. 8–27. Springer, Berlin.

Berrios, G. E. (1991b). Affective disorders in old age: a conceptual history. *International Journal of Geriatric Psychiatry*, **6**, 337–46.

Berrios, G. E. (1993). The psychiatry of old age: a conceptual history. In J. Copeland, M. Abou-Saleh & D. Blazer (eds.) *The Psychiatry of Old Age: an International Handbook*. Wiley, Chichester, in press.

Berrios, G. E. & Hauser, R. (1988). The early development of Kraepelin's ideas on classification: a conceptual history. *Psychological Medicine*, **18**, 813–21.

Berrios, G. E. & Freeman, H. (1991). *Alzheimer and the Dementias*. Royal Society of Medicine, London.

Bianchi, L. (1906). *A Textbook of Psychiatry*. Baillière, Tindall and Cox, London.

Blancard, S. (1726). *The Physical Dictionary wherein the Terms of Anatomy, the Names and Causes of Diseases, Chirurgical Instruments, and their Use, are Accurately Described*. John and Benjamin Sprint, London.

Bleuler, E. (1911). *Dementia Praecox oder Gruppe der Schizophrenien*. Franz Deuticke, Leipzig.

Buffon, M. le Comte, Georges Louis Leclerc (1774). *Histoire Naturelle de l'Homme, de la Vieillese et de la Mort*, vol. 4, *Histoire Naturelle de l'Homme*. De l'Imprimerie Royale, Paris.

Bulbena, A. & Berrios, G. E. (1986). Pseudodementia: facts and figures. *British Journal of Psychiatry*, **148**, 87–94.

Calmeil, L. F. (1835). Démence. In *Dictionaire de Médicine on Repertoire General des Sciences Médicales*, 2nd edition, pp. 70–85. Bechet, Paris.

Charcot, J. M. (1881). *Clinical Lectures on Senile and Chronic Diseases*. The New Sydenham Society, London.

Chereau, A. (1877). Rostan. In A. Dechambre & L. Lereboullet (eds.) *Dictionnaire Encyclopédique des Sciences Médicales*, vol. 84, pp. 238–40. Masson, Paris.

Cicero (1923). *De Senectute, de Amicitia, de Divinatione*. Translated by W. A. Falconer. Loeb, London.

Cohen, G. D. (1983). Historical views and evolution of concepts. In B. Reisberg (ed.) *Alzheimer's Disease*, pp. 29–34. The Free Press, New York.

Cotard, J. (1882). Du délire des négations. *Archives de Neurologie*, **4**, 152–70; 282–96.

Crichton-Browne, J. (1874). Senile dementia. *British Medical Journal*, **i**, 601–3; 640–3.

Cullen, W. (1827). *The Works of William Cullen*. William Blackwood, Edinburgh.

Cullere, A. (1890). *Traité Pratique des Maladies Mentales*. Baillière, Paris.

Darwin, E. (1794–96). *Zoonomia; or the Laws of Organic Life* (2 vols). Johnson, London.

DeFelipe, J. & Jones, E. G. (eds.) (1988). *Cajal on the Cerebral Cortex. An Annotated Translation of the Complete Writings*. Oxford University Press, Oxford.

Démange, E. (1886). *Etude Clinique et Anatomo-Pathologique sur la Vieillese*. Ballière, Paris.

Diderot, D. & d'Alembert, J. (eds.) (1754). *Encyclopédie ou Dictionnaire Raisonné des Sciences, des Arts et des Métieres, par une Societé de Gens de Lettres*, vol. 4, pp. 807–8. Briasson, David, Le Breton, Durand, A Paris.

Dumas, G. (1894). *Les Etats Intellectuals dans la Mélancolie*. Alcan, Paris.

Durand-Fardel, M. (1843). *Traité du Ramollissement du Cerveau*. Baillière, Paris.

Esquirol, E. (1805). *Des Passions*. Didot Jeune, Paris.

Esquirol, E. (1814). Démence. In *Dictionaire des Sciences Médicales, par une Société de Médicins et de Chirurgiens*, pp. 280–93. Panckouke, Paris.

Esquirol, E. (1838). *Des Maladies Mentales*. Baillière, Paris.

Fischer, O. (1907). Miliare Nekrosen mit drusigen Wucherungen der Neurofibrillen, eine regelmaessege Verandaerung der Hirnrinde bei seniler Demenz. *Monatsschrift für Psychiatrie und Neurologie*, **22**, 361–72.

Fox, P. (1989). From senility to Alzheimer's disease: the rise of the Alzheimer's disease movement. *The Milbank Quarterly*, **67**, 58–102.

Fuller, S. C. (1907). A study of the neurofibrils in dementia paralytica, dementia senilis, chronic alcoholism, cerebral lues and microcephalic idiocy. *American Journal of Insanity*, **63**, 415–68.

Fuller, S. C. (1912). Alzheimer's disease (senium praecox): the report of a case and review of published cases. *Journal of Nervous and Mental Disease*, **39**, 440–55; 536–57.

Georget, M. (1820). *De la Folie*. Crevot, Paris.

Gimeno, A. (1910). *La Lucha Contra la Vejez*. Antonio Marzo, Madrid.

Grant, R. L. (1963). Concepts of aging: an historical review. *Perspectives in Biology and Medicine*, **6**, 443–78.

Grmek, M. D. (1958). *On Ageing and Old Age*. W. Junk, Den Haag.

Gruman, G. J. (1966). A history of ideas about the prolongation of life. *Transactions of the American Philosophical Society*, **56**, 1–97.

Guislain, J. (1852). *Leçons Orales sur les Phrénopathies*. L. Hebbelynck, Gand.

Hakkéboutsch, B. M. & Geier, T. A. (1913). De la maladie d'Alzheimer. *Annales Médico-Psychologiques*, **71**, 358.

Hare, E. (1959). The origin and spread of dementia paralytica. *Journal Mental Science*, **105**, 594–626.

Huber, J.-P. & Gourin, P. (1987). Le vieillard dément dans l'antiquité classique. *Psychiatrie Française*, **13**, 12–18.

Hufeland, C. W. (1797). *Die Kunst das menschliche Leben zu Verlängern*. Franz Haas, Wien.

Jackson, J. H. (1875). A lecture on softening of the brain. *Lancet*, **ii**, 335–9.

Johnstone, E., Crow, T. J., Frith, C. D. et al. (1978). The dementia of dementia praecox. *Acta Psychiatrica Scandinavica*, **57**, 305–24.

Kastenbaum, R. & Ross, B. (1975). Historical perspectives on care. In J. Howells (ed.) *Modern Perspectives in the Psychiatry of Old Age*, pp. 421–49. Churchill Livingstone, Edinburgh.

Kiloh, L. G. (1961). Pseudo-dementia. *Acta Psychiatrica Scandinavica*, **37**, 336–51.

Kraepelin, E. (1910). *Psychiatrie: ein Lehrbuch für Studierende und Arzte*. Johann Ambrosius Barth, Leipzig.

Kraepelin, E. (1919). *Dementia praecox and paraphrenia*. (Translation by R. M. Barclay.) Livingstone, Edinburgh.

Krafft-Ebing, R. (1873). De la démence sénile. *Annales Médico-Psychologiques*, **34**, 306–7.

Kral, V. A. (1962). Senescent forgetfulness: benign and malignant. *Canadian Medical Association Journal*, **86**, 257–60.

Lanczik, M. (1988). *Der Breslauer Psychiater Carl Wernicke*. Thorbecke, Sigmaringen.

Lambert, C. I. (1916). The clinical and anatomical features of Alzheimer's disease. *Journal of Mental and Nervous Disease*, **44**, 169–70.

Legrand, M. A. (1911). *La longévité à travers les ages*. Flammarion, Paris.

Lehr, U. (1977). *Psychologie des Alterns*. Quelle und Meyer, Heidelberg.

Levy, M. (1850). *Traité d'Hygiéne Publique et Privée*. Baillière, Paris.

Lucretius (1975). *De Rerum Natura*. Translated by M. F. Smith. Heinemann, London.

Lugaro, E. (1916). La psichiatria tedesca nella storia e nell'attualita. *Rivista di Patologia Nervosa e Mentale*, **21**, 337–86.

Madden, J. J., Luhan, J. A., Kaplan, L. A. & Gibson, N. D. (1952). Non-dementing psychoses in older persons. *Journal of the American Medical Association*, **150**, 1567–70.

Mairet, A. (1883). *De la Démence Mélancolique*. Masson, Paris.

Marc, C. C. M. (1840). *De la Folie*. Baillière, Paris.

Marcé, L. V. (1862). *Traité des Maladies Mentales*. Baillière, Paris.

Marcé, L. V. (1863). Recherches cliniques et anatomo-pathologiques sur la démence sénile et sur les différences qui la separent de la paralysie générale. *Gazette Médicale de Paris*, **34**, 433–5; 467–9; 497–502; 631–2; 761–4; 797–8; 831–3; 855–8.

Marie, A. (1906). *La Démence*. Doin, Paris.

Marinesco, G. (1900). Mécanisme de la sénilité et de la mort des cellules nerveuses. *Comptes Rendus Hebdomadaires des Sciences de L'Académie des Sciences*, **130**, 1136–9.

Metchnikoff, E. (1904). *The Nature of Man. Studies in Optimistic Philosophy*. Heinemann, London.

Meynert, T. (1890). Amentia. In *Klinische Vorlesungen über Psychiatrie auf Wissenschaftlichen Grundlagen, für Studierende und Ärzte, Juristen und Psychologen*. Braumüller, Vienna.

Minois, G. (1987). *Histoire de la Vieillesse. De l'Antiquité à la Renaissance*. Fayard, Paris.

Morel, B. A. (1852). *Etudes Cliniques sur les Maladies Mentales* (2 vols). Masson, Paris.

Morel, B. A. (1860). *Traité des Maladies Mentales*. Masson, Paris.

North, H. M. & Bostock, F. (1925). Arteriosclerosis and mental disease. *Journal of Mental Science*, **71**, 600–1.

Olah, G. (1910). Was kann man heute unter Arteriosklerotischen Psychosen verstehen? *Psychiatrischen und Neurologischen Wochenschrift*, **52**, 532–3.

Perusini, G. (1911). Sul valore nosografico di alcuni reperti istopatologicè caratteristici per la senilità. *Rivista Italiana di Neuropatologia*, **4**, 193–213.

Pick, D. (1989). *Faces of Degeneration*. Cambridge University Press, Cambridge.

Pinel, Ph. (1806). *A Treatise of Insanity*. (Translation by D. D. Davis.) Cadell and Davies, Sheffield.

Pinel, Ph. (1818). *Nosographie Philosophique*, 6th edition. Brosson, Paris.

Postel, J. (1972). Introduction. In E. Georget, *De la Folie*, pp. 7–21. Privat, Paris.

Reveillé-Parise, J. H. (1853). *Traité de la Vieillesse*. Baillière, Paris.

Rostan, L. (1823). *Recherches sur le Ramollissement du Cerveau*, 2nd edition. Bechet, Paris.

Rostan, L. (1833). *Jusqu'à quel Point l'Anatomie Pathologique peut-elle Clairer la Thérapeutique des Maladies*. Thèse de concours, Paris.

Schneider, K. (1959). *Clinical Psychopathology*. (Translation by M. W. Hamilton.) Grune & Stratton, New York.

Simchowicz, T. (1911). Histologische Studien über die Senile Demenz. *Histologische und histopathologischen Arbeiten über der Grosshirnrinde*, **4**, 267–444.

Simchowicz, T. (1924). Sur la signification des plaques séniles et sur la formule sénile de l'écorce cérébrale. *Revue Neurologique*, **31**, 221–7.

Sinclair, Sir J. (1807). *The Code of Health and Longevity*. Constable, Edinburgh.

Sobrino (1791). Aumentado o nuevo Diccionario, 3 vols. Leon, J. B. Delamolliere.

Southard, E. E. (1910). Anatomical findings in 'senile dementia': a diagnostic study bearing especially on the group of cerebral atrophies. *American Journal of Insanity*, **61**, 673–708.

Tomlinson, B. E. & Corsellis, J. A. N. (1984). Ageing and the dementias. In J. H. Adams, J. A. N. Corsellis & L. W. Ducken (eds.) *Greenfield's Neuropathology*, pp. 951–1025. Arnold, London.

von Kondratowitz, H.-J. (1991). The medicalisation of old age. Continuity and change in Germany from the late eighteenth century to the early twentieth century. In M. Pelling & R. M. Smith (eds.) *Life, Death and the Elderly, Historical Perspectives*, pp. 134–64. Routledge, London.

Walton, G. L. (1912). Arteriosclerosis probably not an important factor in the etiology and prognosis of involution psychoses. *Boston Medical and Surgical Journal*, **167**, 834–6.

Woltereck, H. (1956). *Das Alter is das zweite Leben*. Deutsche Verlags-Anstalt, Stuttgart.

Ziehen, T. (1911). Les démences. In A. Marie (ed.) *Traité International de Psychologie Pathologique*, vol. 2, pp. 281–381. Alcan, Paris.

Zilboorg, G. (1941). *A History of Medical Psychology*, Norton, New York.

3

The history of research into dementia and its relationship to current concepts

W. A. LISHMAN

Research into dementia has prospered conspicuously during the past two decades, with the result that we witness now an almost bewildering number of approaches to the subject. Clinicians, epidemiologists, neuropathologists and a host of laboratory workers all see the dementias as prime targets for their activities. Newer disciplines such as cell biology and molecular genetics key quickly into the problem.

Until quite recently, however, things were very different. For much of the present century dementia was neglected, in fact, to a large extent, ignored. It will be interesting perhaps to review the history of the topic and to see what may have shaped this escalation of interest. We will find a changing conception of the nature of dementia, of the relationship between presenile and senile forms, and of the demarcation, if such exists, between dementia and aging processes. Changing views on such issues have by no means come to rest and, by examining their historical perspective, one may hope to derive some leads towards the future. At a more detailed level, neurobiological research has provided us with not one, but several, models which may explain the aetiopathogenesis of Alzheimer's disease, the commonest of all dementing disorders. Changing concepts, in other words, continue to flourish in the context of current advances.

Early twentieth century

As the present century opened, people were certainly interested in dementia. The word and the concept had already been in use for some 200 years, and during the nineteenth century had come to signify progressive cognitive impairment (Berrios (1987); see also Chapter 2).

Dementia and Normal Aging, eds. F. A. Huppert, C. Brayne & D. W. O'Connor.
© Cambridge University Press 1994.

The advent of good histological techniques towards the end of the nineteenth century had allowed a start to be made in defining tissue pathology – general paresis was a continuing focus of interest and cerebral arteriosclerosis was well recognized. Huntington (1872) and Pick (1892) had already described the diseases that were to bear their names. There was also an ill-defined category of 'senile psychosis', sometimes termed 'senile dementia', though this was a broad conception which included much within its remit.

Early descriptions drew an inseparable analogy with the processes to be expected with aging generally. Senile dementia was seen as the parallel, in severe degree, of the bodily decline of old age. Henry Maudsley (1899, p. 168) wrote of senile dementia as 'the pathological term of the natural decay of mind which occurs when nature –

> As it grows again towards earth,
> Is fashioned for the journey, dull and heavy.

Within this concept of dementia lay much of old age mental disorder. Senile melancholia, senile delirium, and states of persecutory insanity were thought to depend on brain pathological changes of a similar nature.

Gowers' 'abiotrophy'

The scientific basis of aging was scarcely speculated upon. But as explanation for an exaggeration of the process, Gowers' concept of 'abiotrophy' became widely influential, certainly in the UK. He proposed that a certain class of disorders – myopathies, Friedreich's ataxia, cerebellar degenerations, even baldness – depended on an inexorable decline in certain cell lines due to premature loss of their viability (Gowers, 1902, 1908). The term was used for cases in which 'certain systems of structure . . . have an essential defect of vital endurance in consequence of which their life slowly fails' (Gowers, 1908, p. 1542). Mental deterioration of late life was suggested as an example.

The conception was applied readily to the dementias. In Bolton's textbook we find dementia attributed to 'deficient durability of higher cortical neurons' (Bolton, 1914, p. 280). Dementia is due to 'natural involution of the cortical neurons, occurring at such individually diverse periods of life as are determined by their inherent capacity of resistance to the processes of decay' (Bolton, 1914, p. 221). In this way, cases even of presenile dementia could fall within the rubric of abiotrophy. Indeed it was fundamental to Gowers' conception that some persons were affected early.

It was during this period that Alzheimer (1906, 1907) described his disease. The description of his first patient, a woman of 51, was followed quickly by further cases. He stressed the presence in the brain of plaques and neurofibrillary tangles, already described by others, also the presence of hyaline material, later identified as amyloid, in the centre of the plaques. Very soon Alzheimer was himself embroiled in debates that were to continue for decades to come (Alzheimer, (1911); translated by Förstl & Levy, (1991)). What was the significance, aetiologically, of these distinctive components revealed by the microscope? And what was the relationship between such presenile cases and senile dementia itself? Fischer (1910) was soon to describe a group of elderly senile dements with well-developed plaques and tangles. The plaques themselves were relabelled 'senile plaques' by Simchowicz (1910), itself a significant development. Thus, there were those who saw an identity between senile dementia and Alzheimer's new disease, and those who regarded the disorders as distinct. Certain clinical features, such as focal signs like language disturbance in younger patients, were adduced in favour of a separation.

These debates were well advanced during the early decades of the present century. They continued thereafter, with the additional observation that senile plaques were found to characterize a large proportion of non-demented elderly brains. Gellerstedt (1933) described them as occurring in 84% of the brains of persons dying over the age of 65 years.

Gradually it became accepted that 'premature senility' was a sufficient explanation for presenile Alzheimer's disease. As McMenemey (1963) pointed out, a host of factors were prejudicial to such a conception. Thus, the very adjective 'presenile' biased one to thinking in terms of senility, though intended only to refer to a period of life. 'Middle-aged dementia' might have been a better term. As a hallmark of the disease, the 'senile' plaque coloured thinking similarly. Abiotrophy, as we have seen, was a prevailing view, implying premature death of tissue. On the clinical front, observation suggested an imperceptible shading from Alzheimer's disease to senile dementia, and thence to the simple memory failure of old age. In analogous fashion the histological features of Alzheimer's disease could be present even in the healthy aged.

Thus, the view gained ground that Alzheimer's disease was a rare and curious entity, representing senility occurring early. The converse view, that it might repay detailed study as a means of clarifying the great mass of senile dementing patients, was voiced rarely. Senile dementia was in any case a rather amorphous conception with indistinct boundaries from natural aging. In this way we entered the 'dark ages'.

The 'dark ages'

During the middle part of the present century, we neglected the dementias seriously. They were a no-man's land, falling between neurology, psychiatry and the barely conceived discipline of geriatrics. In clinical terms they offered little of interest to the diagnostician or therapist. Research workers certainly found more hopeful openings than attempts to reverse a process of aging.

The extent of disinterest is displayed vividly in British text books of the period. Russell Brain's *Diseases of the Nervous System* ran through eight editions between 1933 and 1977; by 1951, dementia still takes up only four of 980 pages. Alzheimer's disease is dealt with in three-quarters of a page and is said to be 'essentially premature senility' (Brain, 1951, p. 962). Walshe's *Diseases of the Nervous System* (1955) does not mention Alzheimer's disease at all.

The psychiatric texts do just a little better. Henderson & Gillespie (1932) devote 10 of 600 pages to the dementias. 'Simple senile deterioration' is the paradigm for senile dementia. Grafted onto this are senile delirium, senile depression and senile paranoid states, all viewed against a background of organic brain degeneration. The edition of 1947 takes new interest in describing the presenile dementias, but there is still no hint that Alzheimer's disease could affect the elderly.

British neuropathologists are likewise rather slow to take an interest. Buzzard & Greenfield's (1921) book on *Pathology of the Nervous System* makes no mention of senile dementia or Alzheimer's disease. But in the first edition of Greenfield et al.'s *Neuropathology* (1958), we find a splendid chapter by McMenemey (McMenemey, 1958). Alzheimer's disease is fully documented, along with arguments for and against the view that it is identical to senile dementia. The concept of abiotrophy is qualified to the extent that environmental factors may yet serve to light up the process. And senile dementia is at last dissected more closely. McMenemey suggests that the term should be applied when dementia occurs over the age of 65 years and cannot be attributed to Pick's disease, cerebral arteriosclerosis, syphilis or any other established condition. He recommends use of the term Alzheimer's disease irrespective of age when abundant tangles and plaques are present in the brain, and the term senile dementia when the patient is elderly and the histological criteria of Alzheimer's disease are incomplete.

With such criteria, things at last became clearer in the neuropathological laboratory. But in the living patient there was a great deal still to be done. There was the need to circumscribe the territory of senile dementia from other mental disorders of old age, and a need to embark in a systematic sense on clinicopathological correlations.

A tighter nosology

In the 1950s, in the UK, a start was made to clarify the nosological status of dementia in the elderly. Here Roth (1955) made a signal contribution, in effect rescuing psychiatry of the elderly from a complacent state of neglect.

Roth (1955) examined all available information on two cohorts of elderly people who were admitted to Graylingwell Hospital. Using 'operational criteria' he divided them into five clinical groupings – affective psychosis, senile psychosis, late paraphrenia, acute confusion and arteriosclerotic psychosis. By examining outcome, in terms of survival or discharge from hospital in the period that followed, distinct nosological groupings were discerned. The affective disorders, in particular, often proved to be remediable, and few progressed to dementia. Paraphrenic patients tended to survive but to remain as in-patients. The arteriosclerotic dements compared to the senile dements showed improved survival, at least during the early follow-up period, and an excess in males compared with the female preponderance in senile dementia.

Old-age mental disorder thus proved to be heterogeneous, with definable conditions, each tending to carry a distinct prognosis. One could no longer readily impute 'underlying dementia' as the cause of all senile mental disturbance. And henceforward the two main forms of dementia in the elderly – the senile and the arteriosclerotic – could be studied more realistically, without their encumbrances of depression, paraphrenia and confusional states. An amorphous conception of senile mental illness had been refined very considerably.

With this new tidiness, senile dementia could be compared properly with presenile Alzheimer's disease. And opinion grew steadily that they were virtually identical except for the matter of age of onset. In fact it was to prove that the presenile cases had greater brain atrophy and more severely developed plaques and tangles than senile Alzheimer's disease (Sourander & Sjogren, 1970). The pathological process differed only in being developed more vigorously when affecting the relatively young.

In the 1950s and 1960s, a start was also made in seeking ties between the clinical picture during life and the histological appearances after death. Corsellis (1962) showed that both parenchymatous and vascular changes became more common in the brain with advancing age, but decidedly more common in those who had shown a progressive dementia. This was an important counter to Rothschild's (1956) suggestion that the structural state of the brain might after all be irrelevant to the dementing process. Roth's group in Newcastle again took a lead by showing that quantitative counts of plaques and tangles correlated well with the severity of dementia as measured prior to death (Roth et al., 1967; Blessed et al., 1968; Tomlinson et al., 1968, 1970). Analogous quantitative estimations showed a relationship between the extent of cerebral softenings and the severity of arteriosclerotic dementia (Tomlinson et al., 1970; Roth, 1971). Altogether, in this era, the dementias began at last to be placed on a firm scientific footing.

It is relevant to note, however, that even in this context there was no clear support for a firm demarcation between dementia and the processes of aging. The quantitative estimations came tantalizingly close to such a separation by showing 'threshold effects' beyond which the development of brain pathology would be reflected regularly in dementia; but tangles, plaques and cerebral softenings in some degree also featured in a proportion of the non-demented elderly. Therefore, continuities could not be disproved decisively.

A third development in the 1950s and 1960s was the start on exploring genetic affinities in the dementias. Kallmann (1956) showed a high concordance of 43% for parenchymatous senile dementia in monozygotic twin pairs, compared with only 8% in dizygotic pairs and 7% in siblings. Larsson et al. (1963) showed a fourfold increase in incidence among the first-degree relatives of patients with the disorder. This did not depend solely on increased longevity in the families concerned. Rather it seemed to point to an inherited susceptibility. This evidence, at last, suggested some process distinct from the mere passing of the years – something that could be viewed in terms of a disease.

An acceleration and intensification of the aging process might well be at work, as reflected in the severity of the tissue pathology, but the cause of such acceleration should be amenable to research.

The medical model

And so we came gradually to the concept of dementia as a problem worthy of being tackled in the light of the 'medical model'. As with other disease states, however baffling, it might yet repay research at a fundamental level.

During the 1970s, arguments were marshalled increasingly to support such a view. Neurobiology was growing steadily in stature, with some impressive achievements in relation to other disorders. Dopamine deficiency was established in the striatum in Parkinson's disease (Vogt, 1970; Hornykiewicz, 1971), leading on to successful replacement therapy. γ-Aminobutyric acid, and its synthesizing enzyme, glutamic acid decarboxylase, were found to be deficient in the basal ganglia in Huntington's dementia (Bird et al., 1973; Perry et al., 1973). Creutzfeldt–Jacob disease proved to be due to a transmissible agent (Gibbs et al., 1968). Such discoveries in relation to other 'degenerative' conditions, even to other dementias, provided a spur for research into Alzheimer's disease. A model was discovered for the induction of neurofibrillary tangles in rabbits by the injection of aluminium salts; and brain aluminium was found to be increased in the Alzheimer brain (Crapper et al., 1976).

Such new-found confidence opened not one but several openings for research into the commonest of all dementing conditions, viz. Alzheimer's senile dementia. Toxic, infective and biochemical perturbations had all emerged as targets for detailed research. Attention to Alzheimer's dementia was spurred on by realization of the numbers of elderly persons afflicted with the condition, and threatening to overwhelm the caring services.

The Medical Research Council (MRC) nominated research into the dementias as a priority area in 1977 (Medical Research Council, 1977), and the Royal College of Physicians commissioned a review of the current state of knowledge in 1981 (Royal College of Physicians, 1981). Moreover, while waiting for the MRC review to appear, three centres in the UK (Edinburgh, Newcastle and London) simultaneously discovered cholinergic depletion of marked degree in the brain, both in presenile and senile Alzheimer's disease (Davies, 1977; Perry et al.,

1977; Spillane et al., 1977; White et al., 1977). From this point onwards research into the dementias gathered pace rapidly.

Figure 3.1 represents a count of the number of publications annually on dementia in the *Cumulated Index Medicus*, representing the British and American literature. We see a quite remarkable uniformity at some 100 publications per year throughout the 1960s and 1970s. The first increases begin to appear in 1977 and 1979, followed by an astonishing escalation from 1980 onwards, climbing to 1500 publications during 1990. Publications on 'aging' begin to rise somewhat earlier in the mid-1970s, then climb in parallel with dementia.

Even a cursory glance at the *Cumulated Index Medicus* shows that the vast majority of this research is devoted to Alzheimer's disease, and the greater part deals with the elderly – 'senile dementia of the Alzheimer type' (SDAT). What was seen formerly only in terms of abiotrophy and senility is now investigaged intensively from multiple points of view.

The many different facets of this research, ranging from clinical, epidemiological and psychological studies to detailed explorations of brain biochemistry and histopathology, are dealt with in other chapters of this volume. All share the common purpose of refining understanding of Alzheimer-type dementia, with the ultimate hope of discovering its nature and pathogenesis.

It is worth noting, however, how quickly concepts can change in

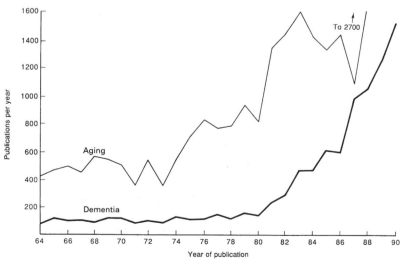

Figure 3.1. Publications per year on aging and dementia listed in the *Cumulated Index Medicus*, 1964–90.

relation to the fundamentals of the disorder. At various times during the past two decades there have been champions for the role of aluminium toxicity, amyloidosis, blood–brain barrier changes, even infective processes. The importance of cortical cell loss, and the significance to be attached to plaques and tangles, have at times been doubted then resurrected strongly.

On the biochemical front, brain cholinergic depletion remains a striking and well-attested finding. There have been changing views, however, about its relationship to cortical or subcortical pathology. The discovery that cells were profoundly depleted in the nucleus basalis of Meynert led, for a time, to the idea that Alzheimer's disease might, after all, represent a focal brain disorder. Whole brain cholinergic function would fail by virtue of losses of input of fibres from this important source. Loss of cells from the locus caeruleus, also well established, might be primary in leading to noradrenergic failure. Thus, Alzheimer's disease was viewed as a disease of subcortical neuronal systems, i.e. of the 'isodendritic core' (Rossor, 1981). What had been seen as a cortical disease process may have had its roots elsewhere. This concept has fallen from favour with realization of the multiplicity of neurotransmitter deficits, and with clearer appreciation of the extent of cortical cell loss. More recent formulations emphasize defects of glutamatergic transmission between the intrinsic cortical neurons themselves in addition to defective inputs into the cortex (Bowen, 1990). And there are those who prefer to conceptualize the problem, not in terms of biochemical systems at all, but as a spreading cortical involvement along defined anatomical pathways (Pearson et al., 1985).

On the genetic front there have been, perhaps, some of the most far-reaching conceptual changes of all. Heston et al.'s (1981) survey showed that the risk to first-degree relatives was increased considerably when the proband was under 70 years of age. Taking data from this and other studies, Mohs et al. (1987) have used life tables to estimate age-specific incidence in relatives, revealing a cumulative risk rising to 46% by the age of 86 years. This seems not inconsistent with an autosomal dominant gene, or genes, with age-dependent gene expression. In other words, it is possible to marshall arguments that Alzheimer's disease is very strongly determined by genetic factors, the evidence being obscured only by the number of persons at risk who die before their disorder has become overt.

Molecular genetics, meanwhile, has focused on familial cases, and with dramatic results. Using markers for chromosome 21, by analogy with Down's syndrome, the familial Alzheimer's gene was cornered quickly (St George-Hyslop et al., 1987). The gene which codes for the A4 amyloid protein precursor was found to be in the same region, on the long arm of the chromosome (Tanzi et al., 1987). Since then we have had hopes raised, lowered and raised again (Goate et al., 1991) that these two genes may be identical with one another, pointing thereby to perhaps the earliest link in an aetiological chain of events.

In the excitement of these fundamental advances, genetic influences have attracted more attention than possible environmental risk factors. The latter are less easy to research with precision, but may exist nonetheless, rendering some individuals vulnerable, or resistant to, the genetic load they bear. As with other disorders there may be close gene–environment interactions which underlie the development of the disease.

Alzheimer's dementia and neural aging

In much of this more recent research, Alzheimer's dementia is conceptualized in terms of the medical model of illness. Like Pick's, Huntington's and Creutzfeldt–Jacob diseases, it is viewed as a dementia with a disease process behind it. The searches for mechanism are based on such a conception. In other words the developments of the past two decades have operated in the main as a vigorous opposition to the idea that Alzheimer's changes are analogous to old age. It seems to have been important to discard this prejudice in order to open up research on a widespread front.

It is perhaps worth pausing, however, to re-evaluate the situation in the light of what we know now. Certain observations remain obstinately to remind us that aging and Alzheimer's dementia are interlinked closely. This, it should be noted, applies only to Alzheimer's dementia – other forms, with perhaps the exception of multi-infarct disease, are absolved from the dilemma.

Thus, it is abundantly obvious that Alzheimer's dementia becomes more common with increasing age. Many of its clinical features are believed widely to be common as age advances, in particular memory impairment. But more strikingly so are changes within the brain – the appearance of plaques and of tangles at least within the hippocampus. On the biochemical front there is decline with age in several neurotransmitters and their synthesizing enzymes, well documented certainly for the cholinergic system. And neuronal loss is now well attested in the aging brain, affecting neocortical and hippocampal neurons, also the nucleus basalis of Meynert and the locus caeruleus. It is hard, indeed, to point to any feature of the brain of an Alzheimer patient which does not also occur with increasing age alone.

Added to this we find a parallel, or rather a paradoxical observation, namely that in Alzheimer's dementia the brain changes tend to be less marked in degree in the more elderly victims of the disorder. Thus, the frequency of plaques and of tangles in the neocortex becomes progressively less in older Alzheimer patients, likewise the percentage cell loss in relation to age-matched controls, and the percentage reduction in nucleolar volume among the cells that remain (Mann et al., 1985). Such erosion of the difference between patients and their healthy peers affects cell counts in many areas – temporal cortex, hippocampus, locus caeruleus, nucleus basalis of Meynert and the raphe nuclei (Mann, 1985). Thus, in the very elderly there may be little in the brain to distinguish Alzheimer patients from non-dements of equivalent age.

Such observations are repeatedly forthcoming. Markers of cholinergic, noradrenergic and serotonergic dysfunction become less divergent from controls in older dements. On the clinical front we find slower rates of progression, less evidence of focal brain failure, and, from Heston et al.'s (1981) study, less evidence over 70 years of age of the operation of genetic influences.

Altogether it would seem that when Alzheimer's dementia affects the elderly it becomes progressively harder to draw firm demarcations between neural aging and the Alzheimer process – to see where the one has ended and the other has begun. The disorder, in effect, appears to approach and coalesce with old age when affecting the very old.

What can underlie this observation? One obvious explanation would be that the elderly normals included in laboratory and clinical studies are not normal after all, but in reality 'subclinical' or 'preclinical' cases. Or it may be, as accepted widely, that the disease process becomes progressively more benign in later life, as happens with some cancers. In genetic terms penetrance may become weaker. A further possibility is that the brains of younger persons require a higher level of exposure to some pathogenic insult before Alzheimer's disease is declared.

A final possibility remains nonetheless, namely that Alzheimer's disease is brain aging after all. Until some definite marker is established – histological, biochemical, viral, behavioural – which separates cases from non-cases in a decisive manner, this conception is not disproved. Continuities between Alzheimer's disease and neural aging processes appear to be more conspicuous in many respects than are discontinuities.

We can conceive of an aging process within the brain which itself accounts for decreased neuronal counts and the accumulation of plaques and tangles. This will lead on to biochemical changes and evidence of cognitive decline. This aging process itself may be under strong genetic and environmental influences, so that it is sometimes considerably accelerated and intensified. In all persons the shift from so-called 'normality' to becoming 'a case of Alzheimer's dementia' will occur when the process has passed a certain threshold in its development.

Some will be affected already in middle life, when examination of the brain will show marked divergences from their peers. But in some the process will be milder and delayed, with 'caseness' appearing only in old age. A smaller augmentation of the aging process will then have been required in order to pass the threshold, since the passing of time will already have done much of the work. Hence, in the very old, differences from age-matched controls may emerge as being barely discernible.

It is hard to judge at the present time whether such a formulation is valid. But the options would seem to be open. It is possible that we have seized on the medical model of Alzheimer's disease too readily, and partly by virtue of analogies with other dementing illnesses. There were other dementias, superficially like Alzheimer's disease, which had an identifiable 'cause' – a gene mutation in Huntington's disease, a transmissible agent in Creutzfeldt–Jacob disease – and there were those like Pick's disease whose pathology did not resemble the aged brain. In Alzheimer's dementia, unlike all the rest, the brain picture seems to point towards that of aging itself.

In the last analysis, of course, the distinction between 'aging process' and 'disease' may melt away – an artificial dichotomy drawn from older concepts. And there will be no need for a return to nihilism if we are obliged to reformulate the problem of Alzheimer's dementia in this fashion. Neurobiology may now have reached the stature when we can tackle head-on the nature of the aging processes within the brain, and the factors – genetic and environmental – which accelerate or retard it. We may no longer have need of the shelter of a formal disease model to provide an impetus to scientific effort.

References

Alzheimer, A. (1906). Über einen eigenartigen, schweren Erkrankungsprozess der Hirnrinde. *Neurologisches Centralblatt*, **xxv**, 1134.

Alzheimer, A. (1907). Über eigenartige Erkrankung der Hirnrinde. *Allgemeine Zeitschrift für Psychiatrie*, **64**, 146–8.

Alzheimer, A. (1911). Uber eigenartige Krankheitsfälle des späteren Alters. *Zeitschrift für die gesamte Neurologie und Psychiatrie*, **4**, 356–85.

Berrios, G. E. (1987). Dementia during the seventeenth and eighteenth centuries: a conceptual history. *Psychological Medicine*, **17**, 829–37.

Bird, E. D., MacKay, A. V. P., Rayner, C. N. & Iversen, L. L. (1973). Reduced glutamic-acid-decarboxylase activity of post-mortem brain in Huntington's chorea. *Lancet*, **i**, 1090–2.

Blessed, G., Tomlinson, B. E. & Roth, M. (1968). The association between quantitative measures of dementia and of senile change in the cerebral grey matter of elderly subjects. *British Journal of Psychiatry*, **114**, 797–811.

Bolton, J. S. (1914). *The Brain in Health and Disease*. Edward Arnold, London.

Bowen, D. M. (1990). Treatment of Alzheimer's disease, molecular pathology versus neurotransmitter-based therapy. *British Journal of Psychiatry*, **157**, 327–30.

Brain, R. (1951). *Diseases of the Nervous System*, 4th edition. Oxford University Press, Oxford.

Buzzard, E. F. & Greenfield, J. G. (1921). *Pathology of the Nervous System*. Constable and Co., London.

Corsellis, J. A. N. (1962). *Mental Illness and the Ageing Brain*. Maudsley Monograph No. **9**, Oxford University Press.

Crapper, D. R., Krishnan, S. S. & Quittkat, S. (1976). Aluminium, neurofibrillary degeneration and Alzheimer's disease. *Brain*, **99**, 67–80.

Davies, P. (1977). Cholinergic mechanisms in Alzheimer's disease. *British Journal of Psychiatry*, **131**, 318–19.

Fischer, O. (1910). *Zentralblatt für die gesamte Neurologie und Psychiatrie*, **3**, 371. (Quoted by W. H. McMenemey (1958), see below.)

Förstl, H. & Levy, R. (1991). On certain peculiar diseases of old age. Translation of A. Alzheimer (1911). *History of Psychiatry*, **ii**, 71–101.

Gellerstedt, N. (1933). Zur Kenntnis der Hirnveranderungen bei der normalen Altersinvolution. *Uppsala Lakareforenings Forhandlingar*, **38**, 193.

Gibbs, C. J., Gajdusek, D. C., Asher, D. M., Alpers, M. P., Beck, E., Daniel, P. M. & Matthews, W. B. (1968). Creutzfeldt–Jakob disease (spongiform encephalopathy): transmission to the chimpanzee. *Science*, **161**, 388–9.

Goate, A., Chartier-Harlin, M. C., Mullan, M., Brown, J., Crawford, F., Fidani, L., Giuffra, L., Haynes, A., Irving, N., James, L., Mant, R., Newton, P., Rooke, K., Roques, P., Talbot, C., Pericak-Vance, M., Roses, A., Williamson, R., Rossor, M., Owen, M. & Hardy, J. (1991). Segregation of a missense mutation in the amyloid precursor protein gene with familial Alzheimer's disease. *Nature*, **349**, 704–6.

Gowers, W. R. (1902). A lecture on abiotrophy. *Lancet*, **i**, 1003–7.

Gowers, W. R. (1908). Heredity in diseases of the nervous system. *British Medical Journal*, **2**, 1541–3.

Greenfield, J. G., Blackwood, W., McMenemey, W. H., Meyer, A. & Norman, R. M. (1958). *Neuropathology*. Edward Arnold (Publishers) Ltd., London.

Henderson, D. K. & Gillespie, R. D. (1932). *A Textbook of Psychiatry for Students and Practitioners*, 3rd edition. Oxford University Press, London.

Henderson, D. K. & Gillespie, R. D. (1947). *A Textbook of Psychiatry for Students and Practitioners*, 6th edition. Oxford University Press, London.

Heston, L. L., Mastri, A. R., Anderson, E. & White, J. (1981). Dementia of the Alzheimer type. Clinical genetics, natural history and associated conditions. *Archives of General Psychiatry*, **38**, 1085–90.

Hornykiewicz, O. (1971). Neurochemical pathology and pharmacology of brain dopamine and acetylcholine: rational basis for the current drug treatment of parkinsonism. In F. H. McDowell & C. H. Markham (eds.) *Recent Advances in Parkinson's Disease*, Chapter 2. Blackwell Scientific Publications, Oxford.

Huntington, G. (1872). On chorea. *Medical and Surgical Reporter (Philadelphia)*, **26**, 317–21.

Kallmann, F. J. (1956). Genetic aspects of mental disorders in later life. In O. J. Kaplan (ed.) *Mental Disorders in Later Life*, pp. 26–46. Stanford University Press.

Larsson, T., Sjogren, T. & Jacobson, G. (1963). Senile dementia: a clinical, sociomedical and genetic study. *Acta Psychiatrica Scandinavica*, (supplement), **167**, 1–259.

Mann, D. M. A. (1985). The neuropathology of Alzheimer's disease: a review with pathogenetic, aetiological and therapeutic considerations. *Mechanisms of Ageing and Development*, **31**, 213–55.

Mann, D. M. A., Yates, P. O. & Marcyniuk, B. (1985). Some morphometric observations on the cerebral cortex and in hippocampus in Alzheimer's presenile dementia, senile dementia of Alzheimer type, Down's syndrome in middle age. *Journal of the Neurological Sciences*, **69**, 139–59.

Maudsley, H. (1899). *The Pathology of Mind*. D. Appleton and Co., New York.

McMenemey, W. H. (1958). The dementias and progressive diseases of the basal ganglia. In J. G. Greenfield, W. Blackwood, W. H. McMenemey, A. Meyer & R. M. Norman (eds.) *Neuropathology*, pp. 475–528. Edward Arnold (Publishers) Ltd., London.

McMenemey, W. H. (1963). Alzheimer's disease: problems concerning its concept and nature. *Acta Neurologica Scandinavica*, **39**, 369–80.

Medical Research Council (1977). *Senile and Presenile Dementias*. A report of the MRC Subcommittee, compiled by W. A. Lishman. Medical Research Council, London.

Mohs, R. C., Breitner, J. C. S., Silverman, J. M. & Davis, K. L. (1987). Alzheimer's disease. Morbid risk among first-degree relatives. Approximates 50% by 90 years of age. *Archives of General Psychiatry*, **44**, 405–8.

Pearson, R. C. A., Esiri, M. M., Hiorns, R. W., Willcock, G. K. & Powers, T. P. S. (1985). Anatomical correlates of the distribution of the pathological changes in the neocortex in Alzheimer's disease. *Proceedings of the National Academy of Sciences, USA*, **82**, 4531–4.

Perry, E. K., Gibson, P. H., Blessed, G., Perry, R. H. & Tomlinson, B. E. (1977). Neurotransmitter enzyme abnormalities in senile dementia. Choline acetyltransferase and glutamic acid decarboxylase activities in necropsy brain tissue. *Journal of the Neurological Sciences*, **34**, 247–65.

Perry, T. L., Hansen, S. & Kloster, M. (1973). Huntington's chorea: deficiency of γ-aminobutyric acid in brain. *New England Journal of Medicine*, **288**, 337–42.

Pick, A. (1892). Ueber die Beziehungen der senilen Hirnatrophie zur Aphasie. *Prager medizinische Wochenschrift*, **17**, 165–7.

Rossor, M. N. (1981). Parkinson's disease and Alzheimer's disease as disorders of the isodendritic core. *British Medical Journal*, **283**, 1588–90.

Roth, M. (1955). The natural history of mental disorder in old age. *Journal of Mental Science*, **101**, 281–301.

Roth, M. (1971). Classification and aetiology in mental disorders of old age: some recent developments. In D. W. K. Kay & A. Walk (eds.) *Recent Developments in Psychogeriatrics*, pp. 1–18. A *British Journal of Psychiatry* Special Publication No. **6**. Headley Bros., Ashford, Kent.

Roth, M., Tomlinson, B. E. & Blessed, G. (1967). The relationship between quantitative measures of dementia and of degenerative changes in the cerebral grey matter of elderly subjects. *Proceedings of the Royal Society of Medicine*, **60**, 254–9.

Rothschild, D. (1956). Senile psychoses and psychoses with cerebral arteriosclerosis. In O. J. Kaplan (ed.) *Mental Disorders in Later Life*, pp. 289–331. Stanford University Press, Stanford.

Royal College of Physicians (1981). Organic mental impairment in the elderly: implications for research, education and the provision of services. Report of the Royal College of Physicians by the College Committee on Geriatrics. *Journal of the Royal College of Physicians of London*, **15**, 141–67.

Simchowicz, T. (1910). *Histologische und Histopathologische Arbeiten*, **4**, 267. (Quoted by W. H. McMenemey (1958), see above.)

Sourander, P. & Sjogren, H. (1970). The concept of Alzheimer's disease and its clinical implications. In G. E. W. Wolstenholme & M. Connor (eds.) *Alzheimer's Disease*, Ciba Foundation Symposium. Churchill, London.

Spillane, J. A., White, P., Goodhardt, M. J., Flack, R. H. A., Bowen, D. M. & Davison, A. N. (1977). Selective vulnerability of neurones in organic dementia. *Nature*, **266**, 558–9.

St George-Hyslop, P. H., Tanzi, R. E., Polinsky, R. J., Haines, J. L., Nee, L., Watkins, P. C., Myers, R. H., Feldman, R. G., Pollen, D., Drachman, D., Growden, J., Bruni, A, Foncin, J. F., Salmon, D., Frommelt, P., Amaducci, L., Sorbi, S., Piacentini, S., Stewart, G. D., Hobbs, W. J., Conneally, P. J. & Gusella, J. F. (1987). The genetic defect causing familial Alzheimer's disease maps on chromosome 21. *Science*, **235**, 885–90.

Tanzi, R. E., Guzella J. F., Watkins, P. C., Bruns, G. A. P., St George-Hyslop, P., van Keuren, M., Patterson, D., Pagan, S., Kurnit, D. M. & Neve, R. L. (1987). Amyloid B protein gene: cDNA, mRNA distribution and genetic linkage near the Alzheimer locus. *Science*, **235**, 880–4.

Tomlinson, B. E., Blessed, G. & Roth, M. (1968). Observations on the brains of non-demented old people. *Journal of the Neurological Sciences*, **7**, 331–56.

Tomlinson, B. E., Blessed, G. & Roth, M. (1970). Observations on the brains of demented old people. *Journal of the Neurological Sciences*, **11**, 205–42.

Vogt, M. (1970). Drug-induced changes in brain dopamine and their relation to parkinsonism. *The Scientific Basis of Medicine Annual Reviews*, (Chapter 16). Athlone Press, London.

Walshe, F. M. R. (1955). *Diseases of the Nervous System*, 8th edition. E. and S. Livingstone, Edinburgh and London.

White, P., Hiley, C. R., Goodhardt, M. J., Carrasco, L. H., Keet, J. P., Williams, I. E. I. & Bowen, D. M. (1977). Neocortical cholinergic neurons in elderly people. *Lancet*, i, 668–70.

4

The relationship between dementia and normal aging of the brain

SIR MARTIN ROTH

The relationship between the circumscribed impairment of memory and other cognitive functions of aged persons and Alzheimer's disease, the commonest form of dementia in later life, has been the subject of debate since Alzheimer published the first clinical and neuropathological report of this condition in 1907. Alzheimer believed that a 55-year-old woman whose illness had begun at the age of 51 years had suffered from a rare form of precocious mental decline caused by the specific cerebral pathology he described in his paper.

The specificity and relevance of the cerebral changes described by Alzheimer were called into question within a short time. Using simple methods of assessment of pathological change, Gellerstedt (1933) reported Alzheimer-type (AD-type) changes, namely senile plaques (SPs) in 84% of aged persons, neurofibrillary tangles (NFTs) in 97% and granulovacuolar degeneration (GVD) in 40%.

Although in most mentally intact subjects the changes were limited, in a proportion, plaque and tangle formation showed a severity and distribution similar to that in demented patients. Similar findings were reported by other investigators in a wide range of cases of mental disorder studied post-mortem (Newton, 1948).

A number of attempts were made to reconcile these conflicting findings. It was pointed out that, since a measure of cognitive decline, usually in the form of impaired memory and recall of recent events, is common though variable in senescence, patients with Alzheimer's disease (AD) were drawn from the extreme end of the normal range of variation of cognitive function in the aged. Such 'continuum' theories, which consider AD to represent an intensified form of the process of aging, are also being advanced at the present time (Brayne & Calloway, 1988).

Dementia and Normal Aging, eds. F. A. Huppert, C. Brayne & D. W. O'Connor.
© Cambridge University Press 1994.

However, although mental functioning is disorganized in AD, other functional systems in the body generally show little or no evidence of impairment. The post-mortem brain may exhibit extensive pathology but the other organs are found to be intact or to show no changes that differentiate AD patients from mentally well-preserved controls. The aging of those with AD is therefore specific and localized; it is the cerebrum alone which is undergoing rapid degeneration.

In contrast, in other disorders which are regarded as parodies of the aging process, mental functioning is unimpaired in the majority of cases. Werner's syndrome is a rare disease due to an autosomal recessive gene (Epstein et al., 1966). It usually presents in the second or third decade with premature greying and thinning of the hair, cataracts, a dwarfed stature and scanty connective tissue. The skin becomes stretched and ulcerated at pressure points. There is hypogonadism and osteoporosis. The arteries become atheromatous at an early age and diabetes mellitus is common. These patients show neither the cognitive impairment associated with normal aging nor cerebral pathology of Alzheimer type. A proportion die in their forties. The example of Werner's syndrome is inconsistent with the theory that AD results from exaggeration or intensification of the general process of aging.

At the opposite extreme, AD has been judged by some investigators to be totally unrelated to the known pathological changes. Plaques and tangles were non-specific epiphenomena. An influential paper by Grünthal (1927) argued that some, as yet unidentified, pathological change or process was the underlying cause of Alzheimer's disease.

Such 'all or none' concepts of AD were refuted when quantified measures of cognitive function and other deficits were undertaken during life and their relationship to reliable measures of SP and NFT density in different areas of cortex and hippocampus were investigated. The relationship between measures of cognitive function, ability to negotiate skills required daily and manifest behaviour on the one hand and quantitative measures of severity of brain changes post-mortem on the other were investigated (Roth et al., 1966, 1967; Blessed et al., 1968; Tomlinson et al., 1968, 1970; Tomlinson, 1972). There were highly significant correlations between scores on cognitive tests and measures of AD-type changes. The presence of abundant tangles in the cerebral cortex proved to be diagnostic of AD. Some NFT were present in the hippocampus of normal elderly persons, but the number in AD was almost twenty times as great (Blessed, 1985).

Turning to differences, according to diagnosis the great majority of patients diagnosed as suffering from AD during life exhibited the

AD-type pathological changes in the cerebral cortex and hippocampus, namely SPs, NFTs and GVD in the pyramidal cells of the hippocampus. SP counts and NFT estimates were much higher in all areas in cases of senile and presenile AD than in controls. The counts in respect of all changes in other forms of psychiatric disorder in aged persons did not differ from counts in control subjects.

However, there was no change in patients with AD that was not also present to some extent in the brains of healthy, mentally intact aged persons. This appears at first sight to be consistent with a continuum concept of the relationship between normal age-specific pathological changes and AD. Observations to be described at a later stage dispose of explanations along these lines. They relate mainly to AD, but the implications for a number of other conditions will be considered.

Normal frequency distributions and threshold effects

A normal distributions of biological variables determined by multiple additive genes and environmental factors may look superficially continuous. But closer investigation has repeatedly revealed discontinuities due to 'threshold' effects. The situation that obtains in relation to AD on the one hand and subjects who are intact in cognitive and personality functioning is as follows. No clinical symptoms are manifest in those for whom mean counts of senile plaques are 15 or below per microscopic field. In the sub-threshold state, NFT are found in the cerebral cortex rarely, being largely restricted to hippocampus and parahippocampal gyrus. At this stage the pathological process is clinically asymptomatic. When plaques and tangles are found to exceed threshold values, clinical dementia has almost invariably been manifest during life.

In the pre-threshold phase, it is possible that the onset of mental deterioration is kept at bay by the reserve capacity of neurons in cerebral cortex which can compensate for the effects of neuronal outfall within certain limits. The concept of 'reserve capacity' is at present hypothetical and requires to be tested by further enquiry. But its plausibility stems from the similarity of the basic data to those of Parkinson's disease (PD) where the threshold theory of causation is supported by considerable evidence. This has been summarized previously as follows (Roth, 1986, p. 45):

There is a preclinical phase of the parkinsonian syndrome in the course of which both the neurons of the nigro striatal system and the total amount of dopamine within it are in decline. In this stage, the specific pathological lesion of parkinsonism, the Lewy body, is already manifest. However, clinical parkinsonism does not appear until 85% of the cells of the nigro striatal system have been depleted and a decrease in levels of dopamine of similar proportions has occurred. In the preclinical phase two compensatory mechanisms help to fend off development of the parkinsonian syndrome. The first of these is an increase in the turnover of dopamine. The second is a heightening of postsynaptic receptor sensitivity in dopaminergic neurons.

When the destruction of dopaminergic neurons has passed beyond threshold point, decompensation occurs. It is manifest in the symptoms of progressively disabling parkinsonism.

Threshold phenomena are incompatible with simple continuum theories. These postulate that a given disorder in question merges insensibly with normal variation in respect of the associated symptoms and deficits and the causes underlying them. When there is a linear relationship of this nature between a disease and normal variation, any significant correlations that are found between measures of behaviour and associated biological variables should make it possible to predict with precision the manifest features as also the biological concomitants at the extreme ends of the distribution. However, neither the cognitive behavioural and other clinical features nor the neuro-pathological characteristics of AD can be forecast in this manner from measures undertaken in normal elderly persons of comparable demographic characteristics. There is a sharp discontinuity at the threshold point; new emergent phenomena are manifest beyond it in clinical profile, course and outcome. As will be seen, novel structural immunological and molecular changes appear in the cerebral pathology of AD which differentiate it from the mentally well-preserved aged.

The threshold concept in AD receives independent corroboration from a number of sources. The presence of plaques and tangles below threshold values may summate with small infarcts also below threshold for the development of multi-infarct dementia (MID). The combined lesions give rise to a special form of dementia of mixed aetiology (Roth, 1971, 1986). It was clear from the measurements that neither of the two types of change could by itself have given rise to dementia. Their combined effect was needed to exceed threshold values and to give rise to a change from quantitative continuous variation to a process of progressive decline in the course of which novel qualitative features appear in the clinical picture.

A similar summation between neuronal damage and Lewy bodies of PD with AD-type changes has been proposed as the explanation for the prevalence of 10–15% of dementia in those with PD (Quinn et al, 1986). This explanation has also been advanced in relation to the dementia associated with parkinsonism in boxers, since there may be a latent period of five years or more after the cessation of a pugilistic career before dementia and/or parkinsonism commence.

The relationship of plaques and tangles to the aetiology of AD continues to be called in question by some investigators. Their views are at variance with much evidence that the changes are closely linked to the degenerative process. With the aid of a Quantimet 720 image analyser, a reduction of neurons ranging between 24% and 40% of the number found in the controls has been recorded in the superior, middle and inferior frontal gyri, the superior and middle temporal tyri and the anterior part of the cingulate gyrus of patients with AD (Mountjoy et al., 1983). Similar findings have been recorded by other workers (Terry et al., 1981).

Furthermore, an inverse correlation was found between the number of neurons on the one hand and numbers of plaques and tangles in the same areas on the other (Mountjoy et al., 1983). The higher the plaque and tangle counts the lower the number of neurons. Hence, a significant though non-linear relationship exists between the aggregation of plaques and tangles, the degenerative process and the cognitive and personality deterioration in AD.

Threshold effects in other disorders

A similar threshold effect has been shown to operate in the case of the form of dementia due to the cumulative aggregation of infarcts in the brain of MD. Small clinically silent infarcts are found commonly in the brains of cognitively intact and normal old persons and also in patients with depressive paranoid and neurotic disorders during life. Progressive mental deterioration does not appear until a total of 75–100 ml of infarction (as estimated in the brain post-mortem) has been exceeded (Tomlinson et al., 1970). Specific neurological signs and symptoms may have been manifest, of course, before this aggregate of infarction has been reached.

The course of events, as observed clinically in patients who suffer a succession of cerebral infarcts, supports the threshold concept. It is very rare for the first one or two strokes to be followed by a progressive mental deterioration. In most cases of MID a longer succession of infarcts have been suffered before impairment of memory and more general cognitive deficits make their appearance.

There is a minority of patients in whom dementia appears following one or two small infarcts followed by minimal and transient neurological defects. In these cases some other cerebral disease (or injury) usually of Alzheimer type has been found to summate with the effects exerted by cumulative infarction. A statement along similar lines can be made about those in whom progressive mental deterioration during life has proved to be associated with sub-threshold values for plaque and tangle counts in the post-mortem brain. Limited cerebral infarctions are present in the great majority of cases. It is the summation of these two or more sub-threshold lesions that causes threshold limits to be exceeded and to initiate clinical dementia.

Such hybrid forms of dementia (usually AD combined with MID) cannot be regarded as being quantitative variants of senescence and continuous in linear fashion with the phenomena of normal aging. The progressive deterioration may commence in abrupt step-wise fashion and advance rapidly following a single small cerebral infarction. In the light of evidence from post-mortem studies of normal controls, 'strokes' that cause such limited damage would have proved to be clinically 'silent' in a previously undamaged brain.

The clinical change in such patients consists of a step-wise shift from a state of normal cognitive and personality functioning to progressive mental deterioration in which the features of AD predominate. The end result is a virtually mindless state with deteriorated habits and double incontinence, unless death from other causes supervenes before such an advanced stage is reached.

The line of demarcation between those who develop an indubitable dementia and the well-preserved aged is relatively sharp. About 10% of those aged 75 years or over develop such a condition (O'Connor et al., 1989). Of these, about half (5%) were diagnosed on the strength of operational criteria as suffering from 'mild dementia' which progressed to an indubitable dementia in a substantial proportion in one- and two-year follow-up investigations (O'Connor et al., 1989). Further investigations are needed in larger samples to determine the long-term outcome of this group of patients and to develop reliable indices of prognosis.

But there is evidence that the distinction between demented and non-demented subjects remains clear even near the end of the life span. In a group of centenarians studied post-mortem by Hauw et al. (1986), nine of twelve subjects studied during life were judged to be not demented. In these patients there were a few tangles in hippocampus and temporal cortex but the remaining cortical areas were almost entirely devoid of pathological change. One of the mentally intact centenarians had not a single plaque in hippocampus or cortex. Of the three demented persons: one had dense and diffuse AD-type changes, another had multiple infarcts; and a third was a 'mixed case' with both AD and MID types of change. Hauw concluded that senile dementia of Alzheimer's type (SDAT) is neither inevitable nor a physiological change; it is a disease merely more common in the elderly.

The interpretation of normal or 'continuous' frequency distributions

The finding of a unimodal smooth distribution cannot be interpreted to mean that there is no break in continuity along any part of the distribution. As Edwards (1963) has pointed out, the extreme ends of normal distributions which represent variation in characteristics such as intelligence, stature, blood pressure and neuroticism, discontinuities due to 'break away' phenomena are found commonly. In the case of intelligence, these discontinuities arise owing to the existence of a number of rare forms of severe mental sub-normality responsible for conditions such as phenylketonuria, homocystinuria and Lesch–Nyhan syndrome, which are due to single mutations, chromosomal abnormalities such as Down's syndrome and fragile X syndrome, and also infantile autism which is of obscure aetiology. These conditions are determined by specific qualitative departures from the norm as distinct from the differences in degree which characterize the majority of the persons who make up the smooth, continuous part of the normal curve. However some of the cases that give rise to such discontinuity arise from post-threshold effects among extreme deviants from the mean.

Other threshold phenomena

There are a number of common diseases of middle and late life which exemplify this change from quantitative to qualitative deviation from the norm. They are due to multiple, additive pathogenetic factors including many genes of small effect and also environmental and exogenous causes. When measurements of biological markers of these conditions, derived from representative samples of the normal population, are plotted they fall on a normal continuous distribution curve. But those who deviate markedly from the mean along such a distribution are liable to manifest pathological states.

Variation in respect of arterial pressure can be delineated over the greater part of the range by a continuous distribution. But those whose blood pressure remains at very high levels for long periods or rises abruptly (in the absence of any new, additional pathological agent) develop malignant hypertension with proteinuria, papilloedema, retinal haemorrhages and encephalopathy. These complications are due to necrotizing changes in the the the arterioles. The disorder has a fatal outcome within months if not treated. Glucose tolerance also varies in continuous manner in the general population, while decreasing overall with advancing age. Those near the lower extreme in respect of tolerance are at risk of being pressed beyond threshold limits in their inability to metabolize glucose normally. Certain forms of diabetes mellitus and its complications can be accounted for along these lines.

Such new emergent properties are commonplace in nature. Minute changes in temperature may give rise to abrupt changes in the character of substances. Water boils to form steam or freezes to produce ice. Metals cooled to very low temperatures suddenly lose all electrical resistance and acquire the other characteristics of a superconducting state.

Edwards (1963) has delineated the causal process which gives rise to such diseases in virtue of extreme deviation through the cumulative effects of multiple genes and exogenous factors by describing it as analogous to the predicament of the camel onto whose back straws are being heaped. The final straw preceding this catastrophe does not differ from the other straws except in respect of being the last. But the effect in this case is irrevocable. This is an apt analogue for common diseases caused by multiple additive genes, such as the commonest forms of AD which also develop when cumulative AD-type changes exceed threshold limits. There is a contribution to causation by heredity (Amaducci et al., 1986) but it is almost certainly polygenic. Exogenous and environmental causes also contribute. In contrast, the rare forms, mainly with an early age of onset determined by single genes, must have specific pathogenetic determinants. The common forms of AD which have an identical pathology are likely to evolve along the same final common neurobiological pathways in their causation. For the present, once the underlying degenerative process has commenced it is irreversible. But this feature may prove to be remediable in the light of advancing knowledge.

A particularly clear and informative example of the production of a severe deformity by a small delay in a developmental process is provided by the harelip–cleft palate syndrome which is determined by polygenic inheritence. The work of C. O. Carter (1965) has shown that, during development in normal subjects, the embryonic layers that are to form the buccal and nasopharyngeal regions are united at a certain stage of development to shut off the nasal cavities from the mouth. If union is delayed by a little, minor degrees of harelip are produced. But if the delay is greater the full harelip syndrome develops. This is therefore an elegant example of quantitative variation producing an all-or-none effect: 'syndrome either present or absent, even though if present variable in degree' (Slater & Cowie, 1971, pp. 8–9). The threshold effects that characterize polygenic inheritance are as common in psychiatry as they are in general medicine.

On the strength of similar considerations, AD has to be regarded as qualitatively apart from normal aging, though continuous with it in certain respects. An aging person either has or does not have AD. In his seventies or eighties he may suffer some impairment of memory recall or retrieval of recent events. In nine persons out of ten in their early seventies, this will change little or not at all in the decade or so that intervenes before life ends. He is unlikely to lose knowledge about his identity before his preterminal illness. In contrast, a person with AD gradually loses all capacity for memory understanding, learning and reasoning. His speech becomes incoherent. The skills he requires to find his way in his own house and in dressing and feeding himself disappear. He cannot recognize his closest relatives or even his own face in the mirror. He is doubly incontinent and in the end reduced to a vegetative existence. He may survive in this state of total oblivion for some years. Yet his life expectation is no more than a quarter of those who have comparable age, sex and demographic features in the general population (Kay, 1962). AD cannot be accounted for in terms of a continuous and predictable extension of normal mental aging.

We are not within sight of any solution to the engima of biological aging in its physical and mental aspects. Scientific investigation of the process needs to be pursued in its own right. Any progress made might shed light on the causation of the degenerative disorders of the nervous system. But progress in medicine has often evolved in the past in an opposite direction from new knowledge of diseases to insights into normal functioning. Advances achieved in knowledge of causation and treatment of diseases of the cardiovascular, respiratory, gastro-intestinal, immunological and central nervous system has transformed understanding of their normal physiology.

The phenomenon is pertinent for AD for a number of reasons. The number of cases of AD in a random population sample would be very small in those aged 75 years and over and would be between 5% and 10%. But this is not the only reason for failure to detect any break in continuity. Brayne & Calloway (1988) have used the Blessed–Roth dementia scale and the information–memory–concentration test to plot the distribution of scores for the samples of patients examined in epidemiological studies with these tests. They obtained smooth, continuous distributions. But these tests are too crude to quantify the differences in mental competence among severe dements. The correlations between the Blessed–Roth dementia scale (as also other measures) and AD-type changes is curvilinear not linear. Further normal distributions can never be interpreted as being conclusive evidence that there is no break in continuity. A small second mode demonstrable by alternative measures may be concealed beneath the continuous distribution. As we will see at a later stage there are indeed some biological measures which demonstrate the existence of qualitative differences between well-preserved elderly persons and those who suffer from AD.

Continuity and discontinuity of the neurobiological changes in the brain in Alzheimer's disease

The differences between the mentally intact aged and Alzheimer's disease are clearly manifest in respect of a wide range of neurobiological parameters.

There is continuity between certain structural and neurochemical characteristics of normal aging and the 'AD type I' and 'AD type II' forms which were previously described less precisely as 'early onset' and 'late onset' forms of AD (Roth, 1986; Bondareff et al., 1987). Cortical plaques are common to all three groups but are below threshold values in the elderly controls. NFTs are also present in the cerebral cortex of those with AD type I and AD type II, but are confined to the hippocampus in normal elderly persons. There is also a decline with age in the concentration of certain neurotransmitters in controls. But the significant deficits in the cholinergic, noradrenergic and serotoninergic transmitter systems of the AD groups set them apart from normal controls. The decline in respect of the important inhibitory neurotransmitter gamma-amino-butyric acid (GABA), as also somatostatin and noradrenaline, is found mainly in AD type II (Rossor et al., 1984) and it represents a qualitative difference from the neurochemistry of normal aging.

NFTs have been described as being completely absent from the cerebral cortex of intellectually well-preserved elderly persons of advanced age (Tomlinson, 1982) and in an earlier study eight out of 26 non-demented elderly had no plaques (Blessed et al, 1968). The paired helical filament is the most specific change of all in AD (Tomlinson, et al., 1970; Tomlinson 1982; Wilcock & Esiri, 1982), and may be packed into dystrophic neurites, neuritic plaques as well as tangles. But these changes may be found in small numbers in the hippocampus of normal old subjects.

The molecular analysis of the structural changes in Alzheimer's disease and in the brains of normal aged

The main non-molecular distinctions between normal aging and AD type I ('late onset' form) comprises extensive proliferation of NFTs in the cortex and circumscribed significant deficits in respect of somatostatin and serotoninergic receptors (Roth, 1986). No significant outfall of pyramidal neurons has been found in this form of AD (Mountjoy et al., 1983, Roth et al., 1985). However, the NFTs in the cerebral cortex and certain types of neurite (both containing paired helical filaments (phf)), in the neuropil, the most specific indices of definite dementia (Braak & Braak, 1991), are present in abundance. These are the AD-type changes most indubitably correlated with the destruction of cortical neurons (Bondareff et al., 1989) for the total number of NFTs, and the extracellular NFTs in particular, are correlated inversely with the total number of remaining neurons. NFTs can be identified with the aid of structural as well as immunochemical techniques (Bondareff et al., 1990, 1993; Harrington et al., 1991; Mukaetova-Ladinska et al., 1992; Wischik et al., 1992) and are among the indices of a qualitative departure from the cerebral pathology of normal aging.

Recent enquiries making use of structural and immunochemical techniques have shown that some of the proteins that have been identified in the AD-type changes in the brains of patients with AD differ in their molecular structure and specificity from those found in the brains of normal aged controls. Tau protein in the normal brain is bound to micro-tubules in axons by its middle repeat region. In Alzheimer's disease, this part of the protein and a part of the C-terminal region is incorporated into the paired helical filaments that make up the neurofibrillary tangle of Alzheimer's disease. These segments of the tau protein have been shown to constitute a substantial part of the paired helical filament (Goedert et al., 1988; Wischik et al., 1988a, b).

Tau protein is present predominantly in an insoluble form in AD in contrast to its soluble state in well-preserved aged persons. With the aid of direct biochemical assay of the phf content of brain tissues, it has proved possible to discriminate unambiguously between AD and normal aging (Harrington et al., 1991; Mukaetova-Ladinska et al., 1992, 1993). In the most affected regions there was an eighteenfold increase in the amount of insoluble tau as compared with the quantity in normal controls.

In AD the tau is also located very largely in the somatodendritic compartment within the cortex whereas in normal elderly controls it is predominantly axonal and in the white matter. Tau proteins in phf are distinguished from normal tau by the fact that they are abnormally phosphorylated although the stage in the formation of phf and tangle formation in which this occurs is uncertain. Further, the use of novel extraction techniques for the isolation of individual phfs has revealed a number of modified bands of tau protein as integral components of phf. These proteins are absent from the brains of controls (Wischik et al., 1992).

A recent molecular analysis of neurofibrillary degeneration in AD utilized antibodies directed against the middle tandem region of tau protein; namely the central repeat region and a short sequence close to the C-terminal. Two largely distinct populations of NFTs could be distinguished with the aid of these antibodies. Intracellular NFTs were immunolabelled exclusively by the antibodies prepared against segments of tau protein located in the fuzzy coat around the central core of the paired helical filaments. Extracellular NFTs were distinguished by selective immunolabelling with an antibody directed against the central repeat region of tau protein. The NFTs were therefore subdivided by these immunological reactions into two populations corresponding to the intracellular and extracellular tangles. The protease digestion to which the tangle is exposed in the process of its transition from intracellular to extracellular compartments is associated with new immunological interactions.

In the course of proteolysis of tangle-bearing cells, the β-amyloid protein precursor is cleaved at first to expose the amino-terminal sequence and then at the carboxy-terminus. This latter step frees β-amyloid protein to be deposited in extracellular space. A small proportion of extracellular NFTs stains with some antibodies against β-amyloid protein as well as antibodies against the central repeat region of tau protein (Bondareff et al., 1990). Some apparently intact NFT-containing neurons constitute an intermediate group exhibiting this interaction with both anti-amyloid and anti-tau antibodies; the tangles are probably in transition from their intracellular site to extracellular space.

There is a third group of NFTs which is intermediate in characteristics between the two other main groups. One is witnessing, in these differences and in the immunochemical changes during the transition of intra into extracellular NFTs, stages in the destruction of neurons, the central feature of Alzheimer's disease. The precise manner in which tau and β-amyloid proteins interact in this process and the nature of the primary causal agent is obscure.

The insoluble tau protein bound intimately to the core of the NFT is present in large amounts in brains of patients with AD. It is found only in a small fraction of these amounts or is absent in the brains of normal aged persons.

One view of its role has been expressed recently in the following terms by Beyreuther & Masters (1991 p. 241): 'We regard Alzheimer's disease (AD) as a unitary disease phenomenon as opposed to "normal aging" in which clinical variables such as age of onset, rate of progression and severity of dementia are the result of the interaction of but a few critical steps in the synthesis and degradation of the amyloid precursor protein (APP)'. The primary causal role given to the amyloid protein in the process of neuronal destruction in this statement is, however, the subject of controversy for reasons which will be discussed at a later stage. But a number of recent developments have established that the APP and its cleavage product, the β-amyloid protein, play a significant part in the development of the disease.

It has been clear for a number of years that, in a proportion of the rare early onset forms of AD, the condition was probably transmitted by a single autosomal dominant gene (St George-Hyslop et al., 1987). Linkage studies which have mapped the gene on the proximal long arm of chromosome 21 have firmly established a specific genetic contribution to the causation of these variants of the disorder, although the mutation has not been found in all familial cases with early onset. The discovery of a mutation entailing the substitution of isoleucine for valine in position 46 of the β-A4 region of the APP in two families (Goate et al., 1991) provided further evidence for the role of amyloid in the pathogenesis of AD in a proportion of the rare early onset cases transmitted by a single gene. In the following year, several teams of workers reported observations in patients with the commonest form of familial AD type II which mapped the gene for transmission of the disease to a locus on chromosome 14 (Schellenberg et al. 1992). This raised the possibility that this mutation bore no functional relationship to the abnormal processing of the β-amyloid protein from its precursor protein, the gene for which is on chromosome 21.

By far the commonest forms of AD are of late onset and the evidence suggests that in most cases the hereditary factors are probably polygenic with no more than a limited role in aetiology. But there are no fundamental differences in structural pathology between the rare early onset cases due to a single mutation and the late onset forms of high prevalence. A similar final common pathway is therefore likely to be followed in the pathogenesis of not only the rare forms of AD determined by specific genes but also the common late-life variants which constitute the great majority of the cases. The fact that the condition can result from a single mutation which must be sharply distinct in its action from the normal aging process therefore provides strong support for the disease concept of AD as opposed to the theory which attributes it to quantitative deviation from the normal aging process.

While deposits of β-amyloid protein have been shown to be an almost invariable feature of AD, the evidence that it is a sufficient condition for the development of the disease is in conflict with a number of lines of evidence. Although the β-amyloid deposits found in the core and corona of neuritic plaques are associated with cognitive deficits, diffuse clumps of amorphous amyloid, common in normal aged, have been shown to have no significant association with the development of cognitive impairment in AD (Delaère, et al., 1989; Braak & Braak, 1991). They are found in abundance in AD in anatomical sites such as the cerebellum and spinal cord where there is neither neuronal damage nor associated clinical signs or symptoms. These diffuse deposits do not correlate with measures of psychological impairment (Tabaton et al., 1989). It is relevant that a mutation in the APP gene has been found in all patients affected by hereditary cerebral haemorrhage with amyloidosis of the Dutch type. The 39 amino acid β-amyloid peptide accumulates very largely in cerebral blood vessels and to some extent in extracellular space. The inheritance of the disorder is related so closely to the APP gene that it is highly probable that both the amyloid change and the familial transmission of the disorder are determined by the same hereditary factor. The mutation causes a substitution of glutamine for glutamic acid. But there are neither neuritic plaques nor tangles. The patients do not develop dementia and die in most cases from cerebral haemorrhage. This syndrome is therefore another qualitative departure from normal variation; its relevance in this context is that it has a clear kinship with AD, despite its very different clinical presentation (van Broeckhoven et al., 1990).

Normal and pathological aging in the cerebrum with special reference to AD changes

The neuropathological picture of normal old age is characterized by diffuse amyloid deposits in the neuropil, small numbers of neuritic plaques, a few NFTs in hippocampus (but very few or none in the cerebral cortex) (Tomlinson et al., 1968; Mountjoy et al., 1983). In contrast, the picture of the cerebrum of AD comprises abundance of NFT and dystrophic neurites in the cerebral cortex, a post-threshold number of neuritic plaques and an outfall of neurons in frontal and temporal cortex and sub-cortical nuclei. Although the diminution of neuronal counts has been found to be statistically significant only in the rapidly progressive, relatively early onset cases of AD, the decline shows the same trend and the same distribution in all cases (Mountjoy et al., 1983). Moreover, NFTs whose increasing proliferation in cerebral cortex and hippocampus proceeds in close parallel with the clinical progression of the disease (Braak & Braak, 1991) show the same regional distribution in all forms of AD. And it is a truncated and insoluble form of tau protein that predominates in a nineteen-fold excess in the brain of patients with AD and not the soluble form that is found in the brains of the well-preserved elderly. Other qualitative differences between tau protein in AD and normal subjects comprise its redistribution from the axons into the somatodendritic compartments of neurons and from the white matter to the cortical grey matter of the cerebral cortex (Mukaetova-Ladinska et al., 1993). Lastly, a substantial proportion of the cerebral tau protein is phosphorylated in AD.

About 90% of these well-preserved elderly aged 75 years and over who exhibited the neurobiological cluster of features described at the beginning of this section can expect to complete their life span with little or no mental impairment. In contrast, that 10% of the population aged 75 years and over with pathological changes diagnostic of AD suffer progressive deterioration of cognitive, emotional and personality functioning terminating in a state of severe mental impairment which reduces them to a vegetative life. They also suffer a marked diminution in life expectation. Hence, in respect of manner of aging and life style and social adaptation and also in respect of structural molecular and neurochemical changes in the brain, those with AD are placed qualitatively apart from normal elderly persons. Benign forms of senescent forgetfulness show little or no progression or extension of deficits to an increasingly wide range of mental faculties.

Recent scientific advances have confirmed, therefore, that there are causal factors qualitatively apart from the processes of normal cerebral aging that account for the disparity between those many aged people who are able, even in their eighties and nineties, to function normally and, in a substantial proportion, to lead intellectually vigorous and creative lives and those on the other side of the divide who, at the age of 50 to 60 years or even earlier, are at an advanced stage of mental deterioration. Such dements cannot recognize their own closest relatives nor their own reflections in the mirror, have lost all traces of their original identity and are reduced to a merely vegetative existence. The paradigm of such dementias is Alzheimer's disease. It is difficult to conceive of any definition of 'disease' which excludes such conditions.

Malignant hypertension, which arises as the result of abrupt or severe and protracted rise of blood pressure, and Parkinson's disease are all 'post-threshold' phenomena in the sense described in earlier sections. In all these disorders there is a break in continuity from normal variation in respect of the underlying physiological functions. The clinical features are unambiguous; they are 'all or none' phenomena. The status of those with AD and multi-infarct dementias is similar. Both are differentiated by clinical presentation, cause and life expectancy from normal aged persons comparable in all relevant respects other than the presence of progressive mental decay.

A central objective of the scientific endeavours of those who work in this field is to emulate the achievements of those who have been enabled by refinement of scientific knowledge of the underlying causal agents and their control, to improve the quality and the duration of life of those with malignant hypertension, late-onset diabetes, multiple strokes due to cerebrovascular disease and parkinsonism.

References

Alzheimer, A. (1907). Über eine eigenartige Erkrankung der Hirnrinde. *Allgemeine Zeitschrift für Psychiatrie und Psychisch-Gerichtlich Medizine*, **64**, 146–8.

Amaducci, L. A., Fratiglioni, L., Rocca, W. A., Fieschi, C., Livrea, P., Pedone, D., Bracco, L., Lippi, A., Gadolfo, C., Bino, G., Prencipe, M., Bonatti, M. L., Girotti, F., Carella, F., Tavalato, B., Feria, S., Lenzi, G. L., Carolei, A., Gambi, A., Grigoletto, F. & Schoenberg, B. S. (1986). Risk factors for clinically diagnosed Alzheimer's disease: a case–control study of an Italian population. *Neurology*, **36**, 922–31.

Beyreuther, K. & Masters, C. L. (1991). Amyloid precursor protein (APP) and beta amyloid-4 amyloid in the etiology of Alzheimer's disease: precursor-product relationships in the derangement of neuronal function. *Brain Pathology*, **1**, 241–52.

Blessed, G. (1985). Measurement in psychogeriatrics. In T. Arie (ed.) *Recent Advances in Psychogeriatrics*, pp. 141–59. Churchill Livingstone, Edinburgh, London.

Blessed, G., Tomlinson, B. E. & Roth, M. (1968). The association between quantitative measures of dementia and of senile change in the cerebral grey matter of elderly subjects. *British Journal of Psychiatry*, **114**, 797–811.

Bondareff, W., Mountjoy, C. Q., Roth, M., Rossor, M. N., Iversen, L. L. & Reynolds, G. P. (1987). Age and histopathologic heterogeneity in Alzheimer's disease: evidence for subtypes. *Archives of General Psychiatry*, **44**, 412–17.

Bondareff, W., Mountjoy, C. Q., Roth, M. & Hauser, D. L. (1989). Neurofibrillary degeneration and neuronal loss in Alzheimer's disease. *Neurobiology of Aging*, **10**, 709–15.

Bondareff, W., Wischik, C. M., Novak, M., Amos, W. B., Klug, A. & Roth, M. (1990). Molecular analysis of neurofibrillary degeneration in Alzheimer's disease: an immunohistorical study. *American Journal of Pathology*, **137**, 711–23.

Bondareff, W., Mountjoy, C. Q., Wischik, C. M., Hauser, D. L., LaBree, L. D. & Roth, M. (1993). Evidence for subtypes of Alzheimer's disease and implications for etiology. *Archives of General Psychiatry*, **50**, 350–6.

Braak, H. & Braak, F. (1991). Neuropathological staging of Alzheimer related changes. *Acta Neuropathologica*, **82**, 239–59.

Brayne, C. & Calloway, P. (1988). Normal ageing, impaired cognitive function, and senile dementia of the Alzheimer's type: a continuum? *Lancet*, **ii**, 1265–6.

Carter, C. O. (1965). The inheritance of common congenital malformations. In A. G. Steinberg & A. G. Bearn (eds.) *Progress in Medical Genetics*, vol. iv. Grüne and Stratton, London.

Delaère, P., Duyckaerts, C., Brion, J. P., Poulain, V. & Hauw, J.-J. (1989). Tau, paired helical filaments and amyloid in the neocortex: a morphometric study of 15 cases with graded intellectual status in aging and senile dementia of the Alzheimer type. *Acta Neuropathologica*, **77**, 645–53.

Edwards, J. H. (1963). The genetic basis of common disease. *American Journal of Medicine*, **34**, 627–47.

Epstein, C. J., Martin, G. M., Schultz, A. L. & Motulsky, A. G. (1966).

Werner's syndrome: a review of its symptomatology, natural history, pathologic features, genetics and relationship to the natural ageing process. *Medicine*, **45**, 177–221.

Gellerstedt, N. (1933). Zur Kenntris der Hirnveranderungen bei der normalen Altersinvolution. *Uppsala Läk Fören Fork*, **38**, 193–408.

Goate, A., Chartier-Harlin, M-C., Mullan, M., Brown, J., Crawford, F., Fidani, L., Giuffra, L., Hayes, A., Irving, N., James, L., Mant, R., Newton, P., Rooke, K., Roques, P., Talbot, C., Pericak-Vance, M., Roses, A., Williamson, R., Rossor, M., Owen, M. & Hardy, J. (1991). Segregation of a missense mutation in the amyloid precursor protein gene with familial Alzheimer's disease. *Nature*, **349**, 704–6.

Goedert, M., Wischik, C. M., Crowther, R. A., Walker, J. E. & Klug, A. (1988). Cloning and sequencing of the cDNA encoding a core protein of the paired helical filament of Alzheimer Disease: identification as the microtubule-associated protein tau. *Proceedings of the National Academy of Sciences, USA*, **85**, 4051–55.

Grünthal, E. (1927). Klinische-anatomische vergleichende Untersuchungen über den Greisenblodsinn. *Zeitschrift für Gesamte Neurologie Psychiatrie*, **111**, 763–818.

Harrington, C. R. Mukaetova-Ladinska, E. B., Hills, R., Edwards, P. C., Montejo de Garcini, E., Novak, M. & Wischik, C. M. (1991). Measurement of distinct immunochemical presentations of tau protein in Alzheimer's disease. *Proceedings of the National Academy of Sciences, USA*, **88**, 5842–6.

Hauw, J.-J., Vignolo, P., Duyckaerts, C., Beck, H., Forette, F., Henry, J. P., Laurent, M., Piette, F., Sachet, A. & Berthaux, P. (1986). Etude neuropathologique de 12 centenaires: la fréquence de la démence sénile de type Alzheimer n'est pas particuliérement élevée dans ce groupe de personnes tres agées. *Revue Neurologique (Paris)*, **142**, 107–15.

Kay, D. W. K. (1962). Outcome and cause of death in mental disorders of old age: a long-term follow-up of functional and organic psychoses. *Acta Psychiatrica Scandinavica*, **38**, 249–76.

Mountjoy, C. Q., Roth, M., Evans, N. F. R. & Evans, H. M. (1983). Cortical neuronal counts in normal elderly controls and demented patients. *Neurobiology of Aging*, **4**, 1–11.

Mukaetova-Ladinska, E. B., Harrington, C. R., Hills, R., Roth, M. & Wischik, C. M. (1992). Regional distribution of paired helical filaments and normal tau proteins in ageing and in Alzheimer's disease with and without occipital lobe involvement. *Dementia*, **3**, 61–9.

Mukaetova-Ladinska, E. B., Harrington, C. R., Roth, M. & Wischik, C. M. (1993) Biochemical and anatomical redistribution of tau protein in Alzheimer's disease. *American Journal of Pathology*, **143**, 565–78.

Newton, R. D. (1948). The identity of Alzheimer's disease and senile dementia and their relationship to senility. *Journal of Mental Science*, **94**, 225–49.

O'Connor, D., Pollitt, P. A., Hyde, J. B., Fellows, J. L., Miller, N. D., Brook, C. P. B., Reiss, B. B. & Roth, M. (1989). The prevalence of dementia as measured by the Cambridge Mental Disorders of the Elderly Examination. *Acta Psychiatrica Scandinavica*, **79**, 190–8.

Quinn, N. P., Rossor, M. N. & Marsden, C. D. (1986). Dementia and

Parkinson's disease – pathological and neurochemical considerations. In M. Roth & L. L. Iversen (eds.) *Alzheimer's Disease and Related Disorders*, vol. **42**, 1, 86–90. Published for British Council for Churchill Livingstone.

Rossor, M. N., Iversen, L. L., Reynolds, G. P., Mountjoy, C. Q. & Roth, M. (1984). Neurochemical characteristics of early and late onset types of Alzheimer's disease. *British Medical Journal*, **288**, 361–4.

Roth, M. (1971). Classification and aetiology in mental disorders of old age: some recent developments. In D. W. K. Kay & A. Walk (eds.) *Recent Developments in Psychogeriatrics*, pp. 1–10. Headley Brothers, Ashford.

Roth, M. (1986). The association of clinical and neurobiological findings and its bearing on the classification and aetiology of Alzheimer's disease. *British Medical Bulletin*, **42**, 42–59.

Roth, M., Tomlinson, B. E. & Blessed, G. (1966). Correlation between scores for dementia and counts of 'senile plaques' in cerebral grey matter of elderly subjects. *Nature*, **200**, 109–10.

Roth, M., Tomlinson, B. E. & Blessed, G. (1967). The relationship between quantitative measures of dementia and of degenerative changes in the cerebral grey matter of elderly subjects. *Proceedings of the Society of Medicine*, **60**, 254–9.

Roth, M., Wischik, C. M., Evans, N. & Mountjoy, C. Q. (1985). Convergence and cohesion of recent neurobiological findings in relation to Alzheimer's disease and their bearing on its aetiological basis. In M. Bergener (ed.) *Thresholds in Aging*, pp. 117–46. Academic Press, London.

Schellenberg, G. D., Bird, T. D., Wijsman, E. M., Orr, H. T., Anderson, L., Nomens, E., White, J. A., Bonnycastle, L., Weber, J. L., Alonson, M. E., Potter, H., Heston, L. L. & Martin, G. M. (1992). Genetic linkage evidence for a familial Alzheimer's disease locus on chromosome 14. *Science*, **258**, 668–71.

Slater, E. & Cowie, V. (1971). *The Genetics of Mental Disorders*, pp. 8–9. Oxford University Press, London.

St George-Hyslop, P. H., Tanzi, R. E., Polinsky, R. J., Haines, J. L., Nee, L., Watkins, P. C., Myers, R. H., Feldman, R. G., Pollen, D., Drachman, D., Gropwdon, J., Bruni, A., Foncin, J.-F., Salmon, D., Foommel, P., Amaducci, L., Sorbi, S., Piacentini, S., Stewart, G. D., Hobbs, W. J., Conneally, P. M. & Gusella, J. F. (1987). The genetic defect causing familial Alzheimer's disease maps on chromosome 21. *Science*, **235**, 885–90.

Tabaton, M., Mandybur, T. I., Perry, G., Onorato, M., Autilio-Gambetti, L. & Gambetti, P. (1989). The widespread alteration of neurites in Alzheimer's disease may be unrelated to amyloid deposition. *Annals of Neurology*, **25**, 771–8.

Terry, R. D., Peck, A., DeTersa, R., Schecter, R. & Horoupian, D. S. (1981). Some morphometric aspects of the brain in senile dementia of the Alzheimer type. *Annals of Neurology*, **10**, 184–92.

Tomlinson, B. E. (1972). The ageing brain. In W. Thomas Smith & J. B. Cavanagh (eds.) *Recent Advances in Neuropathology*, no. 1. Churchill Livingstone, Edinburgh.

Tomlinson, B. E. (1982). Plaques, tangles and Alzheimer's disease. *Psychological Medicine*, **12**, 449–59.

Tomlinson, B. E., Blessed, G. & Roth, M. (1968). Observations on the brains of non-demented old people. *Journal of the Neurological Sciences*, **7**, 331–56.

Tomlinson, B. E., Blessed, G. & Roth, M. (1970). Observations on the brains of demented old people. *Journal of the Neurological Sciences*, **11**, 205–42.

van Broeckhoven, C., Haan, J., Bakker, E., Hardy, J. A., van Hul, W., Wehnert, A., Vegter-Van der Vlis, M. & Roos, R. A. C. (1990). Amyloid beta protein precursor gene and hereditary cerebral hemorrhage with amyloidosis. *Science* (Dutch), **248**, 1120–2.

Wilcock, G. K. & Esiri, M. M. (1982). Observations on the brains of demented old people. *Journal of the Neurological Sciences*, **11**, 202–42.

Wischik, C. M., Novak, M., Thogersen, H. C., Edwards, P. C., Runswick, M. J., Jakes, R., Walker, J. E., Milstein, C., Roth, M. & Klug, A. (1988a). Isolation of a fragment of tau derived from the core of the paired helical filament of Alzheimer disease. *Proceedings of the National Academy of Sciences, USA*, **85**, 4506–10.

Wischik, C. M., Novak, M., Edwards, P. C., Klug, A., Tichelaar, W. & Crowther, R. A. (1988b). Structural characterization of the core of the paired helical filament of Alzheimer disease. *Proceedings of the National Academy of Sciences*, **85**, 4884–8.

Wischik, C. M., Harrington, C. R., Mukaetova-Ladinska, E. B., Novak, M., Edwards, P. C. & McArthur, F. K. (1992). Molecular characterization and measurement of Alzheimer's disease pathology: implications for genetic and environmental aetiology. In D. J. Chadwick & J. Whelan (eds.) *Aluminium in Biology and Medicine*, pp. 268–302. Ciba Foundation Symposium 169. John Wiley & Sons, Chichester and New York.

PART III

The diagnosis of dementia today

5

International criteria and differential diagnosis

A. S. HENDERSON AND N. SARTORIUS

The advent of standardized criteria for the diagnosis of dementia has now brought about the possibility of comparing results of studies undertaken in different countries. This applies to epidemiological, biological and clinical research. In the past, variation in estimates of the incidence or prevalence of mental disorders has been attributable largely to variation in case definition and ascertainment (Henderson, 1986; Jorm et al., 1987). Now the situation has changed, since the diagnostic criteria are specified. Variations attributable to the observer are more likely to lie in the accuracy with which the clinical assessment *applies the criteria* at the time of the examination. This requirement in no way detracts from the magnitude of the advance which the diagnostic criteria have brought about. Rather it emphasizes the responsibility placed on users for their careful application in the conduct of comparative studies. In this chapter we shall consider two sets of diagnostic criteria for dementia: those accompanying the tenth revision of the International Classification of Diseases (Draft ICD-10 (WHO, 1992, 1993) and the revision of the third edition of the Diagnostic and Statistical Manual (DSM-III-R) (American Psychiatric Association, 1987), which, although produced by a national professional organization for use in its own country, has found wide application in other countries as well.

International Classification of Diseases, tenth revision: chapter on mental and behavioural disorders

The tenth revision of the International Classification of Diseases (ICD-10, WHO, 1992, 1993) is different from all those that preceded

Dementia and Normal Aging, eds. F. A. Huppert, C. Brayne & D. W. O'Connor. © Cambridge University Press 1994.

it (Sartorius, 1991). It has three times more categories than the ninth revision. It is accompanied by a 'family' of related classifications and documents – including a classification of disabilities, of reasons for encounter, and a series of classifications for use by medical specialties.

The chapter dealing with mental disorders has been changed in an even more radical manner. First, the greater number of categories has allowed significant expansion of parts of the classification found to be particularly unsatisfactory in the ninth revision (e.g. the parts dealing with mental disorders of children and conditions seen frequently in general health services and in developing countries). Second, while the ninth revision of the classification contained only brief definitions for each category in the mental health chapter, the tenth revision is accompanied by sets of guidelines and criteria contained mainly in two documents, the *Clinical Guidelines to the Classification of Mental Disorders*, and the *Diagnostic Criteria for Research*. The first of these provides for each category: a description of the conditions which should be placed in that category; notes about differential diagnosis; an operationalized description of symptoms of the condition, and a list of synonyms and alternative diagnostic terms which belong to the category. The second document, designed for use in research, is much more peremptory in its definitions of the categories. This should help to reduce the dissimilarity of states labelled by the same diagnosis to a level at which data from different studies can be compared. In addition to these two documents, the World Health Organization (WHO) is also developing a version of the classification of mental disorders adjusted for use in primary health-care services, and a version of ICD-10 which presents its codes along three axes – a clinical syndrome axis, a disability axis and an axis to record environmental circumstances relevant to diagnosis and prognosis.

These documents have been drafted by a large group of clinicians and scientists from different parts of the world, circulated widely and amended to become acceptable to the majority of representatives both of different schools of thought in psychiatry and of different socio-cultural settings in which the classification will be used eventually. In addition, the classification has been piloted in more than 120 centres, in some 40 countries (Sartorius et al., 1988).

The intensive collaboration which WHO has managed to establish with the producers of major national classifications, and in particular with those concerned with DSM-III, DSM-III-R and DSM-IV, justifies hope that the various national classifications will be compatible with ICD-10. In this way, ICD-10 will become the bridge which allows comparison of data and facilitates collaboration between scientists and other mental health workers in different parts of the world.

Agreement between mental health workers and researchers will be improved once ICD-10 is equipped with operationalized criteria and is in wide use. Such agreement will be increased further by the significant progress that has been made in the development of standardized instruments for the assessment of mental states, and instruments for the assessment of other characteristics of people suffering from mental illness, e.g. psychiatric history and personality traits. Some of these instruments have been produced and tested by WHO in major studies involving dozens of centres using a multitude of languages (Sartorius, 1989). Three such instruments have been developed in a programme dealing with diagnosis and classification which WHO has undertaken jointly with the USA Alcohol, Drug and Mental Health Administration (Jablensky et al., 1983), namely the composite international diagnostic interview (CIDI) (Robins et al., 1988), the schedule for clinical assessment in neuropsychiatry (SCAN) (Wing et al., 1990) and the international personality disorder evaluation (IPDE) (Loranger et al., 1991). Other instruments relevant to the diagnostic assessment of dementia that are being tested in WHO-coordinated studies include a battery for the diagnosis of neuropsychiatric damage occurring in the course of HIV-related illnesses (Maj, 1990; Maj et al., 1991) and an instrument to assess dementia and depression in the elderly (Hovaguimian & Junod, 1986). WHO has also produced recommendations concerning the assessment of well-being in the elderly (Fillenbaum, 1984) and supported the exchange of information and publications about instruments suitable for the assessment of mental states in the elderly (e.g. Israel et al., 1984; Häfner et al., 1986; Hovaguimian et al., 1989).

The ICD-10 Diagnostic Criteria for Research

There are four diagnostic criteria for dementia, each having to be fulfilled. These are:

(1) A decline in both memory and intellect, with mild, moderate and severe levels of impairment in each
(2) Absence of clouding of consciousness
(3) Deterioration in emotional control, social behaviour or motivation
(4) Criterion (1) must have been present for at least six months

It should be noted that there is grading of severity separately for memory and for intellect, the overall level of dementia being determined by whichever of the two functions is the more impaired. Impairment of functioning in daily life is not made into a criterion in its own right, but is incorporated into the impairments in memory and intellect, according to their respective severity. In ICD-10, aphasia, apraxia, agnosia and behavioural change are used only to support the diagnosis, whereas this feature counts as a full criterion in DSM-III-R. The criteria recommend the use of brain imaging.

DSM-III-R and DSM-IV

The criteria for dementia in DSM-III-R have now had extensive field use. They will shortly be succeeded by DSM-IV, which will have close similarities to the section on dementia in the ICD-10 *Diagnostic Criteria for Research* (Frances et al., 1990). The DSM-III-R criteria are compared with the ICD-10 research criteria in Table 5.1. This shows the considerable similarity in the areas identified as specific criteria in the two systems. It should be noted that in DSM-III-R no requirement is made about the duration of the syndrome before the diagnosis of dementia can be made; nor are there comments about brain imaging or neuropathology. In ICD-10 on the other hand, social disability is not given as a criterion for diagnosis because of the wide variation in expectations and roles in the countries in which this classification will be used.

Validity of the criteria

Both sets of criteria have been constructed by consensus among experts, principally within the USA for DSM-III-R and among the international scientific community in the case of ICD-10. Although reliability assessments have been made for DSM-III, ICD-10 tests have addressed the acceptability of the criteria, the 'goodness of fit' to the clinical material, and their reliability. It is not yet known if one system has a higher threshold than the other for reaching a diagnosis of dementia, although data about this will be available shortly from several studies (e.g. see Henderson et al., 1994). So far, neither set of criteria for dementia has been validated fully. This validation will have to include a comparison of the diagnosis against clinical information about

Table 5.1. *A comparison of ICD-10 and DSM-III-R*

	ICD-10 (DCR)[a]	DSM-III-R
Impairment of short-term memory	Mild, moderate or severe	No severity grading
Impairment of long-term memory	Mild, moderate or severe	No severity grading
Impaired abstract thinking	Mild, moderate or severe	No severity grading
Impaired judgement	Yes	Yes
Aphasia, apraxia, agnosia	Yes (support diagnosis only)	Yes
Personality change	Emotional control and behaviour	Similar
Interference with work, social activities or relationships	Incorporated in above criteria	Yes
Delirium absent	Yes	Yes
Evidence of a specific organic factor	Yes	Yes
or		
An aetiologic organic factor can be presumed		
Duration	≥ six months	Not specified
Brain imaging	Diagnosis assisted	Not specified
Neuropathology	Diagnosis confirmed	Not specified
Severity		
Mild	Mild memory *and* mild intellectual impairment	Independent living with adequate personal hygiene and relatively intact judgement
Moderate	Moderate impairment of *either* memory *or* intellect, or both	Independent living is hazardous, supervision is necessary
Severe	Severe impairment of *either* memory *or* intellect, or both	Continual supervision is required

[a]DCR, diagnostic criteria for research.

the outcome, as well as against results of non-invasive imaging methods and neuropathological studies using standardized criteria. In a most interesting development, statistical methods have recently been used that enable the properties of different sets of diagnostic criteria to be compared, using latent trait analysis (Grayson et al., 1987; Kay et al., 1987).

The field trials of ICD-10, conducted in all regions of the world, have been designed to generate information on validity of the criteria. The ICD-10 diagnosis of dementia is compared with diagnoses made by experienced clinicians and an attempt is made to assess how well the ICD-10 criteria fit the clinical presentation in diverse cultural settings (WHO, 1992). The diagnosis of dementia in different parts of the world is a specific objective of a WHO multicentric study being conducted currently in Brazil, France, Hong Kong, India, Israel, Korea, Nigeria, Singapore, Spain and Uruguay. Both false-positive and false-negative diagnoses of ICD-10 dementia are being investigated. Another study is focused on the use of clinical methods and special investigations to differentiate dementia of Alzheimer's type (DAT) and vascular dementia as identified by ICD-10 criteria.

Instruments for diagnosing dementia

For research purposes, dementia can be diagnosed satisfactorily only if internationally accepted criteria are used, *and* if appropriate instruments are available for these criteria to be assessed in each individual. Brief screening instruments, such as the mini-mental state examination (Folstein et al., 1975), cannot be used on their own to make a diagnosis. They do not determine the presence or absence of all the elements in the criteria. Several instruments are in use which obtain the necessary information in the course of a systematic interview and mental state examination, together with an interview with a relative or other informant. These instruments vary in the amount of training and clinical experience required. They also vary in how closely they tap each of the elements in the diagnostic criteria.

The instrument with the longest history is the geriatric mental state examination (GMS) (Copeland et al., 1976). The GMS has now been widely used internationally, and a large bank of data is available for it (Copeland et al., 1991). The CAMDEX instrument (Roth et al., 1986) provides DSM-III-R and ICD-10 diagnoses, and has been found to perform well in the field. A recent development is the 'structured interview for the diagnosis of dementia of the Alzheimer type, multi-infarct dementia and dementias of other aetiology according to ICD-10 and DSM-III-R' (SIDAM) by Zaudig et al. (1991). The Canberra interview for the elderly (CIE) was designed for use by lay interviewers, specifically to cover the ICD-10 and DSM-III-R criteria for dementia and depression, and indeed was built upon these criteria (NH&MRC Social Psychiatry Research Unit, 1992; Mackinnon et al., 1993; Henderson et al., 1994). The CIE has computer algorithms for generating these diagnoses. The WHO instruments mentioned above are also likely to find wide application in many countries once they have been fully developed and released.

Dementia: a category or dimension?

Both clinicians and members of the lay public often think of dementia as a disorder that is categorical: it is considered to be either present or absent. For some practical purposes, it may indeed be useful to view dementia in this way. But it is often more fruitful to see it as a continuum of impaired performance, with an underlying continuum of neuropathological changes. It is in this context that the diagnostic criteria of ICD-10 or DSM-III-R, which are explicitly categorical, have to be interpreted: they are convenient specifications for a clinical diagnosis, but they have no more inherent platonic reality than less severe states of the same neuropathological processes. The implication of this for research on dementia is that the syndromes described and specified in the diagnostic criteria are only part of the spectrum of morbidity, and that milder states of impaired memory and thinking are also of scientific and clinical significance.

Differential diagnosis

Dementia is not itself a complete diagnosis, but rather a syndrome whose clinical features are shared by a number of conditions. In ICD-10, the latter include Alzheimer's disease, vascular dementia, multi-infarct (predominantly cortical) dementia, subcortical vascular dementia, dementia in Pick's disease, Creuzfeldt–Jakob disease, Huntington's disease, Parkinson's disease and HIV disease. A summary of the ICD-10 classification is shown in Table 5.2.

In the present context, particular interest is accorded to the territory lying between dementia and normal aging. It is most improbable that a diagnosis of mild dementia by either ICD-10 or DSM-III-R could

Table 5.2. *Classification of the dementias in ICD-10. F0 – Organic including symptomatic mental disorders*

F00	*Dementia in Alzheimer's disease*[a]	
	F00.0	Dementia in Alzheimer's disease, with early onset (type 2)
	F00.1	Dementia in Alzheimer's disease, with late onset (type 1)
	F00.2	Dementia in Alzheimer's disease, atypical or mixed type
F01	*Vascular dementia*[a]	
	F01.0	Vascular dementia of acute onset
	F01.1	Multi-infarct (predominantly cortical) dementia
	F01.2	Subcortical vascular dementia
	(F01.3	Mixed cortical and subcortical vascular dementia)
	(F01.8	Other)
F02	*Dementia in diseases classified elsewhere*[a]	
	F02.0	Dementia in Pick's disease
	F02.1	Dementia in Creutzfeldt–Jakob disease
	F02.2	Dementia in Huntington's disease
	F02.3	Dementia in Parkinson's disease
	F02.4	Dementia in human immunodefiency virus (HIV) disease
	(F02.8	Dementia in other diseases classified elsewhere)
(F03	*Unspecified dementia*[a]	

[a]Fifth character to specify Dementia (F00–F03) with additional symptoms:
.x0 without additional symptoms
.x1 other symptoms, predominantly delusional
.x2 other symptoms, predominantly hallucinatory
.x3 other symptoms, predominantly depressed
.x4 other mixed symptoms.

reasonably be replaced by the term 'normal aging'. The deficits required for the former are not part of normal aging. In ICD-10, the syndrome called mild cognitive disorder (F06.7) is proposed to accommodate the condition characterized principally by subjective complaints of cognitive impairment. The need to introduce such a category was heightened by the appearance of the cognitive motor complex occurring in the course of HIV infection. It has been defined as follows:

(1) For at least two weeks, at least two of the following:

Complaints of memory impairment

Reduced ability to concentrate

Subjective difficulty in attempting new learning

(2) None of these are so severe that dementia or delirium can be diagnosed

(3) Evidence of an infection or physical disorder, cerebral or systemic, closely related in time

(4) No objective evidence of cerebral dysfunction, from neurological or psychological tests

(5) Other mental disorders in ICD-10 are absent

The inclusion of mild cognitive disorder in ICD-10 is deliberate, so that its validity can be assessed and to evaluate how well it can be differentiated from more established and discrete disorders such as dementia, delirium or other changes in behaviour due to brain dysfunction. It has yet to be determined how common this syndrome may be in later life. Since it is essentially a state of subjective dissatisfaction with memory and concentration in the presence of a physical illness, there may be no reason to expect a priori a higher prevalence in the elderly than in younger adults.

In the US, use has come to be made of the term age-associated memory impairment (AAMI) (Crook et al., 1986). This is distinct from benign senescent forgetfulness (Kral, 1962), where memory impairment has to be worse than in comparable elderly persons. It is also distinct from mild cognitive disorder in ICD-10. AAMI appears to be variable in form, according to the composition and source of the samples studied. Unlike AAMI, mild cognitive disorder in ICD-10 has to be associated with an infection or physical disorder (criterion C). It has much in common with the post-infective hyperaesthetic syndrome described by Bonhoeffer (1912).

It is now evident that, for states of cognitive decline falling short of a diagnosable dementia, considerably more information is needed urgently. Such information needs to include non-clinical populations studied prospectively over several years.

Conclusion

The development of standardized criteria and methods for diagnosis has been an essential step for the advancement of knowledge about dementia. The foundation has now been largely laid for ensuring comparability of data within and between countries. It is probable that this advance in method of assessment and the possibility to compare and, above all, to pool data will facilitate significantly the acquisition of knowledge about dementia and related disorders in old age.

References

American Psychiatric Association (1987). *Diagnostic and Statistical Manual of Mental Disorders*, third edition – revised (DSM-III-R). American Psychiatric Association, Washington, DC.

Bonhoeffer, K. (1912). *Die Psychosen im Gefolge von akuten Infektionen, Allgemeinerkrankungen und inneren Erkrankungen*. Vienna.

Copeland, J. R. M., Kelleher, M. J., Kellett, J. M., Gourlay, A. J., Gurland, B. J., Fleiss, J. L. & Share, L. (1976). A semi-structured clinical interview for the assessment of diagnosis and mental state in the elderly: the Geriatric Mental State Schedule. I. Development and reliability. *Psychological Medicine*, **6**, 439–49.

Copeland, J. R. M., Dewey, M. E. & Saunders, P. (1991). The epidemiology of dementia: GMS–AGECAT studies of prevalence and incidence, including studies in progress. *European Archives of Psychiatry and Clinical Neuroscience*, **240**, 212–17.

Crook, T., Bartus, R. T., Ferris, S. H., Whitehouse, P., Cohen, G. D. & Gershon, S. (1986). Age-associated memory impairment: Proposed diagnostic criteria and measures of clinical change. Report of a National Institute of Mental Health Work Group. *Developmental Neuropsychology*, **2**, 261–76.

Fillenbaum, G. G. (1984). *The Well-Being of the Elderly. Approaches to Multidimensional Assessment*. WHO Offset Publication No. 84. World Health Organization, Geneva.

Folstein, M. F., Folstein, S. E. & McHugh, P. R. (1975). 'Mini-Mental State': a practical method for grading the cognitive state of patients for the clinician. *Journal of Psychiatric Research*, **12**, 189–98.

Frances, A., Pincus, H. A., Widiger, T. A., Davis, W. W. & First, M. B. (1990). DSM-IV: work in progress. *American Journal of Psychiatry*, **147**, 1439–48.

Grayson, D. A., Henderson, A. S. & Kay, D. W. K. (1987). Diagnoses of dementia and depression: a latent trait analysis of their perofrmance. *Psychological Medicine*, **17**, 667–75.

Häfner, H., Moschel, G. & Sartorius, N. (1986). *Mental Health in the Elderly: a Review of the Present State of Research*. Springer-Verlag, Berlin.

Henderson, A. S. (1986). The epidemiology of Alzheimer's disease. *British Medical Bulletin*, **42**, 3–10.

Henderson, A. S., Jorm, A. F., Mackinnon, A. J., Christensen, H., Scott, L. R., Korten, A. E. & Doyle, C. (1994). A survey of dementia in the Canberra population: experience with ICD-10 and DSM-IV-R criteria. *Psychological Medicine*, in press.

Hovaguimian, T. & Junod, J. P. (1986). Mental health in old age: a model for concerted action by WHO and university hospitals. *WHO Chronicle*, **40**, 141–8.

Hovaguimian, T., Henderson, S., Khachaturian, Z. & Orley, J. (1989). *Classification and Diagnosis of Alzheimer Disease: an International Perspective.* Hogrefe and Huber Publishers, Toronto.

Israel, L., Kozarevic, D. & Sartorius, N. (1984). *Source Book of Geriatric Assessment, 1 & 2.* S. Karger, Basel.

Jablensky, A., Sartorius, N., Hirschfeld, R. & Pardes, H. (1983). Diagnosis and classification of mental disorders and alcohol- and drug-related problems: a research agenda for the 1980s. *Psychological Medicine*, **13**, 907–21.

Jorm, A. F., Korten, A. E. & Henderson, A. S. (1987). The prevalence of dementia: a quantitative integration of the literature. *Acta Psychiatrica Scandinavica*, **76**, 465–79.

Kay, D. W. K., Henderson, A. S. & Grayson, D. A. (1987). Prospects for epidemiological research on dementia. In B. Cooper (ed.) *Psychiatric Epidemiology: Progress and Prospects*, pp. 257–66. Croom Helm, England.

Kral, V. A. (1962). Senescent forgetfulness, benign and malignant. *Canadian Medical Association Journal*, **86**, 257–60.

Loranger, A. W., Lenzenweger, M. F., Gartner, A. F., Susmann, V. L., Herzig, J., Zammit, G. K., Gartner, J. D., Abrams, R. C. & Young, R. C. (1991). Trait-state artifacts and the diagnosis of personality disorders. *Archives of General Psychiatry*, **48**, 720–8.

Mackinnon, A. J., Christensen, H., Cullen, J. S., Doyle, C. J., Henderson, A. S., Jorm, A. F., Korten, A.E. & Scott, L. R. (1993). The Canberra Interview for the Elderly: assessment of its validity in the diagnosis of dementia and depression. *Acta Psychiatrica Scandinavica*, **87**, 146–51.

Maj, M. (1990). Organic mental disorders in HIV-1 infection. *AIDS*, **51**, 831–40.

Maj, M., Starace, F. & Sartorius, N. (1991). Neuropsychiatric aspects of HIV-1 infection: data collection instrument for a WHO cross-cultural study. *WHO Bulletin*, **69**, 243–5.

NH&MRC (National Health and Medical Research Council) Social Psychiatry Research Unit (1992). The Canberra interview for the elderly (CIE): a new field instrument for the diagnosis of dementia and depression by ICD-10 and DSM-III-R. *Acta Psychiatrica Scandinavica*, **85**, 105–13.

Robins, L. N., Wing, J., Wittchen, H. L., Helzer, J. E., Babor, T. F., Burke, J., Farmer, A., Jablenski, A., Pickens, R., Regier, D. A., Sartorius, N. & Towle, L. H. (1988). The Composite International Diagnostic Interview. *Archives of General Psychiatry*, **45**, 1069–77.

Roth, M., Tym, E., Mountjoy, C. Q., Huppert, F. A., Hendrie, H., Verma, S. & Goddard, R. (1986). CAMDEX: a standardised instrument for the diagnosis of mental disorder in the elderly with special reference to the early detection of dementia. *British Journal of Psychiatry*, **149**, 698–709.

Sartorius, N. (1989). Recent research activities in WHO's mental health programme. *Psychological Medicine*, **19**, 233–44.

Sartorius, N. (1991). The classification of mental disorders in the Tenth Revision of the International Classification of Diseases. *European Psychiatry*, **6**, 315–22.

Sartorius, N., Jablensky, A., Cooper, J. E. & Burke, J. D. (eds.) (1988).

Psychiatric classification in an international perspective. *British Journal of Psychiatry*, **152**, (supplement 1).

WHO (World Health Organization) (1992). *The ICD-10 Classification of Mental and Behavioural Disorders: Clinical Descriptions and Diagnostic Guidelines*. World Health Organization, Division of Mental Health, Geneva.

WHO (World Health Organization) (1993). *ICD-10 Chapter V: Mental and Behavioural Disorders: Diagnostic Criteria for Research*. World Health Organization, Division of Mental Health, Geneva.

Wing, J. E., Babor, T., Brugha, T., Burke, J., Cooper, J. E., Giel, R., Jablensky, A., Regier, D. & Sortorius, N. (1990). SCAN: Schedule for Clinical Assessment in Neuropsychiatry. *Archives of General Psychiatry*, **147**, 589–93.

Zaudig, M., Mittelhammer, J., Hiller, W., Pauls, A., Thora, C., Morinigo, A. & Mombour, W. (1991). SIDAM – a structured interview for the diagnosis of dementia of the Alzheimer type, multi-infarct dementia and dementias of other aetiology according to ICD-10 and DSM-III-R. *Psychological Medicine*, **21**, 225–36.

6

Mild dementia: a clinical perspective

DANIEL W. O'CONNOR

This chapter, which examines mild dementia from a practical, clinical and community-minded perspective, covers a medley of topics: the relationship between 'normal aging', 'cognitive impairment' and 'dementia'; the natural history of dementia in community populations; the role of diagnostic criteria; the difficulties implicit in making assessments of very old people; the relationship between dementia, functional mental disorders and physical handicaps; and the way in which early dementia presents in general and specialist medical practice.

These issues are of little concern to clinicians at present, but matters are likely to change. Elderly people are now better informed about dementia as a result of publicity in newspapers, radio and television; their families want better social and medical services, and general practitioners have a much greater understanding of mental disorder and its consequences. It is perfectly conceivable that forgetful old people will present for help spontaneously and that families will demand a firm diagnosis, practical information, and advice about services as soon as deficits become apparent in everyday life. This will certainly happen if treatments become available but, even if they do not, the spread of information and the rising level of concern in the community have major implications for primary care, psychiatry, neurology and geriatric medicine.

Unfortunately, general practitioners, psychiatrists and epidemiologists have such disparate views of dementia that research findings move slowly, if at all, from one domain to the other. General practitioners see dementia as a hopeless, depressing condition and delay taking action for as long as possible; specialists in hospitals and research centres generalize their findings to all demented persons too quickly, forgetting that their patients are highly selected; while epidemiologists fail to appreciate that dementia (as opposed to cognitive impairment) is a complex clinical syndrome and resort instead to fleeting assess-

Dementia and Normal Aging, eds. F. A. Huppert, C. Brayne & D. W. O'Connor.
© Cambridge University Press 1994.

ments of memory and general knowledge. This chapter looks, or tries to look, at mild dementia through the eyes of all three groups with the aim of promoting understanding and better communication.

Where does dementia begin?

The description by Slater & Roth (1969, pp. 607–8) of the advent of dementia of the Alzheimer's type (DAT) has yet to be equalled:

> The patient's memory usually becomes affected first; he is unable to retain or recall recent events though his memory for remote experiences remains intact . . . There usually appears at the same time some diminution of vitality, a narrowing of interest, a blunting of emotion and a tendency to petulant and irritable behaviour . . . A facade of mastery and full grasp of the situation may be successfully maintained particularly in those of high intelligence and privileged socio-economic status. When combined with the excellent preservation of long-established social responses the presence of a mild or moderate degree of dementia may be effectively concealed.

DSM-III-R (American Psychiatric Association, 1987) and ICD-10 (World Health Organization, 1991) criteria, which depict dementia as an impairment of memory, abstract thought, judgment, personality, higher cortical function and behaviour, spring directly from these writings (see also Chapter 5). This is just as it should be. Diagnostic criteria must be grounded solidly in clinical reality, but inflexible rules which stipulate that dementia comprises features *a*, *b* and *c* but not *d* must be reconciled with the fact that DAT, the commonest form of dementia, progresses slowly. It begins somewhere, but exactly *where* it begins is far from clear. DSM-III (American Psychiatric Association, 1980) and ICD-10 were created with the express intention of isolating distinct, valid and reliable syndromes with a common aetiology, natural history and response to treatment, and yet the world is far more complex. A 'DSM-III' or 'ICD-10' dementia might actually have been present for months or years and have passed in the process from 'normal aging', to 'cognitive impairment', to 'questionable dementia', sometimes quickly and sometimes slowly, sometimes in an unrelenting downward spiral and sometimes with peaks and troughs. While these blurrings of boundaries and outcomes create difficulties for clinicians and epidemiologists, they must be explored as fully as possible if our prognostications (and perhaps treatments) are to prove useful.

The question, 'Where does dementia begin?' can be answered to some extent by the relatives of patients referred to hospitals or specialist centres. However, specialists see such a tiny proportion of all demented people that a prospective approach which asks, 'Which old people will develop dementia?' and 'Which of them will decline to the point where social and medical supports must be deployed?' is of far more interest from a public health perspective. Prospective studies will prove essential should treatments emerge, since, logically, the greatest advantages will accrue to patients with the least neuronal decay. By the same token, early diagnosis and treatment will prove to be worthless if 'mild' degrees of dementias improve or fail to progress. Repeated assessments of cognition, mood and behaviour, informants' reports, and stringent, neuropathological diagnoses are being incorporated into longitudinal studies, but only within strictly delimited research populations and their findings have yet to be synthesized (Berg et al., 1988). In the meantime, little is known of the way in which dementia unfolds in community populations. Is memory failure, of the kind which bedevils many old people, the harbinger of dementia? What factors predict the speed of progression of DAT and other dementias? And how accurate are clinical diagnoses of DAT and multi-infarct dementia (MID) in their embryonic stages?

Is sensecent forgetfulness benign?

Forgetfulness is viewed so commonly as the harbinger of dementia that elderly people feel compelled to cover their lapses with quips and rationalizations, but do minor omissions of memory always lead to progressive cognitive decline? The term 'benign senescent forgetfulness', coined by Kral (1962), implies a tenuous connection. Kral's subjects (all residents of a nursing home) had a patchy recall of incidental details from the recent past; facts or figures were on 'the tips of their tongue' and they recalled them some time later. Malignant forgetfulness, by contrast, comprised a progressive retrograde amnesia, mild disorientation and confabulation. The distinction seemed valid since four-year mortality rates rose from 28% for normal subjects to 38% and 62% respectively for those with benign and malignant dysmnesias. However, Kral's much-vaunted conclusion that benign forgetfulness was a part of the normal aging process, and that malignant forgetfulness stemmed from a discrete pathological process, is perhaps unwarranted, since he acknowledged himself that these two conditions might differ by degree rather than kind. Indeed, minor memory lapses might actually represent an early stage of malignant forgetfulness, and hence dementia, at least in a proportion of cases.

Minor cognitive lapses might be far from innocuous, as shown by Katzman et al. (1989) who followed 434 healthy, independent volunteers aged between 75 and 85 years over a five-year period (subjects with medical or sensory deficits which precluded psychometric testing were excluded). Baseline evaluations consisting of a psychiatric interview, neuropsychological battery and medical examination were followed each year by clinical reviews and further psychometry. Incidence rates of dementia, as defined by DSM-III, were directly proportional to the number of errors on a simple, ten-minute cognitive test administered at the beginning of the study. Respondents with perfect scores out of a maximum of 33 developed dementia at a rate of 0.63 new cases per 100 person-years of observation. By contrast, subjects who made four or fewer errors, and eight or fewer errors, became demented at rates of 4.00 and 26.53 per 100 person-years of observation respectively. While impaired cognition predicted the development of dementia, findings based on groups cannot be applied in a rigid, prescriptive fashion, since not all low-scoring respondents became demented. Factors such as age, sex and histories of stroke, diabetes and left ventricular hypertrophy were also implicated. Thus, the combination of a low cognitive score, extreme old age, stroke, diabetes and heart disease increased the risk that a low initial score would lead to dementia, but none of these factors provided a necessary and sufficient explanation in themselves.

Not all old people with cognitive impairment (i.e. a real or presumed decline in intellectual capacity) become demented, by which is meant a degree of decline which is global in nature and of sufficient severity to interfere with everyday life. This transition is subtle but, perhaps more importantly, it represents a shift in paradigm from the world of psychometry to that of psychiatry. The psychometric model is impersonal: an individual's score x on test y represents a decline of z standard deviations from the norm for persons in this age group. The psychiatric model, by contrast, considers the patient's background, recent history, mental status examination and a range of possible diagnoses (see Chapter 12). These paradigms, or maps of the world, overlap in the sense that the lower the cognitive score the likelier it is that dementia is present, but the two are so fundamentally different that one should never be taken to stand for the other.

The progression of mild dementia

Once this shift occurs – that is, once cognitive impairment assumes a form which is recognized in psychiatric glossaries – what is known of its outcome? Do all old people on the brink of dementia follow a steadily downward path? The answer it seems is no, not in every instance. In fact, the boundaries of 'minimal' or 'questionable' dementia appear to be fluid. O'Connor et al. (1989d, 1990a, 1991c) followed 44 'minimally demented' subjects who were evaluated in detail using the Cambridge Examination for Mental Disorders in the Elderly (CAMDEX) (Roth et al, 1986) in conjunction with standardized diagnostic criteria, as part of a large community survey. None were excluded: subjects were considered irrespective of their backgrounds and specific diagnoses. Of the 24 who survived for two years, five were rated as non-demented, seven as minimally demented, six as mildly demented and six as moderately or severely demented. Thus, only half showed evidence of progression and, significantly, two of the five whose conditions abated were diabetics whose physical and mental health had improved with better diets, regular injections of insulin and more vigilant supervision. Subjects on the brink of dementia, who moved backwards or forwards on repeated examination, also came to light in the Goteborg longitudinal study (Johansson, 1991), although no causes were adduced for this fluctuation. It seems likely that medical, psychiatric and social factors might all be implicated.

The outcome becomes clearer if research populations are cleansed of 'difficult customers'. Reisberg et al. (1986), for example, followed 106 community-resident old people with varying degrees of cognitive decline and dementia. Since those with histories of head injury, stroke, transient ischaemic attack, serious physical illness or functional mental disorder were excluded, the subjects who remained were presumed to suffer from DAT. Twenty-eight were rated at levels 4 or 5 on the Global Deterioration Scale (Reisberg et al., 1982), which approximate to 'questionable dementia' as defined by the Clinical Dementia Rating (CDR) scale (Berg, 1988) and 'minimal dementia' as defined by CAMDEX. Of the 13 persons who remained at home three years later, none had improved, eight showed little change and five had worsened. The removal of subjects with complex medical or psychiatric histories might account for this lack of improvement but, equally, only five of 13 (38%) showed evidence of deterioration compared with 12 of 24 (50%) in the study described above. A three-year review is almost certainly insufficient but, even so, it cannot be assumed that progression is inevitable, especially in non-selected, community populations. Improvements in physical or mental health may produce a shift from 'early dementia' back to 'cognitive impairment' and not all those on the brink of dementia will actually worsen, although their chances of doing so are likely to be very much higher than for persons with intact cognition.

Not surprisingly perhaps, the prognosis of dementia worsens as it moves from 'minimal' to 'mild' to 'moderate' levels but, even here, rigorous selection procedures result in tidier research findings. In a five-year study of 43 volunteers with meticulously documented mild DAT as defined by the CDR, subjects with confounding medical, neurological or psychiatric disorders were rejected so successfully that DAT was confirmed in all 16 cases who came to autopsy (Berg et al., 1988). Prognoses were bleak: mortality rates were nearly four times higher than for healthy, non-demented controls (30% versus 8%) and 17 of the 20 survivors who were traced and re-tested had advanced to moderate or severe degrees of dementia. By contrast, dementia follows a more wayward path in community populations. O'Connor et al. (1989d, 1990a, 1991c) conducted a two-year review of 94 old people who met CAMDEX criteria for mild dementia (see also the previous discussion of these studies). Three of the 56 who survived were rated as non-demented, two were rated as minimally demented, 23 as mildly demented and 28 as moderately or severely demented. As before, a small proportion improved and only half deteriorated substantially. However, even when the focus was narrowed to respondents whose dementia had arisen without obvious cause, at least on clinical grounds, only 14 of 31 subjects had advanced to moderate or severe degrees of diability.

It seems clear that DAT, when defined rigorously on the basis of the history, mental status examination, psychometric testing and computer tomographic (CT) scans, has a poor prognosis in selected patient groups. Equally, outcome is more capricious in representative populations, even when diagnoses are based on detailed clinical evaluations and standardized criteria. There might, however, be factors which help to predict whose status will progress and whose will not. The factors associated with decline, institutionalization or death include senile onset (Huff et al., 1987), a longer duration of symptoms (Thal et al., 1988), impaired parietal function (McDonald, 1969), extrapyramidal signs (Stern et al., 1987) and decreased brain density on CT scans (Naguib & Levy, 1982), but none of these studies focused on mild or early dementia for the simple reason that clinicians encounter few such cases in their day-to-day work. When O'Connor et al. (1991a) reviewed the progress of 31 community-resident, mildly demented old people whose conditions could not be explained by stroke, Parkinson's disease, alcohol abuse and the like, none of a range of possible explanations – age, sex, education, scores on a psychometric battery – discriminated between progressive and non-progressive cases. Only two statistically significant differences emerged from a 'trawl' of the database: subjects whose dementia worsened had been symptomatic for longer (36 months versus 16 months) and a larger proportion had been noted as being demented or possibly demented by their general practitioner (30% compared with none). 'Progression' in this case meant a shift from 'mild' to 'moderate or severe' dementia as defined by CAMDEX. These categories overlap but, to balance this lack of clarity, ratings were based on a vast array of data about cognition, behaviour, everyday function and physical health and were applied in a standardized and reasonably reliable fashion.

Prospective research is hampered by difficulties in ascertaining the cause (or causes) of dementia during life. The DSM-III-R and ICD-10 make it plain that DAT should be diagnosed only in the absence of other causes, as shown by the history, physical examination and laboratory investigations. What should be made, though, of mildly demented persons with histories of alcohol abuse, head injury, hypertension, transient ischaemic attacks or stroke? And what of those who are too deaf, dysphasic or hemiplegic to complete a full mental status examination or psychometric testing? One simple, and perfectly legitimate, solution is to reject all persons with 'messy' backgrounds or disabilities, but such cases exist in abundance. In fact, men who drink to excess and women with transient ischaemic attacks might also have DAT as shown by Ojeda et al. (1986) who reported that 30 out of 44 patients with proven DAT had other conditions (infarctions, haemorrhages, Lewy bodies, subdural haematomas and Wernicke's disease) which might or might not have contributed to their cognitive deficiencies. The chances of identifying successfully all these conditions in life, and of ranking them in order, are remote indeed.

This point might seem obvious and yet, when treatments for DAT or other dementias emerge, they will almost certainly be administered to dementing old people whose conditions cannot always be evaluated in painstaking detail for the reasons described already. Will deafness or dysphasia or physical frailty, which makes transport to hospital for a CT scan impracticable, lead to rejection, and what effects will these omissions have on response rates? Treatment strategies must be applied in the real world, not in the research laboratory, and so studies of the natural history of dementia should be based as close to the coal face as possible.

A general practice perspective

The concept of mild dementia barely figures in medical textbooks or clinical meetings. Doctors have a notion, however poorly defined, of what 'mild diabetes' or 'incipient cataracts' mean in practice but mild dementia cannot be seen or measured in quite the same way. 'Early' cataracts are of much more interest to medical practitioners for the simple reason that a cataract can be removed and replaced with a plastic prosthesis. Doctors are pragmatists at heart. They attach most importance to conditions which respond to treatment and pay much less regard to maladies which cause little overt distress (at least for the present) and which lack effective remedies.

Mild dementia: practical consequences

The fact that we have no treatments for DAT and other common causes of dementia should not in itself give rise to pessimism and inertia. Macular degeneration is untreatable and yet doctors test their patients' eyesight, refer them to specialists and furnish advice on spectacles, magnifying glasses and proper lighting. By contrast, only 3% of the mildly demented elderly persons identified in a British community survey had been referred to the local psychogeriatric service compared with 18% of those with moderate dementia and 33% of those with severe dementia (O'Connor et al., 1988). The point is not that demented old people should always be referred to specialists – psychogeriatric services would be reduced to a shambles if they were – but rather that referral rates provide a rough and ready marker of doctors' interest in dementia and their belief, or lack of belief, that the medical profession has anything to offer. This reluctance to act would make sense if mild dementia were truly innocuous or if general practitioners felt competent to make an assessment, reach a diagnosis (or tentative diagnosis) and provide advice and support but, sadly, none of these conditions apply.

Table 6.1. *Percentage of non-demented and demented community-resident subjects aged 75 years and over who were unable to manage tasks independently*

	Not demented (%) (n = 2095)	Mild dementia (%) (n = 82)	Moderate dementia (%) (n = 64)	Severe dementia (%) (n = 14)
Cannot shop alone	25	70	77	100
Cannot prepare meal	4	16	53	100
Cannot manage housework	5	20	46	100
Needs help to dress	4	17	50	100
Incontinent of urine	2	12	36	93

From O'Connor et al. (1989a).

Table 6.2. *Percentage of non-demented and demented community-resident subjects who were in receipt of personal social services*

	Not demented (%) (n = 2095)	Mild dementia (%) (n = 82)	Moderate dementia (%) (n = 64)	Severe dementia (%) (n = 14)
Home help	17	44	47	43
Meals on wheels	7	27	30	43
Day centre	2	9	22	43

From O'Connor et al. (1989a).

Table 6.1 and Table 6.2, which list data from a recent British survey, show that mild dementia, as defined by CAMDEX, causes appreciable debility (O'Connor et al., 1989a). Mildly demented persons were three to six times more likely than their non-demented peers to have difficulty with shopping, cooking, housework and personal care, and their need for social services was substantially greater. Early dementia also posed problems to families. Table 6.3 lists the ratings made by relatives of the frequency and severity of clusters of behaviours associated with

Table 6.3. *Mean scores of non-demented and demented community-resident subjects on rating scales of problem frequency, problem severity and the emotional strain experienced by relatives*

	Not demented (n = 107)	Mild dementia (n = 58)	Moderate dementia (n = 50)	Severe dementia (n = 12)	Maximum score
Problem frequency					
Physical dependency	3.2	5.2	9.2	18.7	26
Disturbed behaviour	1.0	1.8	4.5	4.9	22
Forgetfulness–inertia	1.8	4.9	10.1	15.9	20
Problem severity					
Physical dependency	2.4	3.3	5.0	13.3	26
Disturbed behaviour	1.8	2.0	3.8	3.8	22
Forgetfulness–inertia	0.9	1.6	3.3	4.8	20
Emotional strain	4.3	7.0	10.3	11.4	26

From O'Connor et al. (1990d). Rating scales taken from Gilleard (1984).

dementia (physical dependency, disturbed behaviour and forgetful-ness–inertia) and of the worries and unhappiness which resulted from their role as carers. Not surprisingly, mildly demented persons were described as more forgetful, less active and more dependent than non-demented subjects, but few were actively disturbed. Relatives saw this loss of function as manageable, judging from their ratings of problem severity, and yet they were under considerably greater strain. In addition, mild dementia resulted in a shortened life expectancy: 6% of non-demented subjects had died within a year of the survey compared with 25% of minimally demented persons and 25%, 22% and 33% of those with mild, moderate and severe degrees of incapacity respectively (O'Connor et al., 1990a).

The recognition of dementia

Williamson et al. (1964) claimed that Scottish general practitioners recognized only 15% of the cases of dementia under their care. How-ever, the fact that as many as 25% of randomly selected patients aged 65 years and over were judged to be demented makes these findings suspect. By contrast, doctors in Cambridge identified successfully 50% of cases of mild dementia, 60% of moderate cases and 78% of severely disabled cases (many of the latter had been admitted to institutions and were actually under the care of other practitioners) (O'Connor et al., 1988). Frequency of contact was of major importance: patients whose condition was identified successfully had been seen by their general practitioners twice as many times in the previous year as those whose dementia was not identified. Presumably, the more frequent the visits, the better the opportunity for doctors to note the practical consequences of the dementing process. Alternatively, the relatives of elderly demented people may call on general practitioners more fre-quently because the patients themselves have difficulty in describing or explaining their symptoms or perhaps because even minor illnesses have a disproportionate effect on patients' level of function in everyday life.

   Despite these successes, doctors' ratings were based more on hunches or suspicions than on hard clinical evidence. Few of the doctors concerned had administered brief cognitive tests or taken histories from relatives and even fewer had committed the word 'dementia' to their records. The doctors concerned made no apologies for this seeming lack of interest. From their point of view, dementia was such a hopeless and depressing condition that the less they said and did about it the better, at least in its early stages.

British general practitioners must now make yearly assessments of the mental, physical and social well-being of all their patients aged 75 years and over. Routine surveillance might uncover early dementias and lead to good, preventive care but, equally, it might simply produce unwarranted distress, multitudes of false-positive diagnoses and wasteful investigations. O'Connor et al. (1993) put this question to the test. A basic screening programme, comprising a brief cognitive test and informant history, was administered to 174 randomly selected general practice patients aged 80 years and over. As it happened, these procedures proved to be acceptable to patients, relatives and the doctors themselves, at least on a one-off basis. A proportion of patients proved to have been diagnosed incorrectly as being demented and some, who were known to be demented, were actually far more handicapped than the doctors had appreciated. Practical responses to this new information included a greater degree of vigilance, more frequent visits, referral to the local social services and requests for practical aids. Annual assessments might not be necessary or even desirable but the fact remains that cognitive tests and informant interviews seem not to be as aversive as doctors suspect.

Families' perceptions

General practitioners are well placed to note subtle changes in memory, intellect and drive but the lack of insight which accompanies dementia makes their task more complex. Patients with painful hips or failing vision complain to their doctors, but not one of the 94 mildly demented persons identified in the Cambridge survey had done so. When questioned directly, two-thirds admitted to memory lapses, half admitted to misplacing items more often than previously, and a third admitted to forgetting the names of family and friends (O'Connor et al., 1990d), but few complained spontaneously and most seemed genuinely unconcerned by their failures on testing. Spouses and children must take responsibility for seeking help, but relatives commonly see mild dementia as a normal, expected part of aging (see Chapter 13). While their reports of changes in memory, orientation and intellectual capacity proved to be consistent with scores on psychometric testing and the observations of research psychiatrists (O'Connor et al., 1989b), only a quarter of those who cared for a mildly demented person had discussed these changes with a doctor (O'Connor et al., 1988). If dementia was accompanied by a stroke or Parkinson's disease, it tended to be the latter conditions which attracted attention. In other cases, spouses 'traded' incapacities ('She doesn't remember what happened this morning, but she can see better than I can') in an attempt to support each other for as long as possible. Families assumed responsibility for paying bills, arranging appointments and making decisions but this shift in the balance of power occurred so gradually that its implications had failed to penetrate. A combination of all these factors (a lack of sophistication, denial, an emphasis on physical as opposed to mental disability, an unwillingness to expose one's spouse to the scrutiny of strangers and the insidious nature of dementia) conspired to keep what was happening within the family.

General practitioners can hardly be blamed if patients and relatives families fail to complain or to ask for assistance, but mild dementia remains submerged for other reasons too. Although DAT remains untreatable, and reversible (or potentially reversible) forms of dementia strike less commonly in aged populations than was previously believed (Larson et al., 1986), preventive strategies should become predominant. Hypnotic and anticholinergic medications should be used minimally, because of their tendency to precipitate falls, excessive sedation and acute confusional states in patients whose mental state is compromised already. Another strategy would be to provide prompt and effective treatments for respiratory and urinary tract infections (which precipitate acute confusional states in vulnerable individuals), and to correct depression, hypothyroidism, diabetes, cardiac failure and a multitude of other conditions which compound the debility produced by dementia (Peters et al., 1989). These benefits must be demonstrated in practice, however, if they are to become an accepted part of clinical lore.

A psychiatric perspective

General practitioners fear that referrals to specialists will precipitate alarm and despondency amongst patients and families and worsen an already fragile state of affairs. It is inconceivable that all mildly demented persons will ever be referred for specialist assessment, but a contact rate as low as 3% means that psychiatrists and neurologists inevitably encounter a highly atypical group of patients. Psychiatrists and researchers whose work is based in clinics or hospitals should be wary therefore of generalizing their observations to all demented persons, and yet the knowledge accumulated through decades of practical experience is relevant both to general practitioners and epidemiologists.

Pseudo-dementia

The notion of 'pseudo-dementia' (a state which resembles dementia but is actually due to a functional mental disorder) has faded somewhat in recent decades as psychiatrists refine their skills in the diagnosis and management of mental disorders in the elderly. What looks to be dementia to the unskilled eye will be recognized immediately as delirium, depression or paranoia by experienced physicians and will be treated accordingly but, even so, the relationship between functional and organic mental disorders is complex. Depression may mimic dementia so closely that even watchful clinicians will be deceived ('true pseudo-dementia'); patients with mild dementias, whose deficits have yet to become apparent, may become confused and disorientated in the face of depression, anxiety or paranoia ('apparent pseudo-dementia') and, finally, depression may complicate established dementias (combined dementia and depression).

Follow-up studies suggest that 'apparent pseudo-dementia' is commonly, but not invariably, the result of a mixture of early dementia and depression. Reynolds et al. (1986) reported that eight out of 16 depressed elderly patients with evidence of cognitive impairment had developed full-blown dementias two years later, while Kral (1983) described a bleak prognosis for 20 out of 22 cases in an eight-year review. In contrast, as many as 16 out of 18 such patients remained well two years later in a study by Rabins et al. (1984). It seems from these and other reports that poor prognoses are associated with lower than average scores on cognitive tests, subtle neurological abnormalities, histories of stroke, and abnormal electroencephalograms (EEGs) and CT scans from the outset (Reding et al., 1985; Reynolds et al., 1986). In addition, depression may complicate established dementias in as many as 20% of the cases referred to specialist clinics and hospitals, although estimates vary widely, presumably because of differences in assessment procedures and diagnostic criteria (Reding et al., 1985). However, the bias implicit in hospital populations becomes apparent when these rates are compared with those from a community survey in which as few as 4% of the mildly demented cases, and 6%

of moderately demented cases, also met DSM-III criteria for major depressive disorders (O'Connor et al., 1990b).

The diagnosis of mild dementia

Most of the demented patients admitted to psychiatric hospitals are disabled so grievously that diagnosis is less of an issue than management. When diagnoses are in doubt, however, clinicians resort to neuroradiology (see Chapter 8) and psychometry to help to clarify the contributions of 'normal aging', functional mental disorder and dementia. Simple cognitive tests, like the mini-mental state examination (MMSE) (Folstein et al., 1975), provide an invaluable, but limited, baseline measure. The MMSE, which taps memory, orientation, recall, language and praxis, is used routinely in clinical and research practice because of its greater than usual scope and its ease of administration. In their initial report, Folstein et al. (1975) recounted that demented hospital patients scored 23 points or less out of a maximum of 30, in contrast to normal volunteers who scored 24 points or more, but the patients admitted to psychiatric hospitals are so highly selected, and severely disabled, that these findings cannot be generalized. Thus, Anthony et al. (1982) reported that 13% of the demented or delirious patients admitted to a large, general teaching-hospital scored in excess of 23 points and that 18% of non-demented patients scored below that. The proportions in a two-stage survey of persons aged 75 years and over were similar at 21% and 9% respectively (O'Connor et al., 1989c). In addition, substantial proportions of elderly people (up to 40% in the latter study) will be labelled in error as demented if diagnoses are based solely on their scores on the MMSE (O'Connor et al., 1989c). The reason is simply that dementia covers a very much wider spectrum in the community, from minimal to severe. The scores of non-demented (but possibly cognitively impaired), minimally demented and mildly demented old people overlap so markedly that the MMSE (in common with all cognitive tests) cannot discriminate between these groups with unerring accuracy (O'Connor et al., 1989c; Storandt & Hill, 1989).

If dementia is judged to be present, psychiatrists seek to determine its cause, paying special attention to remediable conditions like tumours, subdural haematomas and normal pressure hydrocephalus. Little is known, however, about the validity of specific diagnoses in early cases. As noted already, Berg et al. (1988) identified DAT with faultless accuracy, as proven by autopsy, but the patients concerned were selected so rigorously that it seems unlikely that clinicians and epidemiologists, who deal with consecutive patients or respondents, can hope to equal this performance. Clinico-pathological studies have naturally focused on patients admitted to geriatric and psychogeriatric units. While most of the patients concerned have substantial neuro-pathology, many show evidence of more than one disorder (Ojeda et al., 1986), and determining which of these lesions produced the dementia, and which were simply coincidental, may prove to be an impossible task. In addition, the relationship between cognitive dys-function and neuropathology is likely to be much less precise at the borderline between 'normal old age' and 'mild dementia'. Indeed, Crystal et al. (1988) and Katzman et al. (1988) have confirmed that the numbers of plaques and tangles found in the brains of 'normal' (but possibly cognitively impaired) old people overlap with those seen in clinically demented subjects.

Specific diagnoses might also prove to be less valid in early cases in which the clinical picture has yet to solidify. Clinicians have difficulty as it is in distinguishing between DAT and MID, even in conspicuously disabled patients. Wade et al. (1987), for example, found that one of 39 patients diagnosed as having DAT actually had MID, two had a combination of DAT and MID, and three had non-specific conditions such as cortical gliosis. The proportions of cases of DAT identified correctly in life ranged from 55% (Todorov et al., 1975) to 100% (Erkinjuntii et al., 1988), and rates for MID ranged from 17% (Wade et al., 1987) to 92% (Erkinjuntii et al., 1988), but pathological criteria differed so markedly from study to study that the results are hardly comparable (see Chapter 9). Diagnostic 'hit rates' in clinical or com-munity populations of mildly demented people have yet to be examined.

An epidemiological perspective

General practitioners and psychiatrists treat patients and have highly specific goals. Epidemiologists, by contrast, make judgements about the spread of disorders in populations and contend with broader ques-tions of causation and prevention. Indeed, clinicians and epidemiolog-ists have such disparate objectives that their shared terminology – 'cognitive impairment', 'dementia' and the like – merely obscures the gulf between them. Clinicians make diagnoses on the basis of their teaching, reading and practical experience; epidemiologists use structured, standardized assessment instruments. Clinicians have time to review patients' progress, while epidemiologists must rely on a single, snapshot view of the whole of a community. Time is of the essence in research projects and epidemiologists commonly have one opportunity, and one opportunity only, to make an assessment and to reach a diagnosis.

Community assessments: perils and pitfalls

Although complex cases like those described above are much less common in the community at large, the pitfalls involved in epidemiological surveys should never be under-estimated. Many old people have sensory deficits, medical complaints and functional psychiatric disorders which make it difficult, if not impossible, to determine how much of their loss of function is due to physical disability and how much is due to mental incapacity. Accurate assessment requires that subjects hear the questions put to them, express themselves clearly and be patient enough to complete the interview. Unfortunately, 14% of the elderly respondents in a survey in New York spoke a foreign language, 7% were deaf or had some defect of speech and 7% of interviews were subject to noises off-stage, intrusive relatives and other distractions (Gurland et al., 1983). Similarly, 18% of the British respondents aged 70 years and over who were labelled as cognitively impaired on the basis of their scores on a brief cognitive test had a hearing loss in excess of 70 decibels (Herbst & Humphrey, 1980). The implications are clear. Mentally intact old people may be labelled in error as being demented because of deafness or other incapacities, while genuinely demented cases may be passed as normal if failures on testing are attributed solely to sensory or physical deficits (Fillenbaum et al, 1988). Co-morbidity is of particular importance when everyday function is used as a diagnostic benchmark. For example, 84 cognitively intact nonagenarians encountered in the Cambridge survey all had difficulty in one or more of the following areas, even when using aides: sight, vision, walking one block, and managing cooking and housework independently (O'Connor et al., 1989a).

O'Connor et al. (1991b) gauged the impact of mental and physical incapacities using data from a British community survey. It was not their intention to measure the rightness or wrongness of clinical judgements but rather to list the disorders which led research psychiatrists to pull back from attaching the label of 'mild dementia' to persons whose scores on measures of memory and everyday function placed them in the 'mildly demented' range. The conditions responsible for this change in tack included blindness, deafness, dysarthria, dysphasia, mental retardation, physical handicap due to stroke or Parkinson's disease, anxiety, depression, hypomania, chronic schizophrenia, organic personality disorder and delirium. Thus, the sorts of disorders which create uncertainty in clinical practice arise in the community too and tend to be concentrated at the borderland between 'normal old age' and 'mild dementia'. In other words, the better the assessment, the harder it becomes to make a clear distinction between mental and physical abnormalities, not least because dementia, sensory incapacity and physical illness all strike most keenly in advanced old age.

These uncertainties cannot be resolved in the absence of a detailed history. Relatives can often draw distinctions between the limitations imposed by blindness, for example, and those which follow from dementia, but epidemiologists have virtually abandoned informant interviews, partly for reasons of economy and partly through fear that relations view forgetfulness, indecisiveness and a loss of vitality as a normal part of the aging process and fail to report them. Spouses and children interpret the changes produced by dementia in a benign, workaday fashion ('she's good for 85') but, equally, their answers to questions about memory, intellect and behaviour prove to be remarkably consistent with objective measures of cognition and behaviour (Jorm & Korten, 1988; O'Connor et al., 1989b). In the latter study, Pearson correlation coefficients between informants' reports and subjects' scores on a psychometric battery were as high as 0.73 which is highly statistically significant. Thus, informants provide valid reports for the most part and they differ from psychiatrists only in the meaning they attach to these changes. Their accounts deserve to be used more widely.

Diagnostic criteria

Diagnostic criteria are of critical importance in studies of the prevalence or incidence of dementia: the lower the diagnostic threshold, the higher the prevalence rate and vice versa (Black et al., 1990). By common consent, dementia 'begins' as soon as everyday function is compromised, with the result that a 'non-demented' respondent might well be cognitively impaired and at higher than average risk of developing 'dementia proper' in coming months or years. Exactly when dementia begins can be interpreted in various ways. In an intriguing study by Mowry & Burvill (1988), respondents aged 70 years and over were assessed using a range of cognitive tests, a structured interview schedule and an inventory of activities of daily living. Mild dementia was diagnosed by means of scores on the MMSE, DSM-III criteria and the category of 'limited cognitive disturbance' as described by Gurland et al. (1983). The prevalence of mild dementia or its equivalent ranged from 3% using DSM-III criteria, to 15% using the same criteria (excluding social and occupational dysfunction), to 24% using the category of 'limited disturbance'. The study was contrived, and investigations fell short of those employed in clinical practice, but the point is made clearly that diagnoses of mild dementia depend first and foremost on assessment procedures and labelling conventions.

Investigators must also distinguish between mild, moderate and severe degrees of dementia in a reliable and valid fashion. DSM-III-R, ICD-10 and CAMDEX provide descriptions of the level of function expected at each level of dementia. CAMDEX, for example, states that mild dementia entails: 'difficulty in recalling recent information; limited or patchy disorientation to time and place; impaired problem-solving, reasoning and capacity to manage everyday activities; diminished clarity of speech and defective knowledge of the names of prominent figures. The patient's social facade and emotional responsiveness may well be retained but indubitable cognitive deficits are present on testing' (Roth et al., 1988, pp. 50–1). While criteria such as these can be applied with a fair degree of uniformity by the members of a single research team, other teams might apply them quite differently. The Clinical Dementia Rating (CDR) scale (Berg, 1988) provides a partial solution and deserves to be used more widely. It consists of five-point scales of memory, orientation, judgement and problem solving, community activities, home, hobbies and personal care. Ratings of questionable, mild, moderate and severe dementia are reached by scoring each category and applying simple arithmetical rules. Severity ratings are inevitably rather arbitrary, and the CDR can never compensate for deficient assessment techniques, but it offers a structured and replicable solution in an otherwise contentious area.

Assessment schedules

Dementia is a clinical syndrome and diagnoses must always be based on a detailed clinical assessment. Community researchers face constraints of time, staff and funds, but three structured interview schedules provide a rounded view of respondents' backgrounds, their medical and psychiatric histories, current mental status, cognitive function, physical health and competency in everyday life. The Geriatric Mental State schedule (GMS), devised by Copeland et al. (1976) can be administered by trained lay interviewers, and diagnoses are generated, within seconds if necessary, using a computerized algorithm known as AGECAT. Diagnoses of organic mental disorders derive from a limited combination of a brief cognitive test, a few additional memory items and a series of observational ratings. The schedule includes an informant interview but this crucial historical information has yet to be incorporated into the AGECAT programme and it contributes at present just to the distinction between DAT, MID and other dementia subtypes (Copeland & Dewey, 1991). The GMS has the major advantage that data can be collected in an efficient and reliable fashion with the result that identical data will generate identical diagnoses in every instance.

CAMDEX comprises a mental state examination, a medical and psychiatric history, detailed cognitive testing, a brief physical examination and an informant interview which covers changes in memory, intellect, drive, mood and behaviour (Roth et al., 1986). All this information is then collated by clinicians using criteria that are virtually identical to those in ICD-10, although other criteria could be substituted if required. The schedule can be administered reliably (Roth et al., 1986), although a series of 23 joint interviews, conducted as part of a community survey, led to three disagreements, all in the areas of normality, minimal dementia and mild dementia (O'Connor et al., 1991a). CAMDEX was designed to replicate a full clinical assessment, albeit in a structured fashion, and to be capable of detecting mild degrees of cognitive impairment. The interview is lengthy (between 45 and 90 minutes) and the need for skilled professionals makes it essential that screening procedures be applied in very large surveys. O'Connor et al. (1989d) administered CAMDEX to respondents who scored 23 points or less on the MMSE, together with a one-in-three sample of those who scored 24 or 25 points, but sophisticated stratified sampling techniques, of the kind described by Duncan-Jones & Henderson (1978), would be preferable in studies in which substantial numbers of 'cases' are not required for further investigation. A third structured schedule, the Canberra Interview of the Elderly (Social Psychiatry Research Unit, 1992), which is based directly on DSM-III-R and ICD-10 criteria, looks promising and is being tested at present.

Diagnostic validity is just as important an issue in the community as in hospital studies. Post-mortem examination of subjects identified in the course of community surveys is problematic but not impossible as shown by Beardsall et al., (1992) who reported that 85% of normal, community-resident old people consented to autopsy when approached during life and that 75% of the relatives of demented persons consented on the latters' behalf. Over the course of a year, as many as 72% of deaths in these groups were followed by limited post-mortem examinations. This extraordinary success rate required such a major commitment that only substantial research teams could hope to emulate this performance. In the meantime, continued clinical evaluation of surviving subjects has much to offer. Dementia may not progress, at least over a one- to two-year period, but remissions should occur only occasionally and with very good reason.

Both the GMS and CAMDEX have been subject to clinical review. Psychiatrists agreed with AGECAT diagnoses of mild and more advanced dementias in 28 of 31 instances (Copeland et al., 1988), but, in a separate report, only six of 12 subjects diagnosed as mild organic cases using AGECAT were rated as demented by psychiatrists one year later. Two were judged to be depressed, one had developed schizophrenia and three were passed as normal (Copeland et al., 1986). The clinicians' judgements may have been mistaken, but the report included too few details to make sense of these discrepancies. Findings with respect to CAMDEX have been mentioned already. Thirty eight of the surviving 67 mildly demented subjects were identified in a community survey one year later and 25 were rated as moderately or severely demented. Two were graded as minimally demented (both were diabetics whose physical health had improved in the interim) and two were passed as non-demented. While clinical validity appears to be satisfactory, it should be noted that follow-up assessments were not completely independent, since diagnoses were confirmed using identical procedures by members of a single research team.

There have been a multitude of prevalence surveys but few researchers have confirmed their diagnoses, and judgement should be reserved. 'Mild dementia' is still so tenuous a category that reviews should be sought wherever possible to confirm that cognitive and functional disabilities persist. When remissions occur, as they must from time to time, researchers should try to make sense of this change in status by using all the personal, medical and psychiatric data they have to hand. A change in status, for example from 'minimally demented' to 'non-demented', might actually be correct but arguments should be marshalled to justify the initial assessment.

In summary, community assessments require careful thought and planning. Surveys are now so expensive that researchers are tempted frequently to circumvent recognized assessment techniques and to rely instead on brief cognitive tests. These provide a valid measure of cognitive function but 'cognitive impairment', however defined, falls short of a diagnosis of dementia and of mild dementia in particular. Even when studies use detailed, structured assessment schedules, diagnoses of early dementias have yet to be validated with any degree of stringency. Follow-up is essential and reports should also acknowledge that a proportion of the persons encountered are simply too deaf, dysphasic, depressed or uncooperative to be assessed in the detail required.

Summary

Mild dementias, which account for approximately half of all extant cases, are still largely of academic interest. Deliberate attempts to seek them out are unlikely to be of value until treatments for DAT or other common dementias become available, but, once this happens, quick, accurate and reliable forms of detection will become essential. General practitioners are loathe to probe too deeply at present for fear of disturbing stable family relationships, and yet relatives seem to be remarkably tolerant of doctors' inquiries and provide logical and consistent answers.

Epidemiologists have come to rely on brief cognitive tests, despite the fact that normal old age, cognitive impairment and mild degrees of dementia cannot be distinguished on the basis of scores per se. Dementia is a clinical, not a psychometric, entity and diagnoses should be based on the history, mental status examination and physical evaluation. Since dementia may be complicated by other disorders (for example, depression or delirium), follow-up is required to assess the validity of diagnoses. Structured assessment schedules like the GMS and CAMDEX are time consuming and expensive, but have much to offer.

The relationship between cognitive function and neuropathology has yet to be assessed at the borderline of normal old age, cognitive impairment and dementia in community populations. Such studies are likely to prove to be fruitful, provided that sufficient personal, medical and psychiatric information is obtained to make sense of the inevitable discrepancies. Detail, together with painstaking reviews and an honest acceptance of the limitations implicit in all assessment techniques, will mark the way forward.

References

American Psychiatric Association (1980). *Diagnostic and Statistical Manual of Mental Disorders*, third edition. American Psychiatric Association, Washington, DC.

American Psychiatric Association (1987). *Diagnostic and Statistical Manual of Mental Disorders*, third edition – revised (DSM-III-R). American Psychiatric Association, Washington, DC.

Anthony, J. C., LeResche, L., Niaz, U., Von Korff, M. R. & Folstein, M. F. (1982). Limits of the 'Mini-Mental State' as a screening test for dementia and delirium among hospital patients. *Psychological Medicine*, **12**, 397–408.

Beardsall, L., Barkley, C. & O'Sullivan, A. (1992). The response of elderly community residents to request for brain donation: an interim report. *International Journal of Geriatric Psychiatry*, **7**, 199–202.

Berg, L. (1988). Mild senile dementia of the Alzheimer type: diagnostic criteria and natural history. *Mount Sinai Journal of Medicine*, **85**, 87–96.

Berg, L., Miller, J. P., Storandt, M., Duchek, J., Morris, J. C., Rubin, E. H., Burke, W. J. & Cohen, L. A. (1988). Mild dementia of the Alzheimer type: longitudinal assessment. *Annals of Neurology*, **23**, 477–84.

Black, S. E., Blessed, G., Edwardson, J. A. & Kay, D. W. K. (1990). Prevalence rates of dementia in an ageing population: are low rates due to the use of insensitive instruments? *Age and Ageing*, **19**, 84–90.

Copeland, J. R. M. & Dewey, M. E. (1991). Neuropsychological diagnosis (GMS–IIAS–AGECAT package). *International Psychogeriatrics*, **3**, 43–9.

Copeland, J. R. M., Kelleher, M. J., Kellet, J. M., Gourlay, A. J., Gurland, B. J., Fleiss, J. L. & Sharpe, L. (1976). A semi-structured clinical interview for the assessment of diagnosis and mental state in the elderly: the Geriatric Mental State Schedule: development and reliability. *Psychological Medicine*, **6**, 439–49.

Copeland, J. R. M., McWilliam, C., Dewey, M. E., Forshaw, D., Shiwach, R., Abed, R. T., Muthu, M. S. & Wood, N. (1986). The early recognition of dementia: a preliminary communication about a longitudinal study using the GMS–AGECAT package (community version). *International Journal of Geriatric Psychiatry*, **1**, 63–70.

Copeland, J. R. M., Dewey, M. E., Henderson, A. S., Kay, D. W. K., Neal, C. D., Harrison, M. A. M., McWilliam, C., Forshaw, D. & Shiwach, R.

(1988). The Geriatric Mental State (GMS): replication studies of the computerised diagnosis AGECAT. *Psychological Medicine*, **18**, 219–23.

Crystal, H., Fuld, P., Masur, D., Scott, R., Mehler, M., Masdeu, J., Kawas, C., Aronson, M. & Wolfson, L. (1988). Clinico-pathological studies in dementia: non-demented subjects with pathologically confirmed Alzheimer's disease. *Neurology*, **38**, 1682–7.

Duncan-Jones, P. & Henderson, S. (1978). The use of a two-phase design in a prevalence survey. *Social Psychiatry*, **13**, 231–7.

Erkinjuntii, T., Haltia, M., Palo, J., Sulkava, R. & Paetau, A. (1988). Accuracy of the clinical diagnosis of vascular dementia: a prospective clinical and post-mortem neuropathological study. *Journal of Neurology, Neurosurgery and Psychiatry*, **51**, 1037–44.

Fillenbaum, G. G., George, L. K. & Blazer. D. G. (1988). Scoring non-response on the Mini-Mental State Examination. *Psychological Medicine*, **18**, 1021–5.

Folstein, M. F., Folstein, S. E. & McHugh, P. R. (1975). 'Mini-Mental State': a practical method for grading the cognitive state of patients for the clinician. *Journal of Psychiatric Research*, **12**, 189–98.

Gilleard, C. J. (1984). *Living with Dementia: Community Care of the Elderly Mentally Infirm*. Croom Helm, Beckenham.

Gurland, B., Copeland, J., Kuriansky, J., Kelleher, M., Sharpe, L. & Dean, L. L. (1983). *The Mind and Mood of Aging: Mental Health Problems in the Community Elderly in New York and London*. Croom Helm, London.

Herbst, K. G. & Humphrey, C. (1980). Hearing impairment and mental state in the elderly living at home. *British Medical Journal*, **281**, 903–5.

Huff, F. J., Growden, J. H., Corkin, S. & Rosen, T. J. (1987). Age at onset and rate of progression of Alzheimer's disease. *Journal of American Geriatrics Society*, **35**, 27–30.

Johansson, B. (1991). Neuropsychological assessment in the oldest old. *International Psychogeriatrics*, **3**, 51–60.

Jorm, A. F. & Korten, A. E. (1988). Assessment of cognitive decline in the elderly by informant interview. *British Journal of Psychiatry*, **152**, 209–13.

Katzman, R., Terry, R., DeTeresa, R., Brown, T., Davies, P., Fuld, P., Renbing, X. & Peck, A. (1988). Clinical, pathological, and neurochemical changes in dementia: a subgroup with preserved mental status and numerous neocortical plaques. *Annals of Neurology*, **23**, 138–44.

Katzman, R., Aronson, M., Fuld, P., Kawas, C., Brown, T., Morgenstern, H., Frishman, W., Gidez, L., Eder, H. & Ooi, W. L. (1989). Development of dementing illnesses in an 80-year-old volunteer cohort. *Annals of Neurology*, **25**, 317–24.

Kral, V. A. (1962). Senescent forgetfulness: benign and malignant. *The Canadian Medical Association Journal*, **86**, 257–60.

Kral, V. A. (1983). The relationship between dementia (Alzheimer type) and depression. *Canadian Journal of Psychiatry*, **28**, 304–6.

Larson, E. B., Reifler, B. V., Sumi, S. M., Canfield, C. G. & Chinn, N. M. (1986). Diagnostic tests in the evaluation of dementia: a prospective study of 200 elderly outpatients. *Archives of Internal Medicine*, **146**, 1917–22.

McDonald, C. (1969). Clinical heterogeneity in senile dementia. *British Journal of Psychiatry*, **115**, 267–71.

Mowry, B. J. & Burvill, P. W. (1988). A study of mild dementia in the community using a wide range of diagnostic criteria. *British Journal of Psychiatry*, **153**, 328–34.

Naguib, M. & Levy, R. (1982). Prediction of outcome in senile dementia – a computed tomographic study. *British Journal of Psychiatry*, **140**, 263–7.

O'Connor, D. W., Pollitt, P. A., Hyde, J. B., Brook, C. P. B., Reiss, B. B. & Roth, M. (1988). Do general practitioners miss dementia in elderly patients? *British Medical Journal*, **297**, 1107–10.

O'Connor, D. W., Pollitt, P. A., Brook, C. P. B. & Reiss, B. B. (1989a). The distribution of services to demented elderly people living in the community. *International Journal of Geriatric Psychiatry*, **4**, 339–44.

O'Connor, D. W., Pollitt, P. A., Brook, C. P. B. & Reiss, B. B. (1989b). The validity of informant histories in a community study of dementia. *International Journal of Geriatric Psychiatry*, **4**, 203–8.

O'Connor, D. W., Pollitt, P. A., Hyde, J. B., Fellowes, J. L., Miller, N. D., Brook, C. P. B. & Reiss, B. B. (1989c). The reliability and validity of the Mini-Mental State in a British community survey. *Journal of Psychiatric Research*, **23**, 87–96.

O'Connor, D. W., Pollitt, P. A., Hyde, J. B., Fellowes, J. L., Miller, N. D., Brook, C. P. B., Reiss, B. B. & Roth, M. (1989d). The prevalence of dementia as measured by the Cambridge Mental Disorders of the Elderly Examination. *Acta Psychiatrica Scandinavica*, **79**, 190–8.

O'Connor, D. W., Pollitt, P. A., Hyde, J. B., Fellowes, J. L., Miller, N. D. & Roth, M. (1990a). A follow-up study of dementia diagnosed in the community using the Cambridge Mental Disorders of the Elderly Examination. *Acta Psychiatrica Scandinavica*, **81**, 78–82.

O'Connor, D. W., Pollitt, P. A. & Roth, M. (1990b). Coexisting depression and dementia in a community survey of the elderly. *International Psychogeriatrics*, **2**, 45–53.

O'Connor, D. W., Pollitt, P. A., Roth, M., Brooke, C. P. B. & Reiss, B. B. (1990c). Problems reported by relatives in a community study of dementia. *British Journal of Psychiatry*, **156**, 835–41.

O'Connor, D. W., Pollitt, P. A., Roth, M., Brook, C. P. B. & Reiss, B. B. (1990d). Memory complaints and impairment in normal, depressed and demented elderly persons identified in a community survey. *Archives of General Psychiatry*, **47**, 224–7.

O'Connor, D. W., Pollitt, P. A., Hyde, J. B., Fellowes, J. L., Miller, N. D. & Roth, M. (1991a). The progression of mild idiopathic dementia in a community population. *Journal of the American Geriatrics Society*, **39**, 246–51.

O'Connor, D. W., Pollitt, P. A., Hyde, J. B., Miller, N. D. & Fellowes, J. L. (1991b). Clinical issues relating to the diagnosis of mild dementia in a British community survey. *Archives of Neurology*, **48**, 530–4.

O'Connor, D. W., Pollitt, P. A., Jones, B. J., Hyde, J. B., Fellowes, J. L. & Miller, N. D. (1991c). Continued clinical validation of dementia diagnosed in the community using the Cambridge Mental Disorders of the Elderly Examination. *Acta Psychiatrica Scandinavica*, **83**, 41–5.

O'Connor, D. W., Fertig, A., Grande, M. J., Hyde, J. B., Perry, J. R., Roland, M. O., Silverman, J. D. & Wraight, S. K. (1993). Dementia in general practice: the practical consequences of a more positive approach to diagnosis. *British Journal of General Practice*, **43**, 185–8.

Ojeda, V. J., Mastaglia, F. L. & Kakulas, B. A. (1986). Causes of organic dementia: a necropsy survey of 60 cases. *Medical Journal of Australia*, **145**, 69–71.

Peters, D. W., Reifler, B. V. & Larson, E. (1989). Excess disability in dementia. In N. Billig & P. V. Rabins (eds.) *Issues in Geriatric Psychiatry: Advances in Psychosomatic Medicine*, vol. 19, pp. 17–30. Karger, Basel.

Rabins, P. V., Merchant, A. & Nestadt, G. (1984). Criteria for diagnosing reversible dementia caused by depression: validation by two-year follow-up. *British Journal of Psychiatry*, **144**, 488–92.

Reding, M., Haycox, J. & Blass, J. (1985). Depression in patients referred to a dementia clinic: a three-year prospective study. *Archives of Neurology*, **42**, 894–6.

Reisberg, B., Ferris, S. H., DeLeon, M. J. & Crook, T. (1982). The global deterioration scale for assessment of primary degenerative dementia. *American Journal of Psychiatry*, **139**, 1136–9.

Reisberg, B., Ferris, S. H., Shulman, E., Steinberg, G., Buttinger, C., Sinaiko, E., Borenstein, J., de Leon, M. J. & Cohen, J. (1986). Longitudinal course of normal aging and progressive dementia of the Alzheimer's type. *Progress in Neuropsychopharmacology and Biological Psychiatry*, **10**, 571–8.

Reynolds, C. F., Kupfer, D. J., Hoch, C. C., Stack, J. A., Houck, P. R. & Sewitch, D. E. (1986). Two year follow-up of elderly patients with mixed depression and dementia: clinical and electroencephalographic sleep findings. *Journal of the American Geriatrics Society*, **34**, 793–9.

Roth, M., Tym, E., Mountjoy, C. Q., Huppert, F. A., Hendrie, H., Verma, S. & Goddard, R. (1986). CAMDEX: a standardised instrument for the diagnosis of mental disorder in the elderly with special reference to the early detection of dementia. *British Journal of Psychiatry*, **149**, 698–709.

Roth, M., Huppert, F. A., Tym, E. & Mountjoy, C. Q. (1988). *CAMDEX: the Cambridge Examination for Mental Disorders of the Elderly*. Cambridge University Press, Cambridge.

Slater, E. & Roth, M. (1969). *Clinical Psychiatry*. London: Baillière Tindall, pp. 607–8.

Social Psychiatry Research Unit (1992). The Canberra Interview for the Elderly: a new field instrument for the diagnosis of dementia and depression by ICD-10 and DSM-III-R. *Acta Psychiatrica Scandinavica*, **85**, 105–13.

Stern, Y., Mayeux, R., Sano, M., Hauser, W. A. & Bush, T. (1987). Predictors of disease course in patients with Alzheimer's disease. *Neurology*, **37**, 1649–53.

Storandt, M. & Hill, R. D. (1989). Very mild senile dementia of the Alzheimer type: II, psychometric test performance. *Archives of Neurology*, **46**, 383–6.

Thal, L. J., Grundman, M. & Klauber, M. R. (1988). Dementia: characteristics of a referral population and factors associated with progression. *Neurology*, **38**, 1083–90.

Todorov, A. B., Go, R. C. P., Constantinidis, J. & Elston, R. C. (1975). Specificity of the clinical diagnosis of dementia. *Journal of the Neurological Sciences*, **26**, 81–98.

Wade, J. P. H., Mirsen, T. R., Hachinski, V. C., Fisman, M., Lau, C. & Merskey, H. (1987). The clinical diagnosis of Alzheimer's disease. *Archives of Neurology*, **44**, 24–9.

Williamson, J., Stokoe, I. H., Gray, S., Fisher, M., Smith, A., McGhee, A. & Stephenson, E. (1964). Old people at home: their unreported needs. *Lancet*, **i**, 1118–20.

World Health Organization (1991). *ICD-10 Research Diagnostic Criteria*. World Health Organization, Geneva.

7

Neurological aspects of dementia and normal aging

JOHN R. HODGES

Amongst neurologists it is widely believed that dementia is associated with certain abnormal physical signs, the presence of which may aid diagnosis. However, abnormalities on neurological examination are also found with increasing frequency in apparently normal elderly populations. This chapter addresses the issue of whether there really is an increased prevalence of abnormal neurological signs in demented patients. (The term neurological signs here applies to those signs elicited on standard physical examination performed by a clinician using basic standard equipment (reflex hammer, pupil torch, etc.) and does not include abnormalities detected on bedside cognitive testing.) Then, I try to assess the relevance of the findings to the diagnosis of individuals with dementia, and to considerations of the pathogenesis – particularly the issue of whether dementia reflects an exaggeration of the normal aging process. Finally, I attempt to answer the question of whether subgroups of patients with Alzheimer's disease are identifiable on the basis of finding abnormal neurological signs. I have confined myself to dementia of the Alzheimer's type (DAT) and related primary degenerative brain diseases for two reasons: DAT is by far the commonest cause for dementia and the literature on vascular dementia is extremely confused.

Since much of the pertinent literature deal with frontal release signs, also called primitive or developmental reflexes, I have included an appendix describing the most commonly reported of these frontal signs.

Dementia and Normal Aging, eds. F. A. Huppert, C. Brayne & D. W. O'Connor.
© Cambridge University Press 1994.

Is there an increased prevalence of abnormal neurological signs in patients with DAT?

Interest in the neurological features of both dementia and normal aging has a long and illustrious history, but until relatively recently the two aspects have been considered rather separately. McDonald Critchley dedicated his 1931 Goustonian lectures to the topic of the neurology of aging. He provided a detailed and scholarly review of the European literature, which demonstrated clearly that the normal aging process is associated with a wide range of neurological signs; frontal release signs, extrapyramidal and subtle sensory changes were noted to be particularly common in elderly subjects. Despite such observations in normal elderly subjects, the association between certain neurological signs and dementia was, until recently, not questioned. This is illustrated by an influential, and often quoted, review by Paulson & Gottleib in 1968, which discussed the pathological basis of frontal release phenomena in dementia. The reappearance of these developmental reflexes was attributed to diffuse cortical atrophy with resultant weakening of normal higher cerebral inhibition rather than focal frontal disease as was commonly believed. It is interesting to reflect on how much both the methodology of clinical research, and diagnostic concepts of dementia, have evolved since the late 1960s when a retrospective uncontrolled case-note review of patients with 'presenile and senile dementia' was considered to be acceptable.

The general recrudescence of interest in dementia over the past decade together with the development of standardized premorbid diagnostic criteria for Alzheimer's disease, and the realization of the need for strict case–control type methodology has resulted in a critical appraisal of the association of neurological signs and DAT. Initial attempts to examine this association produced conflicting results, perhaps because of the relatively small number of cases studied, but particularly because of the variability in the stages of dementia of the patient groups (e.g. Jenkyn et al., 1977; Koller et al., 1982; Jensen et al., 1983). However, the controversy has now been largely settled as a result of three recent comprehensive studies which have compared large groups of patients with clearly defined DAT and age-matched controls using standardized neurological examinations. Two of these have also related severity of dementia to the prevalence of neurological signs.

Before discussing these studies, two potential sources of bias in all investigations of this type should be considered. Firstly, the presence or absence of neurological signs affects the diagnostic classification of demented patients: those with positive signs (such as exaggerated tendon reflexes) are more likely to be designated as vascular dementia. If some of the patients assigned to this category do, in fact, have DAT then the prevalence of neurological signs in 'DAT' will be lowered artificially. Secondly, the subjects used as normal controls in comparative studies may well be unrepresentative of the general population. The selection of 'supernormal' controls will lead to an underestimation of the prevalence of neurological signs in the control group, and hence a falaciously raised prevalence in the DAT group. Only a large community-based study using a cohort of patients with dementia of various aetiologies (confirmed at post-mortem) and true normal controls will finally answer the questions raised.

Huff et al. (1987) compared 87 age-matched normal controls with 95 patients with DAT, all of whom fulfilled the criteria for probable disease, developed by the National Institute of Neurological and Communication Disorders and Stroke (NINCDS) and the Alzheimer's and Related Disorders Association (ADRDA) (McKhann et al., 1984). They found a significant increase in the following signs: impaired olfaction, frontal release phenomena, parietal sensory signs (astereognosis and graphaesthesia), tremor, cerebellar ataxia and gait disturbance. However, following a multivariate logistic regression analysis, only the first three signs independently predicted the presence of DAT.

In a similar study, Galasko et al. (1990) analysed consecutive patients enrolled into a prospective cohort study at the Alzheimer Disease Research Center at the University of California, San Diego. They compared 135 DAT patients who fulfilled NINCDS–ADRDA criteria and 91 normal controls using a comprehensive and standardized neurological examination. Again, a number of frontal release phenomena (glabellar tap, snout and grasp responses), extrapyramidal features (stooped gait and rigidity) and parietal sensory signs (graphaesthesia) were significantly more common in the DAT patients. All signs increased with disease severity. It is noteworthy, however, that in the mildest DAT group only rigidity and a positive glabellar tap were observed more frequently than in controls.

In the most comprehensive study to date, Franssen and colleagues (1991) from New York studied 135 community-based and nursing home residing elderly subjects, including a wide range of cognitive abilities from normal to severely demented. A complex assessment scale for each neurological sign, with cut-off points of varying sensitivity, was employed. All the signs studied were found to be more frequent in the demented group, but, as in the Galasko et al. (1990) study, very few differences were found between the mildly impaired patients and the controls. They also found an interesting difference between two groups of frontal release phenomena: the so-called 'prehensile' release signs (i.e. sucking, rooting and grasping) were associated only with advanced dementia, whereas the 'nocioceptive' signs (i.e. snout, glabellar tap and palmomental responses) were common at all stages of dementia and did not increase significantly in prevalence with disease severity. Hyperactive tendon reflexes were also extremely common even in mildly affected patients. Extensor plantar responses and paratonia were found only in more advanced stages of dementia.

In addition to the three controlled studies discussed above, a number of investigators have looked at the frequency of neurological signs in relation to severity of dementia in uncontrolled studies. Huff & Growden (1986) reviewed the records of 165 patients with clinically probable DAT divided into four bands of severity according to the Blessed dementia scale (Blessed et al., 1968). Even when adjusted for age, primitive reflexes (snout, suck and grasp responses), abnormal gait and apraxia correlated with severity of dementia. More recently, Burns and colleagues (1991) reviewed the neurological findings in 175 personally examined DAT patients (135 probable and 40 possible by the NINCDS–ADRDA criteria), all of whom came from the local catchment area of the Section of Old Age Psychiatry at the Institute of Psychiatry in South London. Severity of dementia was assessed according to the clinical dementia rating and also CAMCOG, the cognitive component of the Cambridge dementia examination (CAMDEX) (Roth et al., 1986, 1988). Extrapyramidal features, myoclonus, increased muscle tone and grasping (but not other frontal signs) were all associated with a severity of dementia. Similarly, Chui et al. (1985) reported a greater prevalence of extrapyramidal signs and myoclonus in more severely demented DAT patients. Tweedy et al. (1982) found that only snout and grasp reflexes correlated with severity of dementia in a group of patients with mixed aetiologies.

In summary, recent large, controlled studies have been consistent in showing a positive relationship between DAT and certain neurological signs, particularly frontal release signs, extrapyramidal and parietal sensory signs. There may be an interesting difference between prehensile (sucking, rooting and grasping) and nocioceptive (snout, glabellar tap and palmomental responses) frontal signs, the former appearing in advanced dementia. The association with impaired olfaction, cerebellar ataxia, and pyramidal signs is less certain, probably because the studies have employed different assessment examinations and some of these are found in low frequency even in the patient group. Furthermore, it is also clear that the prevalence of most of these signs is related to the severity of cognitive impairment: very demented patients have a very high rate of neurological abnormalities. From this we can conclude provisionally that DAT affects the central nervous system fairly diffusely and causes not just gross cognitive failure, but also eventually dysfunction of pyramidal, extrapyramidal and sensory systems. This leads us now to consider the second question posed in the introduction.

Is an increased prevalence of abnormal neurological signs useful in diagnosing DAT?

As discussed above, two recent studies (Galasko et al., 1990; Franssen et al., 1991) have documented an increased prevalence of neurological signs in DAT, but have also shown that the difference between mildly impaired patients and controls is slight. In the first study, only a positive glabellar tap and extrapyramidal rigidity were common in the mildly demented patients (i.e. 0–8 errors on the Blessed Information Memory and Concentration Scale). Franssen et al. (1991) found only hyper-reflexia and positive nocioceptive signs in their mildly impaired patient group (levels 3 and 4 on the global deterioration scale; approximately 17–28 out of 30 on the Mini-Mental State Examination). However, it is important to emphasize that these particular signs are probably the most difficult to assess, particularly in the setting of an unstandardized clinical examination. Frontal release signs fatigue rapidly on repeated examination, making it important to make a firm judgement about their presence or absence on first testing. This is a problem for an inexperienced examiner. Moreover, it is exactly these same signs which are found with increasing frequency in the normal aging population. In a truly monumental study of more than 2000 current and former employees of a large American company, Jenkyn et al. (1985) found that 37% of normal 80 year olds had an abnormal glabellar blink response, 26% had a positive snout reflex and 21% had increased limb tone. Thus, in a given elderly patient these soft signs have low specificity, making it impossible to distinguish a normal from a mildly demented subject on the basis of a physical examination. However, the rate of these signs rises very rapidly with age. For instance, it is unusual to find frontal release signs below the age of 65 years. Again, in the study by Jenkyn et al., only 3% of normal 60–64 year olds had a positive snout response, 6% showed abnormal glabellar blinking and 6% had abnormal limb rigidity. In other words, neurological findings should always be interpreted on the basis of age and there is no universal cut-off point. The finding of positive frontal release signs is clearly abnormal in a 50 year old, but can be normal in an 80 year old subject.

In conclusion, neurological signs can be diagnostically helpful in the assessment of individual patients, but the assessment of these soft neurological signs requires clinical experience and knowledge of the spectrum of findings in normal elderly subjects.

Could the increased prevalence of abnormal neurological signs in DAT reflect accelerated or abnormal aging?

Since it is well established that there is a progressive increase in the prevalence of neurological signs with advancing years, perhaps the signs found in DAT reflect merely an exaggeration of an aging process rather than resulting from a distinct disease. This argument is difficult to refute and is addressed more fully elsewhere in this book. On the basis of this review, it could be argued that the evidence favours a dichotomous view: certain signs are found with increasing frequency in a normal aging population (e.g. frontal release phenomena), but others present in DAT are not regarded as acceptable sequelae of aging per se (e.g. myoclonus, epilepsy) (Hauser et al., 1986). However, the latter are seen relatively rarely in DAT, except in the very late stages. Equally, it could be argued, therefore, that if normal subjects lived sufficiently long, a proportion would develop even these more drastic neurological features. In other words, it could all be a question of severity – perhaps DAT reflects merely exaggerated aging. Clinical neurological studies cannot, I think, settle this controversy, but in my opinion the dichotomous position is more convincing.

Another confounding factor to consider is the possibility that many apparently normal elderly people who demonstrate abnormal neurological signs may, in fact, have subclinical DAT. The so-called 'normal' subjects attracted to volunteer as normal controls for DAT studies may be at higher risk of DAT. If this were the case then the prevalence of abnormal signs in normal subjects may be exaggerated. To answer this, it would be of interest to know the long-term outcome of normal elderly subjects with and without neurological signs to see whether the presence of frontal release and other signs is a marker for subsequent DAT.

Can subgroups of DAT patients be identified by abnormal neurological signs?

One of the most exciting clinical developments in the area of DAT has been the recognition that there appear to be at least two clearly identifiable subgroups of patients within the broad clinical rubric of DAT; one called variously: diffuse Lewy body disease (DLBD), the Lewy body variant of Alzheimer's disease (Hansen et al., 1990; Armstrong et al., 1991) and senile dementia of Lewy body type (Perry et al., 1990); the other consisting of the focal lobar atrophies. As implied in the various diagnostic terms, there is considerable doubt whether DLBD constitutes a distinct entity, or a variant of Alzheimer's disease with concurrent Lewy body pathology. A full discussion of this condition is beyond the scope of the present chapter. Briefly, DLBD has been identified in several clinicopathological case series affecting up to 25% of those dying with a clinical diagnosis of DAT, even when strict research criteria, such as the NINCDS–ADRDA have been applied (Byrne et al., 1989; Hansen et al., 1990; Perry et al., 1990). Suggested defining criteria for this condition include the presence of extrapyramidal features, prominent visuoperceptual disorders and visual hallucinations early in the course of the disorder. One small study comparing clinical and neuropsychological features of 26 patients with DAT and 13 patients with DLBD, matched for initial severity of dementia, showed that the DLBD group had a higher prevalence of tremor, bradykinesia, neck rigidity and facial mobility as well as greater deficits on tests of attention and visuospatial processing (Hansen et al., 1990). The prognosis for patients with DLBD may be worse than for DAT, but again this is at present based on limited data (Armstrong et al., 1991). Interestingly, there is an existent literature suggesting that the prognosis for DAT patients with extrapyramidal features may be significantly worse than for those without (see Mayeux et al., 1985). It is tempting, therefore, to speculate that these poor prognosis DAT patients, in fact, have DLBD which causes a combination of cognitive dysfunction and extrapyramidal signs. Obviously, this creates problems interpreting the general literature on neurological signs in DAT which have not included post-mortem verification of the diagnosis. Many patients with apparently uncomplicated DAT accompanied by extrapyramidal and other neurological signs may not have straightforward DAT.

Turning to the lobar atrophies, these are not so much newly discovered disorders as a rediscovery of previously well known but subsequently neglected clinical syndromes. Arnold Pick described, in a series of papers between 1892 and 1906, patients presenting with cognitive failure and symptoms suggesting particular focal involvement of one part of the brain, in whom post-mortem showed marked lobar atrophy. His earlier papers dealt with progressive aphasia and the later with progressive frontal lobe dysfunction (Hodges et al., 1992; Hodges, 1993). The histological changes associated with Pick's disease were, in fact, described some years later by Alzheimer, who recognized changes distinct from those later associated with his name. Alzheimer described both argyrophilic intraneuronal inclusions (Pick bodies) and ballooned neurons (Pick cells) in cases with focal lobar atrophy. However, it was soon recognized that focal degeneration confined to the temporal and/or frontal lobes need not be associated with these specific histological changes. The changes in the nosology of the focal atrophies is described elsewhere (Hodges, 1993). For the current discussion, it is sufficient to say that as many as 10–20% of patients dying with primary cerebral degenerative disease, who would fulfil research criteria for DAT such as the NINCDS–ADRDA, may have focal lobar atrophy (Tissot et al., 1985; Brun, 1987; Neary et al., 1988). But, it is important to note that the limited figures available on the epidemiology of the lobar atrophies (Pick's disease) are based entirely on hospital-based series and there is clearly need for a definitive community-based clinicopathological study.

The clinical syndromes associated with the lobar atrophies have become defined increasingly in recent years. Frontal lobe degeneration presents with marked change in personality and behaviour but, in contrast to DAT, there is relative preservation of memory and visuospatial function in the early stages of the disease. Psychiatric phenomena appear to be much more common than in DAT (Orrell & Sahakian, 1991). Frontal release signs are reported in a very high percentage of cases. Since patients with focal atrophy are usually relatively young, the peak age in many series is 45–65 years, the high proportion of cases with frontal signs would not be expected on the basis of normal aging. Lobe atrophy affecting the temporal lobes is associated with a form of progressive fluent aphasia and features of associative agnosia which are explicable in terms of a progressive impairment in semantic memory (Hodges et al., 1992). As the disease progresses, patients may develop the Klüver–Bucy syndrome which consists of a disturbed pattern of sexual activity, over-eating sometimes including inedible material, hyperorality and placidity. These phenomena are seen rarely in DAT (Cummings & Duchen, 1981; Lilly et al., 1983).

In summary, a sizeable minority of patients presenting with dementia may have a non-Alzheimer form of primary cerebral atrophy either DLBD or focal lobar atrophy (Pick's disease). Individual cases should be identifiable after detailed neurological and neuropsychological assessment, but will be included in the general rubric of DAT in large group studies. Since neurological signs are common in both conditions, this may have inflated the prevalence of these signs in studies of DAT patients.

Conclusions

Abnormal neurological signs, particularly frontal release phenomena, extrapyramidal features and parietal sensory deficits, are found more frequently in patients with a clinical diagnosis of DAT than age-matched controls. The prevalence rises in association with worsening dementia. It could be argued that they represent an acceleration of the normal aging process, since their prevalence also rises steeply with advancing years. However, many of the apparently normal controls used in controlled studies may have subclinical DAT. Also some neurological signs, such as myoclonus, found in advanced dementia, practically never occur even in very old age.

Neurological examination may be helpful in clinical assessment when trying to decide whether complaints of cognitive impairment reflect disease, as long as the age of the subject is taken into consideration. However, neuropsychological assessment remains clearly the definitive investigation in such cases.

It is becoming recognized increasingly that a substantial minority of patients diagnosed as DAT in life, even by stringent research criteria, have different pathological disease such as DLBD or lobar atrophy (Pick's disease) which may be identifiable in individual cases, for instance by the presence of very prominent extrapyramidal features in DLBD. These findings may account for the apparent heterogeneity of DAT with differing prognoses related to the presence, or not, of various neurological signs found by some authors. To establish the prevalence of neurological signs in DAT finally, we need a careful study of a community-based cohort which combines clinical and neuro-psychological assessment in life with post-mortem confirmation of pathology.

Appendix

Frontal release signs

A wide range of physical signs have been described under the heading of development or primitive reflexes. The most commonly described are as follows:

(1) Snout (or pout) reflex: this is usually performed using a spatula rested against the patient's lips which is then tapped firmly by the examiner's finger. There should be no response. A pursing or sucking motion of the lips is an abnormal response

(2) Rooting: this refers to involuntary lip movements towards the examiner's finger, or other stimulus, in response to stroking the corner of the mouth

(3) Sucking: when lightly stroked by the examiner's finger, the lips of a normal adult move little or not at all. An abnormal response is the appearance of a definite mouth movement as if sucking or licking

(4) Glabellar tap: after asking the subject to fix his (or her) gaze across the room, the examiner's finger approaches the patient from above the forehead outside the visual field and then taps the glabellar region lightly about 10 times. The normal reflex eye closure habituates after two or three taps, and the eyelids then remain open. More than five partial or complete blinks constitute a positive response

(5) Palmomental reflex: this reflex is elicited by stroking the patient's thenar eminence with a mildly noxious stimulus such as an orange stick. A positive response consists of reflex twitching of the ipsilateral mentalis (chin) muscle

(6) Grasping: whilst engaging the patient in casual conversation, the examiner gently runs his fingers across the patient's palm towards the thenar eminence. There should be no response. Involuntary flexion of the fingers and abduction of the thumb as if to grasp the examiner's hand constitutes a positive response. A parallel reflex, the tonic foot response, can be elicited by stroking the sole which then induces flexion and abduction movement of the toes

(7) Paratonia (*gagenhalten*): an involuntary muscle hypertonia which appears to increase in response to attempted passive limb movements is termed paratonia

References

Armstrong, T. P., Hansen, L. A., Salmon, D. P., Masliah, E., Pay, M., Kunin, J. M. & Katzman, R. (1991). Rapidly progressive dementia in a patient with the Lewy body variant of Alzheimer's disease. *Neurology*, **41**, 1178–80.

Blessed, G., Tomlinson, B. E. & Roth, M. (1968). The association between quantitative measures of dementia and of senile change in the cerebral grey matter of elderly subjects. *British Journal of Psychiatry*, **114**, 797–811.

Burns, A., Jacoby, R. & Levy, R. (1991). Neurological signs in Alzheimer's disease. *Age and Ageing*, **20**, 45–51.

Brun, A. (1987). Frontal lobe degeneration of non-Alzheimer type. I. Neuropathology. *Archives of Gerontology and Geriatrics*, **6**, 192–208.

Byrne, E. J., Lennox, G., Lowe, J. & Godwin-Austen, R. B. (1989). Diffuse Lewy body disease: clinical features in 15 cases. *Journal of Neurology, Neurosurgery and Psychiatry*, **52**, 709–17.

Chui, H. C., Teng, E. L., Henderson, V. W. & Moy, A. C. (1985). Clinical subtypes of dementia of the Alzheimer type. *Neurology*, **35**, 1544–50.

Critchley, M. (1931). The neurology of old age. *Lancet*, **ccxx**, 1119–336.

Cummings, J. L. & Duchen, L. W. (1981). Klüver-Bucy syndrome in Pick's disease: clinical and pathological correlations. *Neurology*, **31**, 1415–22.

Franssen, E. H., Reisberg, B., Kluger, A., Sinaiko, E. & Boja, C. (1991). Cognition-independent neurologic symptoms in normal aging and probable Alzheimer's disease. *Archives of Neurology*, **48**, 148–54.

Galasko, D., Kwo-on-Yuen, P. F., Klauber, M. R. & Thai, L. J. (1990). Neurological findings in Alzheimer's disease and normal aging. *Archives of Neurology*, **47**, 625–7.

Hansen, L., Salmon, D., Mashliah, E., Katzman, R., DeTeresa, R., Thal, L., Pay, M. M., Hofstetter, R., Klauber, M., Rice, V., Butters, N. & Alford, M. (1990). The Lewy body variant of Alzheimer's disease: a clinical and pathological entity. *Neurology*, **40**, 1–8.

Hauser, W. A., Morris, M. L., Heston, L. L. & Anderson, V. E. (1986). Seizures and myoclonus in patients with Alzheimer's disease. *Neurology*, **36**, 1226–30.

Hodges, J. R. (1993). Pick's disease. In A. Burns & R. Levy (eds.) *Dementia*, pp. 737–50. Chapman and Hall, London.

Hodges, J. R., Patterson, K., Oxbury, S. & Funnell, E. (1992). Semantic dementia: progressive fluent aphasia with temporal lobe atrophy. *Brain*, **15**, 1783–1806.

Huff, E. J. & Growden, J. H. (1986). Neurological abnormalities associated with severity of dementia in Alzheimer's disease. *Canadian Journal of Neurological Science*, **13**, 403–5.

Huff, F. J., Boller, F., Lucchelli, F., Querriera, R., Beyer, J. & Belle, S. (1987). The neurologic examination in patients with probable Alzheimer's disease. *Archives of Neurology*, **44**, 929–32.

Jenkyn, L. R., Walsh, D. B., Culber, C. M. & Reeves, A. G. (1977). Clinical signs in diffuse cerebral dysfunction. *Journal of Neurology, Neurosurgery and Psychiatry*, **40**, 956–66.

Jenkyn L. R., Reeves, A. G., Warren, T., Whiting, R. K., Clayton, R. J., Moore, W. W., Rizzo, A., Tuzun, I. M., Bonnett, J. C. & Culpepper, B. W. (1985). Neurologic signs in senescence. *Archives of Neurology*, **42**, 1154–7.

Jensen, J. P. A., Gron, U. & Pakkenberg, H. (1983). Comparison of three primitive reflexes in neurological patients and in normal individuals. *Journal of Neurology, Neurosurgery and Psychiatry*, **46**, 162–7.

Koller, W. C., Glatt, S., Wilson, R. S. & Fox, J. H. (1982). Primitive reflexes and cognitive function in the elderly. *Annals of Neurology*, **12**, 302–4.

Lilly, R., Cummings, J. L., Benson, D. F. & Frankel, M. (1983). The human Klüver–Bucy syndrome. *Neurology*, **33**, 1141–5.

McKhann, G., Drachman, D., Folstein, M., Katzman, R., Price, D. & Stadlan, E. M. (1984). Clinical diagnosis of Alzheimer's disease; report of the NINCDS –ADRDA work group under the auspices of Department of Health and Human Services Task Force on Alzheimer's disease. *Neurology*, **34**, 939–44.

Mayeux, R., Stern, Y. & Spanton, S. (1985). Heterogeneity in dementia of the Alzheimer type. *Neurology*, **35**, 453–61.

Neary, D., Snowden, J. S., Northen, B. & Goulding, P. (1988). Dementia of frontal lobe type. *Journal of Neurology, Neurosurgery and Psychiatry*, **51**, 353–61.

Orrell, M. W. & Sahakian, B. (1991). Dementia of frontal lobe type. *Psychological Medicine*, **21**, 553–6.

Paulson, G. & Gottlieb, G. (1968). Development reflexes: the reappearance of foetal and neonatal reflexes in aged patients. *Brain*, **91**, 37–52.

Perry, R. H., Irving, D., Blessed, G., Fairbairn, A. & Perry, E. K. (1990). Senile dementia of Lewy body type. *Journal of Neurological Sciences*, **95**, 119–39.

Roth, M., Tym, E., Mountjoy, C. Q., Huppert, F. A., Hendric, H., Verma, S. & Goddard, R. (1986). CAMDEX: a standardised instrument for the diagnosis of mental disorder in the elderly with special reference to the early detection of dementia. *British Journal of Psychiatry*, **149**, 698–709.

Roth, M., Huppert, F. A., Tym, E. & Mountjoy, C. Q. (1988). *CAMDEX: the Cambridge Examination for Mental Disorders of the Elderly*. Cambridge University Press, Cambridge.

Tissot, R., Constantinidis, J. & Richard, J. (1985). Pick's disease. In J. A. M. Fredericks (ed.) *Handbook of Clinical Neurology*, vol. 2(46), pp. 233–46. Elsevier Science Publishers, Amsterdam.

Tweedy, J., Reding, M., Garcia, C., Schulman, P., Deutsch, G. & Antin, S. (1982). Significance of cortical disinhibition signs. *Neurology*, **32**, 169–73.

8

Imaging and dementia

C. E. L. FREER

Imaging the brain has a long history extending back to the first macroscopic observations through the nineteenth and early twentieth century clinico-pathological correlations to the sophisticated technology of today allowing many anatomical and functional observations in vivo.

Initially, observations could be made only indirectly through radiographs of the skull. The introduction of air encephalography was the first opportunity to visualize the ventricles and subarachnoid space. Angiography demonstrates the blood vessels and, indirectly, brain structure. The major impetus came with the introduction of computerized tomography (CT) in 1973, allowing safe examinations of structure, and, within the next decade, the groundwork was laid for the subsequent explosion of techniques using magnetic resonance and radionuclides.

Many studies have been performed in the investigation of dementia and the aging effects upon the brain. The techniques, their problems, especially those associated with the aged, and the results are examined to evaluate whether dementia and aging can be separated in the general population.

Study design

Over the years, studies of imaging methods have been used either to gain insight into the disease process or to test for disease in the general population. The difficulties in study design will be presented first so that the results from the various techniques can be assessed critically.

Ideal requirements are an evenly distributed case mix or spectrum, no interobserver variation, no uninterpretable results and a definitive test without verification bias (Begg, 1987).

Dementia and Normal Aging, eds. F. A. Huppert, C. Brayne & D. W. O'Connor.
© Cambridge University Press 1994.

Case mix/spectrum (Ransohoff & Feinstein, 1978)

Initially, a preliminary examination of a test starts with a selected group of severely affected or index cases compared to normals. Even if all other criteria are fulfilled, this study is flawed and cannot be generalized. Many studies of dementia fall into this category, even Neary et al. (1987) in an otherwise well-designed examination of lobar dementia acknowledge this problem. Large studies are required to ensure a case mix relevant to the population on which the test will be used. Pooling of data from multiple small studies can be unreliable.

Observers involved in the development of a study will have special expertise and interest in the technique. They will probably have pre-conceived notions about the inherent efficacy of the test and case mix. Furthermore, individual observers will vary in their response to the images, as they tend to be subjective observations. Many test interpretation biases can be avoided by 'blinding' which is appropriate in the early stages of test efficacy but is unlikely to be continued in everyday clinical practice.

Uninterpretable results should not be rejected, although they are reported rarely. Movement is the usual cause for suboptimal results in dementia studies, especially where the imaging time is long as in magnetic resonance imaging (MRI). Wippold et al. (1991) in a longitudinal study using CT, albeit an instrument of moderate performance by modern standards, had only five technically satisfactory scans at 51 months from the original 30 at the first follow-up examination. Uninterpretability is important, since it may be associated with the disease under study which is likely with dementia patients (Begg et al., 1986).

Dementia poses a particular problem with the lack of a definitive test at the time of the study, although the brain may become available some time later. It may be considered that the examination of cognitive function is the reference against which the imaging is being tested. Underestimation and overestimation of the study test depends on the correlation with the 'definitive' test regardless of the true clinical state. With perfect correlation the test will appear to be accurate regardless of true disease status and likewise if the two tests are independent the study test accuracy will be underestimated.

In many general radiological studies, verification bias is frequent and occurs when the study is confined to those who have had biopsy, surgery or autopsy – unlikely or impossible in dementia. However, if it is assumed that all subjects with unverified normal tests are free from disease, estimates of the efficacy of the test will be overestimated (Greenes & Begg, 1985).

Methods of data analysis

Most investigations of the various imaging tests for the investigation of dementia and aging have used parametric and non-parametric tests of association and correlation. However, the preferred method is sensitivity and specificity of the test and their extension with receiver operating characteristics (ROCs). Sensitivity is the probability of a positive test in a patient with the disease and specificity is the probability of a negative test in a patient without the disease. Few studies use this method of analysis but Bonte et al. (1986), using radioactive Xenon single photon emission computerized tomography (SPECT) with dementia and controls, found with 119 subjects (90 of whom had final diagnoses of possible or protable dementia) 79 true positives, 7 false positives, 22 true negatives and 11 false negatives giving a sensitivity and specificity of 0.88 and 0.76 respectively. Another series used D,L-hexamethylpropyleneamine oxide to which technetium 99m was attached (99mTc-HMPAO; Bonte et al., 1990). It was found that for 39 subjects, of whom 29 were considered to have possible or probable dementia, there were 24 true positives, 4 false positives, 6 true negatives and 5 false negatives with a sensitivity of 0.83 and specificity of 0.6 (Bonte et al., 1990). These figures, however, give little indication of how the test would work in the field, assuming that the test was interpreted with the same skill. As the authors note, the disease prevalence was high. Furthermore, the positive and negative predictive values (probability of disease given a positive test and probability of no disease given a negative test) should be considered. The effect of a reduced prevalence of the disease under examination can be simulated by maintaining the same number of true positives and false negatives but increasing the true negatives and false positives. Sensitivity and specificity will be unchanged but the positive and negative predictive values will be altered substantially. In Table 8.1 true negatives and false positives have been increased by a factor of ten to reduce the disease prevalence. It is not surprising that many observations in studies with high disease prevalence cannot be replicated in practice and do not perform as a useful test.

In addition to sensitivity and specificity, the false positive and false negative fraction can be calculated and can represent the proportion

Table 8.1. *Sensitivity, specificity, predictive values and disease prevalence*

	Xenon	High prevalence	HMPAO	Low prevalence
Sensitivity	0.88	0.88	0.83	0.83
Specificity	0.76	0.76	0.60	0.60
Positive predictive value	0.91	0.53	0.86	0.38
Negative predictive value	0.67	0.95	0.55	0.92
Accuracy	0.85	0.79	0.72	0.65
Prevalence	0.76	0.24	0.74	0.22

HMPAO, D,L-hexamethylpropyleneamine oxide.
From Bonte et al. (1990).

of true negatives and true positives that are assigned incorrectly. The images of the test subjects can be presented to the observers on separate occasions with differing stringencies for deciding whether the variable is present or absent. Therefore, there will be an increase in the sensitivity and false positive fraction as the threshold decreases, from which ROCs, which are independent of disease prevalence, can be compared for different variables, tests and observers (Metz, 1986). In practice, the observers are required to grade the variables to provide the variation in decision thresholds with subsequent retest to evaluate reliability (Swets & Pickett, 1982). Kido et al. (1989) examined 39 demented patients and 29 controls for temporal lobe atrophy in accordance with the hypothesis of Ball et al. (1985). They used subjective and objective observations and whilst there were many highly statistically significant differences, comparison of the ROCs (Hanley & McNeil, 1982) were not significant, suggesting that the observations would not be helpful in practice.

The normal values for biological data can be difficult to define. A sample of presumably normal individuals are examined from which a mean, standard deviation and other conventional statistical parameters are derived, possibly after outliers are removed. However, many diseases, including the dementias, have a significant lead time and there may be difficulty in defining health and disease. In the aging brain, prior insults such as trauma, systemic cancer, alcohol, drug abuse, steroid use and nutritional status might be having an effect along with the natural involutionary changes.

Merkouriou & Dix (1988) have argued that a purely normal population is impossible to achieve and they have proposed a method of
defining typical and atypical values on statistical criteria with at least
120 individuals in each age-group. An alternative is to express the
theoretically normal population in fractiles or percentiles with a minimum of 100 subjects per age-group. The normal range in aging of the
brain poses special problems which have yet to be answered fully (Dix,
1981).

Computerized tomography

Examination of the brain was indirect and invasive by angiography
and air encephalography until the development of CT by Hounsfield
(1974).

Technical aspects

Data are acquired with a single rotating X-ray radiation source and
detectors of varying design and number. A series of projections, or
views, are made and represent the attenuation of the X-ray beam.
The number of data views depends on instrument design and, to a
degree, is under operator control. Acquisition times vary from 1 to
10 seconds and with section thickness from 1 to 10 mm in modern
instruments.

By computation, the raw data are represented as a matrix of attenuation numbers. The matrix varies between 320 by 320 to 1024 by 1024
with a third component, slice thickness, to represent a volume of tissue
– a voxel representing attenuation value visualized by a continuous
grey scale. The attenuation values are expressed in Hounsfield units
(HU) which is the X-ray linear attenuation coefficient relative to water.

Movement and very high attenuation material, such as surgical clips,
create streak artefacts. The middle cranial fossa is degraded by over-
shoot artefacts obscuring the temporal lobe and the cortex is difficult
to visualize owing to the adjacent high density of the inner table of
the calvarium.

The most important problem, which is common to all sectional digi-
tal imaging devices, is the partial volume effect. On an image, the
border between the ventricles and adjacent brain tissue appears to be
well defined but a density across the image will show a slope due to
the HU of the border of the ventricle, for example, being represented

by a voxel which contains variable amounts of cerebrospinal fluid and brain tissue.

Many measurements have been used in the investigation of dementia and aging, including width of the ventricles and sulci, area of the ventricles and the ratio of the bodies of the lateral ventricles to the calvarium. Careful use of these parameters are reliable measurements, although always limited by partial volume effects. A number of automated measurements have been developed (Jernigan et al., 1979; Baldy et al., 1986). The operator isolates the ventricles and a computer program will count all those voxels within and without the defined area to give the ventricular volume and the cerebrospinal fluid (CSF) overlying the brain. The partial volume effect is reduced and less prone to observer error and fatigue.

Clinical applications

Globally, CT is used extensively in the investigation of dementia primarily to detect diseases other than atrophy or involutionary changes. There have been a variety of findings relating to the detection of these diseases: Evans (1982) found that 83% were equivocal or possible and 57% were definite; however, the corresponding figures reported by Tsai & Tsung (1981) were 28% and 26%, respectively, whereas Lawson (1981) reported 5% for both categories. In a group of patients who were very likely to have an abnormality, Jacoby & Levy (1980) found a glioma and a significant subdural haematoma in 40 patients only. However, these variations represent different perceptions of what is a significant or reportable abnormality with varying degrees of sample bias. At Addenbrooke's Hospital (Cambridge, UK), where there is free access to all specialties, the neuroradiology database for the calendar year May 1991 to 1992 failed to reveal any patient with a tumour, subdural haematoma or other significant pathology which might be considered to be a cause of dementia in either those referred by a psychiatrist or those whose primary clinical diagnosis was dementia, without other more relevant clinical signs.

A feature of the wide access of CT is the change in the age distribution of patients examined. Initially, CT was a scarce resource and only patients who were expected to have a high yield were scanned; often there was an age bar at 65 years unless there were exceptional circumstances. Many of these 'old' patients were labelled as having pathological atrophy, since the wide range was not appreciated.

Effect of aging

CT was the first technique to allow the changes within the brain to be examined in vivo. The progressive increase in the ventricles and sulci which had already been noted at autopsy was confirmed. Jacoby and colleagues demonstrated a progressive increase in size with age (Jacoby & Levy, 1980; Jacoby et al., 1980a,b). Zatz et al. (1982) quantified these findings using a computerized method of assessing ventricular, and sulcal, volumes of CSF corrected for head size. In the normal population, there was considerable variation in the volume of CSF, which increased rapidly after the seventh decade. Although a substantial study, the number of subjects was rather low (n = 123) to draw conclusions about gender differences or about the effect of age, since the age range was wide (20–89 years).

By comparison with current technology, the early CT instruments used a coarse matrix and were limited in spatial and contrast resolution. Valentine et al. (1980) noted that 1.6% of the elderly had

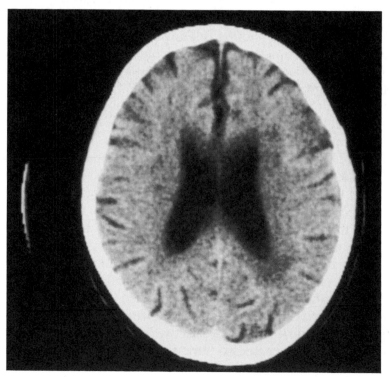

Figure 8.1. Transaxial computerized tomography with posterior paraventricular low attenuation.

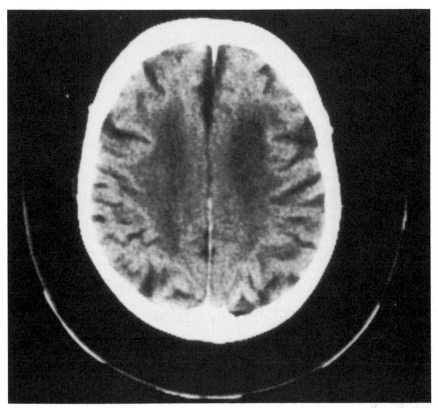

Figure 8.2. Transaxial computerized tomography with low attenuation in the centrum semiovale and atrophy.

low attenuation in the paraventricular regions and centrum semiovale (Figures 8.1 and 8.2). Subsequently, with the technological improvements and increasing number of elderly patients being submitted for examination, this was confirmed to be a frequent finding. George et al. (1986) found normal attenuation in 35 young patients (mean age = 25 years, standard deviation = 2) but low attenuation was present in 14% of the elderly controls (mean age = 69.4 years, standard deviation = 6.5). Lotz et al. (1986) examined at autopsy 82 patients who had a prior CT scan. Demyelination with axonal loss was confirmed in 18 of the 20 positive CT examinations. Seven patients had minor microscopic changes, although the CT was normal. These CT changes were attributed initially to Binswanger's disease (Burger et al., 1976), but, whilst more patients with Alzheimer's disease had low attenuation white matter, there was no clear relationship and cognitive function. 'Leukoariosis' was proposed by Hachinski et al. (1987) as a descriptive term to describe the appearances without any aetiological or pathological connotations. Further studies and the significance of the findings and their relationship to aging and cognition is discussed with magnetic resonance imaging (MRI).

Atrophy and dementia

Many studies have attempted to relate cortical and ventricular changes to dementia. Correlations between cortical atrophy and dementia or cognitive defects have been found in some studies (Earnest et al., 1979; de Leon et al., 1980; Jacoby & Levy, 1980) but were not supported by others (Roberts & Caird, 1976; de Leon et al., 1979; Drayer et al., 1985).

Ventricular size is easier to measure by either planimetry or computerized methods, and some degree of association with dementia has been consistent (Roberts & Caird, 1976; de Leon et al., 1980; Drayer et al., 1985). Jacoby & Levy (1980) and Creasy et al. (1986) found an increase in third ventricular size with dementia. However, in spite of the overall consistency of these findings, there remains the conundrum that a large number of dements have normal cortical and ventricular size and, conversely, many normals have atrophy.

Other psychiatric disorders may be having an effect. Bird et al. (1986) found an increase in lateral ventricle size associated with late-onset depression. Johnstone et al. (1986) showed that 19% of manic depressives had ventricular brain ratios more than two standard deviations greater than patients with neurotic illness and incidentally found a significant association with hypothyroidism. However, these results have not been replicated and their importance is uncertain.

Dementia and Hounsfield units

CT was the first imaging method to provide quantitative data on the structure of tissue. The linear attenuation coefficient is dependent on the physical density, mean atomic number and electron density. It was hoped that this numerical data would provide tissue characterization.

There proved to be many technical, practical and methodological difficulties. The changes between normal and abnormal are small, requiring careful calibration of the system. Any artefacts can cause spurious values. However, the most serious problem is stabilizing the instrument baseline over the study period. Jacobson et al. (1985) showed a considerable drift of up to 17 HU for which correction is difficult and no solution to this problem has been found (Thaler et al., 1979). Owing to beam hardening effects, attenuation values will be distorted when adjacent to bone. Furthermore, this effect is more apparent in the more cranial sections owing to progressive increase in the proportion of the calvarium in the section because of the shape of the skull. In addition, any measurement must be corrected for head and calvarial thickness. The HU may be distorted by the reconstruction algorithm with a 'dishing' and 'doming' effect causing spurious reduction and elevation especially in the centre of the field (Williams & Bydder, 1980). A change of the X-ray tube, inevitable after 20 000 to 60 000 exposures, may alter the values due to the energy dependence of linear attenuation coefficients (Zatz & Alvarez, 1977).

Clinical results

Naeser et al. (1980) found lower HU in the centrum semiovale with presenile and senile dementia patients with an otherwise normal scan appearance. In an examination of 15 separate areas, Bondareff et al. (1981) reported a reduction in the medial temporal lobe, frontal lobe and head of the caudate lobe. Naguib & Levy (1982a, b) suggested that low right parietal HU were associated with an unfavourable prognosis in a longitudinal study, but numbers were too small to be significant. Gado et al. (1983) found some significant changes in the 14 different regions they examined, although the major observation was a loss of grey–white matter discrimination. Albert et al. (1984) suggested that a reduction in the mean density of the whole brain at the level of the body of the lateral ventricles predicted the cognitive status. Colgan (1985) found a significant reduction in HU in the left thalamus, parietal and occipital lobes in those who died in the six-month follow-up period. The relevance of these observations is uncertain considering the technical difficulties. Jacobson (1987), after an extensive examination of alcoholics and normals, concluded that 'great caution should be exercised in the design and interpretation of CT Scan densitometric studies particularly in psychiatric research where the changes are often minor or subtle, if investigations are not to prove worthless'.

Magnetic resonance imaging

Certain nuclei, which, for practical purposes, are protons (1H) for in-vivo imaging, possess a magnetic moment which is arranged randomly in the absence of a magnetic field other than that of the earth. However, when exposed to a magnetic field of 0.02 to 1.5 tesla (1 tesla (T) = 10 000 gauss; earth's magnetic field = 0.05–0.07 gauss), which are used in whole body imaging, they will tend to align along the axis of the external field, although only 15 per million at 1.5 T. When in this state, their magnetic moment can be displaced by radio frequency waves at a given frequency for a nuclear species at a given field strength. When the radio frequency is stopped, the nucleus, or protons, return to their original state and, in so doing, emit radio waves from which signal the image is reconstructed to display tomographic sections in any given plane. Naturally, the image will be dependent on not only the number of protons but also the relaxation parameters (T_1 and T_2). T_1 (longitudinal or spin-lattice relaxation time) describes the time to return to their initial position aligned with the long axis of the applied external field. Displaced protons also have transverse magnetization which will decay gradually as they interact with each other and is described by the T_2 (transverse or spin–spin relaxation time).

In conventional examinations, an image will have varying degrees of these three parameters, spin density, T_1 and T_2 relaxation, which may be varied by alteration in the radio frequency pulse sequences. Images are described as having either T_1 (T_1WI) or T_2 (T_2WI) weighting describing the relative proportions of T_1 or T_2. The images are not simple maps of T_1 or T_2. Furthermore, there is some variation for T_1 and T_2 depending on field strength; white matter increases from about 366 ms at 0.5 T to 687 ms at 1.5 T with T_2 changes being less marked from 72 ms to 82 ms.

MRI is an insensitive technique with an inherently low signal to noise ratio (SNR). Consequently, imaging times are relatively long, 5–8 minutes for T_1WI and as long as 13 minutes for T_2WI, although further technical advances are reducing these times considerably. This poses some difficulty for the elderly and/or demented patient lying in a hostile environment enclosed by the magnet and noise levels reaching 60 dB at 1.5 T. In addition, MRI is sensitive to motion, which is an advantage to detect CSF or blood flow but patient movement will degrade the image quality.

Measurement of T_1 and T_2

Damadian (1971) demonstrated that tumours had different relaxation times compared to normal tissue. These observations were made in vitro with a spectrometer, where there are many technical advantages – a small homogeneous sample, uniform radio frequency and magnetic field, immediate measurements which can be repeated in a short time as SNR is good. T_1 and T_2 have an exponential decay and there should be multiple points to plot the curve. Under these circumstances, measurement of the relaxation parameters are reproducible and accurate. Unfortunately, an imager is far from this ideal. The sample is heterogeneous, i.e. grey/white matter, normal and possibly abnormal. The magnetic field is disturbed by extra gradients to provide tomographic sections, which also delays the measurement of the signal. SNR is poor compared to a spectrometer and more time is required to collect data to provide a good fit for the exponential curve – a 15-point fit with single sections for accurate T_1 can take up to 45 minutes. Clinical imagers can provide a simple two-point fit especially for T_2 as this is the conventional method in acquiring a T_2WI sequence providing also a proton density weighted image. Generally, this is part of a multislice sequence which further impairs radio frequency uniformity and 'cross-talk' between adjacent sections. An examination of 15 different imagers found a 3–50% range of accuracies (Lerski et al. (1988).

Patient movement will also cause variation in T_1 and T_2 although this is difficult to quantify in vivo. Substantial alterations (50–100%) were found when a standardized phantom with different absolute T_2 values in a well-calibrated imager was subjected to regular oscillatory motion to simulate movement from respiration (a frequent artefact in the elderly) and random intermittent movement (C. E. L. Freer & I. Wilkinson, unpublished observations).

There is also variation from the choice of the site of measurement. White matter, such as the centrum semiovale, is larger and easier to identify, but grey matter is more prone to partial volume effects from adjacent CSF. In a random sample of 12 elderly normals and dements (Freer et al. 1990), three experienced observers with prior training measured six different areas (emulating the method of Bondareff et al. (1988) with the same pulse sequences, matrix and manufacturer, although operating at 1.5 T rather than 0.5 T). Using the intraclass correlation coefficient (ICC) with a lower confidence interval (LCL) to test intraobserver effects, the genu of the splenium of the corpus callosum showed least variation (ICC = 0.8; LCL = 0.6) and most in the frontal white matter (ICC = 0.2; LCL = 0.0). Interobserver variation was tested by a fixed effects model ANOVA with an ICC estimate, with which a significant difference was found for the corpus callosum genu, centrum semiovale or frontal white matter but the ICC was only 0.4, 0.2 and 0.4 respectively.

Clinical results

Besson et al. (1986), comparing demented and non-demented patients who had Parkinson's disease with controls, found an overall increase of the white matter T_1 but no difference between the demented and non-demented.

Bondareff et al. (1988) measured T_2 values, with a simple two point fit, in six elderly patients. They chose the genu of the corpus callosum, internal capsule, white and grey matter of the cingulate gyrus and frontal lobe and reported a correlation between T_2 and dementia scores. This was more marked for left hemisphere structures, although there was no significant difference between the two hemispheres.

Clinical imaging

The advent of MRI promised much for the investigation of dementia and the elderly. There is no ionizing radiation, allowing follow-up examinations and volunteer studies, improved contrast resolution compared to CT and multiplanar imaging to examine, for example, the hippocampus in the coronal plane. However, the noise at high field, long examination time and sensitivity to movement pose considerable practical problems.

Linear or area measurements have little to offer beyond that which is known from CT. However, MRI provides data which can separate CSF from brain, facilitating automated computerized methods for volume assessment, which have been shown to be reliable with phantoms and clinical studies (Kohn et al., 1991). However, Wahlund et al. (1990), in demonstrating the increase in CSF volume with age, estimated an inherent measurement error of 12% compared to 3% experimentally. The multiplanar facility allows novel views of the brain to be assessed. Seab et al. (1989) measured the hippocampus in the coronal plane and found a reduction of 40% in their demented patients

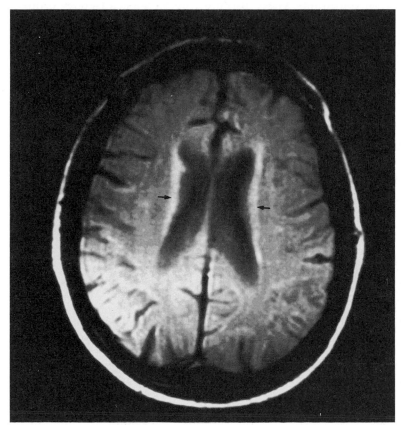

Figure 8.3. Transaxial proton density magnetic resonance imaging with periventricular high signal – a 'rim'.

compared to the controls, with no overlap, although there was no correlation with dementia severity. This appeared to be a local effect, since there was no correlation with overall brain atrophy.

It was soon noted that elderly subjects frequently had focal areas of high signal intensity on T_2WI within the subcortical regions which were thought initially to be areas on infarction. Additionally, it was noted that there were high signal rims to the lateral ventricles and more diffuse high signal areas in the anterior and posterior paraventricular regions, the so-called caps, rims and unidentified bright objects (Keretsz et al., 1988; Figures 8.3 and 8.4).

Awad et al. (1986), in a series of 240 patients, suggested a correlation between cerebrovascular disease, hypertension aging and focal high signal areas. Furthermore, they had the opportunity to examine eight post-mortem brains where the high signal was caused by dilated cerebrospinal CSF spaces which were found around tortuous perforating arteries. Similar appearances were noted by Kirkpatrick & Hayman (1987) with 15 post-mortem 'normal' brains. In these two series there were also five cases of capillary telangectasia, one case of capillary haemangioma and three cases with a diverticulum of the lateral ventricle extending into the adjacent white matter as other causes of focal high signal areas. However, Fazekas et al. (1987) found that the majority of their controls and patients with Alzheimer's disease had focal high signal areas but no association with cardiovascular risk factors such as hypertension. Although a number of studies have described the association of focal high signal areas with hypertension, there are many normotensive subjects with abnormal white matter.

Initially it was suggested that there was a relationship between

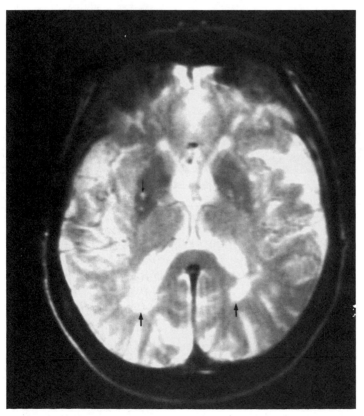

Figure 8.4. Transaxial T$_2$WI (weighted image) magnetic resonance imaging. Posterior paraventricular high signal ('caps' ↑) and focal high signal areas (unidentified bright objects ↓).

dementia and white matter changes. Johnson et al. (1987a) studied 38 patients (28 AD, 8 vascular or mixed and 2 with Parkinson's disease and dementia) and demonstrated a correlation between dementia severity and periventricular white matter changes. Fazekas et al. (1987) found white matter changes with equal frequency in controls and those with AD, although 50% had a prominent high intensity rim around the lateral ventricles. Where there were multiple confluent areas, multi-infarct dementia (MID) and hypertension were also present. Rao et al. (1989) studied 50 middle-aged volunteers with strict exclusions of any cardiac, vascular or brain disease and could not find a relationship between cognitive function and white matter hyperintensities. Hunt et al. (1989), examining 50 patients with a mean age of 78.2 years, found a decline of cognitive function and an increase in white matter hyperintensities with age. However, of the normal patients, 22% had moderate changes and 9% had severe changes. Keretsz et al. (1990) studied 38 dements (27 with AD and 11 vascular) and found periventricular high signal associated with reduced comprehension and attention, but an absence of high signal was associated with impaired memory. These changes can be 'associated with intellectual impairment and somewhat, but not exclusively, with vascular disease' (Hachinski et al., 1987, p. 22).

As with CT, depression may be a confounding factor, since Zubenko et al. (1990) studied 67 depressives, 61 dements and 44 controls and found that leukoariosis could separate depressives from controls. However, leukoariosis was not a distinguishing feature for dementia and controls nor were dementia and depression.

Magnetic resonance spectroscopy

The technology of MRI is now well established, but the problems (physical and practical) associated with spectroscopy remain to be resolved. The goal is to image the relevant area and then to perform in-vivo chemical analysis on a pre-defined volume of tissue.

The fundamental principle of MRI and spectroscopy is the phenomenon of resonance. In descriptions of the physics of conventional imaging the proton (1H) is considered to have a single resonant frequency governed by the external magnetic field. However, the individual protons are affected by adjacent protons or other magnetic dipoles. Spectroscopy enables individual molecules or subcomponents of these molecules to be identified and measured, although the differences (chemical shift) are very small, i.e. 5–30 parts per million. A number of techniques are available to localize volumes: at best they are 1 ml, but are more usually in the 8–27 ml range. Any nucleus to be used by magnetic resonance spectroscopy techniques must be magnetic. The possibilities, inter alia, are P-31, proton, 23-Na and 13-C.

P-31 spectroscopy The P-31 spectra vary from tissue to tissue depending on their energy requirements. Brain has prominent quantities of adenosine triphosphate (ATP) and phosphocreatine (PCr) but only a small quantity of inorganic phosphate (Pi) with phosphomonoesters (PME) and phosphodiesters (PDE). Chemical shift of the various components in the P-31 spectrum can also measure pH with an accuracy of about 0.05 units. The majority of the work has been with tumours where, experimentally, changes in the tumour spectrum are noted with a fall in PCr, ATP and pH: some tumours show Pi peak splitting due to changes in pH reflecting the different chemical environment.

In-vitro analysis of autopsy specimens of brain tissue from those with Alzheimer's disease have been found to contain raised PME in the superior and middle temporal regions and inferior parietal regions compared to controls. Other brain disorders showed an intermediate level. In the demented group, there was an inverse correlation between PME and senile plaques. Brown et al. (1989) examined 17 controls (mean age = 59.5 years; standard deviation (SD) = 12.5), 10 patients with multi-infarct dementia (mean age = 65 years; SD = 10.6) and 17 probable dements (mean age = 67.8 years; SD = 10.6) with P-31 spectroscopy. In the demented patients, there were elevated values of PME and the ratio to PDE in the temporal parietal region; Pi was also elevated in the parietal regions. The ratio of PCr to Pi classified all the multi-infarct dements and 92% of those with Alzheimer's disease.

Proton spectroscopy It would appear, at first sight, that proton spectroscopy would be easier to implement than P-31 or other nuclei. They are present in very high concentration using the same frequency, coils and technology for proton imaging. However, a proton spectrum has a small range of the chemical shift and in biological tissue there are many metabolites which will be dominated by water. In vivo the main component of the spectrum is N-acetyl aspartate, with smaller peaks provided by alanine, creatine and phosphocreatine.

Preliminary results from proton spectroscopy have been unrewarding, but in dementia caused by the acquired immunodeficiency syndrome, complex alterations in the proton spectrum are seen before any changes in images, suggesting that this might be a method of determining axonal loss.

Single photon emission tomography

Extensive investigations have been made with radionuclides to image static and functional aspects of the brain. Extending the initial work of Kety & Schmidt (1948), using nitrous oxide as an agent to measure cerebral blood flow (CBF), radioactive Xenon (113 Xe) with single and multiple probes was developed. Subsequently, dedicated Xenon tomographic scanners have been developed allowing dynamic studies to be performed. However, the majority of the studies on dementia have been with multipurpose instrumentation found in many departments of nuclear medicine. The Gamma camera enabled a large field of view to encompass the whole cranium, although initially as a two-dimensional representation of a complex three-dimensional structure. Subsequently, tomographic sections (single photon emission computed tomography – SPECT) became available using varying ligands.

Technical aspects

To enter freely into the brain across the blood–brain barrier, a radio-labelled compound should have an amine or amine analogue ligand, neutral charge, be lipid soluble with a molecular weight of not more than 500 Daltons. N-isopropyl-p[123]-iodoamphetamine (IMP) and 99 mTc-HMPAO are the main agents. IMP is highly lipophilic, 85% of which is extracted into brain on first pass and fixed by non-specific receptor binding. Peak uptake is seen at 30 minutes with constant grey-to-white matter ratio for two hours. Cortical clearance starts after one hour but is balanced by 'top up' from a pool bound in the lung. Likewise, HMPAO is a highly lipophilic agent with a distribution in the brain according to cerebral blood flow which persists in cerebral tissue, although the mechanism is unclear. Although HMPAO is unstable and should be injected as soon as possible after reconstitution, it is available in kit form with a commonly used radionuclide.

The images from the amine derivatives are qualitative, described as showing alterations in the normal homogeneous distribution, although uptake may be expressed as relative to white matter or the cerebellum

(Figure 8.5). Unfortunately, true quantification is not possible without some absolute reference value (Gemmell, et al., 1990). Xenon studies with the modern dedicated instruments, however, provide a dynamic series with quantification of regional cerebral blood flow in terms of ml per minute per 100 g.

Resolution is dependent on instrument design: 1.0–1.5 cm with conventional Gamma camera systems capable of SPECT, dedicated neuro-SPECT with multiple detectors 5–7 mm and dynamic Xenon 1.5–2.0 cm. Multiple axial, coronal or sagittal sections are available from instruments using the amine derivatives but only three sections with 2 cm intervals are possible with a Xenon system. A typical HMPAO study takes about 45 minutes and may be marred by movement and positioning artefacts.

Xenon CT is a hybrid technique using conventional X-ray CT which detects Xenon due to its high atomic number. Few CT instruments are capable of this technique, but resolution is higher than either radioactive Xenon or amine derivative SPECT, although only semi-quantitative data similar to HMPAO and IMP are acquired. High resol-

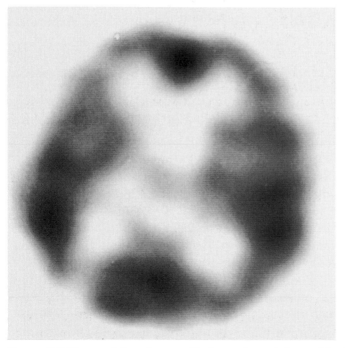

Figure 8.5. Transaxial D,L-hexamethylpropyleneamine oxide single photon emission tomography – normal study (courtesy Dr E. P. Wraight, Addenbrooke's Hospital).

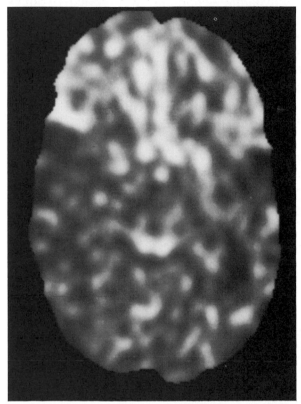

Figure 8.6. Transaxial Xenon computerized tomography. Low perfusion in the posterior temporo-parietal regions bilaterally. Local low perfusion in the (right) anterior Sylvian (courtesy Dr N. M. Antoun, Addenbrooke's Hospital).

ution conventional images can be acquired at the same time to provide an anatomical correlate (Figures 8.6 and 8.7) (D. W. Johnson et al., 1990).

Clinical studies

Many studies have been reported using either dynamic Xenon or static IMP or HMPAO SPECT. The individual studies tend to be with small numbers of well-defined index cases, some without controls and a range of different techniques and methodology of expressing the results. There is, however, a consistent pattern of alterations in the distribution of CBF in the grey matter.

Bonte et al. (1986) used dynamic Xenon and showed that 19 out of 24 patients with probable Alzheimer's disease (AD) had perfusion defects frequently in the temporoparietal region bilaterally (Figure 8.8) and occasionally in the frontal lobes. However, MID patients had patchy bilateral temporoparietal defects. Similarly, other groups of researchers who used IMP also demonstrated bilateral temporoparietal defects with AD patients and a variable pattern with MID patients (Cohen et al., 1986; Sharp et al., 1986; Jagust et al., 1987; Johnson et al., 1987b).

HMPAO studies have shown similar patterns. Neary et al. (1987) examined 21 patients with AD, 9 with dementia of the frontal type

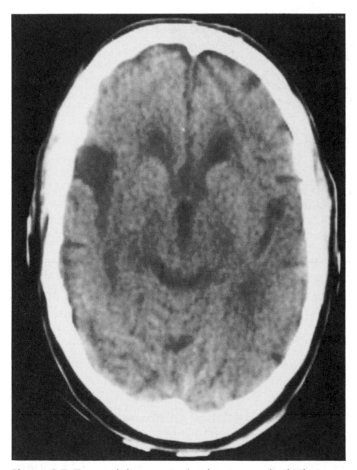

Figure 8.7. Transaxial computerized tomography (CT) corresponding to Xenon CT (Figure 8.6) with local (right) anterior Sylvian atrophy (courtesy Dr N. M. Antoun, Addenbrooke's Hospital).

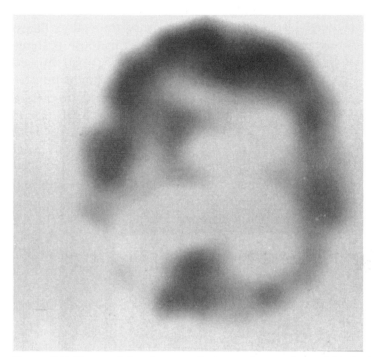

Figure 8.8. Transaxial D,L-hexamethylpropyleneamine oxide single photon emission tomography with bilateral temporoparietal decreased activity more marked on the (right). (See Figure 8.9. Courtesy Dr E. P. Wraight Addenbrooke's Hospital).

and 8 progressive supranuclear palsy patients; there were no controls. They found that 14 with AD had perfusion defects, although these were not necessarily bilateral, and half of these had anterior perfusion defects as well; three had anterior defects only. None of the patients with dementia of the frontal type or progressive supranuclear palsy had bilateral perfusion defects. Gemmell et al. (1987) showed posterior perfusion defects in 13 of their 17 AD patients and only two with MID; there were three controls. Podrecka et al. (1987) (12 AD patients, 11 controls) and Burns et al. (1989a) (20 AD patients, 6 controls) found all their patients with posterior defects. Perani et al. (1988) (16 patients, 16 controls), and Montaldi et al. (1990) (26 patients, 10 controls) found posterior and bilateral frontal defects. The posterior defects may represent the group of dements with late onset, since Jagust et al. (1990) found the usual defects on those 16 AD patients with an onset after 65 years as opposed to a left frontal hypoperfusion in the 10 AD patients younger than 65 years.

SPECT is more sensitive in demonstrating abnormalities in dementia than either CT (Figure 8.9) or MRI, regardless of the cause. Sharp et al. (1986) could not find abnormalities with MRI in those patients who had perfusion defects. The patients of Neary et al. (1987) showed non-diagnostic atrophy without the focal changes that might be predicted by SPECT.

The temporal perfusion defects are not pathognomic of AD. In 18 patients with depression (mean age = 77 years; SD = 7.8) and 14 with AD (mean age = 72.3 years; SD = 8.4), there were almost equal numbers with temporal defects (17 depressed and 16 with AD). The significant differences were an increase in frontal and more than two perfusion defects in AD. Furthermore, five controls had temporal perfusion defects (Upadhyaya et al., 1990).

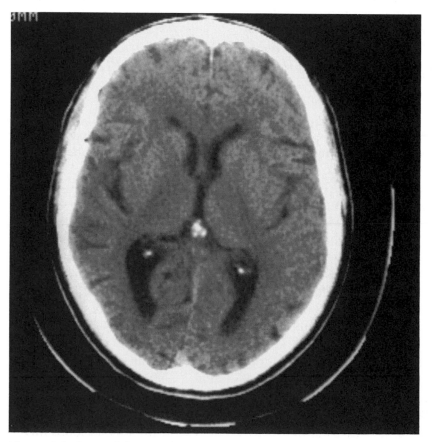

Figure 8.9. Transaxial computerized tomography. Normal study corresponding to Figure 8.8.

Positron emission tomography

A positron emission tomography (PET) scan is a lengthy and arduous examination for patient and physician. Burns et al. (1989b) have outlined the technical difficulties for ^{18}F and ^{15}O. Initially, a plastic mask is constructed for each patient which will provide restraint for the scan. Vascular access is required: intravenous and arterial (or dorsal vein cannulation which, with warming, provides arterialized blood). Before the scan the patient must be deprived of sensory input for at least 45 minutes. The patient is seated with ear plugs and the eyes covered. Neither muscle movement nor sleep should occur; any sensorimotor activity can cause misleading brain activity. When settled, multiple venous and arterial samples are obtained from the lines inserted previously. The radiolabelled agent is injected, or inhaled with ^{15}O, and, after equilibration, scanning is started. The patient lies supine with the restraining face mask for about one hour, or longer for ^{15}O. CT or MRI may be performed at the same time to evaluate any structural change.

The technique has been used to identify and to quantify many brain functions including drug metabolism, receptor analysis, pH, blood volume, cerebral oxygen metabolism ($CMRO_2$) and, most frequently, cerebral glucose metabolism. The method in humans is based on the autoradiographic technique with [^{14}C] deoxyglucose. Glucose and deoxyglucose are transported into the cell with identical kinetics but deoxyglucose does not undergo glycolysis. Using a three-compartment model to describe the uptake and metabolism within the brain, the arterial concentration of glucose and deoxyglucose, rate constants and a correction for a glucose analogue local glucose consumption per unit weight of brain can be derived. Deoxyglucose is labelled with ^{11}C or ^{18}FDG (fluoro-deoxyglucose) produced in a cyclotron with short half-lives, acceptable counting statistics and radiation dose.

Brain metabolism and age

The Kety–Schmidt technique showed a whole brain CBF of 50–60 ml/min/10 g. Subsequent studies before sectional imaging have confirmed these findings, although the relative increase in the frontal lobes have not been confirmed by CT. Kety (1956) suggested a decline of CBF and CMR of oxygen with age, but Dastur (1985) could not confirm these findings in a comparison of young and elderly men, although there was a significant reduction in CBF in a group with atherosclerosis and 'chronic brain syndrome'. However, Shaw et al. (1984) found a reduced CBF with age but this may be related to hypertension rather than aging per se.

PET data is also inconsistent. Kuhl et al. (1982) studied forty volunteers (age range 18–78 years) and found a decline in the cerebral metabolic rate of glucose (CMRgl) most markedly affecting the superior frontal and posterior inferior frontal regions. However, de Leon et al. (1983) and Duara et al. (1984) did not confirm these findings. Subsequently, Chawluk et al. (1987b) showed a reduction in absolute frontal glucose metabolism. Since there is considerable intersubject variation, the values were normalized to the calcarine cortex when further reductions were seen in the inferior parietal, left superior temporal and sensorimotor areas, an effect which was independent of systemic and cardiovascular disease.

Clinical studies

The results follow the same pattern as seen in SPECT with decreased regional glucose metabolism in the temporoparietal regions of patients with AD and further reductions in the frontal lobes with advanced disease (Alavi et al., 1986; Duara et al., 1986). Similarly, global and local reductions in $CMRO_2$ are seen in the same regions with involvement of the frontal lobes with progression of the dementia. (Frackowiak et al., 1981). Reductions in local glucose metabolism are more marked in the left hemisphere (Lowenstein et al., 1989). Multi-infarct dementia shows local defects of glucose metabolism corresponding to areas of infarction (Benson et al., 1983).

The relationship of positron emission tomography to computerized tomography and magnetic resonance imaging

There is no doubt that PET is a very sophisticated method to evaluate brain function in vivo. Haxby et al. (1986) found the usual temporoparietal reductions and left/right asymmetry. However, in five patients with mild dementia cortical reductions, no corresponding neuropsychological defects were found.

The influence of atrophy, as shown by CT or MRI, on the findings with PET (and SPECT) is controversial. Yoshii et al. (1988) found with FDG a reduction in mean CMRgl in the frontal, parietal and temporal regions in older patients, and women had significantly higher values than men. As expected, the degree of brain atrophy was correlated with age. However, after correction of age and sex, there were no longer any significant differences. Covariate analysis showed that atrophy accounted for 21% of the variance. Herscovitch et al. (1986) stressed the need for atrophy correction and Chawluk et al. (1987a) reported a 16.9% and 9% increase in AD patients and controls respectively, using a CT-based technique. Tanna et al. (1991), using an MRI-based whole-brain volumetric method, found that there was an increase of 25% in patients with AD and 15.8% in the controls. These results are, however, for whole-brain metabolic rates and the effect of local atrophy remains to be clarified. Fazekas et al. (1989) examined 30 patients with AD (mean age = 65 years; range = 52–80) and 25 controls by using PET, MRI and CT. They showed a significant difference on CT though with considerable overlap. The dements had more periventricular and white matter high signal on T_2WI but no correlation with PET. Hypometabolic areas were seen with local atrophy, but were also present with normal brain, and cortical high signal areas which might represent the first stages of atrophy. Kobari et al. (1990) examining 14 patients with MID, 19 with AD, 2 with infarcts and 6 controls, found some correlations between CT, MRI and PET. Leukoariosis, as visualized on CT, correlated with atrophy; periventricular high signal areas correlated with MRI; reductions in local CBF and cognitive impairment and those with moderate to severe changes had blood flow reductions in the cortex, basal ganglia and frontal regions. Periventricular high signal correlated only with atrophy and small focal high signal areas were not related to blood flow reductions.

Brain consists of neuronal and non-neuronal tissue and the relative proportions of anatomical loss or reduction in function may give rise to conflicting results. A high neuronal loss could show atrophy, but the local metabolic rate may be preserved by the remaining non-neuronal tissue. Similarly, local metabolism may be lost before any anatomical change which may be a secondary effect. Form and function are not mutually exclusive and have much to learn from each other.

Conclusions

It is clear that, when well-defined index cases are examined by most of the techniques available, some statistically significant differences can be found between patients with AD and controls. Many criticisms could be levelled at these studies with reference to study design, technical or other methodological difficulties. There is no clear evidence that any investigation is sufficiently robust to be a useful test in a population with a case mix found in clinical practice. At worst, the anatomical studies have shown no more than that which is well known from macroscopic autopsy studies and might be considered to be useful only to exclude an underlying organic cause such as a corpus callosum tumour. The functional studies, especially PET, suggest a more promising future to aid our understanding of disease but the total number of examinations is still very small compared to CT and MRI.

Central to imaging the brain in dementia is the separation from the 'noise' of aging. Neither anatomical nor functional studies of presumed normals to date provide sound qualitative or quantitative data. Large longitudinal studies with careful study design are required to provide

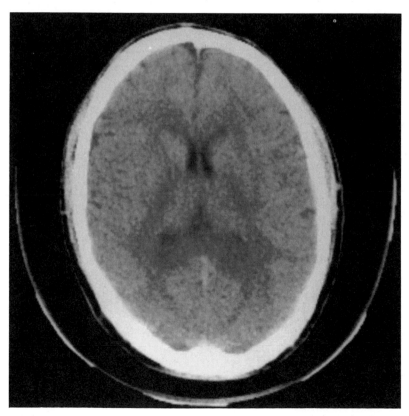

Figure 8.10. Transaxial computerized tomography (male 26 years) with prominence of the anterior interhemispheric fissure and adjacent sulci.

these essential data, although the loss through death, debility, volunteer refusal and suboptimal results make this difficult to achieve (Zimmer et al., 1985; Botwinick et al., 1988; Wippold, et al., 1991). Then it will be possible to generate involution percentile curves similar to growth curves in childhood. A very short or tall child can be identified easily as being abnormal but lesser degrees of abnormality require reference to the mass of sound data that has been acquired. The factors that lead to the varying degrees of aging changes are, by and large, obscure. Consider the young man (Figure 8.10) who had a scan following a minor head injury without any history to account for the relative prominence of the anterior interhemispheric fissure and adjacent sulci: will he preferentially atrophy in the frontal lobes as he ages and confound any imaging method if he develops typical AD?

Unfortunately, imaging the brain is not as easy as measuring height and weight in children. It may transpire that no single imaging examination can separate dementia from aging: the combination of 'noise' from the subject, imaging process, or observer and biological heterogeneity (Friedland et al., 1988) may prove to be insuperable.

References

Alavi, A., Dann, R. & Chawluk, J. et al. (1986). Positron emission tomography imaging of regional cerebral glucose metabolism. *Seminars in Nuclear Medicine*, **16**, 2–34.

Albert, M., Naeser, M. & Levine, H. (1984). CT density numbers in patients with senile dementia of the Alzheimer type. *Archives of Neurology*, **41**, 1264–9.

Awad, I. A., Spetzler, R. F. & Hodak, J. A. et al. (1986). Incidental subcortical lesions identified on magnetic resonance imaging in the elderly. I. Correlation with age and cerebrovascular risk factors. *Stroke*, **17**, 1084–9.

Baldy, R. E., Brindley, G. S. & Ewusi-Mensal, I. et al. (1986). A fully automated computer assisted method of CT brain scan analysis for the measurement of cerebrospinal spaces and brain absorption density. *Neuroradiology*, **28**, 109–17.

Ball, M. J., Fishman, M. & Hachinski, V. et al. (1985). A new definition of Alzheimer's disease: a hippocampal dementia. *Lancet*, **1**, 14–16.

Begg, C. B. (1987). Biases in the assessment of diagnostic tests. *Statistics in Medicine*, **6**, 411–24.

Begg, C. B., Greenes, R. A. & Iglewicz, B. (1986). The influence of uninterpretability on the assessment of diagnostic tests. *Journal of Chronic Diseases*, **39**, 575–84.

Benson, F., Kuhl, D. E. & Hawkins, M. E. et al. (1983). The fluorodexyglucose [23]F scan in Alzheimer's disease and multi-infarct dementia. *Archives of Neurology*, **40**, 711–14.

Besson, J. A. O., Mutch, W. J. & Smith, F. W. et al. (1986). The relationship between Parkinson's disease and dementia. A study using NMR imaging parameters. *British Journal of Psychiatry*, **147**, 380–2.

Bird, J. M., Levy, R. & Jacoby, R. J. (1986). Computed tomography in the elderly: changes over time in a normal population. *British Journal of Psychiatry*, **148**, 80–5.

Bondareff, W., Baldy, R. E. & Levy, R. (1981). Quantitative CT in senile dementia. *Archives of General Psychiatry*, **38**, 1365–8.

Bondareff, W., Raval, J. & Colletti, P. M. et al. (1988). Quantitative magnetic resonance imaging and the severity of dementia in Alzheimer's disease. *American Journal of Psychiatry*, **145**, 853–6.

Bonte, F. J., Ross, E. D. & Chehabi, H. H. et al. (1986). SPECT study of regional cerebral blood flow in Alzheimer disease. *Journal of Computerised Axial Tomography*, **10**, 579–83.

Bonte, F. J., Hom, J. & Weiner, M. F. (1990). Single photon tomography in Alzheimer's disease and the dementias. *Seminars in Nuclear Medicine*, **20**, 342–52.

Botwinick, J., Storandt, M. & Berg, L. et al. (1988). Senile dementia of the Alzheimer type: subject attrition and testability in research. *Archives of Neurology*, **45**, 493–6.

Brown, G. G., Levine, S. R. & Gorell, J. M. et al. (1989). In vivo 32P NMR profiles of Alzheimer's disease and multiple subcortical infarct dementia. *Neurology*, **39**, 1423–7.

Burger, P. C., Burch, J. C. & Kuntze, U. (1976). Subcortical arteriosclerotic encephalopathy (Binswanger's disease): a vascular aetiology of dementia. *Stroke*, **7**, 626–31.

Burns, A., Philpot, M. & Costa, D. et al. (1989a). The investigation of Alzheimer's disease with single photon emission tomography. *Journal of Neurology, Neurosurgery & Psychiatry*, **52**, 248–53.

Burns, A., Tune, L. & Steele, C. et al. (1989b). Positron emission tomography in dementia: a clinical review. *International Journal of Geriatric Psychiatry*, **4**, 67–72.

Chawluk, J. B., Alavi, A. & Dann, R. et al. (1987a). Positron emission tomography in ageing and dementia: effect of cerebral atrophy. *Journal of Nuclear Medicine*, **28**, 431–7.

Chawluk, J. B., Alavi, A. & Jamieson, D. G. et al. (1987b). Changes in local cerebral glucose metabolism with normal ageing, the effects of cardiovascular and systemic health factors. *Journal of Cerebral Blood Flow and Metabolism*, **7**, 411–17.

Cohen, M. B., Grahan, L. S. & Lake, R. et al. (1986). Diagnosis of Alzheimer's disease and multiple infarct dementia by tomographic imaging of iodine-123 IMP. *Journal of Nuclear Medicine*, **27**, 769–74.

Colgan, J. (1985). Regional density and survival in senile dementia. *British Journal of Psychiatry*, **147**, 63–6.

Creasey, H., Schwarz, M. & Frederickson, H. et al. (1986). Quantitative computed tomography in dementia of the Alzheimer type. *Neurology*, **36**, 1563–8.

Damadian, R. (1971). Tumour detection by nuclear magnetic resonance. *Science*, **171**, 1151–3.

Dastur, D. K. (1985). Cerebral blood flow and metabolism in normal human ageing and senile dementia. *Journal of Cerebral Blood Flow and Metabolism*, **5**, 1–10.

de Leon, M. J., Ferris, S. H. & Blau, I. et al. (1979). Correlations between computerised tomographic changes and behavioural deficits in senile dementia. *Lancet*, **ii**, 859–60.

de Leon, M., Ferris, S. & George, A. et al. (1980). Computed tomography evaluation of brain behaviour relationships in senile dementia of the Alzheimer type. *Neurobiology and Ageing*, **1**, 68–79.

de Leon, M., Ferris, S. & George, A. et al. (1983). Computed tomography and positron emission transaxial emission tomography evaluations of normal ageing and Alzheimer's disease. *Journal of Cerebral Blood Flow and Metabolism*, **3**, 391–4.

Dix, D. (1981). On the interpretation of diagnostic test: a common logical fallacy. *Clinical Chemistry*, **21**, 1873–6.

Drayer, B., Heyman, A. & Wilkinson, W. (1985). Early onset Alzheimer's disease: an analysis of CT findings. *Annals of Neurology*, **17**, 407–10.

Duara, R., Grady, C. & Haxby, J. et al. (1984). Human brain glucose utilisation and cognitive function in relation to age. *Annals of Neurology*, **16**, 702–13.

Duara, R., Grady, C. & Haxby, J. et al. (1986). Positron emission tomography in Alzheimer's disease. *Neurology*, **36**, 879–87.

Earnest, M., Heyman, A., Wilkinson, W. et al. (1979). Cortical atrophy, ventricular enlargement and intellectual impairment in the aged. *Neurology*, **29**, 632–7.

Evans, N. J. R. (1982). Cranial computed tomography in clinical psychiatry: 100 consecutive cases. *Comprehensive Psychiatry*, **23**, 445–50.

Fazekas, F., Chawluk, J. B. & Alavi, A. et al. (1987). MR signal abnormalities at 1.5T in Alzheimer's dementia and normal aging. *American Journal of Neuroradiology*, **8**, 421–6.

Fazekas, F., Alavi, A. & Chawluk, J. B. et al. (1989). Comparison of CT, MR and PET in Alzheimer's disease. *Journal of Nuclear Medicine*, **30**, 1607–15.

Frackowiak, R. S. J., Pozzilli, C., Legg, N. J. et al. (1981). A prospective study of regional cerebral blood flow and oxygen utilisation in dementia using positron emission tomography and oxygen 15. *Journal of Cerebral Blood Flow and Metabolism*, **1**, (supplement), S453 4.

Freer, C. E. L., Antoun, N. M. & Baldwin, J. et al. (1990). 'Observer unreliability of T2 measurements in the brain'. XIV Symposium Neuroradiologicum, 17–23 June 1990.

Friedland, R. P., Koss, E. & Haxby, J. V. et al. (1988). NIH conference. Alzheimer disease: clinical and biological heterogeneity. *Annals of Internal Medicine*, **109**, 298–311.

Gado, M., Danziger, W. L. & Chi, D. et al. (1983). Brain parenchymal density measurements in demented subjects and controls. *Radiology*, **147**, 703–10.

Gemmell, H. G., Sharp, P. F. & Besson, J. A. et al. (1987). Differential diagnosis in dementia using the cerebral blood flow agent 99Tc HMPAO: a SPECT study. *Journal of Computerised Axial Tomography*, **11**, 398–402.

Gemmell, H. G., Evans, N. T. & Besson, J. A. et al. (1990). Regional cerebral

blood flow imaging: a quantitative comparison of technetium-99mHMPAO
SPECT with C1502 PET. *Journal of Nuclear Medicine*, **31**, 1595–600.

George, A. E., de Leon, M. J. & Gentes, C. I. et al. (1986).
Leukoencephalopathy in normal and pathological aging: 1. CT of brain
lucencies. *American Journal of Neuroradiology*, **7**, 561–6.

Greenes, R. A. & Begg, C. B. (1985). Assessment of diagnostic technologies:
methodology for unbiased estimation from samples of selectively verified
patients. *Investigative Radiology*, **20**, 751–6.

Hachinski, V. C., Potter, P. & Merskey, H. (1987). Leuko-ariosis. *Archives of
Neurology*, **44**, 21–23.

Hanley, J. A. & McNeil, B. J. (1982). The meaning of the area under a receiver
operating characteristic curve. *Radiology*, **143**, 29–36.

Haxby, J. V., Grady, C. L. & Duara, R. et al. (1986). Neocortical metabolic
abnormalities precede nonmemory cognitive defects in early Alzheimer's
disease. *Archives of Neurology*, **43**, 882–5.

Herscovitch, P., Auchus, A. P. & Gado, M. et al. (1986). Correction of positron
emission tomography data for cerebral atrophy. *Journal of Cerebral Blood
Flow and Metabolism*, **6**, 120–4.

Hounsfield, G. N. (1974). Computerized transverse axial scanning
(tomography). I Description of system. *British Journal of Radiology*, **46**,
1023–47.

Hunt, A. L., Orrison, W. W. & Yeo, R. A. et al. (1989). Clinical significance
of MRI white matter lesions in the elderly. *Neurology*, **39**, 1470–4.

Jacobson, R, R. (1987). 'CT Scan, Psychometric and Clinical studies of the
Wernicke–Korsakoff syndrome'. MD Thesis, Cambridge University,
Cambridge.

Jacobson, R. R., Turner, S. W. & Baldry, R. E. et al. (1985). Densitometric
analysis of scans: important sources of artefact. *Psychological Medicine*, **15**,
879–99.

Jacoby, R. J. & Levy, R. (1980). Computed tomography in the elderly.
3. Affective disorders. *British Journal of Psychiatry*, **136**, 270–5.

Jacoby, R., Levy, R. & Dawson, J. (1980a). Computed tomography in the
elderly: 1. the normal population. *British Journal of Psychiatry*, **136**, 249–55.

Jacoby, R., Levy, R. & Dawson, J. (1980b). Computed tomography in the
elderly: 2. diagnosis and functional impairment. *British Journal of Psychiatry*,
136, 256–9.

Jagust, W. J., Budinger, T. F. & Reed, B. R. (1987). The diagnosis of dementia
with single photon emission computed tomography. *Archives of Neurology*,
44, 258–62.

Jagust, W. J., Reed, B. R. & Seab, J. P. et al. (1990). Alzheimer's disease.
Age at onset and single photon emission computed tomographic patterns of
regional cerebral blood flow. *Archives of Neurology*, **47**, 628–33.

Jernigan, T. L., Zatz, L. M. & Naeser, M. A. (1979). Semiautomated methods
for quantitating CSF volume on cranial computed tomography. *Radiology*, **132**,
463–6.

Johnson, D. W., Stringer, W. A. & Marks, M. P. et al. (1990). Stable Xenon
CT cerebral blood flow imaging: rationale for and role in clinical decision
making. *American Journal of Neuroradiology*, **12**, 201–13.

Johnson, K. A., Davis, K. R. & Buonanno, F. S. et al. (1987a). Comparison of magnetic resonance and roentgen ray computed tomography in dementia. *Archives of Neurology*, **44**, 1127–33.

Johnson, K. A., Mueller, S. T. & Walshe, M. et al. (1987b). Cerebral perfusion imaging in Alzheimer's disease: use of single photon emission computed tomography and iofetamine hydrochloride. *Archives of Neurology*, **44**, 165–8.

Johnson, K. A., Holman, B. L. & Rosen, T. J. et al. (1990). Iofetamine I 123 single photon emission computed tomography is accurate in the diagnosis of Alzheimer's disease. *Archives of Internal Medicine*, **150**, 752–6.

Johnstone, E. C., Owens, D. G. C., Crow, J. J. et al. (1986). Hypothyroidism as a correlate of lateral ventricle enlargement in manic depressive and neurotic illness. *British Journal of Psychiatry*, **148**, 314–17.

Keretsz, A., Black, S. E. & Tokar, G. et al. (1988). Periventricular and subcortical hyperintensities on magnetic resonance imaging. Rims, caps, and unidentified bright objects. *Archives of Neurology*, **45**, 404–8.

Keretsz, A., Polk, M. & Carr, T. (1990). Cognition and white matter changes on magnetic resonance imaging and dementia. *Archives of Neurology*, **47**, 387–91.

Kety, S. S. (1956). Human cerebral blood flow and oxygen consumption as related to ageing. *Journal of Chronic Diseases*, **3**, 426–32.

Kety, S. S. & Schmidt, C. F. (1948). The nitrous oxide method for quantitative determination of cerebral blood flow in man. Theory, procedure and normal values. *Journal of Clinical Investigation*, **27**, 476–83.

Kido, D., Caine, E., Leymay, M. et al. (1989). Temporal atrophy in patients with Alzheimer's disease. *American Journal of Neuroradiology*, **10**, 551–5.

Kirkpatrick, J. B. & Hayman, L. A. (1987). White-matter lesions in MR imaging of clinically healthy brains of elderly subjects: possible pathological basis. *Radiology*, **162**, 509–11.

Kobari, M., Meyer, J. S. & Ichijo, M. et al. (1990). Leukoariosis: correlation of MR and CT findings with blood flow, atrophy and cognition. *American Journal of Neuroradiology*, **11**, 273–81.

Kohn, M. I., Tanna, N. K. & Herman, G. T. et al. (1991). Analysis of brain cerebrospinal fluid volumes with MR imaging: Part I. Methods, reliability and validation. *Radiology*, **178**, 115–22.

Kuhl, D. E., Metter, E. J. & Riege, W. H. et al. (1982). Effect of human aging on patterns of local cerebral glucose utilisation determined by the [^{18}F]fluorodeoxyglucose method. *Journal of Cerebral Blood Flow and Metabolism*, **2**, 163–71.

Lawson, E. B. (1981). Computed tomography in patients with psychiatric illness: Advantages of a 'rule in' approach. *Annals of Internal Medicine*, **95**, 360–4.

Lerski, R. A., McRobbie, D. W. & Straughan, K. et al. (1988). Multi-centre trial with protocols and prototype test objects for the assessment of MRI equipment. *Magnetic Resonance in Medicine*, **6**, 201–4.

Lotz, P. R., Ballinger, W. E. & Quisling, R. G. (1986). Subcortical arteriosclerotic encephalopathy: CT spectrum and pathologic correlation. *American Journal of Neuroradiology*, **7**, 817–22.

Lowenstein, D. A., Barker, W. W. & Chang, J. Y. et al. (1989). Predominant left hemisphere metabolic dysfunction in dementia. *Archives of Neurology*, **46**, 146–52.

Merkouriou, S. & Dix, D. (1988). Estimating reference ranges in clinical pathology: an objective approach. *Statistics in Medicine*, **7**, 377–85.

Metz, C. E. (1986). ROC methodology in radiologic imaging. *Investigative Radiology*, **21**, 720–33.

Montaldi, D., Brooks, D. N. & McColl, J. H. et al. (1990). Measurements of regional cerebral blood flow and cognitive performance in Alzheimer's disease. *Journal of Neurology, Neurosurgery & Psychiatry*, **53**, 33–8.

Naeser, M., Gebhardt, C. & Levine, H. (1980). Decreased computed tomography numbers in patients with presenile dementia. *Archives of Neurology*, **37**, 401–9.

Naguib, M. & Levy, R. (1982a). Prediction of outcome in senile dementia. *British Journal of Psychiatry*, **140**, 263–7.

Naguib, M. & Levy, R. (1982b). CT scanning in senile dementia: a follow up of survivors. *British Journal of Psychiatry*, **141**, 618–19.

Neary, D., Snowden, J. S. & Shields, R. A. et al. (1987). Single photon emission tomography using 99mTc-HMPAO in the investigation of dementia. *Journal of Neurology, Neurosurgery & Psychiatry*, **50**, 1101–9.

Perani, D., Di Piero, V. & Vallar, G. et al. (1988). Technetium-99m HMPAO SPECT study of regional cerebral perfusion in early Alzheimer's disease. *Journal of Nuclear Medicine*, **29**, 1507–14.

Podrecka, I., Suess, E. & Goldenberg, G. et al. (1987). Initial experience with technetium-99m HMPAO brain SPECT. *Journal of Nuclear Medicine*, **28**, 1657–66.

Ransohoff, D. F. & Feinstein, A. R. (1978). Problems of spectrum and bias in evaluating the efficacy of diagnostic tests. *New England Journal of Medicine*, **299**, 926–30.

Rao, S. M., Mittenberg, W. & Bernardin, L. et al. (1989). Neuropsychological test findings in subjects with leukoariosis. *Archives of Neurology*, **46**, 40–4.

Roberts, M. & Caird, F. (1976). Computerised tomography and intellectual impairment in the elderly. *Journal of Neurology, Neurosurgery & Psychiatry*, **39**, 986–9.

Seab, J. P., Jagust, W. J. & Wong, S. T. et al. (1989). Quantitative NMR measurements of hippocampal atrophy in Alzheimer's disease. *Magnetic Resonance in Medicine*, **8**, 200–8.

Sharp, P., Gemmell, H. & Cherryman, G. et al. (1986). Application of iodine-123-labelled isopropylamphetamine imaging in the study of dementia. *Journal of Nuclear Medicine*, **27**, 761–8.

Shaw, T., Mortel, K. & Meyer, J. (1984). Cerebral blood flow changes in benign ageing and cerebrovascular disease. *Neurology*, **34**, 855–62.

Swets, J. A. & Pickett, R. M. (1982). *Evaluation of Diagnostic Systems: Methods from Signal Detection Theory*. Academic Press, New York.

Tanna, N. K., Kohn, M. L. & Horwich, D. N. et al. (1991). Analysis of brain and cerebrospinal fluid volumes with MR imaging: impact on PET data correction for atrophy. *Radiology*, **178**, 123–30.

Thaler, H. T., Rottenburg, D. A. & Pentlow, K. S. et al. (1979). A method of correction for linear drift in computerised brain scans. *Journal of Computerised Axial Tomography*, **3**, 251–5.

Tsai, L. & Tsung, M. T. (1981). How can we avoid unnecessary C.T. scanning in psychiatric patients? *Journal of Clinical Psychiatry*, **43**, 452–4.

Upadhyaya, A. K., Abou-Saleh, M. T. & Wilson, K. et al. (1990). A study of depression in old age using single-photon emission tomography. *British Journal of Psychiatry*, **157**, 76–81.

Valentine, A. R., Moseley, I. F. & Kendall, B. E. (1980). White matter abnormality in cerebral atrophy: clinicoradiological correlation. *Journal of Neurology, Neurosurgery and Psychiatry*, **4**, 788–90.

Wahlund, L. D., Agartz, I. & Almqvist, O. et al. (1990). The brain in healthy aged individuals: MR imaging. *Radiology*, **174**, 675–9.

Williams, G. & Bydder, G. M. (1980). Validity and use of computed tomography attenuation values. *British Medical Bulletin*, **36**, 279–87.

Wippold, F. J., Gado, M. H. & Morris, J. C. et al. (1991). Senile dementia and healthy aging: a longitudinal study. *Radiology*, **179**, 215–19.

Yoshii, F., Barker, W. W. & Chang, J. Y. et al. (1988). Sensitivity of cerebral glucose metabolism to age, gender, brain volume, brain atrophy, cerebrovascular risk factors. *Journal of Cerebral Blood Flow and Metabolism*, **8**, 654–61.

Zatz, L. M. & Alvarez, M. E. (1977). An inaccuracy in computerised tomography: the energy dependence of CT values. *Radiology*, **124**, 91–4.

Zatz, L. M., Jernigan, T. L. & Ahumada, A. J. (1982). Changes on computed tomography with aging: intracranial fluid volume. *American Journal of Neuroradiology*, **3**, 1–11.

Zimmer, A. W., Calkins, E. & Hadley, E. et al. (1985). Conduction of research in geriatric populations. *Annals of Internal Medicine*, **103**, 276–83.

Zubenko, G. S., Sullivan, P. & Nelson, J. P. et al. (1990). Brain imaging abnormalities in mental disorders of late life. *Archives of Neurology*, **47**, 1107–11.

PART IV

Research methodology and population studies

How common are cognitive impairment and dementia? An epidemiological viewpoint

CAROL BRAYNE

This chapter provides a brief overview of population studies of dementia and cognitive impairment and, through these, addresses whether there is any evidence to refute the hypothesis that dementia and its subtypes lie on a continuum with 'normal' aging, such that there is no clear separation of the majority of the population aging without dementia from those with dementia, both cross sectionally and longitudinally. For more detailed reviews of epidemiological surveys the reader is referred elsewhere (Jorm, 1990; Cooper, 1991; Kay, 1991; Jagger 1993). The study of disorders in populations depends crucially on case definition and sample definition and the chapter begins with a brief overview of these. Information available from populations is then presented, starting with mortality and service data, through to prevalence and incidence studies, and finally studies of brain tissue post-mortem.

The components of case definition

Any population study of dementia or cognitive impairment depends on its case definition. For dementia and its subtypes, different sets of diagnostic criteria include different details, although they may appear to be broadly similar. Table 9.1 illustrates this by comparing three sets of diagnostic criteria. The actual criteria vary (see Chapter 5). Deterioration of intellectual, emotional and motivational behaviour is essential to fulfill the criteria of the Cambridge Examination for Mental Disorder in the Elderly (CAMDEX: Roth et al., 1986, 1988); loss of intellectual abilities sufficient to interfere with social functions is essen-

Dementia and Normal Aging, eds. F. A. Huppert, C. Brayne & D. W. O'Connor. © Cambridge University Press 1994.

Table 9.1. *Criteria for dementia, Alzheimer's disease and multi-infarct dementia*

	CAMDEX (Roth et al., 1988)	DSM-III-R (American Psychiatric Association, 1987)	NINCDS–ADRDA (McKhann et al., 1984)
Dementia	Global deterioration of intellectual, emotional, motivational behaviour in clear consciousness for six months. A. Progressive failure in everyday life B. Memory impairment C. Deterioration in one of following: intellectual ability; judgement; higher cortical function; deterioration of personality/general behaviour	A. Loss of intellectual abilities sufficient to interfere with social functions B. Memory impairment C. One of following: impairment of abstract thinking; deterioration in judgement; aphasia/apraxia/agnosia/constructional difficulty; personality change D. Consciousness not clouded E. Other disorders excluded	Decline in memory and other cognitive functions determined by history of decline and abnormalities on examination and tests. Delirium excluded
Alzheimer's disease	Dementia A. Gradual onset B. Absence other aetiological factor C. Early dysphasia, agnosia,	A. Dementia B. Insidious onset with uniformly progressive deteriorating course C. Exclusion of all other	A. Probable Dementia (MMSE, Blessed dementia scale, neuropsych. tests) Deficits 2+ areas cognition

	apraxia; cerebral atrophy; histopathological abnormality Not associated with signs of cerebrovascular disease	specific causes	Progressive decline. Onset 40–90 years. Absence of other disorders which cause decline B. Possible Dementia with other disorder C. Definite Clinical criteria satisfied and histopathological evidence
Multi-infarct dementia	Dementia A. Sudden onset B. Stepwise deterioration C. One or more strokes or transient ischaemic attacks D. Focal signs E. Two of following: patchy psychological deficits; emotional liability; insight loss; depression/anxiety; fits; hypertension; headache/dizziness; gait abnormality	A. Dementia B. Stepwise deteriorating course C. Focal neurological signs D. Evidence of significant cerebrovascular disease related aetiologically	Only as exclusion criterion AD unlikely if: sudden onset; focal signs; gait disturbance

tial for the revised version of the third Diagnostic and Statistical Manual (DSM-III-R) of the American Psychiatric Association (1987). For all sets, and for the tenth revision of the International Classication of Diseases (ICD-10: World Health Organization, 1992), the underlying deterioration is that of intellectual abilities. The operationalization of them will also vary from study to study.

Some population studies have not used diagnostic criteria, but have depended on performance on scales. The proportion of the population identified as abnormal according to a cutpoint is then reported, rather than a proportion actually diagnosed.

Types of diagnosis in populations

The first step in understanding the epidemiology of a disorder is to look at mortality statistics. In this kind of statistic, the cause of death is recorded by the last attending physician. Dementia is seen rarely as a cause of death, although it may be recorded as an underlying disorder. The diagnosis is not made on the basis of internationally agreed criteria, but on the clinician's working knowledge of the patient and internal concept of dementia. It is likely that mild dementia is recorded seldom, and that only the most severe dementia is recorded on a reliable basis. The different codes in the Ninth Edition of the International Classification of Diseases (ICD-9: World Health Organization, 1978) which can be used for dementia are numerous, including many under cerebrovascular disorders as well as vague descriptions such as senility. The validity of the diagnosis of subtypes of dementia in the general setting is unknown. Whilst mortality data is usually considered to be suspect, some have suggested that it can yield useful information (Frecker, 1992).

The next step is to look at other routinely collected records. Contact with health services or social services is recorded in some countries. Health service related records in the United Kingdom depend on the interpretation of a junior doctor's discharge summary by an administrative clerk. Social service records depend on the impression of medically untrained personnel.

Beyond this, there are several options. One is to collect all those individuals who have been identified as demented by whatever system, and then to re-examine their notes or the actual patient and re-assess whether the diagnosis fits the chosen study criteria. Another is to go to the community and identify cases, independently of any contact with services. The final possibility is not to see patients during life at all, but to carry out a post-mortem series, where the amount of pathology held to be consistent with a particular diagnosis is counted, and estimates are derived.

All the approaches above have been used in the attempt to quantify the amount of dementia in the community. All are likely to produce different estimates for the prevalence of dementia.

Validity

The validity of any method is important, and is the ability of the method or measurement to identify the disorder of interest correctly. Dementia is no exception to the difficulties of validation faced in other areas of medicine. There are several types of validity for the diagnosis. These include performance against an agreed concurrent standard, which for a computerized diagnostic algorithm might be comparison with clinical diagnosis, or for a single clinician's diagnosis might be comparison with an independent consensus diagnosis. A further possibility is performance against longitudinal study of either maintained impairment or decline measured in the same way. Finally there is the validity of in-vivo diagnosis against post-mortem findings. There is no single gold standard, since all these methods present some difficulties. It is likely for the time being that we need to use several methods until the search for more accurate diagnostic methods has been successful. Now the most useful are longitudinal study and post-mortem follow-up (as carried out by the Consortium to Establish a Registry for Alzheimer's Disease: Morris et al., 1988; Mirra et al., 1991).

Issues in sample definition

The proportion of people found to be demented, once case definition is agreed, will depend on the type of sample examined. If an institution is sampled, it is likely that a higher proportion of individuals will be demented than if the general population were sampled. If the sample is weighted towards the oldest old, the proportion of people affected will also be higher than in a sample with relatively more younger individuals.

The proportion affected by a disorder depends not only on the number of cases counted, but also on the total population. The mortality rate for any particular same-sex group within a specific age band is defined as the number of people dying (with a given diagnosis) expressed as a proportion of those alive in that group that year. The deaths are based on death certificate returns, and the live population is based on census data projected for the appropriate year. If there are major inaccuracies in the census data this could cause distortion of the rates. A similar situation arises in record-based studies where the denominator population is not examined. If this is smaller than the national level, problems could be caused by migration out of different groups between censuses. Other approaches have involved enumerating the exact numbers in the whole population before sampling – this is particularly useful where it is thought that existing registers are unreliable, such as urban settings. Electoral rolls (e.g. Kay et al., 1964), door to door calling (e.g. Livingston et al., 1990) and Family Health Service Authority lists have all been used as the sampling frame (e.g. Copeland et al., 1987; Brayne & Calloway, 1989; Chadwick, 1992).

Samples may be geographically based, i.e. all or a sample of those living within a specified boundary (e.g. Chadwick, 1992), or based on all those registered with different family doctors, irrespective of residential address (e.g. O'Connor et al., 1989). Institutions have been included in some studies (e.g. O'Connor et al., 1989) and excluded in others (e.g. Morgan et al., 1987). Other studies have been conducted entirely on people living in institutions (e.g. Ames et al., 1988; Heeren et al., 1992). Types of institution have ranged from private retirement homes for the relatively fit elderly, through nursing homes for the physically ill to long-stay psychogeriatric hospitals. These types of study are likely to report widely differing proportions of the population as being demented. The estimates for the whole population will depend partly on whether such institutions are included or excluded from the overall proportions reported. Another factor that is likely to cause bias in the final estimates of the population affected is how communities deal with residents who require long-term care; only some communities can provide such care and these have institutions which may receive individuals from outside their catchment area.

Many investigators have taken complete population samples in a given age range (e.g. Clarke et al., 1984). Others have selected subjects using randomization procedures (e.g. epidemiologic catchment area study: Eaton & Kessler, 1986). Stratification has been used, usually by age, with subselection within strata (e.g. Morgan et al., 1987; Brayne & Calloway, 1989; Copeland et al., 1992). This leads to over-sampling in the older age groups, who would otherwise be under-represented. A less population-based method would be to include all volunteers of a particular age who were attending a general practice (Griffiths et al., 1987).

Differences in sampling techniques are of importance only if systematic biases are introduced which might hamper comparison between studies. If there are differences in the amount of dementia found in one community compared with another, these potential biases must first be examined.

Response rates

All surveys are dependent on the agreement of those contacted to participate. If there is a high refusal rate the very people that the study wishes to identify may be the group refusing to take part. If the prevalence of a disorder is 5%, a refusal rate of 30% could easily hide most of those of interest. It is therefore vital that the response rates of studies are known, and wherever possible some information on refusals reported. Some indication of the effect on estimates of the missed group is also useful.

Routine sources

Mortality

The difficulties in studies of dementia which rely on death certification have been mentioned. Comparison of standardized mortality rates for different areas of the United Kingdom has shown that those areas with the highest rates were those where long-stay institutions were situated (Martyn & Pippard, 1988). This reflects the fact that the most severely demented are those who are likely to be institutionalized and in such a long-stay setting the chance of dementia being included in the death certificate is high, whereas in the normal setting for death (hospital or community) it is much less likely. Furthermore, in a detailed study of a psychogeriatric clinic in England, fewer than 25% of the demented subjects had dementia noted as an underlying cause of death on their death certificates, although dementia or a related condition was noted in 75% elsewhere on the certificate (Martyn & Pippard 1988).

Mortality rates appear therefore to be markedly lower than would be expected if prevalence rates are used as a guide to the amount of dementia in the population (Jordan & Schoenberg, 1986). However, there does appear to have been a secular change in the reporting of dementia and senility, with the former becoming reported more commonly and the latter less commonly (Chandra et al., 1986). One recent paper from Newfoundland is based on mortality statistics and suggests that these could be seen as an accurate reflection of the true occurrence of dementia in the population (Frecker, 1992). In general, however, mortality statistics appear to be of limited value at present in the understanding of dementia.

Rates based on service data

Rates based on patients' contact with services tend to be low, as mentioned above, because those writing discharge summaries are likely to give only the acute reason for contact rather than underlying contributory causes. There is rarely differentiation of types of dementia. Rates based on service records can be flawed because they are based not on individuals but on numbers of episodes. Thus, one person admitted five times in one year would contribute five episodes.

For any understanding of the population distributions of dementia, the rates based on mortality and service contact are too flawed to be useful and field studies are essential.

Field studies

Cognitive scales

Cognitive scales measure current cognitive status. Therefore, they can produce only estimates of cognitive impairment when used in cross-sectional studies. If cognitive scales are used which can detect small changes in function, change from one time point to another can be measured and rates of decline can be estimated (Huppert, 1991). Short scales are unlikely to be sensitive to small changes in higher functions, but will be sensitive to gross changes such as loss of skills of orientation.

Cognitive impairment is not just an indication of dementia, but can be due to many other factors such as educational level, socio-economic group, physical health and depression (Fillenbaum et al., 1988; Brayne & Calloway, 1990a; Colsher & Wallace, 1991). Of these influences on level of cognitive function, education is arguably the most important. Many studies have shown that the distribution of responses on all but the shortest of cognitive scales is influenced by small differences in educational level. In populations where illiteracy is high this can cause problems with interpretation of findings.

Many of the cross-sectional studies of dementia and cognitive impairment have been conducted using short cognitive scales either as the only indicator of dementia or as a screen to be followed by a diagnostic assessment. These cognitive scales are variable in length. The shortest scales include questions such as information and orientation only, e.g. abbreviated mental test (Hodkinson, 1972) and the information–memory–concentration scale (Roth & Hopkins, 1953). Medium-length scales test memory, praxis, calculation and attention (Mini-Mental State Examination (MMSE): Folstein et al., 1975). The longest scales, such as CAMCOG (the cognitive scale of CAMDEX), test most of the cognitive modalities, but in limited detail (Roth et al., 1986). The estimated prevalence of cognitive impairment will depend entirely on the cutpoint chosen. If the scale is being used to identify dementia, the cutpoint will determine the prevalence of dementia unless one is chosen such that all the dementia sufferers are incorporated into the distribution below it (i.e. 100% sensitivity). This is rarely feasible unless the research is aimed only at identifying moderate levels of dementia (Brayne & Calloway, 1990b). The sensitivity and specificity of a scale will depend on: the level of dementia chosen (minimal, questionable, mild, moderate or severe); which set of criteria are chosen for this; and how these criteria are interpreted for a given study.

Figure 9.1 (a–d) shows distributions of four cognitive scales in one community sample (Brayne, 1990). The highest the maximum score, the more closely the distribution approximates to a normal curve, although it remains skewed. If cutpoints are applied to these scales the proportions of the population identified as 'abnormal' varies dramatically, as shown in Table 9.2 (Brayne & Calloway, 1990b). In this table, cutpoints which have been recommended are applied to a population sample of women aged 70 to 79 years. The demented are not contained solely within the tail of a distribution of cognitive scores unless moderate to severe dementia is chosen, but are found over the range of scores.

Behavioural measures

The diagnosis of dementia is not made on the basis of cognitive impairment alone (see Table 9.1). The most important additional components of the diagnosis are impairment in social and living functions caused by the cognitive impairment. It is therefore possible to apply scales measuring function in these areas to identify the amount of disorder in the community. This exercise would require population studies where the informant, but not the subject, would be interviewed at the screening and then the subjects who were identified by informants as declining in function would be assessed clinically. The distribution of scores on well-established scales such as the Blessed dementia scale (Blessed et al., 1968) which could be expected from such an exercise is shown in Figure 9.2 (the results from a population study of women aged 70 to 79 years in which 358 informant interviews were collected). In the scoring of this version of the scale (from CAMDEX), impairment is rated as positive so that most of the population are relatively unimpaired, with a small number of people in the impaired range. These people have a high probability of being diagnosed as demented, in the same way as those in the low scoring range

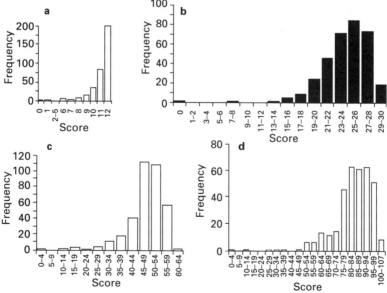

Figure 9.1. Frequency distribution for four cognitive scales (total sample): (a) Information – Memory – Concentration Test (Blessed et al., 1968); (b) MMSE (Mini-Mental State Examination; Folstein et al., 1975); (c) augmented MMSE (Medical Research Council, 1987); (d) CAMCOG (Roth et al., 1988).

Table 9.2. *The percentage of two age-groups of women identified as possible cases by cutpoints on several cognitive scales*

Scales and cutpoints	Percentage of women	
	70–4 years (*n* = 185)	75–9 years (*n* = 180)
Information/Orientation (CAPE)		
7–8 *(maximum score 12)*	0.0	3.3
MMSE (maximum score 30)		
17/18	1.1	10.0
21/22	12.4	25.6
23/24	34.6	37.2
CAMCOG (maximum score 107)		
69/70	6.5	22.2
79/80	24.9	36.1

CAPE, Clifton Assessment Procedures for the Elderly (Pattie & Gilleard, 1979); MMSE, Mini-Mental State Examination (Folstein et al., 1975); Cambridge Cognitive Examination (Roth et al., 1986).
From Brayne & Calloway (1990a).

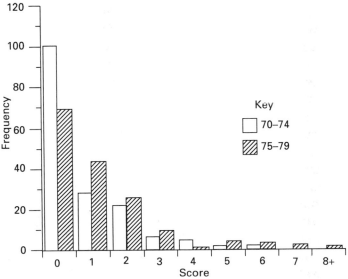

Figure 9.2. Score on Blessed dementia scale (Blessed et al., 1968) by age.

of cognitive scales. A new scale has been developed which is likely to be very useful both in clinical and population settings – the IQCODE (Jorm & Korten, 1988). This contains a series of questions to an informant on whether there has been change in the individual of interest over a specified period of time. Many functions are covered, such as concentration, social and daily activities. Unless instructions are very explicit, physical illness is more likely to influence scores on the Blessed dementia scale (resulting in high scores) compared with the IQCODE.

Dementia

As described above, dementia is a syndrome with many components. This approach has been challenged by some as being outdated and it has been suggested that more specific diagnoses should be made (Ulrich, 1992). For the present, however, the global nature of impairment in dementia is accepted. There is, therefore, no single diagnostic measure. To arrive at a diagnosis of dementia, more than the above scales must be used, since they are influenced by more than the dementia process itself. The only way to improve the estimates provided by single or combined scales is to examine either all the population or a selected group with a full clinical battery to arrive at a clinical diagnosis. A clinical diagnosis can be bypassed or supplemented by clinical algorithms. Clinical algorithms are aids to diagnosis which formalize the decision about which level of response is considered to be sufficient to fulfil a given criterion. The final algorithm is essentially a decision tree; some of the items which contribute to such a tree may be based on observation and some on performance. Where decisions are made according to such algorithms, these can be influenced by small differences in the way that interviewers rate items which have key effects in the algorithm. An example of this is the organicity scale item of the geriatric mental state examination (GMS) in which the single item recall of the date has an important effect on the number of people who are rated as organicity level 03, i.e. case level (C. Brayne, unpublished). Unless very clearly specified, the number of people who fail a particular criterion with a particular clinician will depend on many factors, such as previous experience of dementia, perception of what is normal and acceptable for a given age-group and the nature of professional training. Consensus diagnosis, which is diagnosis including many members of a research group after discussion of all available information, overcomes this to some extent, but does not necessarily improve agreement between research groups.

Levels of dementia

There is a lack of clarity about the way to assign level of severity of dementia, which reflects the uncertainty about questionable and mild dementia. Examination of the set criteria for levels of severity shows considerable variation between sets. The enormous variation and differences in prediction of progression and proportions identified by one interpretation of these criteria were shown elegantly by Rosenman (1991). He operationalized five methods of diagnosing mild dementia. The kappas, a measure of agreement which takes chance into account, averaged 0.15 which is considered to be rather poor agreement. Of the diagnostic deviance, 57% was accounted for by factors thought to be unrelated to dementia, such as depression, limited education and illness. Moreover, prediction of subsequent progression was poor. Interestingly, no single method improved upon the clinician's judgement of the presence of pathological cognitive impairment or a single cutpoint on the MMSE. This agrees well with the longitudinal study of the Hughes Hall Project for Later Life which showed a good prediction of stability of diagnosis or further progression of mild dementia (O'Connor et al., 1991). Post-mortem studies on 10 individuals with very mild dementia registered with the Consortium to Establish a Registry for Alzheimer's Disease also showed considerable accuracy of diagnosis (Morris et al., 1991).

Most studies of minimal dementia show they have a predictive power for subsequent decline for groups (particularly clinical diagnosis), but do not predict an individual's decline well. Variation in the way that an individual moves from the earliest cognitive decline into dementia is based largely on change in functional capabilities. The only way to establish how to predict progression is to follow large unselected populations which have been studied adequately at baseline.

Differential diagnosis

It is only in studies which go further than collecting information on simple scales that a differential diagnosis of dementia can be attempted. In these studies, subtypes of Alzheimer's disease or vascular dementia have been reported. In epidemiological studies, the full investigation which an individual would undergo if in a tertiary centre, such as an Alzheimer's disease research centre, is not feasible. Most studies can attempt some blood tests, and radiography where indicated. Adequate investigation of controls adds extra expense and is included rarely. Studies attempting to do this have considerable attrition between each stage, from screen to clinical interview and from clinical interview to investigation (e.g. Cambridge Project for Later Life: Paykel et al., 1993).

Criteria for Alzheimer's disease exclude other specific conditions which may result in dementia. The degree to which individuals are investigated for these other conditions will vary and affect the numbers left in the final exclusion category, which tends to be the Alzheimer's group. How much the final numbers are affected will depend on the enthusiasm of investigation and the interpretation of abnormal findings. Without imaging, clinical history might point to Alzheimer's disease, but, on imaging, clear evidence of infarction may be present. Does the case become mixed, or remain possible Alzheimer's disease (with an assumption that the lesions seen do not impair cognitive function or have appeared later in the course of the disorder) or does it become vascular? Whatever decision is made, the accuracy of differential diagnosis when carried out in unselected case series is very different from those series where demented subjects fulfil detailed inclusion and exclusion criteria. This is well illustrated by two studies in London. One is based on selected cases fulfilling criteria by the National Institute of Neurological and Communication Disorders and Stroke and the Alzheimer's Disease and Related Disorders Association (NINCDS–ADRDA) (McKhann et al., 1984) and coming to post-mortem with a highly accurate diagnosis of Alzheimer's disease. The other study took all admissions to a psychogeriatric unit and attempted to make full differential diagnosis (with much lower accuracy) backed up by investigation (e.g. cf. Burns et al., 1990; Gilleard et al., 1992). Unfortunately, the most accurate studies are those where case selection is so strict that it does not inform us about how common different types of dementia are in the community.

Prevalence studies

Prevalence studies report the proportion of a given population suffering with dementia or cognitive impairment at the time of interview.

Many of these studies have been carried out over the last 30 years. The studies conducted in the United Kingdom have been carried out mainly in urban areas. Some of these are shown in Table 9.3. The lowest rate reported so far in such studies is 2.5% in Melton Mowbray (Clarke et al., 1984) and the highest (39.7%) in Swansea (Parsons, 1964). Neither of these rates included people living in institutions.

However, as described earlier, variations in methodology (such as differences in sampling with widely differing age structures and differences in case definition) make these rates difficult to compare. Studies of the 65 years and over age-group based on standardized interviews containing either short cognitive scales or the GMS with computerized diagnostic algorithm do provide more consistent results, ranging between 3.2% in Nottingham (Morgan et al., 1987) and 5.2% in Liverpool (Copeland et al., 1987).

Prevalence rates for Europe apart from the United Kingdom are shown in Table 9.4 with rates for several studies carried out more recently at around 5%. The rates shown in Table 9.5 for the United States show wide variation which may be more a function of the different age structures studied than that of a true difference. Table 9.6 shows results from other areas in the world. Again, wide variation is seen, but a figure such as 45% for Korean women is based on failure on cutpoint of the cognitive scale MMSE or other short cognitive scale (i.e. one which has a maximum of around 10 points) and could be due to cultural differences in approaches to such testing, or literacy rates, rather than the dementia syndrome itself. This is a tentative conclusion unless diagnostic information is available.

In all studies where age-specific rates are provided, a sharp increase in the rates of cognitive impairment and dementia have been reported with age. A six-fold difference in the numbers failing a simple information/orientation test is usual between 75–79 year age-group and the 85+ year age-group in these studies. The meta-analysis of European prevalence studies carried out by EURODEM (the European Concerted Action on Dementias) shows the same phenomenon for all types of dementia (Hofman et al., 1991). It could be argued that this increase in the prevalence of apparent dementia with age is merely the result of increasing visual and hearing handicap, along with other illnesses. If this were the case, those studies which have examined these variables also would be expected to find much cognitive impairment, but little Alzheimer's disease, with increasing age. This is not the case as will be discussed later.

Several studies with different case identification methods have found

Table 9.3. *Dementia prevalence (UK)*

Authors	Published	Age group (years)	No.	%	Degree	Comment
Urban						
Sheldon	1948	65+	369	3.9	Severe	
				14.0	All	
Primrose	1962	65+	222	4.5	Severe	Period prevalence/GP
				5.4	All	
Kay et al.	1964	65+	443	5.6	Severe	Psychiatrist
				4.1	Mild	
Williamson et al.	1964	65+	200	8.0	Severe	Psychiatrist
				15.5	Mild	
Parsons	1964	65+	228	14.8	Severe	Psychiatrist
				24.9	Mild	
Kay et al.	1970	65+	461	6.2		Psychiatrist
Herbst & Humphrey	1980	70+	253	16.0		
Clarke et al.	1984	75+	1800	4.5		Included institutions. SCS
				2.5		Community only
Copeland et al.	1987	65+	1070	5.2		GMS–AGECAT

Study	Year	Age	N	Prevalence (%)	Degree	Method
Morgan et al.	1987	65+	1042	3.2		SCS
O'Connor et al.	1989	75+	2616	5.3	Moderate and severe	Included institutions. MMSE and psychiatrist
				10.5	Mild, moderate and severe	
Livingston et al.	1990	65+	813	5.0		Short CARE
Rural						
Griffiths et al.	1987	65+	200	10.0		Community volunteers. SCS
Urban/rural						
Gilmore	1977	65+	300	8.2		Clinical diagnosis
Broe et al.	1976	65+	808	3.8	Severe	Clinical diagnosis
				4.3	All	
Kemp	1985	75–84	1000	4.2		SCS
		85+		7.5		

In the 'Degree' column, 'All' refers to 'all degrees of severity'. GMS–AGECAT, Geriatric Mental State examination, AGECAT is a diagnostic algorithm (Copeland et al., 1986). SCS – Short cognitive scale. Blank spaces in columns signify no information is available.

Table 9.4. *Dementia prevalence (Europe)*

Authors	Published	Country	Age group (years)	No.	%	Degree	Comment
Bremer	1951	Norway	60+	119	2.5	Severe	GP
Essen-Moller et al.	1956	Sweden	60+	443	5.0	Severe	Psychiatrist
					15.8	All	Known to services
Nielsen	1962	Sweden (R)	65+	978	3.1		GP
Jensen	1963	(R)	65+	546	1.1		Psychiatrist
Akesson	1969	Sweden (R)	60+	4198	1.0		Psychiatrist
Hagnell	1970	Sweden	60+	2550	16.1		Psychiatrist
Svanborg	1977	Sweden (U)	70–5	1000	1.3	Severe	
					6.3	All	
Sternberg & Gavrilova	1978	USSR (U)	60+	1020	2.8	All	
Molsa et al.	1982	Finland (U)	65–74 } 75+	421	0.4 1.1		Known to services

Nielsen et al.	1982	Sweden	70+	1683	2.8	F	51% severe dem.
					2.3	M	
Cooper & Sosna	1983	FRG (U)	65+	519	6.0	Severe	Interview
					10.2	All	
Enzell	1983	Sweden (U)	69	4930	1.0	Mild/moderate	
Weyerer	1983	FRG (R)	65+	295	8.8		Psychiatrist
Sulkava et al.	1985	Finland (U/R)	65+	8000	6.7	Severe	Neurologist
Gavrilova et al.	1987	USSR (U)	60+	1704	4.2	All	Psychiatrist
					1.5	Mild	
					3.1	Minimum	
Rocca	1990	Italy	60+	778	6.2		Neurologist
Lobo et al.	1992	Portugal	65+	334	7.4		GMS

In the 'Degree' column, 'All' refers to 'all degrees of severity'; F, female; M, male; R, rural; U, urban; GMS, Geriatric Mental State examination; GP, general practitioner. Blank spaces in columns signify no information is available.

Table 9.5. *Dementia prevalence (USA)*

Authors	Published	Location	Age group (years)	No.	%	Comment
Gruenberg	1961	USA			6.8	
Holzer et al.	1984	USA	65–74	1977	1.1	MMSE
			75+		4.0	
Robins et al.	1984	USA:				MMSE; total, adult population
		New Haven		3058	1.3	
		Baltimore		3481	1.3	
		St Louis		3004	1.0	
Blazer et al.	1985	USA:				
		Baltimore (U)	65+	3921	1.8	MMSE
		Baltimore (R)	65+	3921	2.5	MMSE

Folstein et al.	1985	USA	65–74	564	2.1	Community MMSE, ECA
			75+		11.7	
Kramer et al.	1985	USA	65–74		3.0	
			75+		9.3	
Schoenberg et al.	1985	USA (U)	40+	8994	1.0	
			80+		7.0	
Magaziner	1987	USA	65+	783	10.0	MMSE
Pfeffer et al.	1987	USA	65+	817	15.3	SCS
			80+		35.8	
					12.0	
Bachman et al.	1992	USA	65+		3.1 men	Framingham study
					4.8 women	

R, rural; U, urban; MMSE, Mini-Mental State Examination (Folstein et al., 1975); SCS, short cognitive scale; ECA, Epidemiologic Catchment Area study. Blank spaces in columns signify no information is available.

Table 9.6. *Dementia prevalence in other countries*

Authors	Published	Country	Age group (years)	No.	%	Degree	Comment[a]
Campbell et al.	1983	New Zealand (U)	65+	559	7.7	Inst.	
					2.4	Severe	
					5.3	Mild	
Kay et al.	1985	Australia (U)	70–9	158	3.8	Mild	DSM interview
					2.5	Moderate	
					0.0	Severe	
					10.8	Mild	Psychiatrist
					1.3	Moderate	
			80+	116	17.2	Mild	
					6.9	Moderate	
					0.9	Severe	

Study	Year	Location	Age	N	Prevalence	Severity	Notes
Hagesawa et al.	1986	Japan	65+	1800	4.8	All	No institutional subjects
Shibayama et al.	1986	Japan (U/R)	65+	3105	5.2	Moderate/severe	
					2.2	Mild	
Park & Ha	1988	Korea	65+	549	3.6	Mild	No institutional subjects
					45.0 F	Mild	
					25.0 M	Mild	
					19.0 F	Moderate	
					8.0 M	Moderate	
Jensen & Polloi	1988	Palau (U/R)	90+	31	25.0	Mild	
					42.0	Moderate/severe	

[a]Not all studies include residents in institutions in their estimates.
DSM (see American Psychiatric Association, 1987); F, female; M, male; R, rural; U, urban. Inst. means that subjects in institutions were included.

higher rates for dementia or cognitive impairment in women than in men (Weyerer, 1983; Sulkava et al., 1985; Koukoulik, 1986; Morgan et al., 1987). Others have reported equal rates (Campbell et al., 1983; Weissman et al., 1985; Griffiths et al., 1987). Only a few studies have reported higher rates for men than women (Pfeffer et al., 1987). The comparisons do not use age-standardized rates, i.e. those which take the age structure of the population into account. Since there are more older women than men in many of these populations, even within specific age-groups, age differences could still account for these differences. There are also differences in the pattern of mortality and institutionalization between the sexes, which could produce apparent differences. Men are less likely to survive than women, and men with cognitive impairment have a greater chance of dying because they have a double loading of risk. Men without support in the community may be more likely to be institutionalized than women, since in this age-group they may be less capable of self-care in the early stages of dementia. In the meta-analysis carried out by Jorm and colleagues, there was no differences in overall rates of dementia between men and women (Jorm et al., 1987).

In Jorm's meta-analysis, incorporating most of the prevalence studies for moderate and severe dementia carried out between 1945 and 1985, the authors coded for methodological differences between studies, such as sampling, age grouping, case definition, rural or urban settings, sex and differential diagnosis (Jorm et al., 1987). Surprisingly, refusal rates, sex ratios, inclusion or exclusion of institutionalized patients did not influence rates in this analysis. It is possible that the heterogeneity of the methodology and settings meant that no such systematic effects could be examined. Complete samples tended to report lower rates than stratified samples. The prevalence studies which included the mild category tended to report lower rates for moderate and severe dementia than studies where only moderate and severe dementia were measured. One result was clear – there was a consistent doubling time of 5.1 years in the prevalence rates.

Incidence

Incidence quantifies the number of new cases of disorder that develop in a population of individuals at risk during a specified time interval. Incidence is a better measure when comparison is important, since it removes the effect of survival which is present in prevalence studies.

Table 9.7. *Age-specific incidence of dementia (percentage per annum)*

Age group (years)	Nottingham[a]	Cambridge[b]
65–9	0.23	
70–4	0.70	
75–9	1.30	2.3
80–4	2.25	4.6
85–9	2.18	8.5
90+		8.2

[a]Morgan et al. (1993).
[b]Paykel et al. (1993).

Table 9.8. *Incidence studies of the 65+ age-group (percentage per annum)*

Study	Incidence (%)	Comment
Mann et al. (1992)	2.6	Loose criteria
	1.4	Strict criteria
Copeland et al. (1992)	0.9	GMS–AGECAT
Dartigues et al. (1992)	1.1	Clinical diagnosis

GMS–AGECAT, Geriatric Mental State examination, AGECAT diagnostic algorithm (Copeland et al., 1986).
From Launer et al., 1992.

Incidence studies provide the clearest evidence concerning development of disease in relation to earlier exposures (Hennekens & Buring, 1987).

There have been fewer incidence studies of dementia than prevalence. Prevalence studies have been carried out with the aim of establishing need for levels of service. Incidence studies are more cumbersome, expensive and difficult to carry out. Those rates based on case records from institutions tend to be lower than those based on field studies. Some of the more recent field studies are summarized in Table 9.7 and Table 9.8. These include the Nottingham longitudinal study (Morgan et al., 1992, 1993), the Liverpool study of continuing health (Copeland, et al., 1992), the PAQUID study (*Personnes agés quo vadis*; Dartigues et al., 1992) and the Gospel Oak study (Mann

Table 9.9. *The prevalence of Alzheimer's disease from the EURODEM Group*

Age group (years)	Prevalence (%)	
	Men	Women
60–9	0.3	0.4
70–9	2.5	3.6
80–9	10.0	11.2

From Rocca et al. (1991a).

et al., 1992). These studies report average annual incidence rates of around 1% for the 65 years and over age-group. Very few studies based on large numbers of the very old are available. The Cambridge Project for Later Life (Paykel et al., 1993) is an incidence study of the 75 years and over age-group; its incidence rates are shown in Table 9.7 and show that incidence reflects prevalence very closely with no sparing of the very old. The apparent levelling off in the 90 years and over age-group is unstable because of small numbers. Very similar results were reported from a cohort study of volunteers in the United States (Katzman et al., 1989).

Differential diagnosis in the community

Alzheimer's disease

In studies of Western populations where differential diagnosis has been attempted, the prevalence of clinically diagnosed Alzheimer's disease has usually been found to be higher than that of the main alternative type of dementia – vascular dementia.

The EURODEM meta-analysis provides estimates of Alzheimer's disease based on results combined from European studies, and thus these are rather more reliable estimates than those based on smaller numbers (Table 9.9). Two recent studies from the United States have reported very different estimates of the prevalence of Alzheimer's disease. The East Boston study (Evans et al., 1989) reports markedly higher prevalence of Alzheimer's disease than does the Framingham study (Bachman et al., 1992). The former has also provided high

Table 9.10. *Annual age specific incidence of subtypes of dementia (percentage per annum)*

| Age group (years) | Alzheimer's disease | | Vascular dementia |
	East Boston[a]	Cambridge[b]	(Cambridge[a])
65–9	0.7		
70–4	1.6		
75–9	2.8	1.1	1.1
80–4	9.2	2.5	1.4
85–9		6.8	0.6
90+		3.6	4.5

[a]Hebert et al. (1991).
[b]Brayne et al. (1993).

estimates of the incidence of Alzheimer's disease (Hebert et al., 1991), shown in Table 9.10 in comparison with the incidence study in Cambridge city (Brayne et al., 1993). The main reason for this seems to be the severity of the disorder included. The East Boston study included anyone who fulfilled the NINCDS–ADRDA criteria even at the mildest level. Other studies have included only more severe levels of dementia.

Vascular dementia

Dementia secondary to vascular lesions is thought to be the second most common form of dementia in most populations. The exact nomenclature, concepts and definition of vascular dementia have varied over the years, but the existence of some form of dementia which is related to vascular pathology is accepted generally. It has been suggested that transient ischaemic attacks, reversible stroke and stroke are on a continuum (Koudstaal et al., 1992), and it is therefore possible that, when the means are available to investigate this, vascular dementia may be found to be on a continuum with changes observed in non-demented individuals. Evidence to support this has been presented recently. In a community study of dementia in the Netherlands, over 100 individuals underwent magnetic resonance imaging MRI. All those with current dementia were excluded from the analysis, and

Table 9.11. *The prevalence of vascular dementia by sex from EURODEM studies*

Age group (years)	Prevalence (%)	
	Men	Women
60–9	1.3	0.4
70–9	3.8	2.7
80–9	4.5	4.0

From Rocca et al. (1991b).

despite this a significant correlation between vascular lesions (or leukoaraiosis) and neuropsychological measures was found, such that the more lesions on MRI, the lower the cognitive scores (Breteler et al., 1992).

The prevalence rates of vascular dementia appear to be very variable, and, because few European studies had examined the population in sufficient detail to attempt this diagnosis, no summary rates are given in the EURODEM meta-analysis (Rocca et al. 1991b). The combined rates would be as shown in Table 9.11. A major difficulty is the lack of standardized criteria on which to base the diagnosis. The recent publication of suggested criteria similar to the NINCDS–ADRDA set for Alzheimer's disease (Morris & Heyman, 1992; Chui et al., 1992) address this problem, and, even if flawed, rates based on these criteria will be more similar to one another than those reported previously. It is likely that variability will remain for the same reasons as the variability noted in the studies of Alzheimer's disease – that there is difficulty in setting the degree to which change must be present before the diagnosis of subtype is made.

The rates of vascular dementia do not appear to show quite the same increase with age that is apparent in Alzheimer's disease. This may be due to the shorter survival of individuals with vascular dementia or due to a genuine tailing off in the incidence of vascular dementia with age. This is possible if there is a higher lethality of earlier cerebrovascular disease before any threshold for clinical dementia is reached. In other words, those who are at risk of developing vascular dementia die in the earlier minimal stage, since their mortality rates are high because of old age and vascular risk.

Other types of dementia

Until more is known about the pre-mortem diagnosis of the more recently recognized or resuscitated dementias such as Lewy body dementias or frontal dementias (Perry et al., 1989; see Chapter 7), it will not be possible to give prevalence or incidence rates for the population. Estimates will be possible if an unbiased sample of brain tissue from demented subjects is sought from epidemiological samples.

Population studies and the continuum

The studies noted above have all been based on the premise that dementia is a discrete disorder with normality and disease clearly delineated. However, in the diagnosis of dementia, two major axes must be measured to fulfil the criteria. The fundamental axis is cognitive function, but dementia cannot be diagnosed unless the cognitive impairment is sufficient to cause impairment in activities of daily living, and social functioning. The studies which base their rates on cognitive function demonstrate quite clearly that the prevalence rates are a function of the cutpoint chosen. The cutpoints on cognitive scales are chosen to perform best against a standard, and they vary according to the level of severity of dementia chosen (Brayne & Calloway, 1990b).

The definitions used in the standardized psychiatric interview for the elderly (CAMDEX: Roth et al., 1986) for minimal, mild, moderate and severe dementia show a clear progression through the disorder, with very difficult decisions to be made at the boundaries about the degree of abnormality. Minimal dementia merges with age-associated memory impairment, and there is debate here about whether this should be set against norms from the same cohort or from current peak performance cohorts (Crook et al., 1986; Crook & Ferris, 1992; O'Brien & Levy, 1992). The very real confusion about what is acceptable for so-called 'normal aging' is apparent in this debate.

If the decision for an individual either to be demented or not (i.e. about bimodality of distributions and the search for a perfect cutpoint) is set aside, the axes on which the diagnosis is based can be measured in representative samples from the population. This exercise has shown consistently in many studies that cognitive function is present as a continuous distribution in the community (see Figure 9.1b–d for examples), whether it is measured using short, medium or long cognitive scales and whether it is scaled across functions or within relatively brain-specific regions (Brayne, 1990). Behavioural measures are also distributed continuously in the few studies which have measured them, although smaller numbers of individuals score in the impaired range (Brayne & Calloway, 1988).

If the clearly distinct entity of dementia exists, a separation of the demented population from the rest of the aging population (i.e. a bimodal distribution) should be seen cross-sectionally, and longitudinally, in studies of cognitive function in the elderly. Unfortunately, there are relatively few of these studies which are representative of true populations on which to base conclusions. However, the cohort study in Cambridge city, the Cambridge Project for Later Life (Paykel et al., 1993) shows that there is a decline of one point in MMSE scores over 28 months in the 75 years and over age-group (Brayne et al., 1993). This decline is more marked in older age-groups and for each age-group and sex there is no hint of a bimodal distribution. The phenomenon of increasing incidence of dementia is parallelled by a shift in the whole distribution of cognitive scores downwards (Brayne et al., 1993).

If there is some fundamental bimodal distribution of the latent variables of the dementias, one might expect to see very different patterns of mortality between the non-demented population and that of the demented. These differences are indeed seen, since survival has been found to be reduced in psychiatric illness, and this relationship persists into old age. The mortality is highest in organic syndromes, not just in hospital-based studies but also community-based studies (Bickel & Cooper, 1989; see Chapter 6). Multi-infarct dementia may be associated with poorer survival than Alzheimer's disease, but because of the difficulties of accurate diagnosis in the community this has not yet been proven (Martin et al., 1987). However, on examining the community more closely it has been shown repeatedly that degree of cognitive impairment is associated with a stepwise change in survival. In other words, independently of other confounding variables, survival is shorter for each loss of points on cognitive score (Jagger & Clarke, 1988; Eagles et al., 1990).

Post-mortem studies and the continuum

Post-mortem studies have been mentioned several times in this chapter. Depending on the relationship of the underlying neuropathology of Alzheimer's disease and vascular dementia and others, the frequency of changes in autopsy series could be helpful. A unit increase in plaque, Lewy body or ischaemic lesion, or decrease in synapses would mean a unit decrease in cognitive level. Unfortunately, autopsy series are highly selective, and the appearance of the brain after the terminal illness may not be the same as during the last few years of life. Almost all such series report these lesions increasing with age, and present, to some extent, in most elderly non-demented individuals, as well as being absent in a small number of very elderly individuals, both demented and non-demented (see Chapter 18 for full review). As more clinico-pathological studies are carried out, the lesions causing impairment during life should become clearer and this method will become more likely to yield clues (e.g. Crystal et al., 1988; Arriagada et al., 1992).

It has been noted often that the severity and nature of lesions found in late-onset Alzheimer's disease are different from that found at younger ages. This may be because the presence of cognitive impairment and great age leads to a higher mortality at an earlier stage of the Alzheimer process. Because the dementia is superimposed on a background of neuronal loss and some cognitive decline, the dementia expressed during life may be equivalent to that in younger individuals. That is, there will be a milder spectrum of observed neuropathology as age progresses because the mortality at these milder stages is greater.

Thus, whilst these studies will advance knowledge considerably, the question can be answered only partially until there are techniques to measure accurately the presence of such lesions during life.

Why do clinicians see a dichotomy where epidemiologists do not?

Case series of dementia, in particular Alzheimer's disease, have suggested that there are marked changes in many variables. Those studied include cholinergic, somatostatin, amine, aluminium, parathyroid hormone, glucose, radiological and other neurophysiological measures, but none have been found to be highly sensitive or specific (Blass et al, 1985; Carlsson, 1986; Hollander et al., 1986; Sherman et al., 1986; Elbe et al., 1987; Houck et al., 1988; Love et al., 1989; Kukull et al., 1992). The main reason for finding differences in the clinical setting, which are not confirmed when the measure is made on a wider group, is the selection which occurs before individuals become included in case series.

Clinicians are likely to perceive a dichotomy because the cases they see have passed through multiple filters before being referred. Individuals usually present to services at a level where there is considerable disturbance to themselves or their family or community. People with mild disorder tend not to present to services for any condition. Thus, the physician compares a view of active normality, a culturally determined norm, with what is presented in the clinical setting, and sees a dichotomy. The investigator in the community sees, in addition, the grey area of those who are coping with the abnormality, who may not have perceived or acknowledged it and who are not presenting to the services in need.

Conclusion

Without biological markers of the presence of the particular lesions of Alzheimer's disease in life, it is speculative to assert that there is continuity. However, the measures made during life, and the measures made after death indicate that there is no clear delineation between those without Alzheimer's disease and those with it. This research would be enhanced greatly if it were possible to establish the exact lesions which underly the decline noted during life in both normal aging and dementia.

There is no evidence from epidemiological studies to refute the possibility that the decline noted in cognition in normal aging is on the same continuum as the marked decline seen in dementia. It remains to be seen whether the actual pathologies underlying this decline are the same as those found in the most prevalent dementias – namely Alzheimers' disease, vascular dementia and possibly Lewy body dementia (Perry et al., 1989). Only longitudinal studies on populations with adequate post-mortem examination of brain tissue will clarify this question, unless in-vivo methods of measuring brain abnormalities (such as neuron loss, acetylcholinesterase, tau, β-amyloid, vascular lesions, and Lewy body dementia) which are acceptable to the general elderly population are developed. If, like hypertension, there is a continuous distribution of these underlying lesions in the aging population, it may be possible to improve the prospects for all individuals by shifting the entire distribution away from the pathological end.

References

Akesson, H. O. (1969). A population study of senile and arteriosclerotic psychoses. *Human Heredity*, **19**, 546–66.

American Psychiatric Association (1987). *Diagnostic and Statistical Manual of Mental Disorders*, third edition – revised (DSM-III-R). American Psychiatric Association, Washington, DC.

Ames, D., Ashby, D., Mann, A. H. & Graham, N. (1988). Psychiatric illness in elderly residents of Part III homes in one London Borough: prognosis and review. *Age and Ageing*, **17**, 249–56.

Arriagada, P. V., Growdon, J. H., Hedley-White, R. & Hyman, B. T. (1992). Neurofibrillary tangles but not senile plaques parallel duration and severity of Alzheimer's disease. *Neurology*, **42**, 631–9.

Bachman, D. L., Wolf, P. A., Linn, R., Knoefel, J. E., Cobb, J., Belanger, A., D'Agnostino, R. B. & White, L. R. (1992). Prevalence of dementia and probable senile dementia of the Alzheimer type in the Framingham study. *Neurology*, **42**, 115–19.

Bickel, H. & Cooper, B. (1989). Incidence of dementing illness among persons aged over 65 in an urban population. In B. Cooper & T. Helgason (eds.) *Epidemiology and the Prevalence of Mental Disorders*, pp. 59–76. Routledge, London, New York.

Blass, J. P., Hanin, I., Barclay, L., Kopp, U. & Reding, M. J. (1985). Red blood cell abnormalities in Alzheimer's disease. *Journal of the American Geriatric Society*, **33**, 401–5.

Blazer, D., George, L. K., Landerman, R., Pennybacker, M., Melville, M. L., Woodbury, M., Manton, K. G., Jordan, K. & Locke, B. (1985). Psychiatric disorders: a rural/urban comparison. *Archives of General Psychiatry*, **42**, 651–6.

Blessed, G., Tomlinson, B. E. & Roth, M. (1968). The association between quantitative measures of dementia and of senile change in the cerebral grey matter of elderly subjects. *British Journal of Psychiatry*, **114**, 797–811.

Brayne, C. (1990). 'A study of dementia in a rural population'. MD thesis, London University.

Brayne, C. & Calloway, P. (1988). Normal ageing, impaired cognitive function and senile dementia of the Alzheimer's type: a continuum? *Lancet*, **ii**, 1265–7.

Brayne, C. & Calloway, P. (1989). An epidemiological study of dementia in a rural population of elderly women. *British Journal of Psychiatry*, **155**, 214–19.

Brayne, C. & Calloway, P. (1990a). The association of education and socioeconomic status with the Mini-Mental State Examination and the clinical diagnosis of dementia in elderly people. *Age and Ageing*, **19**, 91–6.

Brayne, C. & Calloway, P. (1990b). The case identification of dementia in the community: a comparison of methods. *International Journal of Geriatric Psychiatry*, **5**, 309–16.

Brayne, C., Huppert, F. A., Gill, C., O'Connor, D. & Paykel, E. S. (1993). Cognitive decline in the 75 and over population in Cambridge, in preparation.

Bremer, A. J. (1951). A social psychiatric investigation of a small rural community in northern Norway. *Acta Psychiatrica Neurologia Scandinavica*, (supplement 62).

Breteler, M. M. B., van Swieten, J. C., van Harskamp, F., van den Hout, J. H. W., van Amerongen, N., Claus, J. J., van Gijn, J. & Hofman, A. (1992). Magnetic resonance imaging in a population sample. *Neurobiology of Aging*, **13**, (supplement 1), S16.

Broe, G. A., Akhtar, A. J., Andrews, G. R., Caried, R. I., Gilmore, A. J. & McLennan, W. J. (1976). Neurological disorders in the elderly at home. *Journal of Neurology, Neurosurgery and Psychiatry*, **39**, 361–6.

Burns, A., Luthert, P., Levy, R., Jacoby, R., Lantos, P. (1990). Accuracy of clinical diagnosis of Alzheimer's disease. *British Medical Journal*, **301**, 1026.

Campbell, A. J., McCosh, L. M., Reinken, J. & Allan, B. C. (1983). Dementia in old age and the need for services. *Age and Ageing*, **12**, 11–16.

Carlsson, A. (1986). Searching for antemortem markers for Alzheimer's disease. *Neurobiology of Aging*, **7**, 400–1.

Chadwick, C. (1992). The multicentre study of cognitive function and ageing: a EURODEM incidence study in progress. *Neuroepidemiology*, **11**, (supplement 1), 37–43.

Chandra, V., Bharucha, N. E. & Schoenberg, B. S. (1986). Patterns of mortality from types of dementia in the United States. *Neurology*, **36**, 204–8.

Chui, H. C., Victoroff, J. I., Margolin, D., Jagust, W., Shankle, R. & Katzman, R. (1992). Criteria for the diagnosis of ischemic vascular dementia proposed by the State of California Alzheimer's Disease Diagnostic and Treatment Centers. *Neurology*, **42**, 473–80.

Clarke, M., Clarke, S., Odeli, A. & Jagger, C. (1984). The elderly at home: health and social status. *Health Trends*, **1**, 3–7.

Colsher, P. & Wallace, R. B. (1991). Epidemiologic considerations in studies of cognitive function in the elderly. Methodologic and nondementing acquired dysfunction. *Epidemiologic Reviews*, **13**, 1–27.

Cooper, B. (1991). The epidemiology of primary degenerative dementia and related neurological disorders. *European Archives of Psychiatry and Clinical Neurosciences*, **240**, 223–33.

Cooper, B. & Sosna, U. (1983). Psychiatric disease in an elderly population. An epidemiologic field study in Mannheim. *Nervenarzt*, **54**, 239–49.

Copeland, J. R. M., Dewey, M. E. & Griffiths Jones, H. M. (1986). Computerised psychiatric diagnostic system and care nomenclature for elderly subjects: GMS and AGECAT. *Psychological Medicine*, **16**, 89–99.

Copeland, J. R. M., Dewey, M. E., Wood, N., Searle, R., Davidson, I. A. & McWilliam, C. (1987). Range of mental illness among the elderly in the community: prevalence in Liverpool using the GMS–AGECAT package. *British Journal of Psychiatry*, **150**, 815–23.

Copeland, J. R. M., Dewey, M. E., Davidson, I. A., Saunders, P. A. & Scott, A. (1992). Geriatric mental state–AGECAT: prevalence, incidence and long-term outcome of dementia and organic disorders in the Liverpool study of continuing health in the community. *Neuroepidemiology*, **11**, (supplement 1), 84–7.

Crook, T. H. & Ferris, S. H. (1992). Age associated memory impairment. *British Medical Journal*, **304**, 714.

Crook, T., Bartus, R. T., Ferris, S. H., Whitehouse, P., Cohen, G. D. & Gershon, S. (1986). Age-associated memory impairment: proposed diagnostic criteria and measures of clinical change – report of a National Institute of Mental Health Work Group. *Developmental Neuropsychology*, **2**, 261–76.

Crystal, H., Dickson, D., Fuld, P., Masur, D., Scott, R., Mehler, M., Masdeu, J., Kawas, C., Aronson, M. & Wolfson, L. (1988). Clinico-pathologic studies in dementia: nondemented subjects with pathologically confirmed Alzheimer's disease. *Neurology*, **38**, 1682–7.

Dartigues, J. F., Gagnon, M., Barberger-Gateau, P., Letenneur, L., Commenges, D., Sauvel, C., Michel, P. & Salamon R. (1992). The Paquid Epidemiological Program on Brain Ageing. *Neuroepidemiology*, **11**, (supplement 1), 14–18.

Eagles, J. M., Beattie, J. A. G., Restall, D. B., Rawlinson, F., Hagen, S. & Ashcroft, G. W. (1990). Relation between cognitive impairment and early death in the elderly. *British Medical Journal*, **300**, 239–40.

Eaton, W. W. & Kessler, G. L. (1986). *Epidemiologic Field Methods in Psychiatry: the NIMH Epidemiologic Catchment Area Program*. Academic Press, New York.

Elbe, R., Giacobini, E. & Scarsella, G. F. (1987). Cholinesterases in cerebrospinal fluid. A longitudinal study in Alzheimer's disease. *Archives of Neurology*, **44**, 403–7.

Enzell, K. (1983). Psychiatric study of 69 year old health examinees in Stockholm. *Acta Psychiatrica Scandinavica*, **67**, 21–31.

Essen-Moller, E., Larsson, H., Uddenberg, C. E., White, G. (1956). Individual traits and morbidity in a Swedish rural population. *Acta Psychiatrica Neurologica Scandinavica*, **100**, (supplement).

Evans, D. A., Funkenstein, H. H., Albert, M. S., Scherr, P. A., Cook, N. R., Chown, M. J., Hebert, L. E., Hennekens, C. H. & Taylor, J. O. (1989). Prevalence of Alzheimer's disease in a community population of older persons higher than previously reported. *Journal of the American Medical Association*, **262**, 2551–6.

Fillenbaum, G. G., Hughes, D. C., Heyman, A., George, L. K. & Blazer, D. G. (1988). Relationship of health and demographic characteristics to mini-mental state examination score among community residents. *Psychological Medicine*, **18**, 719–26.

Folstein, M. F., Folstein, S. E. & McHugh, P. R. (1975). Mini-mental state: a practical method for grading the cognitive state of patients for the clinician. *Journal of Psychiatric Research*, **12**, 189–98.

Folstein, M. F., Anthony, J. C., Parhad, I. & Duffy, B. (1985). The meaning of cognitive impairment in the elderly. *Journal of American Geriatric Society*, **33**, 228–35.

Frecker, M. F. (1992). Dementia in Newfoundland: identification of a geographical isolate? *Journal of Epidemiology and Community Health*, **45**, 307–11.

Gavrilova, S. I., Sudareva, L. O. & Kalin, Y. B. (1987). The epidemiology of dementia in the elderly and old. *Korsakoff Journal of Neuropathology and Psychiatry*, **87**, 1345–52.

Gilleard, C. J., Kellett, J. M., Coles, J. A., Millard, P. H., Honavar, M. & Lantos, P. L. (1992). The St George's dementia bed investigation study: a comparison of clinical and pathological diagnosis. *Acta Psychiatrica Scandinavica*, **85**, 264–9.

Gilmore, A. (1977). Brain failure at home. *Age and Ageing*, Supplement, 56–60.

Griffiths, R. A., Good, W. R., Watson, N. P., O'Donnell, H. F., Fell, P. J., Shakespeare, J. M. (1987). Depression, dementia and disability in the elderly. *British Journal of Psychiatry*, **150**, 482–93.

Gruenberg, E. M. (1961). A mental health survey of older persons. In P. H. Hoch & J. Zubins (eds.) *Comparative Epidemiology of Mental Disorders*, pp. 13–23. Grune and Stratton, New York.

Hagesawa, K., Homma, A. & Imai, Y. (1986). An epidemiological study of age-related dementia in the community. *International Journal of Geriatric Psychiatry*, **1**, 45–55.

Hagnell, O. (1970). Dalbyundersokningorna. 6. Psykiska infufficienser i en totalbefolking incidens och duration. *Lakartidningen*, **67**, 3664–8.

Hebert, L. E., Scherr, P. A., Smith, L. A. & Evans, D. A. (1991). Age-specific incidence of Alzheimer's disease. *American Journal of Epidemiology*, **139**, 786–7.

Heeren, R. J., Lagaay, A. M., Rooijmans, H. G. (1992). Prevalence of the dementia syndrome in the oldest residents of a somatic nursing home. *Nederlands Tijdschrift voor Geneeskunde*, **136**, 695–8.

Hennekens, C. & Buring, J. E. (1987). *Epidemiology in Medicine*. Little, Brown and Co., Boston and Toronto.

Herbst, K. G. & Humphrey, C. (1980). Hearing impairment and mental state in the elderly living at home. *British Medical Journal*, **281**, 903–5.

Hodkinson, H. M. (1972). Evaluation of a mental test score assessment of mental impairment in the elderly. *Age and Ageing*, **1**, 233–8.

Hofman, A., Rocca, W. A., Brayne, C., Breteler, M. M. B., Clarke, M., Cooper, B., Copeland, J. R. M., Dartigues, J. F., Da Silva Droux, A., Hagnell, O., Heeren, T. J., Engedal, K., Jonker, C., Lindesay, J., Lobo, A., Mann, A. H., Molsa, P. K., Morgan, K., O'Connor, D. W., Sulkara, R., Kay, D. W. K. & Amaducci, L. (1991). The prevalence of dementia in Europe: a collaborative study of 1980–1990 findings. *International Journal of Epidemiology*, **20**, 736–48.

Hollander, E., Mohs, R. C. & Davis, K. L. (1986). Antemortem markers of Alzheimer's disease. *Neurobiology of Aging*, **7**, 367–407.

Holzer, C. E., Tischler, G. L., Leaf, P. J. & Myers, J. K. (1984). An epidemiologic assessment of cognitive function in a community population. *Research in Community and Mental Health*, **4**, 3–32.

Houck, P. R., Reynolds, C. F. D., Kopp, U. & Hanin, I. (1988). Red blood cells/plasma choline ratio in elderly depressed and demented patients. *Psychiatry Research*, **24**, 109–16.

Huppert, F. A. (1991). Neuropsychological assessment of dementia. *Reviews in Clinical Gerontology*, **1**, 159–69.

Jagger, C. (1993). The epidemiology of dementia. In A. Burns & R. Levy (eds.) *A Handbook of Dementia*, Chapman Hall, in press.

Jagger, C. & Clarke, M. (1988). Mortality risks in the elderly: five year follow up of a total population. *International Journal of Epidemiology*, **17**, 111–15.

Jensen, K. (1963). Psychiatric problems in four Danish old age homes. *Acta Psychiatrica Scandinavica*, (supplement 169), 411–19.

Jensen, G. D. & Polloi, A. H. (1988). The very old of Palau: health and mental state. *Age and Ageing*, **17**, 220–6.

Jordan, B. D. & Schoenberg, B. S. (1986). Mortality from presenile and senile dementia in the United States. *South Medical Journal*, **79**, 529–31.

Jorm, A. F. (1990). *The Epidemiology of Alzheimer's Disease and Related Disorders*. Chapman Hall, Chichester.

Jorm, A. F. & Korten, A. E. (1988). Assessment of cognitive decline in the elderly by informant interview. *British Journal of Psychiatry*, **152**, 209–13.

Jorm, A. F., Korten, A. E. & Henderson, A. S. (1987). The prevalence of dementia: a quantitative integration of the literature. *Acta Psychiatrica Scandinavica*, **76**, 465–79.

Katzman, R., Aronson, M., Fuld, P., Kawas, C., Brown, T., Morgenstern, H., Frishman, W., Gidez, L., Eder, H. & Ooi, W. L. (1989). Development of dementing illnesses in an 80 year old volunteer cohort. *Annals of Neurology*, **25**, 317–24.

Kay, D. W. K. (1991). The epidemiology of dementing disorders. *Reviews in Clinical Gerontology*, **1**, 55–66.

Kay, D. W. K., Beamish, P. & Roth, M. (1964). Old age mental disorders in Newcastle upon Tyne. Part I: a study of prevalence. *British Journal of Psychiatry*, **110**, 146–58.

Kay, D. W. K., Bergmann, K., Foster, E. M., McKechnie, A. A. & Roth, M. (1970). Mental illness and hospital usage in the elderly: a random sample followed up. *Comprehensive Psychiatry*, **11**, 26–35.

Kay, D. W. K., Henderson, A. S., Scott, R., Wilson, J., Rickwood, D. & Grayson, D. A. (1985). Dementia and depression among the elderly living in the Hobart community: the effect of the diagnostic criteria on the prevalence rates. *Psychological Medicine*, **15**, 771–88.

Kemp, F. (1985). 'The elderly at home'. Report for the East Anglian Health Authority.

Koudstaal, P. J., van Gijn, J., Frenken, C. W. G. M., Hijdra, A., Lodder, A., Vermeulen, M., Bulens, C. & Franke, C. L. (1992). TIA, RIND, minor stroke: a continuum, or different subgroups? *Journal of Neurology, Neurosurgery and Psychiatry*, **55**, 95–7.

Koukoulik, F. (1986). The estimated prevalence of severe dementia due to Alzheimer's disease in the population over 65 years of age in Czechoslovakia in 1983. *Cas. Lek. Cesk.*, **125**, 1289–90.

Kramer, M., German, P. S., Anthony, J. C., von Korff, M. & Skinner, E. A. (1985). Patterns of mental disorders among the elderly residents of Eastern Baltimore. *Journal of the American Geriatric Society*, **33**, 236–45.

Kukull, W. A., Hinds, T. R., Schellenberg, G. D., van Belle, G. & Larson, E. B. (1992). Increased platelet membrane fluidity as a diagnostic marker for Alzheimer's disease: a test in population based cases and controls. *Neurology*, **42**, 607–14.

Launer, L. J., Brayne, C. & Breteler, M. M. B. (1992). Epidemiologic approach to the study of dementing diseases: a nested case-control study in European incidence studies of dementia. *Neuroepidemiology*, **11**, (supplement 1), 114–18.

Livingston, G., Hawkins, A., Graham, N., Blizard, B. & Mann, A. (1990). The Gospel Oak Study: prevalence rates of dementia, depression and activity limitation among elderly residents in inner London. *Psychological Medicine*, **20**, 137–46.

Lobo, A., Dewey, M., Copeland, J., Dia, J. L. & Saz, J. P. (1992). The prevalence of dementia among elderly people living in Zaragoza and Liverpool. *Psychological Medicine*, **22**, 239–43.

Love, S., Burrola, P., Terry, R. D. & Wiley, C. A. (1989). Immunoelectron microscopy of Alzheimer and Pick brain tissue labelled with the monoclonal antibody ALZ-50. *Neuropathology and Applied Neurobiology*, **15**, 223–31.

Magaziner, J., Bassett, S. S. & Hebel, J. R. (1987). Predicting performance on the Mini-Mental State Examination. Use of age and education specific equations. *Journal of the American Geriatric Society*, **35**, 996–1000.

Mann, A. H., Livingston, G., Boothby, H. & Blizard, R. (1992). The Gospel Oak study: the prevalence and incidence of dementia in an inner city area of London. *Neuroepidemiology*, **11**, (supplement 1), 76–9.

Martin, E. M., Wilson, R. S., Penn, R. D., Fox, J. H., Clasen, R. A. & Savoy, S. M. (1987). Cortical biopsy results in Alzheimer's disease: correlation with cognitive deficits. *Neurology*, **37**, 1201–4.

Martyn, C. & Pippard, E. C. (1988). Usefulness of mortality data in determining the geography and time trends of dementia. *Journal of Epidemiology and Community Health*, **42**, 134–7.

McKhann, G., Drachman, D., Folstein, M., Katzman, R., Price, D. & Stadlan, E. M. (1984). Clinical diagnosis of Alzheimer's disease: report of the NINCDS –ADRDA work group under the auspices of Department of Health and Human Services task force on Alzheimer's disease. *Neurology*, **34**, 939–44.

Medical Research Council (1987). 'Report from the Medical Research Council Alzheimer's Disease Workshop'.

Mirra, S. S., Heyman, A., McKeel, D., Sumi, S. M., Crain, B. J., Brownlee, L. M., Vogel, F. S., Hughes, J. P., van Belle, G. & Berg, L. (1991). Consortium to Establish a Registry for Alzheimer's Disease (CERAD). Part II. Standardization of the neuropathologic assessment of Alzheimer's disease. *Neurology*, **41**, 479–86.

Molsa, P. K., Marttila, R. J. & Rinne, U. K. (1982). Epidemiology of dementia in a Finnish population. *Acta Neurologica Scandinavica*, **65**, 541–52.

Morgan, K., Dallosso, H. M., Arie, T., Byrne, E. J., Jones, R. & Waite, J. (1987). Mental health and psychological well-being among the old and the very old living at home. *British Journal of Psychiatry*, **150**, 801–7.

Morgan, K., Lilley, J., Arie, T., Byrne, J., Jones, R. & Waite, J. (1992). Incidence of dementia: preliminary findings from the Nottingham longitudinal study of activity and ageing. *Neuroepidemiology*, **11**, (supplement 1), 80–3.

Morgan, K., Lilley, J. M., Arie, T., Byrne, E. J., Jones, R. & Waite, R. J. (1993). Incidence of dementia in a representative British sample. *British Journal of Psychiatry*, **163**, 467-70.

Morris, J. C. & Heyman, A. (1992). 'Workshop on standardised differential diagnosis of dementia for epidemiological studies: the CERAD approach'. Third International Conference on Alzheimer's Disease and Related Disorders, Padua, Italy, July 12–17 1992.

Morris, J. C., Mohs, R. C., Rogers, H., Fillenbaum, G. & Heyman, A. (1988). Consortium to Establish a Registry for Alzheimer's Disease (CERAD). Clinical and neuropsychological assessment for Alzheimer's disease. *Psychopharmacology Bulletin*, **24**, 641–52.

Morris, J. C., McKeel, D. W., Storandt, M., Rubin, E. H., Price, J. L., Grant, E. A., Ball, M. J. & Berg, L. (1991). Very mild Alzheimer's disease: informant based clinical, psychometric and pathologic distinction from normal aging. *Neurology*, **41**, 469–78.

Nielsen, J. (1962). Geronto-psychiatric period prevalence investigation in a geographically delimited population. *Acta Psychiatrica Scandinavica*, **38**, 307–30.

Nielsen, J. A., Bjorn-Henriksen, T. & Bork, B. R. (1982). Incidence and disease expectancy for senile and arteriosclerotic dementia in a geographically delimited Danish population. In J. Magnussen, J. Nielsen & J. Buck (eds.) *Epidemiology and Prevention of Mental Illness in Old Age*, pp. 52–3. Hellerup, Denmark.

O'Brien, J. T. & Levy, R. (1992). Age associated memory impairment. *British Medical Journal*, **304**, 5–6.

O'Connor, D. W., Pollitt, P. A., Hyde, J. B., Fellows, J. L., Miller, N. D., Brook, C. P. B., Reiss, B. B. & Roth, M. (1989). The prevalence of dementia as measured by the Cambridge mental disorders of elderly examination. *Acta Psychiatrica Scandinavica*, **79**, 190–8.

O'Connor, D. W., Pollitt, P. A., James, B. J., Hyde, J. B., Fellowes, J. L. & Miller, N. D. (1991). Continued clinical validation of dementia diagnosed in the community using the Cambridge Mental Disorders of the Elderly Examination. *Acta Psychiatrica Scandinavia*, **83**, 41–5.

Park, J. H. & Ha, J. C. (1988). Cognitive impairment among the elderly in a Korean rural community. *Acta Psychiatrica Scandinavica*, **77**, 52–7.

Parsons, P. L. (1964). Mental health in Swansea's old folk. *British Journal of Preventive and Social Medicine*, **19**, 43–7.

Pattie, A. H. & Gilleard, C. J. (1979). *Manual of the Clifton Assessment Procedure for the Elderly (CAPE)*. Hodder & Stoughton, Sevenoaks.

Paykel, E. S., Brayne, C., Huppert, F. A., Gill, C., Barkley, C., Gehlhaar, E., Beardsall, L., Girling, D. M., Pollitt, P. & O'Connor, D. (1993). Incidence of dementia in a population older than 75 years in the United Kingdom. *Archives of General Psychiatry*, in press.

Perry, R. H., Irving, D., Blessed, G., Perry, E. K. & Fairbairn, A. F. (1989). Clinically and neuropathologically distinct forms of dementia in the elderly. *Lancet*, **i**, 166.

Pfeffer, R. I., Afifi, A. A. & Chance, J. M. (1987). Prevalence of Alzheimer's disease in a retirement community. *American Journal of Epidemiology*, **125**, 420–36.

Primrose, E. J. R. (1962). *Psychological Illness: a Community Study*. Thomas, Springfield, Illinois.

Robins, L. N., Helzer, J. E., Weissman, M. M., Orvaschel, H., Gruenberg, E., Burke, J. D., Jnr & Regier, D. A. (1984). Lifetime prevalence of specific psychiatric disorders in three sites. *Archives of General Psychiatry*, **41**, 949–58.

Rocca, W. A., Bonaiuto, S., Lippi, A., Luciani, P., Turtu, F., Cavarzeran, F. & Amaducci, L. (1990). Prevalence of clinically diagnosed Alzheimer's disease and other dementing disorders: a door to door survey in Appignano, Macerato Province, Italy. *Neurology*, **40**, 626–31.

Rocca, W. A., Hofman, A., Brayne, C., Breteler, M. M. B., Clarke, M., Copeland, J., Dartigues, J. F., Engedal, K., Hagnell, O., Heeren, T. J., Jonker, C., Lindesay, J., Lobo, A., Mann, A. H., Molsa, P. K., Morgan, K., O'Connor, D. W., da Silva Droux, A., Sulkava, R., Kay, D. W. K. & Amaducci, L. (1991a). Frequency and distribution of Alzheimer's disease in Europe: a collaborative study of 1980–1990 prevalence findings. *Annals of Neurology*, **30**, 381–90.

Rocca, W. A., Hofman, A., Brayne, C., Breteler, M. M. B., Clarke, M., Copeland, J., Dartigues, J. F., Engedal, K., Hagnell, O., Heeren, T. J., Jonker, C., Lindesay, J., Lobo, A., Mann, A. H., Molsa, P. K., Morgan, K., O'Connor, D. W., da Silva Droux, A., Sulkava, R., Kay, D. W. K. & Amaducci, L. (1991b). The prevalence of vascular dementia in Europe: facts and fragments from 1980–1990 studies. *Annals of Neurology*, **30**, 817–24.

Rosenman, B. (1991). The validity of the diagnosis of mild dementia. *Psychological Medicine*, **21**, 923–34.

Roth, M. & Hopkins, B. (1953). Psychological test performance in patients over 60. I: Senile psychosis and affective disorders of old age. *Journal of Mental Sciences*, **99**, 439–50.

Roth, M., Tym, E., Mountjoy, C. Q., Huppert, F. A., Hendrie, H., Verma, S. & Goddard, R. (1986). CAMDEX: a standardised instrument for the diagnosis of mental disorder in the elderly with special reference to the early detection of dementia. *British Journal of Psychiatry*, **149**, 698–709.

Roth, M., Huppert, F. A., Tym, E. & Mountjoy, C. Q. (1988). *CAMDEX. The Cambridge Examination for Mental Disorders of the Elderly*. Cambridge University Press, Cambridge.

Schoenberg, B. S., Anderson, D. W. & Haerer, A. F. (1985). Severe dementia. Prevalence and clinical features in a biracial US population. *Archives of Neurology*, **42**, 740–3.

Sheldon, J. H. (1948). *The Social Medicine of Old Age*. Oxford University Press, Nuffield Foundation London.

Sherman, K. A., Gibson, G. E. & Blass, J. P. (1986). Human red blood cell choline uptake with age and Alzheimer's disease. *Neurobiology of Aging*, **7**, 205–9.

Shibayama, H., Kasahara, Y. & Kobayashi, H. (1986). Prevalence of dementia in a Japanese elderly population. *Acta Psychiatrica Scandinavica*, **74**, 144–51.

Sternberg, E. & Gavrilova, S.(1978). Clinical and epidemiological findings of a psychogeriatric investigation in the Soviet Union. *Nervenarzt*, **49**, 347–53.

Sulkava, R., Wikstrom, J., Aromaa, A., Raitasalo, R., Lehtinen, V., Lahtela, K. & Palo, J. (1985). Prevalence of severe dementia in Finland. *Neurology*, **35**, 1025–9.

Svanborg, A. (1977). Seventy year old people in Gothenburg. A population study in an industrialised Swedish city. II: general presentation of social and medical conditions. *Acta Medica Scandinavica*, **611**, (supplement), 5–35.

Ulrich, G. (1992). Is global equivalent to multifocal? The whole and its parts in psychiatry and neurology. *Nervenarzt*, **63**, 14–20.

Weissman, M. M., Myers, J. K., Tischler, G. L., Holzer, C. E., Leaf, P. J., Orvaschel, H. & Brody, J. A. (1985). Psychiatric disorders (DSM-III) and cognitive impairment among the elderly in a US urban community. *Acta Psychiatrica Scandinavica*, **71**, 366–79.

Weyerer, S. (1983). Mental disorders among the elderly. True prevalence and use of medical services. *Archives of Gerontology and Geriatrics*, **2**, 11–22.

Williamson, J., Stokoe, I. H., Gray, S., Fisher, M., Smith, A., McGhee, A. & Stephenson, E. (1964). Old people at home: their unreported needs. *Lancet*, **i**, 1117–20.

World Health Organization (1978). *International Classification of Diseases, 1975 Revision*. World Health Organization, Geneva.

World Health Organization (1992). *The ICD-10 Classification of Mental and Behavioural Disorders. Clinical Descriptions and Diagnostic Guidelines*. World Health Organization, Division of Mental Health, Geneva.

10

What are the risk factors for dementia?

JAMES A. MORTIMER

Under normal circumstances, neurons in the human brain are incapable of mitosis after early childhood. It is indeed remarkable that an organ composed of such irreplaceable elements can continue to function with relative normality for 100 years or more. While there are various explanations for the maintenance of normal brain function in the face of neuronal damage and loss during the life course, the most important is the very high redundancy of neurons at birth. Results of lesion experiments in animals and clinicopathologic studies of humans suggest that the brain can continue to function without obvious clinical signs, following a very significant amount of cell loss and damage. For example, the clinical signs of Parkinson's disease do not become evident until the dopaminergic deficit in the striatal nuclei reaches 75% or more (Mortimer & Webster, 1982). This observation suggests that the motor disorder of Parkinson's disease is expressed only after a threshold of brain damage is reached, and that this threshold corresponds to loss of function in the great majority of dopaminergic neurons.

A similar model has been proposed to explain the onset of dementia (Mortimer, 1988). In this model, the onset of dementia symptoms is viewed as depending upon two factors: reserve capacity, a hypothetical construct related to the amount of remaining functional brain tissue; and a threshold, which corresponds to the critical amount of brain tissue at which normal cognitive function cannot be sustained. Figure 10.1 depicts three possible scenarios: A: normal brain aging, where the threshold for dementia would not be reached until an age that exceeds life expectancy; B: attainment of the dementia threshold in middle age because of an increased rate of loss of reserve capacity over the life course; and C: attainment of the dementia threshold in middle age because of a decreased reserve capacity present at birth. Of course, these are idealized cases and many other scenarios are

Dementia and Normal Aging, eds. F. A. Huppert, C. Brayne & D. W. O'Connor. © Cambridge University Press 1994.

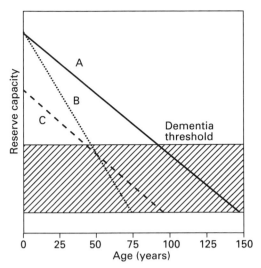

Figure 10.1. Threshold model for dementia. (A) Normal brain aging, where the threshold for dementia is not reached until after normal life expectancy. (B) Attainment of the dementia threshold in middle age because of an increased rate of loss of reserve capacity over the life course. (C) Attainment of the dementia threshold in middle age because of a decreased reserve capacity present at birth.

possible, with variable rates of loss of reserve capacity and different starting points.

The role of risk factors in reducing the reserve capacity of the brain and thereby hastening the onset of clinical dementia has been discussed for over a decade (Mortimer, 1980, 1988; Roth, 1986). Indeed, the concept of a neuropathological threshold for dementia has been around since the prospective clinicopathological studies of Tomlinson et al. (1970), which demonstrated critical levels of brain softening as well as senile plaque and neurofibrillary tangle densities beyond which dementia was usually present. More recently, Katzman et al. (1988) have shown that higher brain weights and greater numbers of large neurons in the cerebral cortex may offer some protection from dementia associated with high densities of senile plaques. The latter finding suggests that either a larger endowment of particular types of neurons at birth or a reduced loss in these neurons over the life course might offer protection from the clinical manifestations of Alzheimer's disease (AD) in old age.

A threshold model of dementia has several implications for the identification of risk factors. First, if dementia is the result of multiple causes, it will likely be difficult to identify any one etiology using case–control studies with small (<100) or even moderate (100–200) numbers of cases. The reason for this difficulty is that, in any series of dementia patients, only a fraction will be demented as a result of any particular etiology. This applies both to dementia in general and to AD in particular, and limits greatly the statistical power to identify risk factors that occur with low frequency in the population, unless they are associated very strongly with the disease under investigation (e.g. family history of AD). This concept is examined below in more detail with regard to case–control studies of AD, and it is argued that the identification of risk factors for AD probably depends very much on the statistical power of studies to identify them. A second implication of the threshold model is that exposures to risk factors should affect not only the frequency of dementia, but also the age at which clinical symptoms first occur. Data relevant to this issue are reviewed. Finally, one might expect to find significant interaction effects between risk factors, since the combination of different exposures, each of which would increase the likelihood of reaching the dementia threshold, should be more powerful than the sum of their independent effects.

Risk factors for Alzheimer's disease

Among risk factors for AD, the ones identified most consistently in research studies are chronological age, the presence of Down's syndrome (DS), family history of dementia and prior head trauma. Other risk factors meriting attention include family history of DS, previous thyroid disease, aluminum exposure, smoking and education.

Chronological age

The association with chronological age is indisputable: the incidence of both dementia and AD increases exponentially, at least through age 85 years (Hagnell et al., 1981). Furthermore, data from 47 studies summarized by Jorm et al. (1987) indicate that the prevalence of moderate to severe dementia doubles on average every 5.1 years. The association of increasing incidence and prevalence of dementia with age can be explained by a relatively simple model based on the concept shown in Figure 10.1. For simplicity, let us assume that all individuals begin life with the same reserve capacity, that reserve capacity is lost at a fixed rate per year which is distributed normally across individuals in the population, and that individuals become demented when a critical reserve capacity (threshold) is reached. Then, an exponential increase in incidence with age would be expected as individuals reach the threshold for manifesting dementia symptoms in increasing numbers, until those with the mean rate of loss of reserve capacity per year become demented. This would be followed by a leveling off and decline in the incidence rate, as the number of individuals with slower rates of decline decreases in accord with the normal distribution. The latter prediction is of some interest, since published data suggesting a leveling off or decline in the risk of dementia after age 85 years (Mortimer et al., 1981) have been interpreted to suggest that those individuals surviving to age 90 years in a non-demented state may not be susceptible. An alternative explanation is that all persons are at risk, but those surviving in a non-demented state into the tenth decade represent a minority of persons with slow rates of decline who have yet to reach the level of neuronal damage sufficient to cause dementia.

Although the size of populations which have been followed for incidence of dementia is insufficient to determine reliably whether the incidence continues to increase, levels off or declines among the very old, indirect evidence from large autopsy studies in which the prevalence of Alzheimer lesions was observed (Tomlinson & Kitchener, 1972; Peress et al., 1973; Matsuyama & Nakamura, 1978) suggests that these lesions may be less prevalent in individuals surviving into the tenth decade of life. However, the latter observation does not address the more important issue: that of changes with age in the incidence of dementia due to all causes.

Down's syndrome (DS)

Studies have shown that almost all individuals with DS who survive to at least age 40 years and come to autopsy have the lesions of AD (Figure 10.2). These data have been interpreted to suggest that all *living* DS cases have the pathological lesions of AD by this age. The observations that only a relatively small fraction of DS individuals have a clinical dementia by age 40 years and that there are many apparently non-demented individuals with DS over age 50 years (Wisniewski et al., 1985) have led to the conclusion that Alzheimer lesions by themselves do not necessarily result in dementia. Although this conclusion may be partially correct, there are two other plausible explanations. First, the density of Alzheimer lesions in some cases of DS is lower than that seen in typical cases of clinical AD (Ball & Nuttall, 1980; Wisniewski et al., 1985), suggesting that a proportion of DS individuals with Alzheimer lesions may be subthreshold for manifesting dementia symptoms. Second, DS individuals who die at a relatively young age and come to autopsy are likely to represent a biased sample. Given the lethality of AD, those individuals who die at an early age may, in fact, be those with more severe Alzheimer lesions.

Individuals with DS appear to have markedly differing susceptibilities to dementia. The expression of a clinical dementia in DS, like that in AD, seems to occur in individuals with more gray matter atrophy (Schapiro & Rapoport, 1988) and selective loss of neurons in the hippocampus (Ball et al., 1986). Thus, a reduced brain reserve capacity (fewer neurons in the hippocampus or forebrain cholinergic nuclei, for example) may be needed to produce the symptoms of dementia in DS in individuals with moderate numbers of Alzheimer lesions.

DS also offers a model for developmental risk factors for dementia. Prior to adulthood, individuals with DS show deficits in the numbers of neurons in the cerebral cortex, hippocampus and the nucleus basalis

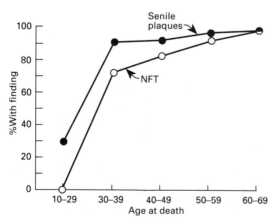

Figure 10.2. Percentage of autopsied Down's syndrome cases with senile plaques and neurofibrillary tangles (NFT) by age at death. (Reprinted by permission of Wiley-Liss, a division of John Wiley and Sons, Inc. From Mortimer & Hutton in *Senile Dementia of the Alzheimer Type.* Copyright © 1985, Wiley-Liss.)

of Meynert (Sylvester, 1983; Casanova et al., 1985; Coyle et al., 1986; Mann et al., 1987). Therefore, it may be not only the loss of such cells secondary to Alzheimer lesions that contributes to dementia in DS, but also the loss or lack of development of these cells during fetal life long before Alzheimer lesions become evident.

Family history of dementia

Together with age and DS, family history of dementia is one of the few established risk factors for AD. Aggregation of dementia of the Alzheimer's type in specific families is well documented (Nee et al., 1983), and the pattern of inheritance in these families is consistent with autosomal dominant transmission with age-dependent penetrance (Foncin et al., 1985). The degree to which these findings in particular families apply to the remainder of Alzheimer cases is unknown. Data from family studies in three clinical series suggest that approximately 50% of first-degree relatives are affected by age 90 years, consistent with autosomal dominant transmission (Breitner et al., 1988; Huff et al., 1988; Martin et al., 1988). Farrar et al. (1989), using a method that weighted likelihood of correct diagnosis of AD, estimated a cumulative risk to first-degree relatives of 24% by age 93 years.

Studies by Heston et al. (1981) and Chandra et al. (1987) suggest that blood relatives of cases with late onset (after age 70 years) may be at no higher risk of AD than the rest of the population. However, these observations are contradicted by two other studies that reported little difference in risk by age of onset (Breitner et al., 1988; Huff et al., 1988).

No population-based twin studies of AD have been completed. Therefore, firm conclusions cannot be drawn regarding concordance and discordance rates for AD in monozygotic and dizygotic pairs. In single-case studies, both concordant and discordant monozygotic twins have been described (Nee et al., 1987). The fact that well-established discordance of monozygotic twins for AD has been demonstrated suggests that factors other than genes may be involved in expression of the disease. However, the relative importance of genetic and environmental factors is unknown.

A collaborative re-analysis of data from 11 case–control studies carried out under the sponsorship of EURODEM provides additional data on the association between family history of dementia and AD (van Duijn et al., 1991b). Re-analysis of seven studies for which data

Table 10.1. *Odds ratios, 95% confidence intervals (CI) and statistical power for family history of dementia in individual studies and pooled analysis*

Study	Odds ratio[a]	95% CI	Statistical power[b]
Heyman et al. (1984)	7.2	2.7–19.1	0.99
Amaducci et al. (1986)	2.6	1.0–7.5	0.92
Chandra et al. (1987)	1.0	0.5–2.2	0.82
Shalat et al. (1987)	4.4	1.8–10.7	0.97
Hofman et al. (1989)	4.8	2.8–8.1	1.00
Broe et al. (1990)	3.8	2.1–6.9	1.00
Graves et al. (1990c)	2.5	1.4–4.4	1.00
Mean statistical power of seven studies			0.96
Pooled analysis	3.5	2.6–4.6	1.00

[a]Adjusted for age, gender, number of siblings and education.
[b]Power to identify an odds ratio of 3.5 ($\alpha = 0.05$).
Adapted from van Duijn et al. (1991a).

were available on family history revealed an adjusted pooled odds ratio for family history of dementia of 3.5 (95% confidence interval (CI): 2.6–4.6) (Table 10.1; van Duijn et al., 1991a).

Head trauma

The contribution of head trauma to Alzheimer's disease has been controversial. Following the initial demonstration of a significant association between antecedent head trauma and AD (Mortimer et al., 1983), two other studies reported a significant positive association between head trauma and AD (Heyman et al., 1984; Graves et al., 1990a) but this association was not confirmed statistically in other studies (Soininen & Heinonen, 1982; Amaducci et al., 1986; Chandra et al., 1987, 1989; Shalat et al., 1987; Broe et al., 1990; Ferini-Strambi et al., 1990).

The examination of head trauma as a risk factor for AD was stimulated initially by several observations. First, severe head trauma by itself can result in a post-traumatic encephalopathy dementia syndrome. Second, several individual-case reports have described pathologically confirmed Alzheimer's disease following a single head trauma

Table 10.2. *Odds ratios, 95% confidence intervals (CI) and statistical power for head trauma with loss of consciousness in individual studies and pooled analysis*

Study	Odds ratio[a]	95% CI	Statistical power[b]
Mortimer et al. (1985)	2.80	0.95–9.93	0.20
Amaducci et al. (1986)	2.00	0.43–12.37	0.13
Chandra et al. (1987)	6.00	0.73–276.01	0.11
Kokmen et al. (1988)	1.43	0.49–4.42	0.21
Hofman et al. (1989)	1.33	0.65–2.80	0.40
Broe et al. (1990)	1.17	0.34–4.20	0.17
Graves et al. (1990a)	2.38	0.99–6.28	0.32
Mean statistical power of seven studies			0.22
Pooled analysis	1.82	1.26–2.67	0.92

[a]Crude odds ratios.
[b]Power to identify an odds ratio of 1.82 ($\alpha = 0.05$).
Adapted from Mortimer et al. (1991).

episode (Claude & Cuel, 1939; Corsellis & Brierly, 1959; Hollander & Strich, 1970; Khaime, 1976; Rudelli et al., 1982). Finally, the syndrome of dementia pugilistica, which is characterized neuropathologically by the accumulation of neurofibrillary tangles in the cerebral cortex and brainstem, can follow a career of professional or amateur boxing (Martland, 1928; Corsellis et al., 1973; Mortimer & Pirozzolo, 1985; Roberts et al., 1990).

The EURODEM re-analysis of 11 case–control studies described above also examined head trauma with loss of consciousness (Mortimer et al., 1991). The pooled results, which were restricted to comparisons between cases and community controls in seven of the 11 studies, strongly support an association between reported severe head trauma and AD (Table 10.2; Mortimer et al., 1991). Despite the absence of significant associations within individual datasets, the pooled data demonstrated an odds ratio of 1.82 with a 95% confidence interval of 1.26 to 2.67. All studies reported odds ratios greater than one; a test for heterogeneity of effect across studies was negative. Adjustment of the odds ratio for family history of dementia, gender, age of onset, education and alcohol consumption had little effect; the odds ratio for head trauma remained positive and significant.

Two explanations for the association between head trauma and AD have been offered (Mortimer et al., 1985). First, head trauma may damage the blood–brain barrier, resulting in loss of immunological protection of brain tissue and entry of toxins and/or viruses that could have a delayed effect. Second, head trauma may damage functioning brain tissue to a degree that does not produce a detectable cognitive loss, but which reduces the functional brain reserve. Such a loss in brain reserve could shorten the time for the threshold for clinically diagnosable dementia to be reached.

Family history of Down's syndrome

The observation of an increased occurrence of DS in the families of Alzheimer patients was made originally by Heston et al. (1981), who reported a significant excess of DS cases only in the families of cases of AD with early age of onset. The association between family history of DS and AD was confirmed in case–control studies of AD by Heyman et al. (1984) and Broe et al. (1990). Other case–control studies which have examined this risk factor have not found significant associations, although this may well be due to the low statistical power of these studies, given the rare occurrence of DS in the general population. The EURODEM pooled analysis of case–control studies found a significantly elevated odds ratio for family history of DS (odds ratio: 2.7; 95% CI: 1.2–5.7), but did not find the expected difference in odds ratios by age of onset (van Duijn et al., 1991a).

Thyroid disease

An increased risk of AD in women with a history of thyroid disease was reported originally by Heyman et al. (1984). However, no other study has confirmed this positive finding, and one found an inverse association (Amaducci et al., 1986). The EURODEM pooled analysis demonstrated that a history of hypothyroidism was associated with AD (odds ratio: 2.3; 95% CI: 1.0–5.4) (Breteler et al., 1991). However, thyroid disease of any kind, hyperthyroidism and goitre had no association (Breteler et al., 1991).

Aluminum

The role of aluminum in causing AD remains controversial more than 25 years after its neurotoxicity in animals was first reported (Klatzo et al., 1965). Although most investigators agree that aluminum accumulates in neurons with neurofibrillary tangles, there is considerable disagreement whether this affinity is associated with cause or effect. Ecologic studies of the associations between aluminum concentrations in drinking water and the occurrence of Alzheimer's disease are suggestive of a possible relationship (Vogt, 1986; Flaten, 1987; Leventhal, 1987; Martyn et al., 1989). However, these studies suffered from a number of weaknesses, including incomplete or biased ascertainment of cases (e.g. based on death certificate data or medical records), reliance on residence at time of death rather than residential history (allowing for the possibility of migration from a region of low aluminum to high aluminum exposure), and limited retrospective information on aluminum concentrations for the years during which most exposure would have occurred.

Data from a recently completed study of miners in Northern Ontario provide additional evidence regarding the role of aluminum exposure in cognitive disorders of aging. Rifat et al. (1990) found a significantly higher incidence of severe cognitive impairment among miners who were exposed to repeated inhalation of aluminum powder to prevent silicosis in comparison to a control group of miners without this exposure. However, the prevalence of AD or dementia in the miners was not determined.

Individual case studies show that extreme occupational exposures to aluminum may (Kobayashi et al., 1987) or may not (McLaughlin et al., 1962) be associated with a dementia with Alzheimer lesions. Few case–control studies have collected information on exposure to aluminum-containing products. Graves et al. (1990b) reported a significantly elevated odds ratio for aluminum-containing antiperspirant use with a trend for higher risk with increased frequency of use.

Smoking

Eight of the 11 case–control studies that were re-analysed in the EURODEM study provided data for a pooled estimate of the effects of smoking (Graves et al., 1991). Although none of these studies had a significant odds ratio for lifetime prevalence of smoking, the pooled odds ratio was significant (odds ratio: 0.78; 95% CI: 0.62–0.98), suggesting that ever having smoked reduces the risk of AD (Graves et al., 1991). This association was supported by a highly significant trend of decreased risk of AD with increasing number of pack-years of smoking. Whether this inverse association with smoking represents a real effect or an artefact due to subject selection is unclear. Nicotinic binding site density, which is markedly reduced in AD patients (Whitehouse et al., 1986; Perry et al., 1987), can be increased experimentally through the administration of nicotine (Schwartz & Kellar, 1985). Conceivably, smoking could increase the number of nicotinic binding sites, delaying expression of the disease. On the other hand, cases of AD contaminated by stroke or other diseases related to smoking are likely to have been excluded from case–control studies, which would increase the possibility of finding a protective effect of smoking for AD.

Education

Recent epidemiologic studies in Shanghai (Zhang et al., 1990), East Boston, Massachusetts, USA (D. Evans, personal communication), and Italy (Bonaiuto et al., 1990) have shown an increase in the prevalence of clinically diagnosed AD with fewer years of formal education. However, this finding has not been confirmed in other populations (Brayne & Calloway, 1990; Beard et al., 1991; Knoefel et al., 1991). It is noteworthy that those populations showing this association had a large number of very poorly educated or uneducated individuals, who appeared to be at much greater risk for the disease. This suggests that factors correlated with very low education and socioeconomic status, such as perinatal nutritional deficiencies, may be responsible for the association, rather than education itself.

It is of interest that low educational attainment in addition to being associated with a higher incidence of AD is also a risk factor for other signs of accelerated aging. In a study of Roman Catholic nuns, Snowdon and coworkers demonstrated that nuns who were more poorly educated had higher rates of severe cognitive impairment, reduced motor function, greater impairment in activities of daily living, and higher mortality rates at all ages after 20 years (Snowdon et al., 1989b, c). Because the adult life style of nuns was fairly uniform regardless of educational attainment, these findings suggest that low educational attainment may be a surrogate for other risk factors present in childhood. A related finding, suggesting that education may be a marker for a risk factor influencing the rate of aging, is an association between educational attainment and age at menopause (D. A. Snowdon, personal communication). More poorly educated women experience menopause earlier, which has been shown to correlate with shorter life expectancy (Snowdon et al., 1989a). Taken together, these studies suggest that the association between education and dementia may represent only one instance of a more general association between education and the rate of biological aging.

Does the identification of risk factors for Alzheimer's disease depend on the statistical power of studies to identify them?

In the EURODEM re-analysis of data from case–control studies, odds ratios for family history of dementia were elevated significantly in six out of seven studies (Table 10.1). As shown in the last column of this table, the mean statistical power of individual studies to identify the pooled odds ratio 3.5 with an α of 0.05 was 0.96 (range: 0.82–1.00). Therefore, it should not be surprising that almost all studies confirmed this association. By contrast, the mean statistical power of individual studies to identify the pooled odds ratio for head trauma (1.82) with an α of 0.05 was only 0.22 (Table 10.2; Mortimer et al., 1991). While none of the studies in the re-analysis of head trauma had a statistically significant odds ratio, in two studies the lower bound of the 95% confidence interval was approximately 1.0. Two out of seven (28.6%) corresponds well to the expected percentage of studies to show a significant association on the basis of the power analyses (22%). A final comparison is available from examination of smoking as a risk factor for AD. Based on the pooled odds ratio of 0.78 found in the EURODEM re-analysis and an α of 0.05, the statistical power to identify this association ranged from 0.09 to 0.20 in the eight studies in which this risk factor was examined, with an average statistical power of 0.14 (Graves et al., 1991). In accord with the low statistical power, none of the studies demonstrated a significant inverse association between smoking and AD, despite the significant pooled odds ratio (Graves et al., 1991).

From these analyses, it can be argued that one of the most important determinants of the identification of risk factors in case–control studies of AD may be the statistical power of such studies to identify these risk factors. For this reason, it is important not to reject prema-

Table 10.3. *Family history of dementia and the relative risk of Alzheimer's disease by onset age*

Age of onset (years)	Relative risk[a]	95% confidence interval
≤59	4.0	2.4–6.1
60–9	5.3	2.8–10.0
70–9	2.3	1.4–3.6
80+	2.6	1.3–5.2

[a]Odds ratio adjusted for age, gender, number of siblings and education. Adapted from van Duijn et al. (1991a).

turely candidate risk factors for which statistical power may be inadequate to confirm the association. The correct conclusion to reach when statistical power is low is not that a particular study could not confirm an hypothesized association, but rather that the study lacked sufficient power either to accept or to reject the hypothesis.

Do certain exposures lower or raise the age of onset of dementia?

With regard to family history of dementia, this question might be re-phrased as follows: 'Do cases with a positive family history have an earlier age of onset than those without such a history?' This question was examined in the EURODEM re-analysis by estimating the relative risk of AD by age of onset (Table 10.3). As shown in this table, the highest relative risk applied to individuals aged 60 to 69 years. Individuals over age 70 years had somewhat lower, though statistically significant, relative risks. These findings are suggestive of a trend towards lower relative risk for family history of dementia with increased age of onset, although the trend is not uniform.

Two recent studies have reported that cases of AD with a history of severe head trauma had a significantly earlier mean age of onset than cases without such a history (Sullivan et al., 1987; Gedye et al., 1989). This observation is consistent with a reduction of brain reserve capacity following the head trauma episode, leading to onset of dementia at an earlier age. However, among the 1059 cases of AD in the EURODEM re-analysis, there was no statistically significant difference in mean age of onset between cases with and without a history of head trauma (Mortimer et al., 1991). For familial cases, the mean age of onset was actually slightly higher for cases with head trauma than without (67.3 vs. 66.1 years, $t = 0.52$, $p = 0.60$). A similar trend was seen for sporadic cases (66.6 vs. 64.5 years, $t = 1.14$, $p = 0.25$).

In the EURODEM re-analysis, no difference in relative risk of AD by family history of Down's syndrome was seen when cases were stratified by age of onset (<65 years, >65 years) (van Duijn et al., 1991a), suggesting that blood relatives of DS cases do not necessarily experience an earlier onset of disease, contrary to previous observations (Heston et al., 1981). The EURODEM re-analysis of case–control studies also showed that smokers on average had an earlier age of onset than non-smokers (Graves et al., 1991), in the opposite direction from that expected from the hypothesis that smoking offers protection by increasing the number of nicotinic receptor sites.

In general, the findings regarding modification of age of onset by specific risk factors (familial susceptibility to dementia and DS, severe head trauma, smoking) are either negative or mixed. These findings offer little support for a simple threshold model in which the age of onset is decreased or increased by exposures with hypothesized effects on brain reserve capacity.

Is there evidence for an interaction between risk factors in increasing the risk of Alzheimer's disease?

If AD is due to a combination of risk factors, one might expect to find significant interactions between these risk factors. Such a finding would support a threshold model in which each risk factor exposure would move an individual closer to the threshold, making dementia more likely to occur following another exposure. An alternative possibility is that AD is caused by a variety of risk factors, which act independently rather than in concert.

The EURODEM re-analysis of the association between head trauma and AD (Mortimer et al., 1991) provides some insight into this issue. When AD cases were divided into those with a positive family history (familial cases) and those without such a history (sporadic cases), analyses of these strata showed odds ratios for head trauma of 1.42 (95% CI: 0.76–2.71) for familial cases and 2.31 (95% CI: 1.17–4.84) for sporadic cases. Although the difference in these odds ratios was not statistically significant ($\chi^2 = 1.17$, $p = 0.30$), the trend was for head trauma to have a larger effect among individuals without a family history of dementia. The possibility that a family history of dementia may increase or decrease the susceptibility to AD following a head trauma episode was then investigated by including an interaction term for family history and head trauma in a conditional logistic regression model together with the main effects of family history and head trauma. In this analysis, the main effects of both family history of dementia and head trauma remained significant, and no further variance was explained by the interaction ($\chi^2 = 0.00$, $R^2 = 0.00$, p = 0.98). The findings that head trauma and family history of dementia explain individual components of the variance, and that family history of dementia does not increase the susceptibility to AD following a head trauma episode, suggest that these risk factors represent independent causal pathways. Little support is provided for a cumulative effects model.

Cognitive decline and vascular risk factors

That vascular and Alzheimer lesions overlap frequently is evident from the clinicopathologic study of Tomlinson et al. (1970). Nineteen of their 25 cases receiving a final pathologic diagnosis of AD had mild to moderate vascular lesions. In 10% of the demented cases in this study, there were insufficient numbers of lesions to satisfy pathologic criteria for either Alzheimer's disease or vascular dementia. The dementia in these cases apparently resulted from a summation of the effects of both types of lesions. The contribution of vascular lesions to Alzheimer dementia is also evident in studies relating computerized tomography (CT) findings to clinical severity. Steingart et al. (1987) reported that the presence of white matter lucency of leukoaraiosis on CT was predictive of more severe dementia in patients with clinically diagnosed AD. Leukoaraiosis is correlated strongly with a history of hypertension (Steingart et al., 1987) and stroke (Inzitari et al., 1987), both risk factors for vascular dementias. Thus, there is ample evidence suggesting that Alzheimer and vascular lesions may combine to increase the risk and severity of dementia, as one would expect from a threshold model.

Conclusions

Dementia is likely to be the result of several different causes, some of which may not have been identified as yet because of low statistical power of extant case–control studies. In most case–control studies of Alzheimer's disease, cases were selected to comply with rigorous criteria, and therefore may be poorly representative of dementia cases in general, where multiple disease processes are likely to contribute to the cognitive impairment. For AD itself, existing data suggest that several risk factors are involved, but simple extrapolations from a threshold model, such as reduction in age of onset by specific exposures or a cumulative effect of risk factors manifested by significant inter-action effects, are not well supported by the data. One possibility is that there may be different types of AD. Because of the manner in which cases were selected in case–control studies, the type seen in very old age (when a threshold model may be more applicable) has not been well studied. The mean age of onset in most case–control studies is in the early 70s. At this age or earlier, one or another risk factor may play a dominant role. A better test of the threshold model of dementia would be provided by a study restricted to cases with age of onset over 80 years where rigorous exclusion criteria were not applied. Such a study has not yet been performed.

References

Amaducci, L. A., Fratiglioni, L., Rocca, W. A., Fieschi, C., Livrea, P., Pedone, D., Bracco, L., Lippi, A., Gandolfo, C., Bino, G., Prencipe, M., Bonatti, M. L., Girotti, F., Carella, F., Tavalato, B., Ferla, S., Lenzi, G. L., Carolei, A., Gambi, A., Grigoletto, F. & Schoenberg, B. S. (1986). Risk factors for clinically diagnosed Alzheimer's disease: a case–control study of an Italian population. *Neurology*, **36**, 922–31.

Ball, M. J. & Nuttall, K. (1980). Neurofibrillary tangles, granulovacuolar degeneration, and neuron loss in Down syndrome: quantitative comparison with Alzheimer dementia. *Annals of Neurology*, 7, 460–5.

Ball, M. J., Schapiro, M. B. & Rapoport, S. I. (1986). Neuropathological relationships between Down syndrome and senile dementia Alzheimer type. In C. J. Epstein (ed.), *The Neurobiology of Down Syndrome*, pp. 45–58. New York, Raven Press.

Beard, C. M., Kokmen, E., Offord, K. P. & Kurland, L. T. (1991). Lack of association of Alzheimer's disease with education, occupation and marital status. *Neurology*, **41**, (supplement 1), 307.

Bonaiuto, S., Rocca, W. A. & Lippi, A. (1990). Impact of education and occupation on the prevalence of Alzheimer's disease (AD) and multi-infarct dementia (MID) in Appignano, Macerata Province, Italy. *Neurology*, **40**, (supplement 1), 346.

Brayne, C. & Calloway, P. (1990). The association of education and socioeconomic status with the Mini Mental State Examination and the clinical diagnosis of dementia in elderly people. *Age and Ageing*, **19**, 91–6.

Breitner, J. C. S., Silverman, J. M., Mohs, R. C. & Davis, K. L. (1988). Familial aggregation in Alzheimer's disease: comparison of risk among relatives of early- and late-onset cases, and among male and female relatives in successive generations. *Neurology*, **38**, 207–12.

Breteler, M. M. B., van Duijn, C. M., Chandra, V., Fratiglioni, L., Graves, A. B., Heyman, A., Jorm, A. F., Kokmen, E., Kondo, K., Mortimer, J. A., Rocca, W. A., Shalat, S., Soininen, H. & Hofman, A. (1991). Medical history and the risk of Alzheimer's disease: a collaborative re-analysis of case–control studies. *International Journal of Epidemiology*, **20**, (supplement 2), S36–S42.

Broe, G. A., Henderson, A. S., Creasey, H., McCusker, E., Korten, A. E., Jorm, A. F., Longley, W. & Anthony, J. C. (1990). A case–control study of Alzheimer's disease in Australia. *Neurology*, **40**, 1698–707.

Casanova, M. F., Walker, L. C., Whitehouse, P. J. & Price, D. L. (1985). Abnormalities of the nucleus basalis in Down's syndrome. *Annals of Neurology*, **18**, 310–13.

Chandra, V., Philipose, V., Bell, P. A., Lazaroff, A. & Schoenberg, B. S. (1987). Case–control study of late onset 'probable Alzheimer's disease'. *Neurology*, **37**, 1295–300.

Chandra, V., Kokmen, E., Schoenberg, B. S. & Beard, C. M. (1989). Head trauma with loss of consciousness as a risk factor for Alzheimer's disease. *Neurology*, **39**, 1576–8.

Claude, H. & Cuel, J. (1939). Démence pre-sénile post-traumatique après fracture de crane: considérations médicos-légales. *Annales Médico-Légales*, **19**, 173–84.

Corsellis, J. A. N. & Brierly, J. B. (1959). Observations on the pathology of insidious dementia following head injury. *Journal of Mental Science*, **105**, 714–20.

Corsellis, J. A. N., Bruton, C. J. & Freeman-Browne, D. (1973). The aftermath of boxing. *Psychological Medicine*, **3**, 270–303.

Coyle, J. T., Oster-Granite, M. L. & Gearhart, J. D. (1986). The neurobiologic consequences of Down syndrome. *Brain Research Bulletin*, **16**, 733–87.

Farrar, L. A., O'Sullivan, D. M., Cupples, A., Growdon, J. H. & Myers, R. H. (1989). Assessment of genetic risk for Alzheimer's disease among first-degree relatives. *Annals of Neurology*, **25**, 485–93.

Ferini-Strambi, L., Smirne, S., Garancini, P., Pinto, P. & Franceshi, M. (1990). Clinical and epidemiological aspects of Alzheimer's disease with presenile onset: a case–control study. *Neuroepidemiology*, **9**, 39–49.

Flaten, T. P. (1987). 'Geographical association between aluminum in drinking water and registered death rates with dementia (including Alzheimer's disease) in Norway'. In Proceedings from the Second International Symposium on Geochemistry and Health, Science Reviews.

Foncin, J. F., Salmon, D., Supino-Viterbo, V., Feldman, R. G., Macchi, G., Mariotti, P., Scoppetta, G., Caruso, C. & Bruni, A. C. (1985). Démence présénile d'Alzheimer transmise dans une famile entendue. *Revue Neurologique*, **141**, 194–202.

Gedye, A., Bettie, B. L., Tuokko, H., Horton, A. & Korsarek, E. (1989). Severe head injury hastens age of onset of Alzheimer's disease. *Journal of the American Geriatrics Society*, **37**, 970–3.

Graves, A. B., White, E., Koepsell, T. D., Reifler, B. V., van Belle, G. & Larson, E. B. (1990a). The association between aluminum-containing products and Alzheimer's disease. *Journal of Clinical Epidemiology*, **43**, 35–44.

Graves, A. B., White, E., Koepsell, T. D., Reifler, B. V., van Belle, G., Larson, E. B. & Raskind, M. (1990b). A case–control study of Alzheimer's disease. *Annals of Neurology*, **28**, 140–8.

Graves, A. B., White, E., Koepsell, T. D., Reifler, B. V., van Belle, G., Larson, E. B. & Raskind, M. (1990c). The association between head trauma and Alzheimer's disease. *American Journal of Epidemiology*, **131**, 491–501.

Graves, A. B., van Duijn, C. M., Chandra, V., Fratiglioni, L., Heyman, A., Jorm, A. F., Kokmen, E., Kondo, K., Mortimer, J. A., Rocca, W. A., Shalat, S., Soininen, H. & Hofman, A. (1991). Alcohol and tobacco consumption as risk factors for Alzheimer's disease: a collaborative re-analysis of case–control studies. *International Journal of Epidemiology*, **20** (supplement 2), S48–S57.

Hagnell, O., Lanke, J., Rorsman, B. & Ojesjo, L. (1981). Does the incidence of age psychosis decrease? A prospective, longitudinal study of a complete population investigated during the 25-year period 1947–1972: the Lundby study. *Neuropsychobiology*, **7**, 201–11.

Heston, L. L., Mastri, A. R., Anderson, V. E. & White, J. (1981). Dementia of the Alzheimer type: clinical genetics, natural history, and associated conditions. *Archives of General Psychiatry*, **38**, 1085–90.

Heyman, A., Wilkinson, W. E., Stafford, J. A., Helms, M. J., Sigmon, A. H. & Weinberg, T. (1984). Alzheimer's disease: a study of the epidemiological aspects. *Annals of Neurology*, **15**, 335–41.

Hofman, A., Schulte, W., Tanja, T. A., van Duijn, C. M., Haaxma, R., Lameris, A. J., Otten, V. M. & Saan, R. J. (1989). History of dementia and Parkinson's disease in first-degree relatives of patients with Alzheimer's disease. *Neurology*, **39**, 1589–92.

Hollander, D. & Strich, S. J. (1970). Atypical Alzheimer's disease with congophilic angiopathy presenting with dementia of acute onset. In G. E. W. Wolstenholme & M. O'Connor (eds.) *Alzheimer's Disease and Related Disorders*, pp. 105–24. Churchill, London.

Huff, F. J., Auerbach, J., Chakravarti, A. & Boller, F. (1988). Risk of dementia in relatives of patients with Alzheimer's disease. *Neurology*, **38**, 786–90.

Inzitari, D., Diaz, F., Fox, A., Hachinski, V. C., Steingart, A., Lau, C., Donald, A., Wade, J., Mulic, H. & Merskey, H. (1987). Vascular risk factors and leuko-araiosis. *Archives of Neurology*, **44**, 42–7.

Jorm, A. F., Korten, A. E. & Henderson, A. S. (1987). The prevalence of dementia: a quantitative integration of the literature. *Acta Psychiatrica Scandinavica*, **76**, 456–79.

Katzman, R., Terry, R., DeTeresa, R., Brown, T., Davies, P., Fuld, P., Renbing, X. & Peck, A. (1988). Clinical, pathological, and neurochemical changes in dementia: a subgroup with preserved mental status and numerous neocortical plaques. *Annals of Neurology*, **23**, 138–44.

Khaime, T. S. B. (1976). Role of craniocerebral trauma in the development of Alzheimer's disease. *Zhurnal Nevropatogii i Psikhaitrii*, **76**, 1028–32.

Klatzo, I., Wisniewski, H. & Streicher, E. (1965). Experimental production of neurofibrillary degeneration. Light microscopic observations. *Journal of Neuropathology and Experimental Neurology*, **24**, 187–99.

Knoefel, J. E., Wolf, P. A., Linn, R. T., Bachman, D. L., Cobb, J., Belanger, A. & D'Agostino, R. (1991). Education has no effect on incidence of dementia and Alzheimer's disease in the Framingham study. *Neurology*, **41**, (supplement 1), 322–3.

Kobayashi, S., Hirota, N., Sito, K. & Utsuyama, M. (1987). Aluminum accumulation in tangle-bearing neurons of Alzheimer's disease with Balint's syndrome in a long-term aluminum refiner. *Acta Neuropathologica*, **74**, 47–52.

Kokmen, E., Chandra, V. & Schoenberg, B. S. (1988). Trends in incidence of dementing illness in Rochester, Minnesota, in three quinquennial periods, 1960–1974. *Neurology*, **38**, 975–80.

Leventhal, G. H. (1987). 'Alzheimer's disease and environmental aluminum in Maryville and Morristown, Tennessee'. Unpublished doctoral dissertation, University of Tennessee.

Mann, D. M. A., Yates, P. O., Marcyniuk, B. & Ravindra, C. R. (1987). Loss of neurones from cortical and subcortical areas in Down's syndrome patients at middle age: quantitative comparisons with younger Down's patients and patients with Alzheimer's disease. *Journal of the Neurological Sciences*, **80**, 79–89.

Martin, R. L., Gerteis, G. & Gabrielli, W. F. (1988). A family-genetic study of dementia of Alzheimer type. *Archives of General Psychiatry*, **45**, 894–900.

Martland, H. S. (1928). Punch drunk. *Journal of the American Medical Association*, **91**, 1103–7.

Martyn, C. N., Osmond, C., Edwardson, J. A., Barker, D. J. P., Harris, E. C. & Lacey, R. F. (1989). Geographical relation between Alzheimer's disease and aluminum in drinking water. *Lancet*, **1**, 59–62.

Matsuyama, H. & Nakamura, S. (1978). Senile changes in the brain in the Japanese; incidence of Alzheimer's neurofibrillary change and senile plaques. In R. Katzman, R. D. Terry & K. L. Bick (eds.) *Alzheimer's Disease: Senile Dementia and Related Disorders*, pp. 287–97. Raven Press, New York.

McLaughlin, A. I. G., Kazantzis, G., King, E., Teare, D., Porter, R. J. & Owen, R. (1962). Pulmonary fibrosis and encephalopathy associated with the inhalation of aluminum dust. *British Journal of Industrial Medicine*, **19**, 253–63.

Mortimer, J. A. (1980). Epidemiologic aspects of Alzheimer's disease. In G. J. Maletta & F. J. Pirozzolo (eds.) *The Aging Nervous System*, pp. 307–32. Praeger, New York.

Mortimer, J. A. (1988). Do psychosocial risk factors contribute to Alzheimer's disease? In A. S. Henderson & J. H. Henderson (eds.) *Etiology of Dementia of Alzheimer's Type*, pp. 39–52. John Wiley and Sons, Chichester.

Mortimer, J. A. & Webster, D. D. (1982). Comparison of extrapyramidal motor function in normal aging and Parkinson's disease. In J. A. Mortimer, F. J. Pirozollo & G. J. Maletta (eds) *The Aging Motor System*, pp. 217–41. Praeger, New York.

Mortimer, J. A. & Hutton, J. T. (1985). The epidemiology and etiology of Alzheimer's disease. In J. T. Hutton & A. D. Kenny (eds.) *Senile Dementia of the Alzheimer Type*, pp. 177–96. Alan R. Liss, Inc., New York.

Mortimer, J. A. & Pirozzolo, F. J. (1985). Remote effects of head trauma. *Developmental Neuropsychology*, **1**, 215–29.

Mortimer, J. A., Schuman, L. M. & French, L. R. (1981). Epidemiology of dementing illness. In J. A. Mortimer & L. M. Schuman (eds.) *The Epidemiology of Dementia*, pp. 3–23. Oxford University Press, New York and Oxford.

Mortimer, J. A., French, L. R., Hutton, J. T., Schuman, L. M., Christians, B. & Boatman, R. A. (1983). Reported head trauma in an epidemiologic study of Alzheimer's disease. *Neurology*, **33**, (supplement 2), 85.

Mortimer, J. A., French, L. R., Hutton, J. T. & Schuman, L. M. (1985). Head trauma as a risk factor for Alzheimer's disease. *Neurology*, **35**, 264–7.

Mortimer, J. A., van Duijn, C. M., Chandra, V., Fratiglioni, L., Graves, A. B., Heyman, A., Jorm, A. F., Kokmen, E., Kondo, K., Rocca, W. A., Shalat, S., Soininen, H. & Hofman, A. (1991). Head trauma as a risk factor for Alzheimer's disease: a collaborative re-analysis of case–control studies. *International Journal of Epidemiology*, **20**, (supplement 2), S28–S35.

Nee, L. E., Polinsky, R. J., Eldridge, R., Weingartner, H., Smallberg, S. & Ebert, M. (1983). A family with histologically confirmed Alzheimer's disease. *Archives of Neurology*, **40**, 203–8.

Nee, L. E., Eldridge, R., Sunderland, T., Thomas, C. B., Katz, D., Thompson, K. E., Weingartner, H., Weiss, H., Julian, C. & Cohen, R. (1987). Dementia of the Alzheimer type: clinical and family study of 22 twin pairs. *Neurology*, **37**, 359–63.

Peress, N. S., Kane, W. C. & Aronson, S. M. (1973). Central nervous system findings in a tenth decade autopsy population. In D. H. Ford (ed.) *Neurobiological Aspects of Maturation and Aging*, pp. 473–83. Elsevier, Amsterdam.

Perry, E. K., Perry, R., Smith, C. J., Dick, D. J., Candy, J. M., Edwardson, J. A., Fairbairn, A. & Blessed, G. (1987). Nicotinic receptor abnormalities in Alzheimer's and Parkinson's disease. *Journal of Neurology, Neurosurgery and Psychiatry*, **50**, 806–9.

Rifat, S. L., Eastwood, M. R., McLachlan, D. R. & Corey, P. N. (1990). Effect of exposure of miners to aluminum powder. *Lancet*, **336**, 1162–5.

Roberts, G. W., Allsop, D. & Bruton, C. (1990). The occult aftermath of boxing. *Journal of Neurology, Neurosurgery and Psychiatry*, **53**, 373–8.

Roth, M. (1986). The association of clinical and neuropsychological findings and its bearings on the classification and aetiology of Alzheimer's disease. *British Medical Bulletin*, **42**, 42–50.

Rudelli, R., Strom, J. O., Welch, P. T. & Ambler, M. W. (1982). Posttraumatic premature Alzheimer's disease. Neuropathologic findings and pathogenetic considerations. *Archives of Neurology*, **39**, 570–5.

Schapiro, M. B. & Rapoport, S. I. (1988). Alzheimer's disease in premorbidly normal and Down's syndrome individuals: selective involvement of hippocampus and neocortical associative brain regions. *Brain Dysfunction*, **1**, 2–11.

Schwartz, R. D. & Kellar, K. J. (1985). In vivo regulation of (3H) acetylcholine recognition sites in brain by nicotinic cholinergic drugs. *Journal of Neurochemistry*, **45**, 427–33.

Shalat, S. L., Seltzer, B., Pidcock, C. & Baker, E. I. (1987). Risk factors for Alzheimer's disease: a case–control study. *Neurology*, **37**, 1630–3.

Snowdon, D. A., Kane, R. L., Beeson, W. L., Burke, G. L., Sprafka, J. M., Potter, J., Iso, H. & Jacobs, D. R. (1989a). Is early natural menopause a biological marker of health and aging? *American Journal of Public Health*, **79**, 709–15.

Snowdon, D. A., Ostwald, S. K. & Kane, R. L. (1989b). Education, survival, and independence of elderly Catholic sisters, 1936–1988. *American Journal of Epidemiology*, **130**, 999–1012.

Snowdon, D. A., Ostwald, S. K., Kane, R. L. & Keenan, N. L. (1989c). Years of life with good and poor mental and physical function in the elderly. *Journal of Clinical Epidemiology*, **42**, 1055–66.

Soininen, H. & Heinonen, O. P. (1982). Clinical and etiological aspects of senile dementia. *European Neurology*, **21**, 401–10.

Steingart, A., Hachinski, V. C., Lau, C., Fox, A. J., Fox, H., Lee, D., Inzitari, D. & Merskey, H. (1987). Cognitive and neurologic findings in demented patients with diffuse white matter lucencies on computed tomographic scan (leuko-araiosis). *Archives of Neurology*, **44**, 36–9.

Sullivan, P., Petitti, D. & Barbaccia, J. (1987). Head trauma and age of onset of dementia of the Alzheimer type. *Journal of the American Medical Association*, **257**, 2289.

Sylvester, P. E. (1983). The hippocampus in Down's syndrome. *Journal of Mental Deficiency Research*, **27**, 227–36.

Tomlinson, B. E. & Kitchener, D. (1972). Granulovacuolar degeneration of hippocampal pyramidal cells. *Journal of Pathology*, **106**, 165–85.

Tomlinson, B. E., Blessed, G. & Roth, M. (1970). Observations on the brains of demented old people. *Journal of the Neurological Sciences*, **11**, 205–42.

van Duijn, C. M., Clayton, D., Chandra, V., Fratiglioni, L., Graves, A. B., Heyman, A., Jorm, A. F., Kokmen, E., Kondo, K., Mortimer, J. A., Rocca, W. A., Shalat, S., Soininen, H. & Hofman, A. (1991a). Familial aggregation of Alzheimer's disease and related disorders: a collaborative re-analysis of case–control studies. *International Journal of Epidemiology*, **20**, (supplement 2), S13–S20.

van Duijn, C. M., Stijnen, R. & Hofman, A. (1991b). Risk factors for Alzheimer's disease: overview of the EURODEM collaborative re-analysis of case–control studies. *International Journal of Epidemiology*, **20**, (supplement 2), S4–S12.

Vogt, T. (1986). 'A study of the relationship between aluminum in drinking water and Alzheimer's disease in southern Norway'. Presented at the Second Conference of the Society for Human Ecology. Bar Harbor, Maine.

Whitehouse, P. J., Martino, A. M., Antuono, P. G., Lowenstein, P. R., Coyle,

J. T., Price, D. L. & Kellar, K. J. (1986). Nicotinic acetylcholine binding sites in Alzheimer's disease. *Brain Research*, **371**, 146–51.

Wisniewski, K. E., Wisniewski, H. M. & Wen, G. Y. (1985). Occurrence of neuropathological changes and dementia of Alzheimer's disease in Down's syndrome. *Annals of Neurology*, **17**, 278–82.

Zhang, M., Katzman, R., Jin, H., Cai, G., Wang, Z., Qu, G., Grant, I., Yu, E., Levy, P. & Liu, W. T. (1990). The prevalence of dementia and Alzheimer's disease (AD) in Shanghai, China: impact of age, gender, and education. *Annals of Neurology*, **27**, 428–37.

11

How do risk factors for dementia relate to current theories on mechanisms of aging?

THOMAS B. L. KIRKWOOD

The aim of this chapter is to review current ideas about the mechanisms that cause human aging, and to examine what these ideas can tell us about the relationship between dementia and 'normal' aging. At the outset, we might note that there is considerable uncertainty about what precisely defines aging. In the 1950s, Medawar commented: 'Nothing is clearer evidence of the immaturity of gerontological science than the tentative and probationary character of its system of definitions and measurements' (Medawar (1955), p. 4). Many authors have addressed this issue subsequently (e.g. Medawar, 1955; Maynard Smith, 1962; Strehler, 1977; Kirkwood, 1985; Arking, 1991), yet, in spite of considerable clarification, there remains sufficient lack of consensus that the author of a recent textbook of gerontology preferred to avoid the use of the word 'aging' altogether (see Finch (1990) p. 5). It is hardly surprising, therefore, that the relationship between aging and disease remains a matter for ongoing debate (e.g. Brody & Schneider, 1986; Evans, 1988; von Drass & Blumenthal, 1992).

A definition that serves our purposes here is to regard aging as a 'process of progressive, generalized impairment of function, resulting in an increasing age-specific death rate'. An advantage of this definition is that it combines the ideas of aging as both a process and an attribute. The definition touches on those aspects of the process of aging that conform most closely to everyday experience, namely, the association of aging with degenerative change resulting eventually in death, yet it leaves open the details of the process, especially its underlying causes. As an attribute, aging is identified through possession of an increasing age-specific death rate. This is an attribute of populations, since it is best seen when the survival curve for the population is plotted as a

Dementia and Normal Aging, eds. F. A. Huppert, C. Brayne & D. W. O'Connor. © Cambridge University Press 1994.

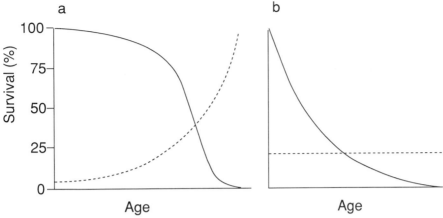

Figure 11.1. (a) Typical survival curve for a population that exhibits aging: the continuous line shows the percentage who survived expressed as a function of age, the dashed line shows the increasing age-specific death rate (scale not defined). (b) Survival curve for a population that does not show aging; the age-specific death rate is constant and survival declines exponentially. In practice, many species exhibit the a-type survival curve only when raised in protected environments; in the wild, survival resembles typically the b-type curve.

function of chronological age (see Figure 11.1). For the individual, the effect is an increasing probability of death. The value of this actuarial definition of aging is that it provides a diagnostic criterion by which to judge whether or not a species exhibits aging, and to compare the rates of aging among different populations (species, genotypes, etc). Some species (e.g. sea anemones) do not show an increase in age-specific death rates (see Comfort, 1979; Finch, 1990), and, apparently, these species do not senesce. This is important when we consider the reasons why aging occurs in other animals, for it tells us that senescence is not due to some wholly unavoidable process of biological wear-and-tear. If a sea anemone can maintain its tissues indefinitely through processes of renewal and repair, why not a human?

Why aging occurs

It is important to understand why aging occurs because there are in principle many ways in which it might be caused, and this plurality of possible causes has spawned a bewildering array of mechanistic theories. During aging, almost every character of the body undergoes some form of change. Many of these changes will be secondary rather than primary events, and a major problem is to devise ways of disentangling causes from consequences. The way that we answer the 'why?' question will influence the types of mechanisms we should look for experimentally. For instance, should we seek genes that regulate the aging process actively, like the genes that govern development of an embryo, or does aging occur merely because the organism is not programmed for long-term survival? To answer the 'why?' question satisfactorily requires that we approach the problem from an evolutionary point of view and attempt to understand the ways through which natural selection has shaped a process that, from the standpoint of the individual, is clearly disadvantageous.

A popular explanation for the evolution of aging is that senescence provides a mechanism for a species to guard against overcrowding and to provide living space for new generations (e.g. Wynne-Edwards, 1962; Beutler, 1986). This adaptive view supports the notion that senescence is a programmed process under active genetic control, and that genes have evolved specifically to cause aging. Despite the popularity of this view, there are compelling reasons why it is unsound. First, mortality in wild populations is usually so great that individuals rarely live long enough to show clear signs of senescence (Medawar, 1952). Secondly, for aging to have arisen in this way would have required that selection for advantage to the species or group was stronger than selection at the level of the individual for the advantages of a longer life. The conditions under which selection at the group level can outweigh selection at the level of the individual are stringent (Maynard Smith, 1976), and it is unlikely that they apply to the evolution of aging (Kirkwood, 1985).

If aging is not directly beneficial, then its evolution needs to be understood in terms of the indirect action of natural selection. Two broad approaches to this problem can be distinguished (see Kirkwood & Rose, 1991). The first delineates the way in which selection acts on genes with age-specific times of action to produce an accumulation of late deleterious effects. The second examines the optimum investment in the maintenance of somatic (i.e. non-reproductive) parts of the organism and demonstrates that this optimum is less than is required for indefinite survival.

The force of natural selection (that is, its ability to discriminate between alternative genotypes) weakens progressively with advancing age (Haldane, 1941; Medawar, 1952; Williams, 1957; Hamilton, 1966; Charlesworth, 1980). This happens because, at older ages, fewer individuals remain alive, whether or not the species exhibits senescence.

The upshot is that there is only loose genetic control over the later stages of the life span. If germ-line mutations occur which give rise to deleterious effects late in life, there is little or no selection to eliminate the mutations from the population. Similarly, if genes have pleiotropic effects such that they produce favourable effects early in life, but have deleterious consequences later, they will be selected for on the basis of their early benefits with scant regard to their delayed side-effects. Either or both of these types of genes can accumulate within the genome, and, in individuals who escape earlier death from accidental causes or in protected populations, aging and death may result from the combined expression of the late-acting deleterious gene effects (Medawar, 1952; Williams, 1957). This defines a general route by which senescence is expected to arise within a population, although the theory is not specific about the kinds of deleterious processes which may be involved.

The second evolutionary approach is more specific about the nature of aging processes. In a fundamental sense, organisms can be regarded as objects that take up resources from their environment and utilize these resources both to survive and to reproduce. This poses the problem of how best to divide the resources between, on the one hand, keeping the individual alive through ongoing maintenance, and, on the other hand, producing genetic copies to secure continuance of the genes when individuals die. Given the hazard of accidental death, to which no species is entirely immune, each individual has only a finite expectation of life, even in the absence of senescence. When the individual dies, the resources invested in the maintenance of its soma are lost. Too low an investment in the prevention or repair of somatic damage is obviously a mistake because then the individual may disintegrate too soon. However, too high an investment in maintenance is also wasteful because there is no advantage in maintaining the soma better than is necessary to survive the expected lifetime in the wild environment in reasonably sound condition. Therefore, fitness is maximized at a level of investment in somatic maintenance which is less than would be required for indefinite survival.

This conclusion is the basis for the disposable soma theory of aging (Kirkwood, 1977, 1981; Kirkwood & Holliday, 1979), named for its analogy with disposable goods that are manufactured with limited investment in durability on the principle that they have a short expected duration of use. The disposable soma theory has important implications concerning the mechanisms of aging for it supports strongly the view that aging results from the accumulation of random somatic defects (see below). In this sense, the theory reconciles the apparent wear-and-tear nature of senescence with the action of genetic factors, for it suggests that aging results from selection to tune the investments in key cell-maintenance processes to levels that are high enough to ensure that the organism remains in sound condition through its natural expectation of life in the wild environment, but not so high as to be wasteful.

Genetic factors in aging

The evolutionary theories give broad insights into the genetic factors that control lifespan. In the disposable soma theory, selection acts on the genes that regulate the key mechanisms of somatic maintenance in such a way as to secure the optimum balance between surviving long enough and spending too much on maintenance. A simple model illustrates how this results in the control of the rate of aging.

Consider a specific type of maintenance, e.g. DNA repair, and suppose that the rate of incidence of DNA damage is a constant. By increasing or decreasing the rate at which new DNA defects are corrected, the rate at which DNA damage accumulates is altered correspondingly. This, in turn, influences the time taken for defects to build up to a level that causes cellular dysfunction, and eventually senescence and death. The more active the DNA repair process, the more energy is expended (Galas et al., 1986).

Now if we recall that in the disposable soma theory it is the presence of environmental mortality that makes it not worthwhile to invest in better maintenance than is needed to preserve somatic functions through the normal expectation of life in the wild, we see that it is the level of environmental mortality that imposes the selection for a longer or shorter lifespan. A species subject to high environmental mortality will do better not to invest heavily in somatic maintenance, and should concentrate instead on more rapid and prolific maintenance. A species subject to low environmental mortality may profit by doing the reverse.

An important feature of this argument is its generality. Each somatic maintenance function that requires metabolic energy for its operation is subject to similar tuning. This conclusion is important, for it tells us that we should not expect to find a single cause of aging. Rather, we must anticipate that the evolutionary process will tune the network of somatic maintenance functions so that each component mechanism secures roughly the same duration of life.

So far, we have considered only the disposable soma theory in relation to genetic control of aging. The more general theories of Medawar (1952) and Williams (1957) admit the possibility of other genetic factors, in addition to those regulating somatic maintenance. In the case of Williams' theory, these would be pleiotropic genes that have beneficial effects early in life at the expense of deleterious effects later. In the case of Medawar's theory, these might simply be deleterious genes that act so late as to be beyond the reach of selection. Since neither theory specifies the nature of the genes in any detail, it is not possible to make further inference at this stage about their implications for mechanisms of aging.

Mechanisms of aging

A wide variety of specific mechanisms of aging postulating damage to cells and tissues has been proposed (for reviews, see Warner et al., 1987; Finch, 1990; Arking, 1991). Much interest has focused recently on the role of oxygen radicals as a source of widespread damage to cells, and in particular to mitochondria (e.g. see Saul et al., 1987; Linnane et al., 1989). The role of DNA damage has also been studied extensively (e.g. see Hanawalt, 1987; Vijg, 1990), as has the role of abnormal proteins (e.g. see Adelman & Roth, 1983; Rosenberger, 1991). While evidence has been adduced in support of each of these (and other) theories, their precise contributions (if any) to the aging process have not yet been established.

A long-standing debate about aging has been concerned with the relative importance of programmed events versus the kinds of stochastic damage just considered. The absence of evolutionary support for the idea that aging is programmed as an overall process to terminate the life of an organism weakens the case for programme theories at the mechanistic level. Nevertheless, it is known that programmed cell death (apoptosis) is essential in development and during haemopoiesis, and it appears that active genetic controls on DNA synthesis and cell division play a part in the limited cell proliferation of fibroblast cultures that are used commonly as a model of cell aging (Smith, 1990; Ning & Pereira-Smith, 1991). It is difficult to sustain the argument that apoptosis or programmed cell aging are primary causes for the aging of the organism, but it is quite possible that they contribute, perhaps extensively, to senescence as secondary consequences of stochastic damage to cells. For instance, a cell that is normally prevented from apoptosis by a signal from outside will die if the ability to receive and transduce the signal appropriately is compromised by damage. Such a process could even be adaptive if it serves to bring about the suicide and replacement of a defective cell, though this is less likely to be of benefit in a post-mitotic organ (e.g. the brain), than in a tissue with cell turnover. Taken to an extreme, one could imagine a scenario where active cell death is the major, outward sign of senescence, while stochastic damage is the pervasive, underlying cause (see Kirkwood, 1991).

Timing of senescent changes

The coordinate development of senescent changes in the various organs of the body is seen often as evidence for the existence of a pacemaker organ or clock that regulates the overall process of aging (e.g. see Warner et al., 1987). The case for a central clock is weakened, however, by the evolutionary arguments that point to the gradual loosening, and eventual disappearance, of genetic control over the late stages of the lifespan. Note that there is a sharp distinction here between iteroparous (repeatedly reproducing) organisms with which we are concerned principally in this chapter, and semelparous organisms like octopus and Pacific salmon which reproduce once only and die soon afterwards, and for which the force of natural selection remains high right up to the time of reproduction. In these species, programmed endocrine changes play a central, pacemaking role that contributes, though perhaps only incidentally, to the fairly rapid post-reproductive death (Robertson, 1961; Wodinsky, 1977; see also Kirkwood, 1985). By contrast, in iteroparous species the tailing-off in the force of selection means that the biological relevance of a central pacemaker becomes less and less as time goes by.

The synchronicity of age-related changes in different organs is explained most satisfactorily by the fact that, in so far as selection works against the occurrence of senescence in the wild, any organ that failed consistently before the others would be subject to selection to improve its durability. On the other hand, if any organ failed long after the others this would be a luxury with no real advantage in terms of survivorship, and the resources invested in the maintenance of this organ should be trimmed, therefore, bringing its rate of senescence in line with that of other organs.

For all organs it is to be expected that selection will have favoured the evolution of a measure of reserve capacity, such that most organs remain in good condition when the organism dies a natural death. As noted earlier, for most species, natural death results usually from some kind of accident. (Humans are exceptional in the extent to which aging is seen, and this presumably reflects the recent low mortality to which our species is now exposed, through social living, agriculture and medicine; see Kirkwood & Holiday (1986) for further discussion.) In organs that are subject to variable and unpredictable stresses during the lifetime (e.g. haemopoietic system, skin), a larger reserve capacity might have been selected for.

Aging and disease

We are now in a position to consider the relationship between aging and disease. Several general observations can be made. First, the view suggested by theory is that aging is due primarily to the accumulation of defects. This results in progressive deviation from the more ordered condition of young cells and tissues, and is likely to involve damage both to DNA and also to the cellular machinery for regulating gene expression, synthesizing gene products, and maintaining the cell, e.g. by turning over cell constituents. This process is 'normal', and yet by its very nature involves the production of abnormality. During aging, there is a gradual broadening of cell phenotype, coupled with some corruption of the somatic genotype.

Secondly, the process of aging is driven primarily by stochastic events and it is therefore not surprising that in monozygotic twin pairs, or in genetically homogeneous populations of inbred laboratory animals, there is variation both in lifespan and also in age-related pathology. Some changes are nearly universal, like those that affect elasticity of skin. These result presumably from stochastic events which are both so numerous, and individually so minor, that their aggregate effect is highly reproducible. Other changes, such as those that give rise to cell proliferative disorders like cancer, vary greatly between individuals. The triggering events for the latter changes are presumably rare, but of major consequence, and the element of chance is revealed much more clearly. Yet, in spite of the differences in the statistical distributions of common and sporadic age-associated conditions, it is possible (even probable) that some of the same fundamental mechanisms are at work. In mice, cancer incidence rates rise much faster with age than in humans, so that in spite of the thirty-fold difference in lifespan between the two species, the lifetime risks of developing a malignant tumour are similar. This is not really surprising, for many of the same mechanisms that guard against the general accumulation of DNA damage (and other damage) also guard against the mutations which may activate oncogenes and/or inactivate tumour suppressor genes.

Thirdly, in outbred populations, individuals are likely also to be genetically variable in the levels at which specific cell maintenance functions are set from conception. The disposable soma theory indicates that, in the population, natural selection will direct these levels in the direction of the evolutionary optimum. As individuals approach the optimum, however, the differences on which selection acts grow smaller, and some genetic polymorphism is to be expected. There are likely to be several alleles at which such polymorphism occurs, reflecting the fact that longevity is probably regulated by a network of cell maintenance functions, and so the potential for genetic variability is considerable. Some individuals may be genetically less well protected against certain types of somatic damage than others, thus predisposing them to show particular kinds of disorders during aging.

Finally, lifestyle factors (diet, stress, heavy manual work, sun exposure, etc.) may contribute differentially to the rates at which defects may accumulate.

The upshot is that theories of aging lead to a picture in which there is a progressive, roughly synchronous decline in function of many different organs, but where the rate of decline may be influenced by chance and/or heredity and/or lifestyle (Figure 11.2). Longitudinal studies of human aging reveal increasing heterogeneity in many physiological functions, coupled with an overall average decline, consistent with this picture. If a disease state is defined when a critical function declines below a certain level, or falls outside some defined 'normal' range, then Figure 11.2 illustrates how certain diseases become more common with age. Should it be true, as appears increasingly likely, that the aging process is indeed neither more nor less than the progressive accumulation of somatic damage resulting in abnormal or impaired function, there is no reason conceptually to separate these conditions from the spectrum of states that define 'normal' aging, although in practice the labelling of a condition as a 'disease' may correspond to the decision that clinical action is required.

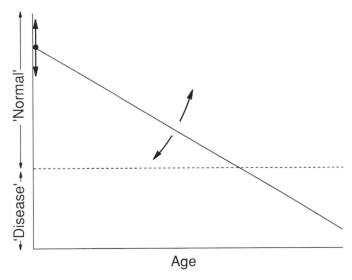

Figure 11.2. The level of function of an organ may decline progressively with increasing age, until a level is reached where a disease condition is defined. Both the starting level and the rate of decline may vary, as indicated by the arrows, because of chance and/or heredity and/or lifestyle (see text). Thus, different trajectories may be observed within a population for a specific organ, and, within an individual, different organs may decline at different rates. A linear decline is shown for illustrative purposes only: in practice, the decline will often be non-linear.

Dementia and Aging

Identifying risk factors can sometimes give important clues to the aetiology of disease. In the case of dementia, several risk factors show consistent statistical significance (see Chapter 10 and Jorm (1990)). The leading risk factor is chronological age. This applies, as far as we know, to all human populations. As a risk factor, however, age is informative only to the extent that it tells us that whatever causes dementia does so over a fairly long period of time.

Apart from age, the other risk factors that are demonstrated consistently for dementia, principally Alzheimer's disease (AD), are family history, especially of early onset disease, Down's syndrome, and head trauma. Even when these specific risk factors are present, dementia typically takes many years to develop. Thus, the actions of these risk factors are of interest for the ways they might accelerate the normal, slow development of disease. Various additional risk factors, such as thyroid disease and high aluminium exposure have been proposed, but the evidence for these remains inconclusive (see Chapter 10).

From studies of risk factors for dementia, the conclusions support the 'functional reserve' hypothesis (see Chapter 10). Formally, this is very similar to the general scheme, suggested by current theories on the mechanisms of aging, that is depicted in Figure 11.2.

Conclusions

Neither the mechanisms of dementia nor the mechanisms of senescence are yet known. Nevertheless, theories of aging have developed to a point where we can now delineate rather clearly the kinds of mechanisms that are likely to be involved in aging, and it is possible to see how these might be related to the mechanisms responsible for dementia.

Theory suggests that aging occurs because, in evolutionary terms, the optimum allocation of resources to somatic maintenance is less than is required for indefinite somatic survival. This leads to three clear predictions. First, aging is due to unrepaired cellular and molecular defects. Secondly, the genetic control of lifespan is effected through selection to raise or to lower the efficiency of key maintenance processes in relation to the prevailing level of accidental mortality. Thirdly, the argument applies with equal force to different maintenance processes operating within the body, and therefore we must expect to find a number of interacting, possibly synergistic mechanisms at work. An important aspect of cell maintenance that interacts with all other mechanisms is the accurate synthesis and processing of new proteins and the removal of faulty molecules by proteolysis. During aging, proteins can be damaged by mutations in the DNA that codes for their sequences, by errors arising during transcription and translation, or by oxidative damage or glycation. The maintenance of a balance between the rates of generation and removal of abnormal proteins is an essential requirement for dividing and post-mitotic cell alike. Disturbance of this balance may be particularly relevant to age-related disorders of the brain.

Molecular genetic approaches have recently given a particular impetus to the study of amyloid in relation to AD by the discovery that, in a subset of families with hereditary predisposition to AD, specific point mutations in the β-amyloid precursor protein (APP) cosegregate with the AD phenotype (Chartier-Harlin et al., 1991;

Goate et al., 1991; Murrell et al., 1991; Naruse et al., 1991). Progress-ive cerebral deposition of β-amyloid is a characteristic feature of AD, and the suggestion from these studies is that the mutations affect APP translation and/or processing in a way that leads to increased β-amyloid deposition. The APP gene is located on human chromosome 21, and the presence of an extra copy of this chromosome in Down's syndrome individuals is consistent with the involvement of APP in the aetiology of AD in Down's syndrome cases (Tanzi & Hyman, 1991). In spite of these important clues to the involvement of β-amyloid in AD, the majority of families with a history of predisposition to AD do not show defined mutations in the APP gene, suggesting multiple aetiologies for the disease. These multiple aetiologies may converge via a common pathway involving APP metabolism, but as yet little is known about the processing and normal function of APP.

Eventually, the biological processes causing dementia and aging will be discovered, and it will then be possible to establish definitively whether the pathogenesis of dementia shares common pathways with other age-associated dysfunctions, or whether dementia may be a time-dependent disorder distinct from normal aging with a separate causa-tive mechanism at work. Whatever the relationship between dementia and aging turns out to be, it will be surprising if normal brain aging, presumably affecting the same cells that are involved in dementia, does not at least interact with the processes that cause dementia.

Acknowledgement   I thank Louise Bottomley for helpful discussion.

References

Adelman, R. C. & Roth, G. S. (1983). *Altered Proteins and Aging*. CRC Press, Boca Raton.

Arking, R. (1991). *Biology of Aging: Observations and Principles*. Prentice Hall, Englewood Cliffs.

Beutler, E. (1986). Planned obsolescence in humans and other biosystems. *Perspectives in Biology and Medicine*, **29**, 175–9.

Brody, J. A. & Schneider, E. L. (1986). Diseases and disorders of aging – an hypothesis. *Journal of Chronic Diseases*, **39**, 871–6.

Charlesworth, B. (1980). *Evolution in Age-Structured Populations*. Cambridge University Press, Cambridge.

Chartier-Harlin, M.-C., Crawford, F., Houlden, H., Warren, A., Hughes, D., Fidani, L., Goate, A., Rossor, M., Roques, P., Hardy, J. & Mullan, M. (1991). Early-onset Alzheimer's disease caused by mutations at codon 717 of the β-amyloid precursor protein gene. *Nature*, **353**, 844–6.

Comfort, A. (1979). *The Biology of Senescence*, 3rd edition. Churchill Livingston, Edinburgh.

Evans, J. G. (1988). Aging and disease. In D. Evered & J. Whelan (eds.) *Research and the Ageing Population*, pp. 38–57. John Wiley and Sons, New York.

Finch, C. E. (1990). *Longevity, Senescence and the Genome*. Chicago University Press, Chicago.

Galas, D. J., Kirkwood, T. B. L. & Rosenberger, R. F. (1986). An introduction to the problem of accuracy. In T. B. L. Kirkwood, R. F. Rosenberger & D. J. Galas (eds.) *Accuracy in Molecular Processes: Its Control and Relevance to Living Systems*, pp. 1–16. Chapman and Hall, London.

Goate, A., Chartier-Harlin, M.-C., Mullan, M., Brown, J., Crawford, F., Fidani, L., Giuffra, L., Haynes, A., Irving, N., James, L., Mant, R., Newton, P., Rooke, K., Roques, P., Talbot, C., Pericak-Vance, M., Roses, A., Williamson, R., Rossor, R., Owen, M. & Hardy, J. (1991). Segregation of a missense mutation in the amyloid precursor protein gene with familial Alzheimer's disease. *Nature*, **349**, 704–6.

Haldane, J. B. S. (1941). *New Paths in Genetics*. George Allen and Unwin, London.

Hamilton, W. D. (1966). The moulding of senescence by natural selection. *Journal of Theoretical Biology*, **12**, 12–45.

Hanawalt, P. C. (1987). On the role of DNA damage and repair processes in aging: evidence for and against. In H. R. Warner, R. N. Butler, R. L. Sprott & E. L. Schneider (eds.) *Modern Biological Theories of Aging*, pp. 183–98. Raven Press, New York.

Jorm, A. F. (1990). *The Epidemiology of Alzheimer's Disease and Related Disorders*. Chapman and Hall, London.

Kirkwood, T. B. L. (1977). Evolution of ageing. *Nature*, **270**, 301–4.

Kirkwood, T. B. L. (1981). Repair and its evolution: survival versus reproduction. In C. R. Townsend & P. Calow (eds.) *Physiological Ecology: an Evolutionary Approach to Resource Use*, pp. 165–89. Blackwell Scientific Publications, Oxford.

Kirkwood, T. B. L. (1985). Comparative and evolutionary aspects of longevity. In C. E. Finch & E. L. Schneider (eds.) *Handbook of the Biology of Aging*, pp. 27–44. Van Nostrand Reinhold, New York.

Kirkwood, T. B. L. (1991). Genetic basis of limited cell proliferation. *Mutation Research*, **256**, 323–8.

Kirkwood, T. B. L. & Holliday, R. (1979). The evolution of ageing and longevity. *Proceedings of the Royal Society, London, B*, **205**, 531–46.

Kirkwood, T. B. L. & Holliday, R. (1986). Ageing as a consequence of natural selection. In A. J. Collins & A. H. Bittles (eds.) *The Biology of Human Ageing*, pp. 1–16. Cambridge University Press, Cambridge.

Kirkwood, T. B. L. & Rose, M. R. (1991). Evolution of senescence: late survival sacrificed for reproduction. *Philosophical Transactions of the Royal Society, London, B*, **332**, 15–24.

Linnane, A. W., Marzuki, S., Ozawa, T. & Tanaka, M. (1989). Mitochondrial DNA mutations as an important contributor to ageing and degenerative diseases. *Lancet*, **i**, 642–5.

Maynard Smith, J. (1962). Review lectures on senescence. I. The causes of ageing. *Proceedings of the Royal Society, London, B*, **157**, 115–27.

Maynard Smith, J. (1976). Group selection. *Quarterly Review of Biology*, **51**, 277–83.

Medawar, P. B. (1952). *An Unsolved Problem of Biology*. H. K. Lewis, London.

Medawar, P. B. (1955). The definition and measurement of senescence. In G. E. W. Wolstenholme & M. P. Cameron (eds.) *Ciba Foundation Colloquia on Aging 1*, pp. 4–15. Churchill, London.

Murrell, J., Farlow, M., Ghetti, B. & Benson, M. D. (1991). A mutation in the amyloid precursor protein associated with hereditary Alzheimer's disease. *Science*, **254**, 97–9.

Naruse, S., Igarashi, S., Aoki, K., Kaneko, K., Iihara, K., Miyatake, T., Kobayashi, H., Inuzuka, T., Shimizu, T., Kojima, T. & Tsuji, S. (1991). Missense mutation Val-Ile in exon 17 of amyloid precursor protein gene in Japanese familial Alzheimer's disease. *Lancet*, **337**, 987–9.

Ning, Y. & Pereira-Smith, O. M. (1991). Molecular genetic approaches to the study of cellular senescence. *Mutation Research*, **256**, 303–10.

Robertson, O. H. (1961). Prolongation of the lifespan of Kokanee salmon (*Oncorhynkus nerka kennerlyi*) by castration before the beginning of gonad development. *Proceedings of the National Academy of Sciences, USA*, **47**, 609–21.

Rosenberger, R. F. (1991). Senescence and the accumulation of abnormal proteins. *Mutation Research*, **256**, 255–62.

Saul, R. L., Gee, P. & Ames, B. N. (1987). Free radicals, DNA damage, and aging. In H. R. Warner, R. N. Butler, R. L. Sprott & E. L. Schneider (eds.) *Modern Biological Theories of Aging*, pp. 113–29. Raven Press, New York.

Smith, J. R. (1990). DNA synthesis inhibitors in cellular senescence. *Journal of Gerontology*, **45**, B32–5.

Strehler, B. L. (1977). *Time, Cells and Aging*, 2nd edition. Academic Press, New York.

Tanzi, R. & Hyman, B. T. (1991). Alzheimer's mutation (scientific correspondence). *Nature*, **350**, 564.

Vijg, J. (1990). DNA sequence changes in aging: how frequent? How important? *Aging*, **2**, 105–23.

von Dras, D. D. & Blumenthal, H. T. (1992). Dementia of the aged: disease or atypical-accelerated aging? Biopathological and psychological perspectives. *Journal of the American Geriatrics Society*, **40**, 285–94.

Warner, H. R., Butler, R. N., Sprott, R. L. & Schneider, E. L. (1987). *Modern Biological Theories of Aging*. Raven Press, New York.

Williams, G. C. (1957). Pleiotropy, natural selection and the evolution of senescence. *Evolution*, **11**, 398–411.

Wodinsky, J. (1977). Hormonal inhibition of feeding and death in *Octopus*: control by optic gland secretion. *Science*, **198**, 948–51.

Wynne-Edwards, V. C. (1962). *Animal Dispersion in Relation to Social Behaviour*. Oliver and Boyd, Edinburgh.

12

A method for measuring dementia as a continuum in community surveys

A. F. JORM

The view that dementia is categorically distinct from normal aging runs into problems when applied in epidemiological field surveys. For example, studies of prevalence produce rather different results depending on where the dividing line is placed for distinguishing dementia from normal aging. While this type of problem has been acknowledged in the literature (Jorm et al., 1987; Brayne & Calloway, 1988), the alternative view that dementia is continuous with normal aging has had remarkably little impact on the conduct of field surveys. One reason for this is that methods for measuring dementia as a continuum have not been developed. While there are a large number of tests which provide a continuous measure of cognitive functioning in the elderly (e.g. Mini-Mental State Examination: Folstein et al., 1975; CAMCOG: Roth et al., 1988), these are not really continuous alternatives to categorical diagnoses.

To see why, consider the process involved in making a diagnosis of dementia, as illustrated in Figure 12.1. The diagnostic process begins with the observation of poor cognitive performance, usually to a degree which interferes with social or occupational functioning. The poor performance can be life-long or recently acquired. Only the recently acquired cases proceed to the next step. Their cognitive impairment can be due to a number of sources and, in diagnosing dementia, alternatives such as delirium and depression have to be ruled out. Basically, dementia is the residual category after these alternatives have been excluded. The diagnostic process can continue further to classify the type of dementia. The clinical diagnosis of Alzheimer's disease (AD) is made by excluding vascular dementia, alcohol abuse and other rarer causes.

Cognitive impairment is a sensitive indicator of dementia but is

Dementia and Normal Aging, eds. F. A. Huppert, C. Brayne & D. W. O'Connor. © Cambridge University Press 1994.

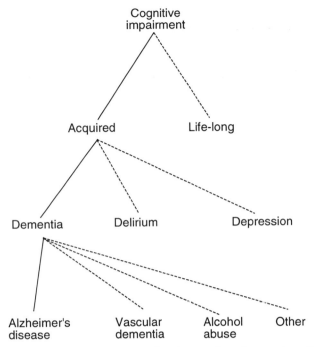

Figure 12.1. Decision tree for diagnosing dementing diseases. The influences which must be excluded in diagnosing dementia and Alzheimer's disease are shown with dashed lines.

non-specific, so exclusion criteria need to be applied to improve specificity. Such exclusion criteria are easy to apply to a categorically distinct group with cognitive impairment, but continuous measures of cognitive functioning do not allow for the exclusion of other influences from an individual's score.

The purpose of the present chapter is to describe a simple method of data analysis which can be used to adjust for extraneous influences on cognitive test performance and so derive continuous alternatives to categorical diagnoses of dementia and AD in field surveys.

Description of the method

The method begins with a continuous measure of cognitive functioning. This measure will be correlated with certain other variables which correspond to the exclusion criteria of categorical diagnoses. The influence of these variables is portrayed by the dashed lines in

Figure 12.1. For example, cognitive performance will be correlated with pre-morbid (life-long) ability, depressive symptoms and delirium symptoms. The contribution of these variables to cognitive perform-ance is not of interest to a researcher studying the underlying con-tinuum running from successful cognitive aging to severe dementia. Such variables will here be referred to as 'covariates'.

The relationship between the cognitive score and the covariates can be examined using multiple linear regression, where the cognitive score (Y) is predicted from the covariates (X_1 . . . X_k). In studying dementia as a continuum, we are interested in that component of the cognitive score not accounted for by the covariates. To isolate this dementia component, the predicted cognitive score for each subject ($\hat{Y}$) can be subtracted from the actual score (Y) to yield the residual score ($Y - \hat{Y}$). This residual score represents the original cognitive functioning score purged of the influence of the covariates and can be regarded as being a continuous dementia score.

This analysis can be extended further to produce a continuous measure of AD by adding other covariates (e.g. a scale of alcohol use, and a scale of vascular dementia). By calculating $\hat{Y}$ using the additional covariates, the residual score can be regarded as a continuous measure of AD.

The number of covariates used is decided by the investigator. In principle, it would be possible to consider a large number of variables, but in practice most of these will be of so little importance in a field survey that they can be ignored, e.g. tests for syphilis or niacin deficiency. There is also choice in how the covariates are measured. Many can be considered appropriately to be continuous and could be measured as such, but the method also applies where the covariates are categorical.

Illustration of the method

The method of developing continuous measures of dementia and AD could be applied potentially to any field survey data in which standard diagnostic instruments are used with all subjects. As an illustration, it is applied here to data from a study of dementia and depression in the Hobart community carried out by Kay et al. (1985; called the 'Hobart study') using a version of the Geriatric Mental State examina-tion (GMS) (Copeland et al., 1976). The Hobart study is not ideal for the purpose because of the lack of informant data and the exclusion

Table 12.1. *Illustrative regression analysis predicting cognitive performance (Y) from education (X_1), English fluency (X_2) and depressive symptoms (X_3)*

Variable	Coefficient	Standard error	t-value	Significance
X_1	0.57	0.10	5.55	0.00
X_2	−0.06	1.69	−0.03	0.97
X_3	−0.15	0.03	−5.36	0.00
Constant	26.63	0.80	33.10	0.00

of institutionalized subjects. Nevertheless, the data are quite adequate for purposes of illustration. The aim of the present exposition of the method is to stimulate others who have carried out field surveys to apply it to their own existing data.

The sample consisted of 274 non-institutionalized persons aged 70+ years who were interviewed with the GMS and tested on the Mini-Mental State Examination (MMSE). To produce a continuous measure of cognitive functioning for the present analysis, the MMSE items (including both WORLD backwards and serial sevens) were added to four GMS cognitive items to give a score from zero to 39 (the Y score). Cognitive test scores could, of course, be influenced by pre-morbid ability. Two variables were selected to measure this: number of years of education (X_1) and the interviewer's rating of fluency in English (X_2). A better measure of pre-morbid ability would have been the National Adult Reading Test (Nelson & O'Connell, 1978), but this was not used in the Hobart study. Another possible influence on cognitive functioning is depression, which was measured in the Hobart study by a depressive symptom scale (X_3). If the influence of these variables is removed from the cognitive score, the result can be regarded as being a continuous measure of dementia. (Ideally, the influence of delirium should also be removed at this stage, but was not measured in the Hobart study.)

The first step is a regression analysis predicting cognitive score ($\hat{Y}$) from each of the exclusion variables (X_1, X_2, X_3). The results of this analysis are shown in Table 12.1. It can be seen that years of education and depressive symptoms both have a significant influence on cognitive performance, whereas English fluency does not. The influence of these variables can be removed from each subject's cognitive score by calcu-

Table 12.2. *Examples to show how cognitive scores are adjusted for the influence of years of education and depressive symptoms*

Subject characteristics	Actual cognitive score	Predicted score	Residual (dementia score)
Well educated			
Few depressive symptoms	30	35.02	−5.02
Many depressive symptoms	30	28.87	1.13
Poorly educated			
Few depressive symptoms	30	31.02	−1.02
Many depressive symptoms	30	24.87	5.13

lating the residual score $(Y - \hat{Y})$. This residual score becomes the continuous measure of dementia.

To see how the residual score adjusts for the covariates, it is useful to consider specific examples of subjects having the same cognitive score but differing on the covariates. Table 12.2 shows results from four hypothetical subjects who are either well or poorly educated (5 or 12 years of education) and have either few or many depressive symptoms (-10 or 30 on a scale constructed by summing standard scores). Each subject has a cognitive score of 30 and is fluent in English. The first subject, who is categorized as being well educated and with few depressive symptoms, is predicted to have a cognitive score of 35.02. The actual score is 5.02 points lower than this, implying that the subject does more poorly than expected for someone in this category. The next subject is also well educated but with many depressive symptoms. The predicted cognitive score of 28.87 is lower than the actual cognitive score, giving a positive residual of 1.13. Relatively speaking, this subject is performing well. The third subject, with poor education and few depressive symptoms, performs slightly more poorly than expected, while the final subject, who is poorly educated and has many depressive symptoms, performs much better than expected. From these examples it can be seen that the subjects' cognitive scores are adjusted up or down depending on values of the covariates. Sub-

Table 12.3. *Illustrative regression analysis predicting cognitive performance (Y) from education (X_1), English fluency (X_2), depressive symptoms (X_3), stroke symptoms (X_4) and alcohol abuse (X_5)*

Variable	Coefficient	Standard error	t-value	Significance
X_1	0.58	0.10	5.63	0.00
X_2	−0.19	1.69	−0.11	0.91
X_3	−0.15	0.03	−5.29	0.00
X_4	0.16	0.40	0.40	0.69
X_5	−1.21	0.69	−1.74	0.08
Constant	26.63	0.81	32.97	0.00

jects who would be excluded by conventional diagnostic criteria have their scores adjusted upwards relative to other subjects.

The above analysis can be extended to yield a continuous measure of AD. To illustrate the method with the Hobart data, two additional covariates were constructed: a four-point scale of stroke symptoms (X_4) and a five-point scale of alcohol abuse (X_5). The resulting regression analysis is shown in Table 12.3. Again, education and depressive symptoms have a significant influence, while English fluency and stroke symptoms have little influence (stroke symptoms were rare in this non-institutionalized sample), and alcohol abuse has an influence approaching statistical significance at the 0.05 level. In this case, the residual score $(Y-\hat{Y})$ can be regarded as being a continuous measure corresponding to the clinical diagnosis of AD.

Subjects who have low scores on the continuous measures are those who would generally be diagnosed by clinicians as being demented. This can be illustrated in the Hobart study, where subjects were rated by a psychiatrist on a scale from normal to severe dementia. Table 12.4 shows the scores of the normals and the various demented groups. As expected, the subjects diagnosed as being demented tended to score lower on the continuous measures of dementia and AD.

The present illustration of the method has used a cross-sectional community survey, but, potentially, it could be applied to longitudinal studies. With longitudinal data, cognitive functioning at the first time point studied would be the most important covariate. Such an analysis

Table 12.4. *Scores on continuous measures as a function of a psychiatrist's diagnosis*

Diagnosis	Dementia score		Alzheimer's disease score	
	M	SD	M	SD
No dementia (n = 222)	0.51	4.01	0.50	3.95
Mild dementia (n = 35)	−0.64	5.41	−0.59	5.40
Moderate dementia (n = 7)	−10.23	4.39	−10.41	4.50
Severe dementia (n = 1)	−18.31	—	−18.36	—

M, mean; SD, standard deviation.

would provide a continuous alternative to the traditional study of incident cases.

Some limitations of the method

The use of multiple linear regression to adjust for the influence of covariates involves the critical assumption that the covariates are related linearly to the cognitive scores. If any of the relationships are non-linear, the method should not be used, although in some cases suitable transformations could be carried out to make them linear. An important case of non-linearity is if the cognitive score has a ceiling such that many subjects score at the maximum possible. Many dementia screening tests have this characteristic. In such cases, the cognitive score may change linearly with values of a covariate, but only up to the maximum score, at which point the relationship must flatten out. It is therefore important to use a cognitive test which discriminates over the whole range of cognitive ability in the population being studied.

The proposed method leaves the choice of covariates to the researcher. This choice is not simple and has considerable implications for what questions can be sensibly asked regarding the resulting score. For example, age was not entered as a covariate in the illustrative analysis of the Hobart data on the grounds that age differences still require explanation. If, however, an investigator was interested in the role of factors other than age, the influence of this variable could be removed from the cognitive score. As another example, there has been controversy about whether education is related to the incidence of dementia. Kittner et al. (1986) have argued that scores on dementia screening tests should be adjusted to eliminate educational differences on the presumption that such differences are due to test bias. By contrast, Berkman (1986) has argued that such an adjustment might prevent the investigation of real differences in dementia incidence. In the illustrative analysis using the Hobart data, the influence of education was removed, which would mean that no education difference was found in dementia scores. If a decision had been made not to have education as a covariate, a different outcome would have resulted. The arbitrariness of results depending on choice of covariates might seem a limitation of the method, but the same limitation applies to traditional diagnostic criteria. For example, DSM-III-R criteria for dementia (American Psychiatric Association, 1987) require the presence of memory *impairment*, while the draft research criteria for ICD-10 (World Health Organization, 1990) require memory and intellectual *decline*. The ICD-10 criteria are implicitly taking pre-morbid memory ability into account, whereas the DSM-III-R criteria are not. This subtle difference between the criteria might well influence whether a relationship is found with education. The proposed method makes such decisions explicit for the researcher.

In adjusting cognitive scores, the regression method derives the average effect of a covariate in the population and applies this average effect to adjust each individual's score. In the Hobart study, for example, each year of education is associated with an average increase of 0.58 points in the cognitive score, and each symptom of alcohol abuse is associated with an average decrease of 1.21 points (see Table 12.3). However, variables like education and alcohol abuse will have greater effects on some individuals and lesser effects on others. In a field survey, where the interest is on average effects, these individual inaccuracies will not be of great consequence. However, if the method were applied to give information about particular individuals, sometimes it could give an inaccurate picture.

Finally, the method treats the measurement of dementia purely as a process of adjusting cognitive performance for covariates. However, there may be more to dementia than impaired cognitive performance. For example, if behavioral changes are regarded as an important component, they need to be included as well. In principle, such additional features of dementia could be combined with the cognitive score, perhaps using a technique like canonical correlation. Such possibilities merit exploration.

Some advantages of the method

Since exclusion criteria are easy to apply when making categorical diagnoses, it might be asked whether there is any advance in using a more complex statistical method to apply them to continuous measures. In fact, the application of exclusion criteria in making categorical diagnoses has considerable limitations which the new method overcomes. Exclusion criteria eliminate individuals from further consideration if they have certain characteristics. Thus, a person who is depressed might be precluded from a diagnosis of dementia or a person who has had a stroke might be excluded from a diagnosis of AD. What this procedure ignores is multi-morbidity, which becomes increasingly common as people age. People can be impaired in several different ways simultaneously, but exclusion criteria tend to force them into one category only. The result is that people who are given a diagnosis involving many exclusion criteria (e.g. AD) will be a very atypical group with less co-morbidity than usual. By contrast, the continuous method does not exclude anybody, but simply adjusts cognitive scores depending on the individual's scores on the covariates.

In epidemiological field studies, it is often necessary to assess a large sample in order to find a comparatively small number of 'cases'. Much of the data on the 'normals' is of limited interest, despite the large investment of resources involved in gathering it. Multi-stage sampling procedures involving the progressive screening of subjects have been developed in an attempt to increase the yield of cases, but, inevitably, may lead to higher non-participation rates. However, if all subjects in a survey receive a score on a continuous measure, they all provide equally valuable data.

Perhaps the most important advantage of the method is to move the focus of dementia research beyond the simple distinction between diseased and normal aging. Rowe & Kahn (1987) have argued that this distinction is limited because it ignores the substantial variability within the normal elderly. They proposed a further distinction, within the normal group, between 'usual' and 'successful' aging. Consistent with this proposal, the method described here provides a means of researching the full continuum from severe dementia to successful cognitive aging.

Acknowledgements   Thanks to Scott Henderson and Ailsa Korten for comments on an earlier draft of this chapter, and to David Kay who kindly allowed access to the Hobart data.

References

American Psychiatric Association (1987). *Diagnostic and Statistical Manual of Mental Disorders*, third edition – revised (DSM-III-R). American Psychiatric Association. Washington, DC.

Berkman, L. F. (1986). The association between educational attainment and mental status examinations: of etiologic significance for senile dementias or not? *Journal of Chronic Diseases*, **39**, 171–4.

Brayne, C. & Calloway, P. (1988). Normal ageing, impaired cognitive function, and senile dementia of the Alzheimer's type: a continuum? *Lancet*, **ii**, 1265–7.

Copeland, J. R. M., Kelleher, M. J., Kellett, J. M., Gourlay, A. J., Gurland, B. J., Fleiss, J. L. & Sharpe, L. (1976). A semi-structured clinical interview for the assessment of diagnosis and mental state in the elderly: the Geriatric Mental State Schedule: I. Development and reliability. *Psychological Medicine*, **16**, 89–99.

Folstein, M. F., Folstein, S. E. & McHugh, P. R. (1975). 'Mini-Mental State': a practical method for grading the cognitive state of patients for the clinician. *Journal of Psychiatric Research*, **12**, 189–98.

Jorm, A. F., Korten, A. E. & Henderson, A. S. (1987). The prevalence of dementia: a quantitative integration of the literature. *Acta Psychiatrica Scandinavica*, **76**, 465–79.

Kay, D. W. K., Henderson, A. S., Scott, R., Wilson, J., Rickwood, D. & Grayson, D. A. (1985). Dementia and depression in the Hobart community: the effect of the diagnostic criteria on the prevalence rates. *Psychological Medicine*, **15**, 771–88.

Kittner, S. J., White, L. R., Farmer, M. E., Wolz, M., Kaplan, E., Moes, E., Brody, J. A. & Feinleib, M. (1986). Methodological issues in screening for dementia: the problem of education adjustment. *Journal of Chronic Diseases*, **39**, 163–70.

Nelson, H. E. & O'Connell, A. (1978). Dementia: the estimation of premorbid intelligence levels using the New Adult Reading Test. *Cortex*, **14**, 234–44.

Roth, M., Huppert, F. A., Tym, E. & Mountjoy, C. Q. (1988). *CAMDEX: the Cambridge Examination for Mental Disorders of the Elderly*. Cambridge University Press, Cambridge.

Rowe, J. W. & Kahn, R. L. (1987). Human aging: Usual and successful. *Science*, **237**, 143–9.

World Health Organization (1990). *ICD-10 Draft of Chapter V: categories F00 –F99, Mental and Behavioural Disorders (Including Disorders of Psychological Development). Diagnostic Criteria for Research*. World Health Organization, Division of Mental Health, Geneva.

PART V

Behaviour and cognition in dementia and normal aging

13

The meaning of dementia to those involved as carers

P. A. POLLITT

> I'm coping better because I've accepted that Mum has dementia . . .
> whereas a year ago I couldn't accept it. My family hasn't accepted it.
> My brothers think she's being awkward or bloody-minded and if I say,
> 'Well, it's her dementia', they say, 'Don't be daft'. I try to say it's a
> disease, she can't help it, but they won't have it, they still thinks she's
> just being awkward, which I find quite sad . . . (daughter of a woman
> with moderate dementia).
>
> The consultant told me it was 'SD'. I said, 'Do you mean senile
> dementia?' and he said yes, it was. I just couldn't believe it. My husband
> knew something was wrong, he'd say 'Look after me, Mary, don't let
> anything happen to me' and I'd say, 'Don't worry, darling, it's only
> your eyes', but, of course, I knew it wasn't . . . but I'd never met
> anybody with it which in itself was a godsend because I didn't know
> what was going to happen. I was worrying about that moment but I
> wasn't worrying about the future because I didn't know what was going
> to happen (wife of a man with moderate dementia).

Stereotyped views of mental disorders such as dementia distort and
exaggerate the condition and thus make it difficult for people to recognize early and borderline cases (Townsend, 1978). While 'dementia'
is used clinically as a value-free description, society attaches meanings
to it which are pejorative and stigmatizing, and this may also be a
factor in the resistance to perceiving or defining somebody as
demented.

As the two comments quoted above imply, resistance to acknowl-
edging the meaning of changes and to accepting the condition may
continue to a late stage in the illness, even, as the first example indicates, after a diagnosis has been made. There may also be a desire to

Dementia and Normal Aging, eds. F. A. Huppert, C. Brayne & D. W. O'Connor.
© Cambridge University Press 1994.

remain in ignorance of the likely course of the illness, as the second example illustrates.

Much of the existing literature on caring for people with dementia is based on cases where the condition is already considerably advanced and a clinical diagnosis has been made. This chapter is about people who were found to be dementing by a community survey but who, in the majority of cases, had not been given a diagnosis of dementia; and about the ways that relatives and those most closely involved perceived and explained the changes that take place with a dementing illness. It also looks at the implications of a discrepancy in viewpoint between carers and professionals, and at the extent to which the data support the thesis that information and assistance offered early in the course of a dementing illness help to prevent carer stress and crises.

The Hughes Hall Project for Later Life

The material presented here is from the Hughes Hall Project for Later Life: a study, carried out in Cambridge, of the prevalence and course of dementia in which not only the individuals identified as dementing, but also their relatives, were followed up over a two-year period. There were three objectives in relation to this last aspect:

(1) To examine the *experience* of dementia for relatives of sufferers and to study their problems, rewards (if any) and ways of coping
(2) To examine the involvement of services, and the adequacy of formal assistance, at the time of entry into the study
(3) To examine the effectiveness of early and/or extra assistance from a multi-disciplinary specialist team in terms of easing the burden on carers and delaying or preventing admission into residential care

Comparison was made with those also identified by the project as dementing but who lived outside the catchment area of the specialist team (the Cambridge community resource team for the elderly, henceforth referred to as the 'CRT').

Thus, the group described here consisted of all those found to be dementing who lived north of the river but within the city boundaries (the area served by the CRT) and their carers. Some had a co-resident carer, some lived alone, some were in sheltered accommodation; none were in residential care. Identification of dementia was by means of a screening survey administered to approximately one third of the population of Cambridge aged 75 years and over, using the Mini-Mental State Examination (MMSE) (Folstein, et al., 1975). Those falling below an agreed cut-off point on the MMSE were then investigated by research psychiatrists using the Cambridge mental disorders in the elderly examination (CAMDEX): a comprehensive test of mental function which included an interview with an informant about changes in memory, intellect, personality, drive and behaviour (Roth, et al., 1986).

The initial testing was carried out in the context of a general study of the elderly: their health, family and social contacts; ability to carry out the activities of daily living; their use of services. The CAMDEX interview has been designed for use in the community. Although concerned primarily with cognitive function, it also enquires into general health, activities of daily living, and family medical history. Dementia ratings were allocated on the basis of the criteria given below. It was recognized that within each category there was a wide range of disability and that the boundaries between levels were not absolute.

> Mild dementia: loss of short-term memory, together with difficulties in reasoning and acquiring new information; some disorientation in time and place; and some impairment of skills of daily living
> Moderate dementia: clear loss of cognitive skills and inability to carry out simple everyday tasks without guidance and supervision
> Severe dementia: total loss of cognitive skills and of the ability to carry out everyday tasks

On the basis of these criteria, 50% (38/76) of the group were identified as being mildly demented, 43% as being moderately demented and 7% as being severely demented. (For a more detailed description of the method and of the diagnostic criteria see O'Connor et al., (1989a).)

The relative or friend closest to the elderly person was interviewed between four and six weeks after the CAMDEX. This was a semi-structured, open-ended interview designed to find out how the elderly person managed, and about his or her needs and problems; about how relatives saw these problems, what help they and others were providing, and whether or not they felt that more assistance was needed.

The great majority of the people we describe here had not been diagnosed as dementing prior to contact with the research team. Information about the existence or possible existence of dementia was not passed on unless requested (which happened rarely, for reasons which are described in this chapter). Extra assistance was offered on the basis of need or potential need, not on the basis of a diagnosis.

It was possible, therefore, to examine attitudes to and explanations for the deterioration in function and changes in behaviour of the dementing person, and to observe whether and why perceptions changed as the illness progressed.

Perceptions of dementia

An early and striking discovery was that the majority of relatives did not see themselves as 'the carer' of a dementing person. Only 40% saw the elderly person's problem as being one of mental impairment and only half of these would have considered the term 'dementia' to be appropriate. The daughter and wife quoted above made these comments two years after the person had been identified by the project as suffering from moderate dementia.

Although aware of the changes and deterioration in the elderly person (O'Connor et al., 1989b), the majority of relatives discounted or minimized the significance of these changes. They saw themselves as looking after, or simply helping, someone who was old, or as caring for someone suffering from physical, rather than mental, problems. These included almost all cases of mild dementia and a third of cases of moderate dementia.

In perceiving their elderly relatives as 'normal for their age', these informants revealed both an expectation of decline in old age ('She forgets occasionally but I think she's really good for her age' was a typical comment) and an understanding of 'sound mind' which did not correspond to our own. They were often quite sanguine about the symptoms of dementia. For example, a loss of short-term memory seemed less important than recall of childhood years which was seen as evidence of an especially good memory. Partial memory was seen as deliberate forgetfulness, even perversity ('She can remember if she wants to'). Loss of function was minimized, while retained faculties were seized on as evidence of normality. There was also a tendency to deny the significance of other changes in mental functioning, such as the ability to handle money.

In some cases, changes were explained in terms of physical problems. Deafness or speech impairment was held to account for inability to communicate and appeared to mask confusion and memory loss. A partner's own deafness sometimes helped to maintain the belief in, or appearance of, an unchanged personality. For example, an 81-year-old man whose markedly demented wife was virtually without coherent speech said: 'I can't have a very good talk with her because I can't always hear what she says, apart from the fact that she mumbles'.

Explanations for abnormal behaviour

Even where behaviour was seen clearly to be abnormal, there was resistance to seeing it as being a loss of intellectual function. It was seen as being perverse or intentionally obstructive: 'He could do it but he won't try' (the wife of moderately demented man); manipulative: 'She puts on an act . . . a real Oscar-winning performance' (the son of a moderately demented woman); or attention seeking: 'She has always cried and become upset in order to get her own way' (the son of a mildly demented woman).

Sometimes, the difficulties were presented not so much as a change in behaviour but as part of a familiar pattern, either intrinsic to the character of the affected individual or reflecting long-standing problems in the relationship: 'She has always been aggressive and difficult and suspicious' (the daughter of a moderately demented woman). Some informants saw the elderly people as bringing their loss of mental capacity upon themselves. It was as if they had not been sufficiently vigilant. When people made statements such as 'We must keep her doing things for herself' it was in order to prevent the unspoken alternative: 'senility'. Some were blamed explicitly for their problems: 'There are other things open to her, she could talk to people, she *chooses* not to. You have to make that little bit of effort sometimes' (the daughter of a mildly demented woman). Attitude of mind was seen to be very important and some elderly people were criticized for their lack of motivation: 'She won't do anything to help herself, she won't try to do her knitting or her tapestry' (the daughter of a moderately demented woman). This implied that recovery depended on the ability of the individual to *want* to get better. It had not occurred to these respondents that the will itself might be affected. Even those who had been diagnosed clinically as dementing were sometimes expected to be rational and to have insight and control over their behaviour: 'She's her own worst enemy, if only she would *realise* how difficult and aggressive she can be' (the daughter of a moderately demented woman).

Relatives not only expected rational thinking but also normal emotional responses. Many found the lack of normal responses such as gratitude very difficult to accept, and new responses such as suspiciousness and hostility even more so. 'She used to say dreadful things to my father that he couldn't come to terms with. He couldn't relate to the illness at all. He just thought it was her suddenly not loving him' (daughter of a moderately demented woman). Again this indicated the difficulty that relatives experienced in accepting the reality of the disorder. For some, this called into question the relationship itself. An elderly woman who lived alone was unable to remember visitors who had come five minutes before, and therefore felt almost constantly lonely. She was criticized by her nephew and niece for her insensitivity: 'I don't think she's got any feelings . . . she's always saying, "nobody cares about me, nobody loves me", it gets through to us . . . it hurts . . . We *are* looking after her'.

Explanation for seeing changes as being normal

The reasons for seeing dementia as being a normal part of aging may be partly due to the way old age is perceived in our society. There is a general expectation of decline with age, often with little distinction between 'normal' and 'abnormal' loss of function. Sankar suggests that 'the cultural meaning of old age as a time of sickness is shared and further elaborated by the medical profession', and she points out that old age is often given as a diagnosis (Sankar, 1984, p. 251).

The reasons for 'normalizing' the symptoms of dementia may be partly due to the commonly held views of dementia as a form of madness. This was implicit in some of the descriptions given to us: 'He's not mental, you know . . . he's not going to go around hitting people' (wife of a moderately demented man); 'My aunt is only half way to being mental, they don't have to dope her up' (nephew of mildly demented woman). While such images of dementia may be misleading, the clinical diagnosis is not much more encouraging, for it implies the fragmentation of the mind, the destruction of personality and the likelihood of deterioration. For the carer, to deny, or fail to recognize, that the changes are abnormal is thus to deny their personal and social implications, implications which call into question the integrity of the personality itself.

In her work on lay perceptions of illness, Pollock found that the essence or the substance of the person is identified with the functions of the mind. This may, at least in part, account for why mental illness 'signifying a deranged or damaged mind is felt to be more alarming than a defective or deformed body' (Pollock, 1984, p. 262). Seeing the problem in terms of physical, rather than mental, difficulties kept such fears at bay and also allowed for hope of improvement or even recovery, particularly in the case of stroke-related dementia where the severity of the physical problems could be allowed to mask the presence of mental impairment. Thus, when relatives made statements such as 'Her mind's not too bad, it's just the forgetfulness' (the sister of a mildly demented woman) or 'He can talk sense, he's not senile' (the wife of a moderately demented man), they were resisting the move across the threshold from normal to abnormal, from 'just old age' to 'senile dementia'. There was a natural desire to 'hold on' to the person, the spouse or the parent for as long as possible.

Explanation of cause

In the absence of medical diagnoses and information, relatives produced their own explanations and theories of cause. There was a need to make sense of the changes, to find meanings and reasons for what had happened to their parents, spouses, or siblings. These were not always revealed in explicit statements, but were implied in less direct ways. The changes were often invested with a moral significance or extended into the past to become part of the elderly person's biography. Blaxter, in her work on disabled people, found that 'the major feature of patients' accounts . . . was their strenuous attempts to see their medical condition *as a whole*' – contrary to the medical system which treats different physiological systems separately (Blaxter, 1976, p. 221). Sheldon, in her work with relatives of dementia sufferers, found that they sometimes saw 'illness as retribution for past misdeeds and wondered why a loved and respected parent should suffer' (Sheldon, 1982, p. 185). Gilhooly also found that relatives speculated about dementia in terms of morality (cited in Gilleard (1984)).

Blaxter also found that affected individuals were more likely to attribute causes to the environment and behaviour (e.g. overwork, stress) than to physiology (Blaxter, 1976). In the accounts given by the relatives in our study, precipitating factors included: experiences of death and desertion; severe disappointment; retirement; loss of role when grandchildren had grown up; moving house or locality. The illness was sometimes seen as a form of retreat from the world, as an escape from painful situations and experiences: 'It happens to you when you give up on life', said a woman who believed her sister's dementia had been caused by the suicide of a close relative.

Some saw the elderly person as having invited the problems because of past laxity or selfish behaviour: 'There were 12 of us and she was the most difficult one of all. She wasn't happy-go-lucky, no sense of humour . . . My mother used to say, "you're the most willing, you do it, Amy's a bit awkward . . ."' (the sister of a moderately demented woman). Others saw the changes in their elderly relatives as revealing 'true character'. They seemed to feel that a layer or facade had been stripped away revealing the 'true self' or hidden self. This was believed to be either the result of advancing age or of illness such as a stroke. One daughter described her moderately demented mother as 'nasty . . . she says wicked things . . . she didn't used to . . . but looking back maybe it was there but controlled, but now she's had these strokes the aggression has been released'; another said of her mother who was also moderately demented, 'the aggressive side towards me has stayed, she doesn't forget *me*, while J. was her favourite and she's forgotten her. The nasty side has stayed'.

Changes in perception at the two-year follow-up

We found, in reviewing these cases, that at the end of two years just over half of those who remained in the community continued to be seen by their relatives as being essentially normal for a person of that age. The observed changes continued to be regarded as common features of aging. Accommodation to and normalization of the sufferers' disabilities had continued despite what was often marked deterioration (as evidenced by CAMDEX testing and relatives' own accounts), sometimes accompanied by bizarre behaviour. Moments of lucidity were seized on as signs that the 'person' was not lost. Comfort was drawn from inconsistencies in behaviour: 'He was a bit more "with it" yesterday' (wife of moderately demented man); 'He seemed to come to himself when Mum died' (son of a moderately demented man); 'At times he's almost like himself – but you can't rely on it' (wife of a moderately demented man).

Some, however, had moved towards an acceptance of the condition as being irreversible and likely to get worse. In several of these cases, the CRT (to which sufferers and relatives had been referred) were gently encouraging relatives to recognize the implications of increasing difficulties. Others had undergone a sudden shift in perception which was not always because of a decline in the elderly person's mental state. Sometimes, a break from usual routines had made the extent of the deficit apparent: 'I first noticed the change when we got a new car, my husband couldn't adjust to it' (the wife of a moderately demented man). In another case, a woman noticed the change in her mildly demented husband when the couple went on holiday and he was unable to remember where their hotel room was.

The redefinition of the problem

Once dementia was acknowledged formally, together with the recognition of its effect on the mind and the will, there was much less expectation on the sufferer to exercise control or to show insight. A similar tendency to redefine the same symptoms as illness once they are *perceived* as being abnormal has been noted in relation to other conditions (for example, schizophrenia) (Yarrow, 1955; Mills, 1962; Pollock, 1984).

Kreisman & Joy identified 'definite stages of response' to mental illness, moving from denial or minimization of symptoms to gradual acceptance of them as being part of an illness (Kreisman & Joy, 1974). We were also able to identify a series of stages from denial to acceptance, and each of our respondents could be located at one or other of these stages. We found that some people moved through each stage, while others made a 'conceptual leap' from 'normal', 'just old age', to a redefinition of the condition as 'abnormal', as 'dementia'.

The first stage in this progression was one where change was seen as simply being consonant with old age: 'She's pretty good for an 83-year-old, she's still got all her buttons' (sister of mildly demented woman). At the second stage, changes in behaviour were seen as being abnormal but were blamed on physical impairments such as deafness, or on perversity or contrariness. The third stage was marked by implicit acknowledgement: 'He's 88 and I'm 85 . . . we expect it don't we? . . . we mustn't grumble' but, later in the interview, this elderly wife of a mildly demented man revealed her underlying anxiety when she asked, 'What will happen if *I* can't manage?' When a man noted for never contradicting his mildly demented wife, and for consistently denying that she had any problems, expressed concern about his own health and his wife said, 'I'll look after you, dear', his sharp retort was revealing, '*You* couldn't'.

The fourth stage was marked by explicit suspicion but needing confirmation: 'Mother's getting very strange but I feel too embarrassed to discuss it with the doctor' (the daughter of a moderately demented woman). 'I tried to talk to the GP but, you see, everything, according to him, was "just old age"' (the niece of a mildly demented man). The son of a 98-year-old man with moderate dementia became worried when his father failed to recognize familiar faces and became frightened of his own clothes hanging on the back of the bedroom door. He tried to discuss these problems with the GP but reported the doctor as saying, 'Don't worry, that's usual at his age'. Here, the son (like the niece in the previous example) was seeking confirmation of a suspicion which might have led to a reassessment of the problem, but found instead that he had been rerouted back to stage one.

Finally, at the fifth stage, there was explicit acknowledgement of dementia. Sometimes this had been arrived at gradually: 'Mother's getting a bit woolly in her thinking', so this moderately demented woman's son had started to look for permanent residential care. 'He wasn't listening . . . I kept saying "you don't listen to a word I say" and then I began to realize that he didn't understand or know how to respond, so then I took him to the doctor' (the wife of a moderately demented man). Sometimes this change in perception could be attributed to the involvement of the CRT. Our involvement as interviewers may also have played a part. Although we were careful not to refer to 'dementia', we may have made respondents more aware of the implications of their difficulties.

A sudden shift in perception usually occurred when something out of the ordinary had happened, causing a relative to reassess the situation and redefine it (Zola, 1964; Robinson, 1971). For example, an elderly person's admission to hospital for a physical illness might result in dementia being recognized, or the illness of a protective spouse might bring the helplessness of the other to light. 'What's an old lady like that doing living on her own?' This accusing enquiry from the police after a mildly demented woman had had a fall resulted in her family realizing that not all was well with her. The temporary change in the condition of an 89-year-old woman with mild dementia led to a permanent shift in the perception and attitudes of her son and daughter-in-law. The woman had a 'funny turn', her words were jumbled and her laughter was unnatural. Although this passed quickly and she returned to her former state, her daughter-in-law was alarmed:

'You don't think she is going senile, do you? We're OK looking after physical things but we don't want her to go mental'. Despite regaining her former state, this woman's son and daughter-in-law, had decided she was 'mental' and revised their plans about having her come to live with them.

Implications of discrepancies between lay and professional views of mental illness

Discrepancies between lay and professional views in relation to health and illness behaviour have been explored extensively (Blaxter, 1976; Stacey, 1977). Relatives of schizophrenic patients, for example, have been found to regard quite bizarre behaviour as being normal (Pollock, 1984; Teusink & Mahler, 1984). In the case of dementia, we need to ask whether it matters if there is a divergence in perception between professionals and carers. Is it likely to result in requests for help being ignored or in offers of help being refused?

This chapter has indicated the ways in which those who were involved closely with sufferers ignored, discounted and minimized the implications of the changes that had taken place. The question then arises of whether efforts should be made to reverse this tendency. The desire to remain in ignorance of the illness or of its likely course runs contrary to views expressed by carers' groups, such as the Alzheimer's Association. These groups are often critical of the delay in making diagnoses and advocate giving information in the early stages of the disease process so that relatives may receive earlier assistance from services, and access to benefits and to information about the nature of the illness, as well as help with managing the dementing person.

Carers themselves, in looking back, are often reported as expressing regret about their own lack of information and understanding. For example, in collecting retrospective accounts from daughters who had cared for their mothers, Lewis & Meredith (1988, p. 45) found that 'the onset of senile dementia often went unrecognised by the carer' and these daughters expressed sadness about not reaching an understanding of the condition sooner. Levin et al. (1989), in their study of carers of the confused elderly, found that it was common for carers to feel guilty about their initial lack of understanding and their resulting behaviour. Our study found that understanding and forgiveness sometimes did not come until after death. Comments such as 'He couldn't help it, poor love, his mind had gone' (the wife of a moderately demented man) and 'It wasn't her that was speaking, it was the illness' (the daughter of a moderately demented woman) made after the person had died, contrasted sharply with those made about people who were still alive, as indicated above. We found that expressions of regret, remorse and guilt were more likely to be made – as with Lewis & Meredith's (1988) informants – after the death of the elderly person. This suggests that hindsight may play a part in accounts given *after* diagnosis, or death, of the situation *before* these events have taken place.

It can be argued that lack of understanding of the condition may mean that relatives base their interpretations of the affected person's behaviour on inappropriate models of illness and hold unrealistic expectations of recovery. They may experience excessive frustration and anger because they continue to expect rational behaviour. This can be detrimental to family relationships and crises may become unavoidable. It may also be the case that reversible conditions go undetected and depressive illness remains untreated. On the other hand, earlier awareness of dementia and earlier diagnoses may also be detrimental. For the sufferer it means loss of status as a person and 'social death' (Sweeting, 1991). For the carer it means a re-evaluation of that person, of the relationship and of the future. Many of the relatives persisted in seeing the changes that stemmed from dementia as belonging to the realm of the normal for as long as possible in order to preserve or to retain a beloved spouse or parent. In some cases, coping strategies were premised on an assumption of the normality or perversity of the condition. Furthermore, such re-evaluations were sometimes unnecessary. Our follow-up study showed that the condition did not always deteriorate beyond the mild stages, that some elderly people died first. In such cases, earlier awareness could have created problems where problems did not exist, and could have created needs where needs were not felt.

However, it was also the case that some people were worried and were having difficulties, and might well have benefited from an earlier diagnosis. The obvious source of help and information for such cases was the general practitioner (GP). But GPs can help only if they are asked. Ways would have to be found of overcoming the reluctance to discuss intellectual failing that many of our informants manifested. This was partly because they did not perceive the problem as being *medical*, as illness, but as a normal aspect of aging. Others were uncertain: 'I don't like to bother the doctor with my mum's problems' (the daughter of a mildly demented woman). Some GPs who had been approached appeared to collude with the view that the changes were normal: 'The GP said to us, "What do you expect when they're both over 80?"' (the son of a moderately demented man and a minimally demented woman). In other cases, it seemed that mental problems were felt by relatives to be almost a taboo subject, something they had to protect the doctor against: 'I've never discussed my husband's [memory] problems with the doctor . . . I always feel they don't want to hear too much' (80-year-old wife of a mildly demented man). And in the absence of treatment or a cure, especially before the advent of the CRT, it is possible that GPs felt there was little that they could do.

Where a diagnosis of dementia had been given, it had not always been well received. One wife rejected the term: 'It's making them into a totally different person'. Some felt being told the nature of the condition was unhelpful: 'People should be left in ignorance for as long as possible. We do expect a slowing down as we get older' (wife of a moderately demented man). Another wife took the opposite view, however, saying she liked to have things confirmed, that it was 'uncertainty that worries me'. Thus, as the quotes at the beginning of the chapter indicate, earlier diagnosis may be positive or negative in its effect.

We also found that, in a minority of cases, diagnosis did not always lead to a reassessment, to a crossing of the threshold from 'normal' to 'abnormal'. One woman granted that her mildly demented mother's memory was bad, 'She's got what they call "something senility" but it's not that far advanced', and continued to refer to her mother as a 'silly old fool' who had never been 'all that bright . . . and always lived in her own little world'. One man, although told his father had dementia, insisted that there was no real impairment or problems that could be distinguished from those of any other 90-year-old; and another son said, 'Dad's so-called senility was because he was deaf. He just gave up. He couldn't hear anything so he just went into himself. He was never funny with it, not like my mother'.

Conclusion

This chapter has attempted to give an idea of the complexity and multiplicity of attitudes and perceptions of the people who are involved most closely with cognitively impaired elderly people. Understanding these views has implications for treatment and for services. It is important, to quote Sheldon (1982, p. 185), to 'determine what the illness actually means to the carers. Otherwise professional helpers can exhaust themselves trying inappropriate methods, when a simpler but appropriate intervention will improve coping dramatically'. This point was illustrated by the work of the Cambridge CRT whose own interventions were based on their assessment of functional incapacity rather than on a specific diagnosis. Some GPs, too, had a discriminating approach to their dementing patients, giving to relatives the amount of information that they saw as being appropriate and offering the sort of help which they thought would be acceptable without necessarily shifting perceptions at all.

Recognition of the divergence in views between lay and professional people can, in the broadest sense, contribute to a greater understanding of the realities of living with dementia, as well as of help-seeking and coping behaviour generally; and, in a narrower sense, it can help to avoid situations where people do not seek, or are not offered, help to which they are entitled. And while many studies have rightly emphasized the stress and strain and unremitting burden of caring for somebody with dementia, we should be careful about generalizing from known, advanced cases to all demented people, many of whom will not be identified as being impaired and whose relatives may prefer it that way.

References

Blaxter, M. (1976). *The Meaning of Disability: A Sociological Study of Impairment.* Heinemann, London.

Folstein, M. F., Folstein, S. E. & McHugh, P. R. (1975). 'Mini-mental state': a practical method for grading the cognitive state of patients for the clinician. *Journal of Psychiatric Research*, **12**, 189–98.

Gilleard, C. J. (1984). *Living with Dementia: Community Care of the Elderly Mentally Infirm.* Croom Helm, London and Sydney.

Kreisman, E. E. & Joy, V. D. (1974). Family response to the mental illness of a relative: a review of the literature. *Schizophrenia Bulletin*, **10**, 34–57.

Levin, E., Sinclair, I. & Gorbach, P. (1989). *Families, Services and Confusion in Old Age.* Gower, Aldershot.

Lewis, J. & Meredith, B. (1988). *Daughters Who Care.* Routledge, London.

Mills, E. (1962). *Living with Mental Illness: a Study in East London.* Routledge and Kegan Paul, London.

O'Connor, D. W., Pollitt, P. A., Hyde, J. B., Fellows, J. L., Miller, N. D., Brook, C. P. B., Reiss, B. B. & Roth, M. (1989a). The prevalence of dementia as measured by the Cambridge Mental Disorders of the Elderly Examination. *Acta Psychiatrica Scandinavica*, **79**, 170–8.

O'Connor, D. W., Pollitt, P. A., Roth, M., Brook, C. P. B. & Reiss, B. B. (1989b). The validity of informant histories in a community study of dementia. *International Journal of Geriatric Psychiatry*, **4**, 203–8.

Pollock, K. (1984). 'Mind and matter: a study of conceptions of health and illness among three groups of English families, with particular reference to multiple sclerosis, schizophrenia and "nervous breakdown" '. Unpublished PhD thesis. University of Cambridge, Cambridge, UK.

Robinson, D. (1971). *The Process of Becoming Ill*. Routledge and Kegan Paul, London.

Roth, M., Tym, E., Mountjoy, C. Q., Huppert, F. A., Hendrie, H., Verma, S. & Goddard, R. (1986). CAMDEX: a standardised instrument for the diagnosis of mental disorder in the elderly with special reference to the early detection of dementia. *British Journal of Psychiatry*, **149**, 698–709.

Sankar, A. (1984). 'It's just old age'. In D. I. Kertzer & J. Keith (eds.) *Age and Anthropological Theory*. University of Cornell Press, Ithaca, New York.

Sheldon, F. (1982). Supporting the supporters: working with relatives of patients with dementia. *Age and Ageing*, **11**, 184–8.

Stacey, M. (1977). 'Concepts of health and illness: a working paper on the concepts and their relevance for research'. In Social Science Research Council, *Health and Health Policy – Priorities for Research: the Report of an Advisory Panel to the Research Initiatives Board*. London.

Sweeting, H. (1991). 'Caring for a relative with dementia: anticipatory grief and social death'. Paper presented at a Workshop on Research Methods in the Study of Carers of Dementing Elderly People, University of Dundee, March 1 1991.

Teusink, J. P. & Mahler, S. (1984). Helping families cope with Alzheimer's disease. *Hospital and Community Psychiatry*, **35**, 152–6.

Townsend, J. M. (1978). *Cultural Conceptions and Mental Illness: a Comparison of Germany and America*. University of Chicago Press, Chicago, London.

Yarrow, M. R., Clausen, J. A. & Robbins, P. R. (1955). The social meaning of mental illness. *Journal of Social Issues*, **11**, 33–48.

Zola, I. K. (1964). Illness behaviour of the working class: implications and recommendations. In A. B. Shostak & W. Gomberg (eds.) *Blue Collar World*. Prentice-Hall, New York.

14

Personality and behaviour in dementia and normal aging

TONY HOPE

The changes which take place in the behaviour of people with dementia are important clinically and interesting theoretically (Fairburn & Hope, 1988; Burns et al., 1990). They are important clinically because behavioural changes can be a major cause of distress for carers (Rabins et al., 1982; Argyle et al., 1985) even in only moderately impaired individuals (Teri et al., 1989) and they are a common reason for demented people requiring institutional care (Sanford, 1975; Margo et al., 1980; Chenoweth & Spencer, 1986; Steele et al., 1990). They are of theoretical interest because they raise the question of what the causal mechanisms might be.

The purpose of this chapter is to review the literature on the behavioural and personality changes which take place in dementia with specific interest in the relationship between dementia and normal aging.

What is meant by 'behaviour'?

The term behaviour is being used here to refer to what can be observed directly. It will not include mood disorders such as depression and anxiety, nor delusions and hallucinations, nor changes in cognitive functioning.

In general, the definition of any behaviour should be clear, complete and objective (Barlow & Hersen, 1984). By *clear* is meant that the definition is unambiguous and understood easily. By *complete* is meant that the boundaries of the behaviour are well specified. By *objective* is meant that the behaviour is observable and can be identified with a minimum of subjective interpretation.

Dementia and Normal Aging, eds. F. A. Huppert, C. Brayne & D. W. O'Connor. © Cambridge University Press 1994.

Behaviour may be identified at many different levels. At one extreme, one could specify simple movements such as raising the right arm. At the other extreme are complex types of behaviour in which the purpose and the agent's intention must be known. The problem with studying simple movements is that they are unlikely to prove interesting. The problem with studying complex behaviour is that the observer needs to make sophisticated judgements and assumptions. In the context of dementia this can be particularly problematic, since it can be unclear whether the subject is capable of forming an intention. On the whole it seems most fruitful to identify behaviour between these extremes. The ideal would be 'units' of behaviour which have aetiological significance.

What is meant by 'change in personality'?

Consider a man who has never been particularly aggressive. He becomes demented. He is often angry and abusive. His wife says that he is generally more irritable. Should we describe what has happened as a change in personality, or should we say that his behaviour has changed?

The concept of personality is usually used to refer to an individual's enduring and persistent responses across a variety of situations (Harré & Lamb, 1983). Therefore, we might call it 'personality' change if the aggressive behaviour occurs in a variety of situations and is persistent, and a 'change in behaviour' if the aggression occurs only in a few specific settings or is less consistent. On this view, personality change is simply one end of a spectrum of changes in behaviour – it is behaviour change which occurs over a wide range of settings. Thus, change in behaviour is the more general term which includes personality change. These are the senses in which the terms will be used in this chapter.

Methods for assessing behaviour

The main purpose of this chapter is to review change in behaviour and personality in the light of the 'continuum hypothesis'. However, it is important first to consider the methods for assessing such changes.

One of the attractions in studying behaviour is that it is observable. However, in order to capitalize on the objective nature of behaviour, it is necessary to use methods of assessment which are reliable. This is by no means as easy as one might think at first, because of the difficulty in defining exactly what is to count as each unit of behaviour.

The choice of what method to use will depend on the purpose for the assessment. There are a large number of rating scales available which are designed to help in predicting the type and amount of care needed; in contrast, little attention has been given to designing measures appropriate to the detailed study of behavioural abnormalities.

First, the general methods for the assessment of abnormal behaviour will be reviewed; instruments designed to cover a wide range of behaviour will then be considered, followed by measures for specific types of behavioural abnormality. Finally, the assessment of personality will be considered.

Direct observation

Although direct observation has been widely used in the study of behavioural disturbance in children, it has been little used in the context of dementia. It is not suitable as a method for rating a wide range of behaviour because the sampling frame needs to be appropriate to the way in which each behaviour is distributed in time. However, the paucity of studies using direct observation is disappointing.

Snyder et al. (1978) observed a number of 'wanderers'. Cohen-Mansfield et al. (1989) developed an observation method ('the agitated behaviour mapping instrument') which they used to examine the distribution of 'agitated behaviour' through the day. Hope and colleagues have used direct observation in two single-case studies of the effect of medication on 'hyperactivity' (Hope et al., 1991b) and excessive eating (Hope & Allman, 1991). A good use of direct observation would be in the validation of less direct methods of assessment such as rating scales.

Objective measurement of specific behaviour

Some types of behavioural abnormality could be measured using a mechanical or electronic device rather than through observation. However, there has been very little development of such methods. Rindlisbacher & Hopkins (1992) used a motion sensor sewn into a short-sleeved shirt to investigate the distribution of activity over time. Electroencephalogram (EEG) recordings have been used extensively in the study of sleep. The development and use of further methods would be an interesting and important area for future research.

Collecting information from carers

By far the most common way in which behavioural data have been collected is indirectly from those who are in close contact with the demented person. This can be done by using a semi-structured interview, a fully structured interview, or written questions. With semi-structured interviews, the interviewer makes the ratings in the light of the description obtained from the informant. Although some questions are mandatory, the interviewer can pursue the questioning until in a position to make the rating. In a fully structured interview the interviewer cannot deviate from the specified questions. When written questions are used, the informant makes the ratings in the light of the instructions given (rating scale).

The principal value of the semi-structured interview is that it is more likely to be valid in the collection of complex data. The principal drawback is that it is time consuming. The main problem with structured interviews and written questionnaires is that the informant may not mean the same thing by a particular concept as does the research worker. This problem becomes particularly important with detailed studies which involve making precise distinctions between different types of behaviour.

The only semi-structured interview covering a wide range of behaviour in detail and developed for use with people suffering from dementia is the present behavioural examination (PBE) (Hope & Fairburn, 1992). This interview is designed to be administered to the principal carer. The questions are grouped into seven domains as follows: abnormal behaviour concerning walking; eating abnormalities; sexual abnormalities; aggressive behaviour; sleep and diurnal rhythm changes; incontinence; and odd behavioural abnormalities. In addition, there are sections devoted to mental and physical health. The aim of the PBE is to give a profile of the current behaviour of the subject. It covers the four weeks immediately prior to the time of the interview. In total, there are 121 main questions and a further 66 'nested' questions (i.e. questions which are relevant only if a specific main question is rated positively). The test–retest, and inter-rater reliabilities of the PBE are similar to those of the present state examination (Kendell et al, 1968).

Both the geriatric mental state (GMS; Copeland et al., 1976) and the comprehensive assessment and referral evaluation (CARE; Gurland et al., 1977) are semi-structured interviews. They are concerned mainly with mental state rather than behaviour. CAMDEX (Roth et al., 1986) is a semi-structured interview developed specifically for the assessment of people with dementia. It is concerned mainly with diagnosis and the cognitive impairments and contains few behavioural items.

The majority of measures of behaviour in dementia are structured interviews or self-rated scales. Most of these have been designed to help to decide what level of care is required. These instruments are of limited value for the scientific study of the nature of behavioural changes in dementia. A useful source book of such rating scales is Israel et al. (1985). Woods & Britton (1985) provide a valuable review.

A number of rating scales have been developed recently which focus in more detail on the behaviour itself. However, none has been validated against an interview measure or direct observation. Because the information being gathered is complex, it remains questionable whether the informant understands the same thing by each item as the investigator.

The behavioral pathology in Alzheimer's disease rating scale (BEHAVE-AD) by Reisberg et al. (1987) has been developed principally as a measure of outcome for treatment studies. It consists of 25 ratings: 12 are concerned with delusions and hallucinations, and six relate to mood. Seven questions address behaviour in the sense used in this chapter. Three are to do with aggressiveness, one with diurnal rhythm disturbance and three are concerned with activity disturbances. The psychometric properties of BEHAVE-AD have not been evaluated in detail. Patterson et al. (1990) have provided some inter-rater reliability data but no information on test–retest reliability.

Greene et al (1982) have developed the behavioural and mood disturbance scale. This is designed to measure such disturbance in subjects living at home and is completed by the main carer. Its purpose is to give a measure of those types of behaviour which are likely to cause difficulties and stress for the carer.

Swearer et al. (1988) developed the behavior severity rating scale in order to examine the relationships between disruptive behaviour, disease severity and diagnosis. This has nine behavioural items (and two items relating to mood). The psychometric properties of this scale have not been examined. In addition to these measures, there are a number of rating scales which focus on one, or a limited number, of behavioural abnormalities. These are summarized in Table 14.1.

The question of the validity of rating scales for behaviour is an important one, although it has received little research attention. The rating scale for aggressive behaviour in the elderly (RAGE; Patel & Hope, 1992), which was designed to be used by nursing staff, was subjected to a small validity study in which ratings were compared with the results of direct observation. This confirmed the validity of the nurse ratings. However, for this validity study the rating scale was adapted to cover one nursing shift (eight hours) rather than the three days which the standard scale covers. The assessment, by carers, of *cognitive* decline has been compared with a direct measure of cognitive function (Jorm & Korten, 1988; Jorm et al., 1989). These studies show that carers can assess changes in various aspects of cognitive functioning accurately. However, carer reports of behaviour (such as hitting or shouting) may be less accurate than reports of changes in cognitive function (such as whether the ability to understand newspaper articles has changed).

Assessment of personality

Most personality measures are not applicable to people with cognitive impairment because they involve self-assessment. Blessed et al. (1968) developed a dementia scale in order to relate clinical and pathological features. This scale consists of 35 items (with a maximum score of 65) of which 11 items (with a score of one each, if present) are concerned with changes in personality. In completing these items, information is to be obtained from close relatives. Brooks & McKinlay (1983) developed a personality inventory for use with victims of head injury, which was designed to be completed on the basis of information provided by an informant. This measure has been applied to subjects with dementia by Petry et al. (1988, 1989) (see below).

The continuum hypothesis

A central theme of this book is the relationship between normal aging and dementia, and the light that this sheds on the *continuum hypothesis*, i.e. the hypothesis that dementia is on a continuum with normal

Table 14.1. *Some standardized measures of behaviour and personality changes in dementia*

Scale	Authors	Date	Behaviour included	Further comments
Present behavioural examination (PBE)	Hope & Fairburn	1992	Wide selection	Detailed semi-structured interview with carer
Behavioural pathology in Alzheimer's disease rating scale (BEHAVE-AD)	Reisberg et al.	1987	Seven items covering aggressiveness, diurnal rhythm disturbance and activity disturbance. Further items on delusions, hallucinations and mood	Rating scale
Behavioural and mood disturbance scale	Greene et al.	1982	Various – from the perspective of what is likely to cause difficulties and stress on carer	Rating scale
Behaviour severity rating scale	Swearer et al.	1988	Nine items covering a range of behaviour; two items on mood	Rating scale
Rating scale for aggressive behaviour in the elderly (RAGE)	Patel & Hope	1992	Twenty items covering specific types of physical and verbal aggression	Rating scale designed to be used by nursing staff for patients on psychogeriatric ward
Ryden aggression scale	Ryden	1988	Twenty-five items covering physical and verbal aggression, including item on sexual aggression	Rating scale designed for community subjects

Cohen-Mansfield agitation inventory	Cohen-Mansfield et al.	1989	Twenty-nine items covering aggressive behaviour, activity disturbances, shouting, hoarding and abnormal eating	Rating scale
Disruptive behaviour rating scale	Mungas et al.	1989	Four items (two concerned with aggressive behaviour) and a checklist of 13 specific aggressive items	
Staff observation aggression scale	Palmstierna & Wistedt	1987	Structured way of describing individual acts of aggressive behaviour with severity rating	
	Nilsson et al.	1988		
Overt aggression scale	Yudovsky	1986	Severity rating of single aggressive act	
	Kay et al.	1988		
Dementia scale	Blessed et al.	1968	Eleven out of 35 items concern personality change. Other items cover activities of daily living and cognitive abilities	Not designed specifically for the elderly or people with dementia
Personality inventory	Brooks & McKinlay	1983	Eighteen pairs of personality characteristics	Developed for patients with head injury. Applied to subjects with dementia by Petry et al. (1988, 1989)

aging. In the context, therefore, of behavioural and personality changes, the questions arise:

(1) How do changes seen in dementia relate to changes found in normal aging?
(2) To what extent is there a continuum in such changes from normal aging to mild dementia to severe dementia?
(3) What is the relationship between such changes and premorbid personality and behaviour?

These questions can only be answered partially and tentatively in the current state of knowledge.

I will consider personality changes first. I will then review changes in sleep and changes in eating, since there are sufficient data concerning these two areas to allow comparison between normal aging and dementia. Finally, I will consider other behavioural changes briefly.

Personality changes and normal aging

There have been many studies of personality changes in normal aging which are reviewed well by Schaie & Willis (1991). A major problem with such studies is distinguishing true changes in personality from cohort effects. For example, it appears that data which were interpreted initially as suggesting that people become more reserved as they grow older is better accounted for as a generational effect.

The overwhelming result of studies of personality change with age is that there is an exceptional amount of stability in personality characteristics. The two changes which do appear to be genuinely a result of aging are an increase in excitability (the inability to keep emotions on an even keel) and a decrease in general activity (Schaie & Willis, 1991).

Personality changes and dementia

Rubin and colleagues (1987), using the Blessed scale (Blessed et al., 1968), found that passive behaviour (inertia) was observed in about 90% of patients with mild dementia and agitated and irritable behaviour occurred in about two thirds of cases. It is possible that this passive behaviour is a more extreme form of the decreased activity seen in normal aging; and that the agitated behaviour is related to the increase in excitability referred to in the preceding section.

Petry et al. (1988, 1989) used the personality inventory of Brooks & McKinlay (1983) to compare personality characteristics before and after onset of dementia using a control group of healthy people before and after retirement. The patients with dementia were followed-up three years after the initial study. Petry et al. (1989) propose four patterns of personality change:

(1) Marked change in personality at the onset of dementia with little change as the dementia progresses
(2) A continuous progression of the personality change with the progression of the dementia
(3) No change
(4) An initial change in personality at the onset of dementia which then tends to return to the premorbid state

The second of these patterns is that most clearly consistent with the continuum hypothesis. Petry et al. observed this pattern with regard to listlessness, insensitivity and being emotionally cold. The first and the fourth patterns, which were observed in the majority of personality items including irritability, do not support the continuum hypothesis (although they do not disprove it – see below). Other studies suggest that there are more kinds of personality or behaviour change which follow pattern 2. For example, O'Connor et al. (1990) found, in a community sample of people with dementia, that the levels of disturbed behaviour and inertia increased with increasing severity of dementia.

The other question of relevance to the continuum hypothesis is whether the personality changes which take place in dementia can be seen to be exaggerations of premorbid personality. On the view that dementia is a disease quite separate from normal aging, one might predict that the personality changes reflect the disease rather than the premorbid personality; whereas, if the continuum hypothesis is correct, one might expect to see some continuity between the personality characteristics before and after the onset of dementia. Petry et al. (1988, p. 1189) conclude that 'The behavioral changes observed were similar from case to case. The uniformity of direction of change of behavior indicates that the alterations are not primarily a release of premorbid personality traits but represent a uniform behavioral profile produced by the illness'. However, as is discussed below, the question of the relationship between premorbid personality and behaviour change in dementia is not straightforward. In some cases the dementia does seem to 'release' or exaggerate premorbid personality characteristics.

Sleep disturbance and electroencephalogram recordings

Sleep disturbance is one of the most troublesome behavioural abnormalities in dementia (Sanford, 1975). It is a common reason for admission to an institution because carers cannot cope without adequate sleep themselves. Furthermore, the demented person who is up at night is at high risk of injury through falling.

There has been a considerable amount of good research on sleep patterns in dementia making use of EEG recordings. This work has been reviewed comprehensively by Vitiello & Prinz (1989). Because EEG recordings allow precise quantitative studies to be carried out, and because there are exactly comparable data for normal aging and Alzheimer's disease, it is possible to test the continuum hypothesis more adequately than in relation to other types of behavioural disturbance. The results can be summarized as follows: the changes in sleep patterns which occur in Alzheimer's disease are exaggerations of the changes which occur in normal aging; and the more advanced the Alzheimer's disease the greater these changes. As we grow older so we wake more often at night, and the amount of stage 4 sleep decreases (Regestein, 1980; Feinberg & Floyd, 1982; Reynolds et al., 1983). These effects are increased even in mild dementia (Prinz et al., 1982; Vitiello et al., 1990). As the dementia progresses, so there are significant losses in REM sleep and there is increasing daytime sleep. This daytime sleep is principally of stages 1 and 2 and therefore does not compensate for the nighttime loss of REM and stage 4 sleep (Vitiello & Prinz, 1989). In advanced dementia, there can be a complete breaking up of the normal sleep/wake cycle: short periods of sleep and wakefulness follow each other throughout the night and day. Thus, the evidence from EEG recordings is in line with predictions from the continuum hypothesis.

Other markers of the circadian rhythm are also affected by aging, for example, plasma melatonin (Nair et al., 1986) and body temperature (Touitou et al., 1986). Whether Alzheimer's disease affects these other rhythms is still unclear (van Gool & Mirmiran, 1986).

The changes in sleep observed in normal aging and Alzheimer's disease might be related to cell loss in: the reticular formation, the basal nucleus of Meynert (Vitiello & Prinz, 1989); the locus coeruleus (Mann & Yates, 1983); or the suprachiasmatic nucleus (Swaab et al., 1985, 1987).

Abnormalities in eating and weight

There is a tendency towards decreased food intake and loss of weight in the normal elderly. There are likely to be many causes for this and these have been reviewed comprehensively by Morley & Silver (1988) and Silver (1991). Amongst the causes suggested are: effects on the central control of feeding through, for example, a reduction of various neurotransmitters; decreased taste sensation and decreased olfaction.

Of all the changes in eating seen in dementia (reviewed by Hope et al. (1991a)), decreased food intake is probably the most common. Morris et al. (1989) found that 63% of a community sample of people with dementia ate substantially less, at some stage in their illness, than prior to the onset of dementia. This decrease in intake appeared to be associated normally with weight loss. Many other studies have documented weight loss as a common feature of dementia (Rheaume et al., 1987; Sandman et al., 1987; Tavares & Rabins, 1987; Singh et al., 1988; Franklin & Karkeck, 1989; Renvall et al., 1989). The weight loss which is seen in dementia, and particularly in Alzheimer's disease (Sandman et al., 1987), could be interpreted as an exaggerated form of what is seen in the normal elderly. This is particularly the case if one considers the possible causes mentioned above. For example, the decrease in olfaction observed in normal aging is seen, to an even greater extent, in dementia (Knupfer and Spiegel, 1986; Serby 1986; Doty et al., 1987).

The continuity with normal aging is also evident in so far as reduction in cortical neurotransmitters can account for the changes in eating and weight. A reduction in opioid peptides, noradrenaline and 5-hydroxytryptamine is seen in normal aging, and to a greater degree in Alzheimer's disease (Hardy et al, 1985; see Chapter 19, this book). The reduction in opioid neurotransmitters and noradrenaline could cause reduced eating and loss of weight. A reduction in 5-hydroxytryptamine could underlie the increase in eating and gain in weight which is seen in as many as a quarter of people with dementia at some stage in their illness (Morris et al., 1989).

Other types of abnormal behaviour

There are many types of abnormal behaviour which have been described in dementia and which have not been discussed so far, for example activity disturbances (wandering), aggressive behaviour, incontinence, shouting, screaming and hoarding. Many of these, it is thought, tend to occur at later stages of dementia and do not relate clearly to behaviour seen in normal aging. However, there are some data concerning such behaviour which relate to the continuum hypothesis. In particular, it is pertinent to ask: firstly, whether there is evidence that a particular behaviour becomes increasingly severe as the dementia progresses; and, secondly, whether the behaviour can be seen as being an exaggeration of premorbid functioning.

There has been little research using good measures which relates behaviour to the degree of dementia. In general, more behavioural problems are reported in those who are more severely demented (Teri & Logsdon, 1990) and behavioural problems tend to get worse as the dementia progresses (Petry et al., 1989). There is evidence that sleep apnoea (Reynolds et al., 1985), incontinence (Berrios, 1986), and high levels of 'pacing' and physical aggression (Cohen-Mansfield et al., 1990) are seen more frequently the more severe the cognitive impairment. And, indeed, incontinence increases with age amongst the normal population so that a continuum can be traced from normal aging to dementia. In contrast, hiding and hoarding of objects, and verbal complaints tend to occur more in the mildly than in the severely demented (Cohen-Mansfield et al., 1990).

If a change can be seen to be an exaggeration of premorbid personality, then this provides some continuity between the person before and after the onset of dementia, and gives prima facie support to the continuum hypothesis.

There are data on this point for only two types of behaviour: aggressive behaviour and activity disturbance (wandering). Hamel et al. (1990) found, in a study of community-based patients, that premorbid patient aggression and a more troubled premorbid relationship between the caregiver and the subject were both associated with higher levels of aggressive behaviour. Ware et al. (1990), in another community-based study reported that, in 61% of subjects, aggressive behaviour was seen as an exaggeration of premorbid personality; in the remaining 39%, however, the carer viewed the behaviour as being quite new.

With regard to activity disturbance, McDonald et al. (1982) proposed that persistent wandering behaviour was caused by the dementing process disinhibiting an existing personality trait. However, in a community sample of 'wanderers', Hope & Fairburn (1990) found little connection between premorbid personality and the 'wandering' behaviour.

Thus, data on these points are conflicting. It appears that in some people there is a connection between the abnormal behaviour and their premorbid functioning, but much disturbed behaviour seems to arise new as a result of the dementia.

Conclusions

At the phenomenological level, some changes in personality and behaviour which are observed in dementia form a continuum with normal aging whereas others do not. However, the fundamental test of the continuum hypothesis is at the level of continuity in aetiology (the underlying cause) rather than the continuity of the phenomena (i.e. the behavioural changes themselves). Although continuity in the phenomena is most likely to be accounted for by continuity in the cause, the reverse is not necessarily the case. Thus, if the cognitive impairment seen in dementia is on a continuum with normal aging (see Chapter 15), then any behaviour which is a direct result of the cognitive impairment does not provide evidence against the continuum hypothesis, even if the behaviour appears, phenomenologically, to be quite different from what is seen in normal aging. For example, a person might 'wander off' and get lost only when his spatial memory falls below a particular level of functioning. His behaviour might, therefore, change suddenly but as a result of continuous changes in both the pathology and cognitive abilities. The same argument holds for behaviour which results from neurotransmitter changes which are on a continuum with those seen in normal aging (see Chapter 19).

Unfortunately the aetiologies of the various behavioural changes which take place in dementia are largely unknown. In the present state of knowledge it is simply unclear to what extent the behavioural abnormalities relate to causes which themselves are on a continuum with normal aging.

Acknowledgements   I am grateful to many people for stimulating discussions on the topics in this chapter. I would particularly like to acknowledge Christopher Fairburn, Vikram Patel, Peter Allman,

Christopher Ware, Hugh Series, Janet Keene and Kathy Gedling. Sandra Cooper helped to prepare the typescript. The research I have carried out in this area has been possible only through a Wellcome Trust Training Fellowship and a Medical Research Council Special Project.

References

Argyle, N., Jestice, S. & Brook, C. P. B. (1985). Psychogeriatric patients: their supporters' problems. *Age and Ageing*, **14**, 355–60.

Barlow, D. H. & Hersen, M. (1984). *Single Case Experimental Designs: Strategies for Studying Behaviour Change*. Pergamon Press, Oxford.

Berrios, G. E. (1986). Urinary incontinence and the psychopathology of the elderly with cognitive failure. *Gerontology*, **32**, 119–24.

Blessed, G., Tomlinson, B. E. & Roth, M. (1968). The association between quantitative measures of dementia and of senile change in the cerebral grey matter of elderly subjects. *British Journal of Psychiatry*, **114**, 797–811.

Brooks, D. N. & McKinlay, W. (1983). Personality and behavioral change after severe blunt head injury. *Journal of Neurology, Neurosurgery and Psychiatry*, **46**, 336–44.

Burns, A., Jacoby, R. & Levy, R. (1990). Psychiatric phenomena in Alzheimer's disease. IV. Disorders of behaviour. *British Journal of Psychiatry*, **157**, 86–94.

Chenoweth, B. & Spencer, B. (1986). Dementia: the experience of family caregivers. *Gerontologist*, **26**, 267–72.

Cohen-Mansfield, J., Watson, V., Meade, W., Gordon, M., Leatherman, J. & Emor, C. (1989). Does sundowning occur in residents of an Alzheimer's unit? *International Journal of Geriatric Psychiatry*, **4**, 293–8.

Cohen-Mansfield, J., Marx, M. S. & Rosenthal, A. S. (1990). Dementia and agitation in nursing home residents: how are they related? *Psychology and Aging*, **5**, 3–8.

Copeland, J. R. M., Kelleher, M. J., Kellett, J. M. & Gourlay, A. J. (1976). A semi-structured clinical interview for the assessment of diagnosis and mental state in the elderly; the Geriatric Mental State Schedule. I. Development and reliability. *Psychological Medicine*, **6**, 439–49.

Doty, R. L., Reyes, P. F. & Gregor, T. (1987). Presence of both odor identification and detection deficits in Alzheimer's disease. *Brain Research Bulletin*, **18**, 597–600.

Fairburn, C. G. & Hope, R. A. (1988). Changes in behaviour in dementia: a neglected research area. *British Journal of Psychiatry*, **152**, 406–7.

Feinberg, I. & Floyd, T. C. (1982). The regulation of human sleep. *Human Neurobiology*, **1**, 185–94.

Franklin, C. A. & Karkeck, J. (1989). Weight loss and senile dementia in an institutionalized elderly population. *Journal of the American Dietetic Association*, **89**, 790–2.

Greene, J. G., Smith, R., Gardiner, M. & Timbury, G. C. (1982). Measuring behavioural disturbance of elderly demented patients in the community and its effects on relatives: a factor analytic study. *Age and Ageing*, **11**, 121–6.

Gurland, B., Kuriansky, J., Sharpe, L., Simon, R., Stiller, P. & Birkett, P. (1977). The Comprehensive Assessment and Referral Evaluation (CARE) – rationale, development and reliability. *International Journal of Aging and Human Development*, **8**, 9–42.

Hamel, M., Gold, D. P., Andres, D., Reis, M., Dastoor, D., Grauer, H. & Bergman, H. (1990). Predictors and consequences of aggressive behavior by community-based dementia patients. *Gerontologist*, **30**, 206–11.

Hardy, J., Adolfsson, R., Alafuzoff, I., Bucht, G., Marcusson, J., Nyberg, P., Perdahl, E., Wester, P. & Winblad, B. (1985). Transmitter deficits in Alzheimer's disease. *Neurochemistry International*, **7**, 545–63.

Harré, R. & Lamb, R. (eds.) (1983). *The Encyclopedic Dictionary of Psychology*. Blackwell, Oxford.

Hope, R. A. & Fairburn, G. C. (1990). The nature of wandering in dementia: a community-based study. *International Journal of Geriatric Psychiatry*, **5**, 239–45.

Hope, R. A. & Allman, P. (1991). Hyperphagia in dementia: fluvoxamine takes the biscuit. *Journal of Neurology, Neurosurgery and Psychiatry*, **54**, 88.

Hope, T. & Fairburn, C. G. (1992). The development of an interview to measure current behavioural abnormalities: the Present Behavioural Examination (PBE), *Psychological Medicine*. **22**, 223–30.

Hope, R. A., Morris, C. H. & Fairburn, C. G. (1991a). Eating abnormalities in dementia. *Clinics in Applied Nutrition*, **1**, 55–62.

Hope, R. A., Patel, V. & Series, H. (1991b). Dexamphetamine may reduce hyperactivity in dementia – a case study using direct observation. *International Journal of Geriatric Psychiatry*, **6**, 165–9.

Israel, L., Kozarevic, D. & Sartorius, N. (1985). *Source Book of Geriatric Assessment*, vols. 1 and 2. Karger S. in association with WHO, Basle.

Jorm, A. F. & Korten, A. E. (1988). Assessment of cognitive decline in the elderly by informant interview. *British Journal of Psychiatry*, **152**, 209–13.

Jorm, A. F., Scott, R. & Jacomb, P. A. (1989). Assessment of cognitive decline in dementia by informant questionnaire. *International Journal of Geriatric Psychiatry*, **4**, 35–9.

Kay, S. R., Wolkenfeld, F. & Murrill, L. M. (1988). Profiles of aggression among psychiatric patients. I. Nature and prevalence. *The Journal of Nervous and Mental Disease*, **176**, 539–46.

Kendell, R. E., Everett, B., Cooper, J. E., Sartorius, N. & David, M. E. (1968). The reliability of the 'Present State Examination'. *Social Psychiatry*, **3**, 123–9.

Knupfer, L. & Spiegel, R. (1986). Differences in olfactory test performance between normal aged, Alzheimer and vascular type dementia individuals. *International Journal of Geriatric Psychiatry*, **1**, 3–14.

Mann, D. M. A. & Yates, P. O. (1983). Patterns of sleep and the noradrenergic neurotransmitter system in the elderly and the demented. *Journal of the American Geriatrics Society*, **31**, 450–1.

Margo, J. L., Robinson, J. R. & Corea, S. (1980). Referrals to a psychiatric service from old people's homes. *British Journal of Psychiatry*, **136**, 396–401.

McDonald, C., Behl, N. & Sudhaker, P. (1982). Recalcitrant behaviour problems. In R. G. McCreadie (ed.) *Rehabilitation in Psychiatric Practice*, pp. 57–66. Pitman, London.

Morley, J. E. & Silver, A. J. (1988). Anorexia in the elderly. *Neurobiology of Aging*, **9**, 9–16.

Morris, C. H., Hope, R. A. & Fairburn, C. G. (1989). Eating habits in dementia. A descriptive study. *British Journal of Psychiatry*, **154**, 801–6.

Mungas, D., Weiler, P., Franzi, C. & Henry, R. (1989). Assessment of disruptive behavior associated with dementia: the disruptive behavior rating scales. *Journal of Geriatric Psychiatry and Neurology*, **2**, 196–202.

Nair, N. P. V., Hariharasubramanian, N., Pilapil, C., Isaac, I. & Thavundayil, J. X. (1986). Plasma melatonin – an index of brain aging in humans? *Biological Psychiatry*, **21**, 141–50.

Nilsson, K., Palmstierna, T. & Wistedt, B. (1988). Aggressive behavior in hospitalized psychogeriatric patients. *Acta Psychiatrica Scandinavica*, **78**, 172–5.

O'Connor, D. W., Pollitt, P. A., Roth, M., Brook, C. P. B. & Reiss, B. B. (1990). Problems reported by relatives in a community study of dementia. *British Journal of Psychiatry*, **156**, 835–41.

Palmstierna, T. & Wistedt, B. (1987). Staff observation aggression scale, SOAS: presentation and evaluation. *Acta Psychiatrica Scandinavica*, **76**, 657–63.

Patel, V. & Hope, R. A. (1992). A rating scale for aggressive behaviour in the elderly – the RAGE. *Psychological Medicine*, **22**, 211–21.

Patterson, M. B., Schnell, A. H., Martin, R. J., Mendez, M. F., Smyth, K. A. & Whitehouse, P. J. (1990). Assessment of behavioral and affective symptoms in Alzheimer's disease. *Journal of Geriatric Psychiatry and Neurology*, **3**, 21–30.

Petry, S., Cummings, J. L., Hill, M. A. & Shapira, J. (1988). Personality alterations in dementia of the Alzheimer type. *Archives of Neurology*, **45**, 1187–90.

Petry, S., Cummings, J. L., Hill, M. A. & Shapira, J. (1989). Personality alterations in dementia of the Alzheimer type: a three-year follow-up study. *Journal of Geriatric Psychiatry and Neurology*, **2**, 203–7.

Prinz, P. N., Vitaliano, P. P., Vitiello, M. V., Bokan, J., Raskind, M., Peskind, E. & Gerber, C. (1982). Sleep, EEG and mental function changes in senile dementia of the Alzheimer's type. *Neurobiology of Aging*, **3**, 361–70.

Rabins, P. V., Mace, N. L. & Lucas, M. J. (1982). The impact of dementia on the family. *Journal of the American Medical Association*, **248**, 333–5.

Regestein, Q. R. (1980). Insomnia and sleep disturbances in the aged. Sleep and insomnia in the elderly. *Journal of Geriatric Psychiatry*, **13**, 153–71.

Reisberg, B., Borenstein, J., Salob, S. P., Ferris, S. H., Franssen, E. & Georgotas, A. (1987). Behavioral symptoms in Alzheimer's disease: phenomenology and treatment. *Journal of Clinical Psychiatry*, **48**, (supplement), 9–15.

Renvall, M. J., Spindler, A. A., Ramsdell, J. W. & Paskvan, M. (1989). Nutritional status of free-living Alzheimer's patients. *American Journal of the Medical Sciences*, **298**, 20–7.

Reynolds, C. F., Spiker, D. G., Hanin, I. & Kupfer, D. J. (1983).

Electroencephalographic sleep, aging, and psychopathology: new data and state of the art. *Biological Psychiatry*, **18**, 139–55.

Reynolds, C. F., Kupfer, D. J., Taska, L. S., Hoch, C. C., Sewitch, D. E., Restifo, K., Spiker, D. G., Zimmer, B., Marin, R. S., Nelson, J., Martin, D. & Morycz, R. (1985). Sleep apnea in Alzheimer's dementia: correlation with mental deterioration. *Journal of Clinical Psychiatry*, **46**, 257–61.

Rheaume, Y., Riley, M. E. & Volicer, L. (1987). Meeting nutritional needs of Alzheimer patients who pace constantly. *Journal of Nutrition for the Elderly*, **7**, 43–52.

Rindlisbacher, P. & Hopkins, R. W. (1992). An investigation of the sundowning syndrome. *International Journal of Geriatric Psychiatry*, **7**, 15–23.

Roth, M., Tym, E., Mountjoy, C. Q., Huppert, F. A., Hendrie, H., Verma, S. & Goddard, R. (1986). CAMDEX. A standardised instrument for the diagnosis of mental disorder in the elderly with special reference to the early detection of dementia. *British Journal of Psychiatry*, **149**, 698–709.

Rubin, E. H., Morris, J. C. & Berg, L. (1987). The progression of personality changes in patients with mild senile dementia of the Alzheimer type. *Journal of the American Geriatrics Society*, **35**, 721–5.

Ryden, M. B. (1988). Aggressive behavior in persons with dementia who live in the community. *Alzheimer Disease and Associated Disorders*, **2**, 342–55.

Sandman, P-O., Adolfsson, R., Nygren, C., Hallmans, G. & Winblad, B. (1987). Nutritional status and dietary intake in institutionalized patients with Alzheimer's disease and multiinfarct dementia. *Journal of the American Geriatrics Society*, **35**, 31–8.

Sanford, J. R. A. (1975). Tolerance of debility in elderly dependants by supporters at home: its significance for hospital practice. *British Medical Journal*, **3**, 471–3.

Schaie, K. W. & Willis, S. L. (1991). *Adult Development and Aging*, 3rd edition, Harper Collins, New York.

Serby, M. (1986). Olfaction and Alzheimer's disease. *Progress in Neuro-Psychopharmacology and Biological Psychiatry*, **10**, 579–86.

Silver, A. J. (1991). Eating disorders in the elderly. *Clinics in Applied Nutrition*, **1**, 63–7.

Singh, S., Mulley, G. P. & Losowsky, M. S. (1988). Why are Alzheimer patients thin? *Age and Ageing*, **17**, 21–8.

Snyder, L. H., Rupprecht, P., Pyrrek, J., Brckhus, S. & Moss, T. (1978). Wandering. *Gerontologist*, **18**, 272–80.

Steele, C., Rovner, B., Chase, G. A. & Folstein, M. (1990). Psychiatric symptoms and nursing home placement of patients with Alzheimer's disease. *American Journal of Psychiatry*, **147**, 1049–51.

Swaab, D. F., Fliers, E. & Partiman, T. S. (1985). The suprachiasmatic nucleus of the human brain in relation to sex, age and senile dementia. *Brain Research*, **342**, 37–44.

Swaab, D. F., Roozendaal, B., Ravid, R., Velis, D. N., Gooren, L. & Williams, R. S. (1987). Suprachiasmatic nucleus in aging, Alzheimer's disease, transsexuality and Prader–Willi syndrome. *Progress in Brain Research*, **72**, 301–10.

Swearer, J. M., Drachman, D. A., O'Donnell, B. F. & Mitchell, A. L. (1988).

Troublesome and disruptive behaviors in dementia. Relationships to diagnosis and disease severity. *Journal of the American Geriatrics Society*, **36**, 784–90.

Tavares, A. R. & Rabins, P. V. (1987). Weight loss in Alzheimer's disease: a longitudinal study. *Zeitschrift für Alternsforschung*, **42**, 165–7.

Teri, L. & Logsdon, R. (1990). Assessment and management of behavioral disturbances in Alzheimer's disease. *Comprehensive Therapy*, **16**, 36–42.

Teri, L., Borson, S., Kiyak, H. A. & Yamagishi, M. (1989). Behavioral disturbance, cognitive dysfunction, and functional skill. Prevalence and relationship in Alzheimer's disease. *Journal of the American Geriatrics Society*, **37**, 109–16.

Touitou, Y., Reinberg, A., Bodnan, A., Auzeby, A., Beck, H. & Touitou, C. (1986). Age-related changes in both circadian and seasonal rhythms of rectal temperature with special reference to senile dementia of Alzheimer type. *Gerontology*, **32**, 110–18.

van Gool, W. A. & Mirmiran, M. (1986). Aging and circadian rhythms. *Progress in Brain Research*, **70**, 255–77.

Vitiello, M. V. & Prinz, P. N. (1989). Alzheimer's disease. Sleep and sleep/wake patterns. *Clinics in Geriatric Medicine*, **5**, 289–99.

Vitiello, M. V., Prinz, P. N., Williams, D. E., Frommlet, M. S. & Ries, R. K. (1990). Sleep disturbances in patients with mild-stage Alzheimer's disease. *Journal of Gerontology*, **45**, M131–8.

Ware, C. J. G., Fairburn, C. G. & Hope, R. A. (1990). A community-based study of aggressive behaviour in dementia. *International Journal of Geriatric Psychiatry*, **5**, 337–42.

Woods, R. T. & Britton, P. G. (1985). *Clinical Psychology with the Elderly.* Croom Helm, New York.

Yudofsky, S. C., Silver, J. M., Jackson, W., Endicott, J. & Williams, D. (1986). The Overt Aggression Scale for the objective rating of verbal and physical aggression. *American Journal of Psychiatry*, **143**, 35–9.

15

Memory function in dementia and normal aging – dimension or dichotomy?

FELICIA A. HUPPERT

The increase in public awareness of Alzheimer's disease (AD), and dementia in general, has led many older adults to express concern that their memory failures might indicate they are developing dementia. The problem arises because memory impairment is the most prominent early feature in dementia and it is also extremely common, if not universal, among older adults.

Is it possible to distinguish the memory decline seen in normal aging from the progressive memory deficit characteristic of dementia? Such differentiation would be of value not only to basic neuroscience, but also to reassure those elderly people whose forgetfulness is benign. There are several approaches to differentiating normal and abnormal memory problems: one is to invoke diagnostic criteria for dementia; another more empirical approach is to examine the findings of clinical and experimental studies of memory performance in demented and elderly control subjects; and a third approach is to use the techniques of epidemiology to examine how memory changes over time in population samples of the elderly, including those who develop dementia. This chapter will assess the contribution of all three approaches.

Diagnostic criteria for memory impairment in dementia

Currently, the two most widely used sets of diagnostic criteria for mental disorders are DSM-III-R, DSM-IV (American Psychiatric Association, 1987, 1993) and ICD-10 (World Health Organization, 1992).

Although there are some differences between the two sets of criteria, they are alike in requiring, for a diagnosis of dementia:

(1) demonstrable evidence of memory impairment (i.e. self-report is not enough)

Dementia and Normal Aging, eds. F. A. Huppert, C. Brayne & D. W. O'Connor.
© Cambridge University Press 1994.

(2) an additional cognitive deficit (e.g. thinking, judgement, language, perception, constructional ability) and/or personality problems

(3) no other obvious cause for these difficulties

This implies that it is reasonable to reassure individuals who are worried that their memory problems mean incipient dementia, if they show any of the following:

(1) no objective evidence of memory impairment

(2) some memory impairment but no other cognitive deficit or personality change

(3) their memory impairment is attributable to some other cause e.g. depression

Although this approach seems straightforward and is probably used quite widely among clinicians, there are some problems. Since AD, the most common form of dementia, is a gradually progressive disorder, we would expect symptoms to appear before diagnostic criteria are satisfied. In particular, we would expect a gradual progression of memory failure of which the individual may be aware, before memory impairment is demonstrable on objective tests or confirmed by an informant. We might also find memory deficit to be evident prior to impairment of other cognitive functions or prior to personality change. In addition, the presence of factors associated with cognitive impairment (e.g. delirium, depression, some forms of medication) may mask a co-existing or incipient dementia. Thus, close adherence to the diagnostic criteria is of little assistance in differentiating the memory impairment in normal aging from that seen in the early stages of dementia.

Framework for analysing memory

There is an immense diversity of memory tasks and processes. An understanding of memory impairment requires an appreciation of this diversity. To attempt a full description is beyond the scope of this chapter and, in any case, such descriptions follow fashions which change so rapidly they are out of date by the time they are published. Rather, a simple, pragmatic framework will be presented as a basis for drawing together some of the extensive data on memory impairment in dementia and normal aging.

In considering disorders of memory, we can look at the content of what is being remembered, the age of the memory and the processes involved in remembering. Content may include the type of material (e.g. whether verbal or pictorial information is being assessed) and also whether the information refers to a particular episode or event ('episodic memory') or whether it is of a more general kind ('semantic memory') assessing knowledge of objects, words and facts. Learning a word list and recalling a recent item of news are typical examples of episodic memory; giving word definitions or generating a list of animal names are typical ways of assessing semantic memory. In the context of dementia and normal aging, the episodic/semantic distinction has played an important role in research and theory and is described in more detail below.

The age of a memory, or the time when the information was learnt, is a major determinant of retrieval. In general, memory impairment is associated with the relative preservation of remote memories compared with memory for recently acquired information. However, there is a danger in confusing the recent/remote distinction with the episodic/semantic distinction. Tests of recent memory assess episodic memory almost invariably. For example, in tests of word list recall, the subject is not acquiring new knowledge, but simply learning that a few words which are already part of their general knowledge need to be recalled. This requires the subject to associate the individual words with the specific learning context, and to recall them on request. On the other hand, tests of semantic memory nearly always assess remote memory, i.e. knowledge acquired a long time ago. When the focus is on assessing remote memory, clinicians ask questions like 'When did the second world war begin?', which is clearly a test of semantic memory or general knowledge. It has been suggested that even questions which appear to assess remote episodic memory (e.g. 'Where were you married?') may not do so. Either contextual detail fades or the stories become so well rehearsed that these memories take on the character of semantic memory (Cermak, 1984).

With regard to memory processes, the mental operations which are required for successful performance are very different in different tasks. Tasks which involve new learning place high requirements on attentional resources to organize, to encode and to store the information, prior to the retrieval operations needed to utilize it at the time of recall. In contrast, tasks which assess memory for information learnt outside the assessment situation require only retrieval processes, regardless of whether the information is episodic or semantic in character and whether it was acquired recently or in the remote past.

Of course, retrieval processes vary, depending on the nature of the retrieval task. Recall tasks place high demands on search processes, whereas recognition tasks may require only familiarity judgements. Both recall and recognition require conscious recollection of the information and are called explicit or direct tests of memory. Other tasks require only evidence of a change in behaviour to show that learning has taken place; the subject may have no conscious recollection of the learning experience. These other tasks include priming and procedural learning tasks and are called implicit or indirect tests of memory. An example of priming is the ability to identify incomplete information more quickly when the information has been presented recently. An example of procedural or skill learning is keeping a pointer on the track of a moving target (e.g. the pursuit rotor task). Such tasks place few demands on retrieval processes, which may explain why memory-impaired subjects often show normal performance on such tasks (see below).

This brief account of the content and age of memories, and the processes required for successful performance on different memory tasks, provides the background for the research findings discussed below.

Experimental comparisons of memory in demented and control subjects

The goal of many experimental studies is to establish whether differences between memory performance in demented and control subjects are qualitative or quantitative. If qualitative differences are found, such as one group being influenced by an experimental variable while the other is not, then differentiation between normal and abnormal memory impairment should be easy. The fact that there is as yet no diagnostic memory test, i.e. one which provides a definite diagnosis of dementia, suggests either that no qualitative differences have been found, or that any such effects reflect group differences and are not useful at the level of individuals. Where there is evidence for quantitative differences in memory performance, differentiation between normal and abnormal memory may nevertheless be possible by using cutpoints (see below).

Selection of subjects

Before describing some of the main findings in the literature, it should be noted that the value of the experimental studies depends critically on the way in which subjects and controls are selected. First, only comparisons with mild or early-stage cases are informative in this context. Second, the controls should obviously be as similar as possible to the experimental subjects in everything except the presence of dementia. Matching for age, sex and education are routine and it is usual to apply to controls the exclusion criteria applied to the demented group. Since most studies restrict cases to those with AD or probable AD, the main exclusion is the absence of disorders that in and of themselves could account for the progressive deficits in memory and cognition (McKhann et al., 1984). However, one suspects that most normal controls vary from the demented group in ways which are rarely specified. Since the normal controls are usually community volunteers, they are less likely to have mobility problems and sensory deficits and are more likely to have good general health. The patients, too, are usually selected in ways not specified by diagnostic criteria. All have been referred to specialists, which means: (1) the dementia is of sufficient severity or duration that it has come to specialist attention and may therefore be less mild or less early than one might wish; and (2) patients who see specialists may not be representative of all demented subjects. Thus, in the interpretation of findings, great care needs to be taken in generalizing from these selected patient and control groups to the population at large. One implication of these considerations is that observed differences are likely to be an exaggeration (if not a distortion) of the performance which would be seen in a genuinely representative sample.

Similarities and differences in memory performance

The history of science shows us that it is risky to make generalizations, but at this stage it seems fairly safe to say that demented subjects are impaired on any task which requires the conscious recollection of newly learnt information, i.e. on all direct tests of recent memory, including short-term memory (e.g. digit span) (see review by Nebes, 1992). This deficit is apparent even in the mild or early stages of dementia (Table 15.1). Virtually all direct tests of recent memory employ episodic memory tasks, although theoretically they do not

Table 15.1. *Mean scores on tests of recently acquired information*

Tests	Mean score		
	Normals (n = 56)	Minimal dementia (n = 12)	Mild/moderate dementia (n = 9)
Clinical items			
Recall of six objects (6)	3.40	2.0	1.0
Recall of name and address (5)	4.55	4.2	2.6
Recall of three words (3)	2.05	1.5	1.0
Psychometric tests of memory			
Free recall (16)	4.00	1.8	0.6
Cued recall (16)	3.45	1.3	0.1
Recognition (16)	12.75	10.1	6.6
Behavioural tests of memory			
Story (immediate) (21)	3.65	2.5	0.4
Story (delayed) (21)	2.45	0.3	0.1
Route (immediate) (5)	4.00	3.3	2.0
Route (delayed) (5)	4.05	2.7	0.8
Name (4)	2.90	1.4	0.1

Adapted from Huppert & Beardsall (1991).
Numbers in brackets indicate the maximum score for each test.

have to. Recalling vocabulary learnt recently in a foreign language would presumably qualify as a direct test of recent semantic memory, although it is likely that normal subjects would use episodic/contextual information to aid recall, e.g. visualizing the words on the page.

Recall of recently acquired information is impaired in all subjects when they are required to divide their attention during learning, e.g. performing a digit span test while keeping a stylus on target in a pursuit rotor task. The impairment produced by dual task performance is relatively greater in demented than in control subjects (e.g. Morris, 1984; Baddeley et al., 1986; Grober & Sliwinski, 1991). This has been termed a defect in 'working memory' which is the ability to hold information in a short-term store while carrying out other processing operations.

Although laboratory tests of dual-task performance seem rather contrived, much of our everyday memory is of this kind, e.g. having a conversation while driving or preparing a meal. Such tasks place high demands on processing resources and are therefore quite likely to be sensitive even to small reductions in processing capacity.

Memory researchers have recently begun to take an interest in another complex, everyday type of task, known as prospective memory. Prospective memory is remembering to carry out an action at the appropriate time, e.g. remembering to mail a letter or turn off the cooker before the food burns. Prospective memory can be regarded as an example of performing under conditions of divided attention, since other events intervene between the intention to act and the carrying out of the action.

The Rivermead Behavioural Memory Test (Wilson et al., 1985) contains three measures of prospective memory: remembering to make an appointment when a buzzer sounds; remembering to ask for a personal belonging to be returned at the end of the assessment session; and remembering to deliver a message in the course of retracing a route around the room. Huppert & Beardsall (1993) administered these tests to normal and demented subjects from a population sample, and found that subjects with dementia, even those with minimal severity, were disproportionately impaired on prospective memory compared to retrospective memory (conventional measures of retrieval of newly acquired information). Table 15.2 presents the percentage of individuals in each group who showed adequate performance on these tasks. Further analyses will be required to determine whether the vulnerability of prospective memory tasks reflects the high processing demands of keeping the intention in mind while carrying out other activities, the lack of specific cues at the time of retrieval, or the element of planning which is involved in the successful performance of a prospective memory task. What is clear, however, is that very simple prospective memory tasks are sensitive even to the very early stage of dementia.

While most studies show impaired memory for newly acquired information in demented subjects, regardless of the type of information being examined, there are recent reports of material-specific impairment in dementia. Material-specific memory loss can occur following focal brain lesions (e.g. selective inability to retrieve verbal material

Table 15.2. *Percentage of subjects attaining the maximum score on tests of prospective memory*

	Normal (n = 27)	Low scoring normal (n = 26)	Minimal dementia (n = 12)	Mild/moderate dementia (n = 9)
Appointment	82	58	8	0
Belonging	79	68	0	22
Message (immediate)	93	54	25	22
Message (delayed)	78	58	8	11

From Huppert & Beardsall (1993).

or to recognize faces) but we would not expect it to be present in age-related memory impairment or most cases of dementia, where the pathology is diffuse and bilateral. However, in a group of 55 mild AD patients, Baddeley et al. (1991) report two with a material-specific memory deficit, one of these showing relatively greater impairment on verbal (list learning) compared with spatial (block tapping) material, the other showing the reverse pattern. Becker et al. (1992), in a series of 190 AD patients, report that 13% had a material-specific memory disorder. On the other hand, 10% (10 out of 102) of the normal controls showed the same pattern. Thus, the apparent material-specific deficit of some AD patients may simply reflect normal variation in performance which may have been present prior to the development of the disorder. Indeed, failure to take account of normal variation may lead to misinterpreting apparent dissociations on cognitive tests in demented subjects.

Direct vs. indirect measures of episodic memory in dementia

While mildly demented subjects are impaired on virtually all direct measures of episodic memory, a very different picture emerges in relation to indirect tests of memory. Indirect memory tests look for evidence of prior learning by assessing whether behaviour has changed, but without requiring the subject consciously to recollect the learning experience. For example, in word-stem completion priming, subjects are shown the first three letters of words and asked simply to say the first word that comes to mind beginning with the three letters. Each stem can be completed by several words, so if the subjects produce words from the learning list this provides evidence of memory. Several studies have demonstrated that demented subjects perform normally on this task (e.g. Miller 1975; Christensen & Birrell 1991; Partridge et al., 1990), suggesting that the information was learnt and stored, but the difficulty observed in recall testing arose from inability to gain conscious access to it. The few studies which have failed to find normal priming in demented patients used an incidental learning procedure, e.g. they asked subjects to judge how much they liked each of the words in the list, rather than asking them to remember the words (Shimamura et al., 1987; Salmon et al., 1988; Heindel et al., 1989). This procedure would have led to a poor level of initial encoding which may have affected the demented subjects differentially compared to the controls. Normal performance in demented subjects has also been shown on other indirect measures of memory, such as perceptual priming, where a word or object has to be identified from a fragmented form. Even moderately demented subjects identify items more easily if they have seen them in the learning session (e.g. Huppert & Beardsall, 1988). Demented subjects may also show normal learning and retention on tasks such as motor skill learning (e.g. Eslinger & Damasio, 1986; Heindel et al., 1989), despite having no conscious recollection of doing the test before.

The finding that at least some forms of memory are intact in demented subjects has implications both for our understanding of memory processes and for patient management. Further research is required to determine whether there are two separate memory systems as suggested by Mishkin and colleagues (Mishkin et al., 1984; Mishkin & Appenzeller, 1987), one for 'memories' and one for 'habits', or whether there is a single system which may be accessed in a conscious way or in a more automatic way.

With respect to patient management, there is evidence that even patients with a moderately severe dementia are capable of learning (e.g. Wertheimer et al., 1992). But are they also capable of retaining information over a long period?

Rates of forgetting

There have been a few studies of the ability of demented subjects to retain information over long intervals. On a test of picture recognition,

Kopelman (1985) found a normal rate of forgetting over a one-week retention interval in patients with AD. Similar results have been reported by Corkin et al. (1984). To avoid the difficulty inherent in comparing forgetting rates when groups start at different levels, both studies equated the initial level of learning in the AD and control groups using the titration procedure developed by Huppert & Piercy (1978). Knopman (1991), using a serial reaction-time task, also reports normal retention. Subjects had to press one of four keys corresponding to one of four locations on a screen, when an asterisk appeared. Subjects were unaware that a 10-item sequence was repeated randomly. Demented subjects learnt the sequence and showed normal retention over a two-week interval.

Perhaps the most surprising thing about this set of findings is that retention was normal not only on indirect testing (the serial reaction-time task) but also on direct testing (recognition memory). The explanation may be that in the recognition memory tasks, subjects had to choose between items they had seen before and items they had never seen. To succeed on such tasks, they did not need to recollect where or when they had seen the items (episodic information) but simply had to make a familiarity judgement. Further work is required to determine whether long-term retention is normal in demented subjects on tests such as verbal recognition, which requires episodic information.

Remote versus recent memory

While recent events are very poorly recalled by individuals with dementia, the ability to recall remote events may be retained until dementia has progressed to a moderate or severe stage. Tests of autobiographical memory have been used to determine whether there is a temporal gradient in the recall of events in one's life. For example, Kopelman (1989) has developed a test of cued autobiographical memory and a personal events interview in which subjects are asked to recall specific information from various decades in their life (e.g. where they have lived, names of schools attended), and recall accuracy is verified independently. While AD patients perform more poorly than normals in all time periods, they also show a different pattern of results. Normals are better at recalling recent time periods compared with remote time periods, while for AD patients, the older the information the better their performance. The same pattern of performance is shown by AD patients when memory for remote public information is assessed; for example when subjects are asked questions about public events or famous faces, where the event or individual became famous at a particular point in the past. While AD patients perform more poorly than normals, they recall proportionately more information from the more remote past than the more recent past (Sagar et al., 1988; Kopelman 1989).

The temporal gradient seen in dementia is not simply the consequence of impaired encoding or storage of information. In his review of the area, Sagar (1990) makes the important point that the temporal gradient covers events which took place long before the onset of the dementia. There are alternative explanations for the gradient. One is that memory traces are strengthened over time due to reminiscence and/or to the formation of associations with newly acquired information, thus enriching the set of retrieval cues available for older memories (Sagar, 1990). The other explanation is that over time the memory trace of an episode loses its associations with time and context, and assumes the character of semantic memory (Cermak, 1984). We need then to ask whether semantic memory is less vulnerable to the ravages of dementia than is episodic memory.

Semantic memory

In a seminal paper, Weingartner et al. (1983) showed that a small group of patients in the early stages of dementia were severely impaired on four tests of semantic memory. They included: verbal fluency; completing highly structured sentences (e.g. some say 'a dog is man's best . . .'); deciding which of two common actions occurs first (e.g. eating in a restaurant and reading the menu); and generating ideas in response to a question (e.g. 'What are things you would do after getting up in the morning?'). It could be argued that this last task is not a valid test of semantic memory, since normals can succeed by accessing their episodic memory for the activities they carried out in the recent past. However, in this study Weingartner et al. showed that Korsakoff patients, whose episodic memory deficit was as severe as that of the demented patients, performed normally on this task. The authors conclude that demented individuals 'have little access to previously acquired knowledge and therefore face great difficulty in organizing and encoding ongoing events' (Weingartner et al., 1983, p. 380). However, they also note that the errors made by demented subjects were related semantically to the context, indicating that the impairment in semantic memory is not absolute.

In the intervening decade, there has been continual debate about the presence and extent of semantic memory impairment in dementia. The debate has been summarized in excellent reviews by Nebes & Brady (1988, 1990). Semantic information about concepts appears to be organized hierarchically, with the supraordinate category at the top of the hierarchy (e.g. 'animal'), its more specific attributes (e.g. four-legged, can fly) further down the hierarchy, followed by lower order categories (exemplars such as dog, insect), and so on. It has been suggested that, early in the course of dementia, knowledge of specific attributes and examplars is lost or becomes inaccessible, while category knowledge is retained until later in the disease. Such a loss of specific information would effectively strip concepts of much of their meaning, making it difficult to name pictures, understand language or encode information into memory. However, while some authors find evidence for a loss of specific attributes in AD (e.g. Martin & Fedio, 1983; Chertkow et al., 1989), others do not (e.g. Grober et al., 1985; Nebes & Brady, 1988). According to Nebes & Brady (1990), the key lies in the demands placed on subjects by the experimental task. When AD subjects are asked a direct question about an object's attributes (e.g. 'Is it made of metal?'), they perform poorly. If they are asked merely to decide whether an item is related to an attribute, they perform comparatively normally.

Thus, the distinction between direct and indirect tests of memory is as important in relation to understanding deficits in semantic memory as it is in understanding deficits in episodic memory. Nebes & Brady (1990) conclude that the problem for AD patients is more that of searching consciously for the appropriate level of attributes than it is a loss of knowledge of attribute information.

Another way to approach the question of whether semantic knowledge is lost or merely difficult to access is to examine whether subjects make consistent errors when their knowledge of items is tested across a range of tasks and across modalities. Huff et al. (1986) and Chertkow & Bub (1990) have demonstrated a significant item-to-item correspondence on tests of naming and comprehension using the same examples. In a very comprehensive study, Hodges et al. (1992) analysed the errors made by individual patients across tests of category fluency, picture naming, spoken word-to-picture matching, picture sorting and generation of verbal definitions, and found a significant correspondence between the individual items. They also found a relative preservation of supraordinate knowledge (e.g. demented patients were normal at deciding whether pictures represented living things or man-made objects), as well as a disproportionate reduction in the generation of examples from lower-order categories (e.g. breeds of dog). They concluded that their finding 'offers compelling evidence that the semantic breakdown in DAT is caused by storage degradation' (Hodges et al., 1992, p. 301). Elegant as this study is, all the tests employed *direct* measures of semantic knowledge. A final decision about whether semantic knowledge is lost from store or only difficult to access must await a similarly elegant study using indirect measures of knowledge.

Are there memory tasks which can discriminate between dementia and normal aging?

All studies of memory to date have shown only quantitative differences between mildly demented and normal elderly subjects. Generally, demented groups perform in a similar fashion to normals, but at a lower level, and there is always overlap between scores. This suggests that there is a continuity in memory performance. There do not appear to be any tests which discriminate with 100% accuracy between early or mild dementia and normal aging.

Nevertheless, it may be possible to find tests which discriminate with a reasonable degree of effectiveness. Such tests would undoubtedly be of value to clinicians. Suitable tests must not only show large differences in mean scores between groups, but also they must discriminate at the level of individuals. Among the investigations which have undertaken the appropriate analysis on the appropriate groups, Welsh et al. (1991) have examined the relative efficacy of the memory measures adopted by CERAD (Consortium to Establish a Registry for Alzheimer's Disease). Table 15.3 is a summary of their data on a group of 49 mild AD cases and 49 matched controls who were either community volunteers or informants for the patients. The best discriminator was the delayed recall of a 10-word list which was tested five to eight minutes after recall of the third learning trial. Use of a cutting score of 2SD below the control mean showed that delayed recall correctly classified 94% of the controls and 86% of the mildly demented. It is unlikely that discrimination would be as high in unselected groups of controls and demented subjects. No other measure approached this level of discrimination.

Huppert & Beardsall (1991) compared performance on 11 tests of

Table 15.3. *The efficacy of CERAD memory measures*

	Mean score			Classified correctly (%)	
	Control (n = 49)	Mild dementia (n = 49)	Dementia score as proportion of control value	Control	Mild dementia
Learning					
Trial 1	4.8	2.8	0.6	96	41
Trial 2	7.0	4.2	0.6	94	49
Trial 3	7.9	4.7	0.6	98	41
Delayed recall	6.8	1.8	0.3	94	86
Recognition					
Correct 'Yes'	9.7	8.2	0.8	96	39
Correct 'No'	9.7	7.7	0.8	98	25
Intrusions					
Trial 1	0.3	0.6	2.0	96	14
Trial 2	0.2	0.4	2.0	78	33
Trial 3	0.1	0.3	3.0	94	20
Delay	0.4	0.9	2.3	90	27

Adapted from Welsh et al. (1991).

memory for newly acquired information, in normal and demented subjects taken from a general population sample. Results of the discriminant function analysis are presented in Table 15.4. The tests which showed the best discrimination were: (1) recall of six objects presented initially as a naming test (without specific instructions to remember them); and (2) recalling the name associated with the photograph of a face, an item from the Rivermead Behavioural Memory Test (Wilson et al., 1985). The test of recalling three words (from the Mini-Mental State Examination of Folstein et al. (1975)) was one of the poorest measures for detecting dementia. Summing the scores on the two best items was shown to produce a high level of discrimination even

Table 15.4. *Percentage of subjects classified correctly as normal or demented using discriminant function analysis on individual memory tests*

	Correct classification (%)		
	Normal (n = 56)	Demented (n = 21)	Total
Clinical items			
Recall of six objects	84	91	86
Recall of name and address	91	57	82[a]
Recall of three words	79	57	73[a]
Psychometric tests of memory			
Free recall	75	86	78
Cued recall	66	86	71[a]
Recognition	86	71	82
Behavioural tests of memory			
Story (immediate)	61	81	66[a]
Story (delayed)	68	91	74
Route (immediate)	70	67	69
Route (delayed)	84	62	78[a]
Name	91	76	87

[a]Classification not significantly different from chance for either group.
From Huppert & Beardsall (1991).

between two groups on the borderline of cognitive decline and dementia. They were: a 'low-scoring normal' group who scored 21 or less on the MMSE but were normal when assessed by the CAMDEX diagnostic interview (Roth et al., 1986, 1988); and a group of subjects diagnosed as having minimal dementia, i.e. they did not meet DSM-III-R or equivalent criteria for dementia, but appeared to be in the very early stages of dementia as defined by CAMDEX operational criteria. The category 'minimal dementia' is roughly equivalent to 'questionable dementia' on the Clinical Dementia Rating (CDR=0.5) of Hughes et al. (1982). Correct classifications were made for 89% of the low-scoring normals and 92% of the minimal dementia subjects. However, the number of demented subjects in this study was small (n=21), and the finding needs to be replicated.

Storandt & Hill (1989) administered an extensive test battery with a large memory component to 66 mild AD patients, 41 with questionable AD and 83 controls. They carried out a discriminant analysis to determine the measures and their weights that would correlate maximally with group membership. The analysis showed that a single canonical variable accounted for 86% of the variation in scores. Using a cutoff point on this variable, they found that no control subjects and only three of the mild AD patients were misclassified. They also reported: 'there is no cutoff point, however, that allows good discrimination of the questionably demented group' (Storandt & Hill, 1989, p. 385). The scores of the questionable AD group completely overlapped those of the other two groups. This is particularly interesting in view of the fact that the controls were volunteers with the usual selection biases, and therefore differences are more likely to be seen than in the general population. One would expect that normal elderly people with a range of physical illnesses and sensory deficits would perform below the level of the control group, overlapping extensively with the demented groups. Thus, data such as those of Storandt & Hill (1989) provide evidence in support of the continuity hypothesis. The contradictory findings of Huppert & Beardsall (1991) may be due either to the small sample or to the use of more sensitive measures.

Can memory impairment predict dementia?

The above studies have examined cross-sectional associations between memory performance and diagnostic groups. However, a key question is whether memory performance on one occasion can predict the subsequent development of dementia. While many ongoing longitudinal studies are actively exploring this question, there are few published findings to date. Katzman et al. (1989) followed 434 normal volunteers over five years and found that 56 developed dementia. The best predictor was poor performance (5–8 errors) on the information-memory-concentration tests of Blessed et al. (1968). The incidence of dementia among poor performers was almost four times higher than for the entire sample (12% vs. 3.5% per year). However, the poor performers had a lower level of education, and this effect does not appear to have been taken into account in the incidence analysis.

Tuokko et al. (1991) followed a group of patients who had all been referred to specialist services to establish whether they had dementia. Of 45 who did not meet diagnostic criteria at intitial assessment, 18 were diagnosed as demented 12–18 months later. The group which developed dementia was found to have significantly lower scores on a cued recall test at initial assessment, and also showed a significant decline in scores compared to the stable scores of the group which remained non-demented. The results of this study should be treated with caution however, because, although the authors report no significant differences in age, education or gender between the 'change' and 'no change' groups, the group which became demented were in fact older, less well educated and contained a higher proportion of women (55% vs. 37%), and all these factors are associated with an increased risk of AD (Chapter 9 this volume). Future studies need to consider the combined effect of such variables, and not just their individual effects.

There is an additional problem in determining whether poor memory performance is a predictor of dementia. Several longitudinal studies have found that rapid decline in memory performance is associated with increased mortality (Scherr et al., 1988; Colsher & Wallace, 1991a), but these studies have not established the diagnostic status of these individuals before death. This may result in an underestimate of the strength of the association between memory impairment and dementia. On the other hand, given the multiplicity of causes of memory impairment (e.g. Huppert, 1991a), poor memory performance at one point in time, or longitudinal memory decline, are likely to be non-specific symptoms of incipient dementia.

Are dementia-related and age-related memory impairments similar to one another?

The main findings concerning memory function in the early stages of dementia may be summarized as follows:

(1) There is a severe impairment of recently acquired information when memory is assessed by conscious recollection (recall, recognition)
(2) The impairment is exacerbated in divided attention tasks
(3) There is evidence of new learning when memory is assessed by indirect tests
(4) Remote memory for early time periods may be relatively preserved
(5) Semantic memory is impaired, apart from supraordinate knowledge, when assessed by conscious recollection

(6) Indirect tests suggest that the structure of semantic memory remains intact
(7) Rate of forgetting is normal, at least for material which does not require retrieval of contextual information

If the memory impairment seen in early dementia lies some way along a continuum of an age-related decline in memory, then the elderly controls with whom demented subjects have been compared may not be 'normal' in terms of their memory performance compared to young adults.

Similarities and differences in memory performance of younger and older adults

There have been several recent reviews of the mushrooming literature on age differences in memory (Huppert, 1991b; Craik & Salthouse, 1992). This section focuses on those findings which are most relevant to the relationship between dementia and normal aging.

The age range studied and the method of selecting older and younger age-groups can have a profound effect on the conclusions which are drawn. Few studies include the very old (age 75 years and over) and some stop at age 69 years. Yet Schaie and his colleagues (Schaie, 1983) have shown that cognitive function begins to decline sharply only around age 67 years. Most studies match younger and older adults in terms of education and health, which usually means that both groups are well educated and healthy. The main reason for this selection is the assumption that significant differences in performance are more likely to reflect genuine age differences and cannot be attributed to the 'confounding' effect of poor health, sensory impairment, poor education, etc. Clearly, however, such studies cannot rule out cohort or generational differences in ability or task performance, and this issue will be discussed in more detail below.

A major finding is that careful matching of older and younger subjects greatly reduces age differences in memory for recently acquired information, and, in some studies, age differences are eliminated. Attempts have been made to establish why some tasks show age differences while others do not and hence to identify the processes responsible for these differences.

On standard tests of recognition memory, the results consistently indicate no age differences in well-educated or high IQ groups (see

Poon, 1985). This contrasts with the impaired recognition memory of groups with mild dementia, although recognition tests are not good at discriminating between demented and control subjects at the individual level (see above). Measures of free recall and paired-associate learning generally demonstrate age differences in performance even when groups are matched. In order to improve the recall of older subjects, some investigators have given instruction in the use of verbal elaboration strategies or visual imagery but the results do not consistently show a reduction in age differences.

In general, age differences are magnified when there is little contextual information provided at the time of retrieval (Craik, 1986). Recognition tasks provide a great deal of contextual information and the subject has to decide only whether or not the item is familiar or was in the learning list. Recall tasks provide little contextual information and rely on the subject initiating a mental search. Recall tasks therefore place greater demands on processing resources and are likely to be impaired if processing resources are compromised. In a classic study, Craik & McDowd (1987) demonstrated that recall deficits are not simply the result of recall tests being more difficult than recognition tests. They showed that the recall of older adults was impaired relative to recognition even when a difficult recognition task was compared with an easy recall task.

Memory performance is affected not only by the processing demands of the retrieval task, but also by the amount of processing resources which a subject can devote to the learning task. Under conditions of dual-task performance, where subjects have to divide their attention between tasks (e.g. learning a list of spoken words while carrying out a visual reaction-time task), subsequent recall is impaired. Studies have shown that this impairment is relatively greater for older compared with younger subjects, and indeed that, following divided attention tasks, the recall of young subjects resembles that of older subjects whose attention was not divided (Craik, 1982). Data of this type have been interpreted by Craik and others as demonstrating that normal elderly people have a reduction in their processing capacity.

Several other deficits shown by older adults can also be interpreted in this way. These include: age differences in 'working memory'; the ability to carry out processing operations while holding information in a short-term store (e.g. Morris et al., 1988); and prospective memory, where an instruction to carry out an action is retained while the subject performs other activities. Reliable age differences in prospective memory have been reported in laboratory tests where subjects have to keep the instruction in mind and are not able to use memory aids (e.g. Cockburn & Smith, 1988; West, 1988). Age differences are usually absent, or may even favour older adults, in naturalistic situations such as being instructed to make telephone calls or to send postcards at predetermined times (e.g. Moscovich, 1982). In the Moscovich studies, all the older subjects and the few young subjects who performed well reported using external memory aids such as notes in diaries or calendars, i.e. in fact, they did not rely on their memories.

Learning involves acquiring specific information as well as integrating the information or event with its context. For example, as well as taking in the gist of a news item, noting whether the newsreader was male or female and whether it was on radio or television. Schacter et al., (1984) have suggested that the process of integrating events with their context, demands a considerable amount of processing resources. Consistent with this, several studies show that, compared with young adults, older adults are relatively more impaired on context recall than on item recall (e.g. McIntyre & Craik, 1987). McIntyre & Craik showed that, whereas young people recalled the source of newly acquired facts after a one-week delay, older adults remembered the facts but showed 'source amnesia', i.e. they attributed the facts to the wrong source (not to the experiment) or to the wrong modality (auditory versus visual presentation).

Turning to the distinction between direct and indirect tests of memory, indirect tests (response facilitation) place fewer demands on processing than do direct tests (recall, recognition) and, therefore, we may expect to find minimal age differences on indirect memory tasks. Most studies confirm this prediction (e.g. Light & Singh, 1987). However, one study, using a wider than usual age range, showed significant deficits on a word-stem completion test among individuals in their 70s and 80s (Davis et al., 1990). It is interesting that the method and stimuli used by these investigators were identical to those used by Shimamura et al. (1987) and co-workers, who are among the few investigators to have shown impaired performance on indirect testing in AD patients.

In addition to the evidence above that there are age-related deficits in remembering recently acquired information, it appears that the retrieval of remote memories may also suffer some impairment in older adults. Sagar et al. (1991) asked subjects aged 50 years and over to relate an autobiographical memory from any period of their lives in response to each of 10 words (e.g. bird, flag, car). They found that older subjects produced significantly older memories even when memories were divided into two time periods (0–20 years ago; more than 20 years ago). The same trend was found in AD patients, i.e. older AD patients produced older memories. The memories produced by AD patients aged 50 to 69 years were significantly older than those produced by age-matched controls, but there were no significant differences between AD patients and controls aged 70 years and over. The authors conclude: 'The alteration in age distribution of episodes produced by dementia has qualitatively similar, but lesser, effects to those of advancing age in normal subjects' (Sagar et al., 1991, p. 243).

To determine whether newly acquired information is stored as effectively by adults of different ages, investigators have examined the effect of varying the retention interval. In his review of the literature, Salthouse (1991) concludes that the loss of information across short periods of time (seconds to hours) does not appear to vary as a function of age. The picture is far less clear when the retention interval is extended to 24 hours or more. Salthouse cites a roughly equal number of studies reporting no age differences, and greater loss among older adults (see Salthouse, 1991, p. 236). One of the problems may be that rates of change are difficult to compare unless groups start at a comparable level – where performance must be less than 100% accurate to ensure that ceiling effects do not obscure underlying differences. One study which circumvented this problem was a study of picture recognition memory (Huppert & Kopelman, 1989). Older subjects, whose performance was equivalent to that of younger subjects at a 10-minute retention interval, showed faster forgetting over the subsequent 24-hour and one-week retention intervals. It was mentioned above that, on the same task, the forgetting rates of demented subjects did not differ from normal controls (Kopelman, 1985). Therefore, we appear to have an instance where age-related changes alone are associated with impairment, and dementia, at least in mild form, does not significantly exacerbate this impairment.

Semantic memory

The evidence that verbal ability and general knowledge tends to be preserved in old age, has led some investigators to suggest that episodic, but not semantic memory, shows age-related impairment (Mitchell, 1989). However, this does not take account of the name-finding difficulty of which elderly people frequently complain, nor of the age-related deficit on word fluency tasks, which has been shown in both cross-sectional and longitudinal studies (Schaie, 1980). This is seen in Figure 15.1, along with evidence that performance on a vocabulary test also declines with age, whether one uses cross-sectional or longitudinal data. The surprisingly steep decline in word fluency as individuals age (longitudinal data) probably reflects the fact that subjects were required to write the words, rather than the more usual procedure of saying them aloud.

In one of the rare investigations of very old people, Poon et al. (1992), as part of their study of centenarians, have shown a dramatic age-related decline in WAIS vocabulary (Figure 15.2). The very poor performance of the oldest old appears in spite of sampling criteria which included only subjects who were community-dwelling, cognitively intact (not demented or disoriented) and in reasonable health.

Since evidence of memory impairment plays a key role in the diagnosis of dementia, the findings of severe memory problems among the very old make it clear that the diagnosis of dementia is extremely difficult to make in this age group. This conclusion is reflected in the widely used criteria for Alzheimer's disease (NINCDS–ADRDA; McKhann et al., 1984) which state that the diagnosis can be made only if onset of dementia is between the ages of 40 and 90 years.

Difficulty in name finding is a frequent complaint of individuals as they grow older. Age-related problems in the retrieval of well-known

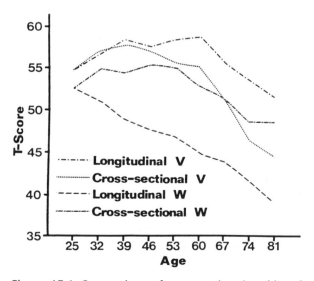

Figure 15.1. Comparison of cross-sectional and longitudinal data on age changes and differences on verbal meaning (V) and word fluency (W), from the Seattle Longitudinal Study. (From Schaie, 1980.)

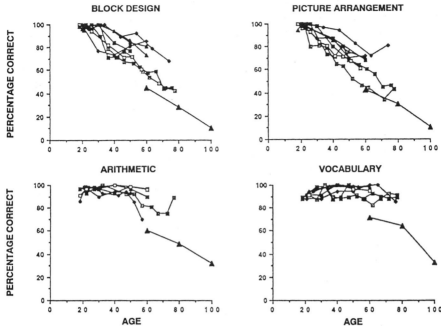

Figure 15.2. Performances of centenarian study participants (solid triangle) compared with normative data on subtests of the WAIS-R. (From Poon et al., 1992. Copyright © 1992 by the Baywood Publishing Company, Inc. Amityville, New York.)

words have been demonstrated both in laboratory studies and in naturalistic studies, where subjects record in a diary every occurrence of a 'tip-of-the-tongue' (TOT) experience (Burke et al., 1991).

Burke & Laver (1990) propose that to understand semantic memory deficits in the elderly it is necessary to distinguish between tests which involve language comprehension (e.g. the verbal subtests of the WAIS) and those which involve language production, e.g. name finding, verbal fluency. They suggest it is language production only which is impaired as a result of age differences in the retrieval of phonological information. To be confident of this conclusion, one would need to establish that the comprehension and production measures are of equal difficulty. However, it remains to be established whether or not phonological retrieval (or the tasks which measure it) are more demanding than comprehension measures. For example, in comprehension measures, such as WAIS vocabulary, a range of possible responses indicates good comprehension in tasks, but in production measures, such as retrieving a specific name, there is one correct response only.

At present, however, neither the comprehension/production distinction nor the direct/indirect distinction provides an adequate conceptualization of the specific name-finding impairment shown by the normal elderly. In a study using fictitious mini-biographies, Cohen & Faulkner (1986) have shown that the age-related retrieval difficulty is relatively greater for proper names than for other words. Subjects heard for example 'James Gibson is a policeman who lives in Glasgow and wins prizes for ballroom dancing' and later attempted to fill in blanks in a written version. There were no significant age differences in the retrieval of occupations, hobbies and place names, only in the retrieval of first names and surnames.

Findings such as these demonstrate that semantic memory is not a single entity, and some forms of semantic knowledge are spared in old age while others are impaired.

Memory performance in elderly population samples

While experimental and clinical studies have produced much valuable information about memory functions and processes in elderly normal and demented subjects, participants in these studies are not representative of the elderly population as a whole. The effect of using a non-representative sample can be seen in Figure 15.3 from Huppert (1991a). Subjects from a representative community sample performed

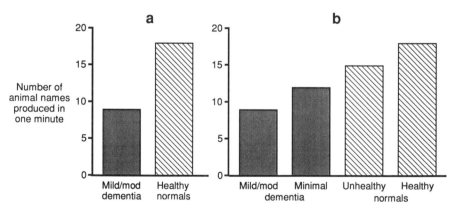

Figure 15.3. Mean number of correct animal names produced in a one-minute fluency test. Subjects were aged 75+ years, from a representative community sample. (a) Compares the scores of subjects with dementia and a selected group of healthy normal subjects; (b) includes scores for unhealthy normal subjects (75% of the normal population) and those with very early stage or minimal dementia. (From Huppert, 1991a.)

a word fluency task (naming as many different animals as possible in one minute). Subjects meeting clinical criteria for dementia (nearly all mild severity) were compared with a group of normal elderly subjects selected to resemble the usual volunteer control group, i.e. they were mobile and relatively healthy. Their mean scores are shown in Figure 15.3a. There was a highly significant difference between groups, with relatively little overlap: 90% of the demented subjects produced fewer than 15 words while 78% of the normals produced 15 words or more. However, the discrimination broke down, as shown in Figure 15.3b, when the full sample was considered, i.e. including normal subjects who were not in good health or not mobile (three-quarters of the normal sample) and those diagnosed as having minimal dementia. Once again, these findings are more consistent with there being a spectrum of memory function, rather than a normal/demented dichotomy.

Clearly the best way to examine the relationship between memory impairment and dementia is to study memory performance and memory processes in large, representative population samples, including individuals in institutions. Cross-sectional studies allow an examination of the variables which are correlated with memory performance, while longitudinal studies enable an examination of the rate and predictors of memory decline, as well as a separation of age and cohort effects.

It is reasonable to assume that the normalization samples for standard memory tests such as the revised Wechsler Memory Scale (WMS-R; Wechsler, 1987) are representative of the population. However, this is not the case. The following exclusion criteria were applied to the normalization sample: 'Only nonimpaired individuals were included in the standardization sample. Examiners were instructed to screen potential examinees for a list of several medical risk factors that might affect performance on the WMS-R, such as excessive use of alcohol, neurological disease, and psychiatric disorders' (Wechsler, 1987, p. 45). Not only are these criteria poorly specified, and appear to have been applied at the discretion of lay interviewers, they almost certainly excluded a high percentage of normal (non-demented) older individuals, particularly if sensory deficits were also an exclusion. This has serious consequences for the use of these norms in assessing whether or not an individual's memory performance is below that expected for their age. The effect will be to overestimate the number of elderly people with clinically significant memory impairment. Rather than excluding individuals with risk factors which might affect performance, normalization samples should be based on unselected population samples and the effects of these risk factors should be examined.

Cross-sectional studies

There have been a few studies of memory in unselected population samples. Scherr et al. (1988) studied 3682 (82.1%) of the non-institutionalized residents aged 65 years and over of a geographically defined community in East Boston. They employed tests of orientation, digit span and recall of a simple story. Age-related performance is shown in Figure 15.4. In addition to the strong inverse relationship between age and performance on these tasks, education, socio-economic index and level of disability on an ADL scale were all related independently to memory performance. This report does not separate groups with and without dementia, but it is clear from their findings that the prevalence of dementia cannot account for the very high levels of memory impairment in this elderly population.

A British study, the Health and Lifestyle Survey (Cox et al., 1987), administered a 10-word recall test to a nationally representative sample of 7414 community residents aged 18 years and over assessed in their own homes. Age was the main variable which influenced performance but other variables which exerted significant effects included education, physical health, socio-economic group, reasoning ability,

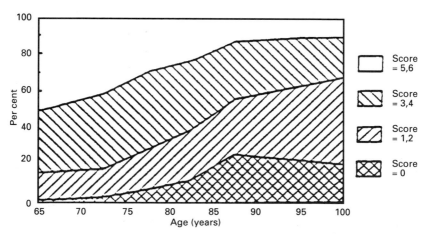

Figure 15.4. Distribution of immediate memory test (recall) scores by age in participants in the East Boston study. (From Scherr et al., 1988.)

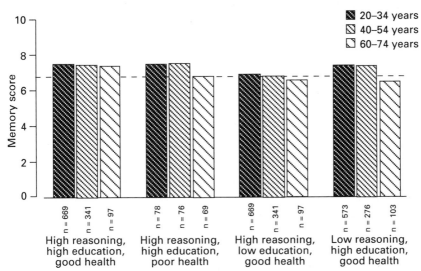

Figure 15.5. Mean number of items recalled in an incidental memory test of respondents in three discrete age-groups matched for health, educational qualifications and performance on a reasoning test. The numbers at the bottom of the columns are the number of individuals in each group. (From Huppert & Elliott, 1988.)

sex (females performed better than males) and participation in leisure activities. Further analyses were undertaken to establish whether, by matching on key variables, age differences in memory could be eliminated. Figure 15.5 shows the results of such an analysis. Matching young, middle-aged and older adults on education, IQ (measured by a test of reasoning ability) and health, resulted in the elimination of age differences for subjects who obtained high scores on all three variables. Matching on any two of these variables was not sufficient to offset age differences in this non-institutionalized population sample (Huppert & Elliott, 1988; Huppert, 1991b). Although education had the largest effect within an age group, high participation in leisure activities (excluding sport) offset the adverse effect of attaining no educational qualifications. This can be seen in Figure 15.6 showing performance of all retired subjects aged 60 to 74 years, in relation to the number of leisure activities in the past two weeks, which they endorsed from a standard list. Analysis of variance revealed that the effect of leisure activities was significant only for the group without educational qualifications. Moreover, the poorly-educated group with high participation in leisure activities did not differ significantly from the well-educated group. It is interesting that in this study there was no association between memory performance and sport or other physical activity.

Rather similar findings have been reported in a Canadian study of 484 community residents aged 55 to 85 years, although participants in this study were volunteers. Hultsch et al. (1993) tested subjects on a variety of cognitive variables including measures of semantic and episodic memory. They found that self-reported health and an active lifestyle contributed to performance and moderated the effects of age on their cognitive measures. Data such as those obtained in the British and Canadian studies highlight the importance of a range of individual difference variables, including aptitude, health and lifestyle variables, in determining memory performance. Given the increased range of cognitive performance with advancing age, it is likely that individual difference variables play a greater role in determining performance among older compared with younger adults.

Longitudinal studies

Longitudinal studies enable us to determine whether age differences in performance found in cross-sectional studies are related to the aging process or whether they reflect cohort or generational differences. There have been a few population-based longitudinal studies which

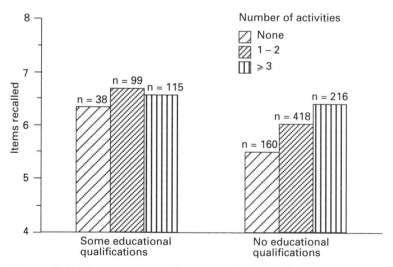

Figure 15.6. Mean number of items recalled in an incidental memory test by retired respondents aged 60 to 74 years, showing the relationship between leisure activities, education and memory. (From Huppert & Elliott, 1988.)

have investigated changes in memory. Three subtests of the Wechsler Memory Scale (story recall, paired associates, visual reproduction) were administered to community volunteers (aged 63 to 87 years) participating in the second wave of the Duke longitudinal study (Siegler, 1983). The results showed significant decline across the three time-periods only for reproduction of a visual design, suggesting that verbal memory was retained better than non-verbal memory. However, as individuals participated for longer periods of time, the level of decline was reduced even as participants became older. Further analyses showed selective dropout (from refusal or death) of individuals with low baseline scores on the verbal memory tasks (Siegler et al., 1982). This suggests that the apparent long-term stability of verbal memory was a spurious result, and it remains to be determined whether there are genuine differences in the rates of decline for verbal and non-verbal memory tasks. Although the cross-sectional baseline data showed that level of formal education was the variable related most strongly to all the memory tests, the investigators do not report whether education was also related to the extent of change over time. This could be because they did not have the statistical power to test this association due to the surprisingly small sample size. All three tests were completed by 172 subjects at baseline, and longitudinal performance was evaluated after four years (n = 116), 10 years (n = 62) and 16 years (n = 26).

The most influential longitudinal study of aging and cognitive function is the Seattle longitudinal study of Schaie and his colleagues (summarized in Schaie, 1983). They selected subjects born between 1889 and 1952 from a group health cooperative, and followed them longitudinally for up to 21 years, as well as recruiting a new sample every seven years. This enabled them to compare longitudinal data, with its problems of selective dropout, with data from independently drawn aging samples, to establish the relative magnitude of age-related differences in cognitive decline versus cohort (birth year) differences. Their cognitive assessment consisted of the so-called 'primary mental abilities' (verbal meaning, spatial ability, reasoning, numerical ability, word fluency). Unfortunately, this does not include any measures of learning or retrieval of new information, but it does contain two measures of semantic memory – verbal meaning (a multiple-choice vocabulary test) and word fluency (writing as many words as possible beginning with the letter S in a five-minute period). Their detailed analyses showed that there were large cohort effects: later born cohorts performed better than earlier born cohorts on verbal meaning, independently of their age at the time they were tested; in contrast, earlier born cohorts performed better than later born cohorts on word fluency. However, on both tasks, older individuals showed a greater decline than younger individuals, independently of cohort and selective drop-out effects.

Although this work has had a profound impact on the methodology and interpretation of age differences in cognitive function, it is important to be aware of the limitations of the study. Of the original 2816 subjects contacted, only 910 (32%) agreed to take part. This would certainly have introduced a sampling bias, although it is difficult to know what effect it had. In addition, the small number of survivors (n = 128) at the 21-year follow-up, means that these data are less reliable than the seven-year (n = 1602) and 14-year (n = 617) follow-up data.

More recently, Colsher & Wallace (1991b) have reported longitudinal data from the Iowa 65+ Rural Health Study. This was a study of a large geographically defined population, in which over 80% of the target population participated. The memory task was a 20-word list, tested by immediate and delayed (15 minute) recall. The number of subjects who completed the test at baseline and at both the three-year and six-year follow-up was 1768, representing 90% of all participating survivors. Advanced age was associated with poorer immediate and delayed recall and more rapid decline on immediate recall. However, age was not associated with rate of decline on delayed recall. More educated subjects recalled significantly more words on both immediate and delayed tests, but education did not predict differential rates of decline. The fact that the oldest groups in this sample (age 85+ years) declined at the same rate as younger groups (65–74 years, 75–84 years) on delayed recall, adds weight to the cross-sectional evidence of Welsh et al. (1991) that delayed recall is a good discriminator between normal elderly and mild dementia cases.

The main drawbacks with existing studies of large population samples are: (1) that few use genuinely representative samples with high response rates and the inclusion of testable, institutionalized subjects; and (2) that memory performance is assessed by relatively crude tests, shedding little light on memory processes. The latter has been partly the result of testing people in their own homes, where considerations of test brevity and acceptability are paramount, to retain high participation rates. However, with the advent of portable computers, it has become possible to employ more sophisticated, process-oriented tests, which, with imaginative programming and simple responses (e.g.

via a touch screen), are enjoyed by elderly people and provide more sophisticated data. A new generation of longitudinal studies of cognitive aging is under way and will provide more definitive conclusions about the ways in which memory changes across the full spectrum of cognitive and physical ability.

The concepts of age-associated memory impairment (AAMI) and aging-associated cognitive decline

From the foregoing review, there can be no doubt that the aging process is associated with memory impairment. Older adults complain about their failing memories and there is objective evidence of age-related impairment of memory from both longitudinal and cross-sectional studies. It is not possible at present to ascertain to what extent this impairment is an inevitable part of the aging process, and to what extent it is the consequence of other age-related problems such as sensory deficits, illness, medication, incipient dementia or terminal drop. Longitudinal studies show that poor memory performance is a predictor of mortality. The Duke longitudinal study (Siegler, 1983) showed that rates of memory decline decreased in long-term survivors, suggesting that decline may not be inevitable except in the terminal drop stage. On the other hand, cross-sectional studies using optimally healthy old people show significant deficits when memory tasks become quite demanding, e.g. involving divided attention or the retrieval of contextual information.

The term 'age-associated memory impairment' (AAMI) has been used as a diagnostic label to categorize individuals on the basis of the following criteria (Crook et al., 1986):

(1) At least 50 years of age
(2) Complaints of memory loss reflected in everyday tasks; gradual onset
(3) Memory test performance at least one standard deviation below the mean of young adults on standardized tests of recent memory with adequate normative data
(4) Adequate intellectual function (e.g. scale score of at least 9 on WAIS vocabulary)
(5) Absence of dementia as determined by a score of 24 or higher on the Mini-Mental State Examination
(6) Exclusion criteria: delirium, neurological disorder, cerebral

vascular pathology, head injury, current psychiatric disorder, alcoholism or drug dependence, any medical disorder that could produce cognitive deterioration, use of any psychotropic drug that may affect cognitive function

Since vast numbers of elderly people would meet these criteria, such diagnostic labelling has been severely criticized (e.g. O'Brien & Levy, 1992). A decision has recently been made not to include AAMI as a diagnostic category in DSM-IV (American Psychiatric Association, 1993), despite considerable pressure from those who would gain by offering treatment for this 'disease'. However, it was felt that there should be some formal recognition in DSM-IV of the cognitive impairment or decline which is seen commonly among the elderly. This new approach acknowledges the important point that old age is associated with a greater range of cognitive performance and, because of this, it is not helpful to express abnormality simply in terms of the norms for young adults. The new nomenclature and the assumptions underlying it are depicted in Figure 15.7 from Caine (1992). 'Aging-associated cognitive decline' is defined as a condition (not a disease or diagnosis) which describes age-related deterioration in cognitive performance that is 'normative' or usual and is not associated with any defined pathological process. On the other hand, some individuals have documented cognitive decline which is associated with systemic disease or disease of the central nervous system, e.g. head trauma, early progressive dementia, effects of alcohol abuse. This is termed 'mild cognitive disorder' and it may be within the normative range or below this range, and it may be transient or persistent. Cognitive disorder which is moderate or severe, and is below the normative range, is classified as dementia if both memory and other cognitive functions are impaired.

This new approach acknowledges the dimensional nature of cognitive performance and cognitive impairment. Indeed, Caine (1992) makes the point that the threshold for diagnosing dementia has to change across the age-course reflecting the increase in age-associated cognitive decline.

Further development of the concepts of 'aging-associated cognitive decline' and 'mild cognitive disorder' will depend on the outcome of the new generation of representative, population-based longitudinal studies of memory and other aspects of cognitive function.

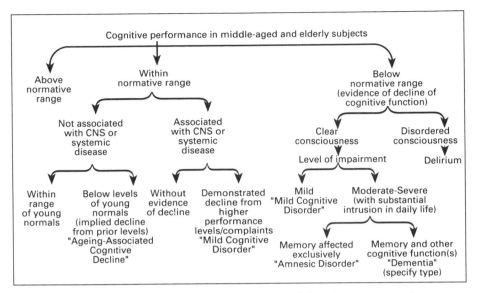

Figure 15.7. Classification of cognitive function and disorders. (From Caine, 1992.)

Conclusions

In distinguishing between normal and abnormal memory impairment and decline, three main approaches have been discussed in this chapter, namely the diagnostic, the experimental and the epidemiological approaches. The main conclusions are as follows:

(1) The diagnostic approach is problematic when attempting to differentiate normal aging and the early stages of dementia, since the progressive nature of the disorder may mean that symptoms of memory impairment appear before the criteria are satisfied

(2) Clinical and experimental studies of memory play an important role in the analysis of memory processes and the nature of memory impairment. In general, memory performance is impaired in relation to the processing demands placed on the individual by the memory task: the greater the demands, the greater the impairment

(3) Clinical and experimental studies show that the deficits seen in mildly demented individuals compared to control subjects, are similar in kind, if not in magnitude, to the deficits shown by

older compared to younger subjects. (A summary of these findings is given in Table 15.5)

(4) There are no reliable reports of qualitative differences in memory performance between demented (other than severely demented) and control subjects, nor between younger and older subjects

(5) There appears to be a continuity in the memory performance of normal elderly subjects and those with mild dementia or whose dementia is in the early stages

(6) Although clinical and experimental studies of memory are useful in the analysis of memory processes, they are of little assistance

Table 15.5. *Summary of dementia-related compared with age-related differences on memory test performance*

	Demented vs. normal	Old vs. young
Episodic memory		
Direct tests		
Recall	x	x
Recognition		
Item	x	√ (? – very old)
Context	x	x
Dual task	x	x
Rate of forgetting	√	x
Indirect		
Priming	√	√ (x – very old)
Skill learning	√	x
Semantic memory		
Direct		
Vocabulary	x	√ (x – very old)
Fluency	x	x
Name finding	x	x
Indirect		
Semantic priming	√	√ (? – very old)

x indicates impairment; √ indicates no impairment.

in distinguishing between age-related and dementia-related memory impairment in individuals

(7) The aging process is associated with a wide variety of conditions which decrease health and fitness, and, because of this, the range of performance on memory and other cognitive tests increases with age. This means that population-based studies of unselected samples are required to establish normal or normative levels of functioning, so that abnormality can be detected reliably

(8) Longitudinal studies of population-based samples show that advanced age is associated with impaired memory at each time of testing, and more rapid decline in memory performance over time. This makes the differentiation between age-associated decline and dementia-related decline particularly difficult to establish among very elderly people

(9) Future advances in our understanding of memory function in relation to dementia and normal aging depend upon the dimensional approach to cognitive function being merged with a dimensional approach to the neurobiological changes which take place in dementia and normal aging

References

American Psychiatric Association (1987). *Diagnostic and Statistical Manual of Mental Disorders*, third edition – revised (DSM-III-R). American Psychiatric Association, Washington, DC.

American Psychiatric Association (1993) DSM-IV *Draft Criteria*. American Psychiatric Association (Task Force on DSM-IV), Washington, D.C.

Baddeley, A. D., Logie, R., Bressi, S., Della Sala, S. & Spinnler, H. (1986). Dementia and working memory. *Journal of Experimental Psychology*, **38**, 603–18.

Baddeley, A. D., Della Sala, S. & Spinnler, H. (1991). The two-component hypothesis of memory deficit in Alzheimer's disease. *Journal of Clinical and Experimental Neuropsychology*, **13**, 372–80.

Becker, J. T., Lopez, O. L. & Wess, J. (1992). Material specific memory loss in probable Alzheimer's disease. *Journal of Neurology, Neurosurgery and Psychiatry*, **55**, 1177–81.

Blessed, G., Tomlinson, B. E. & Roth, M. (1968). The association between quantitative measures of dementia and of senile change in the cerebral grey matter of elderly subjects. *British Journal of Psychiatry*, **114**, 797–811.

Burke, D. M. & Laver, G. D. (1990). Aging and word retrieval: selective age deficits in language. In E. A. Lovelace (ed.) *Aging and Cognition: Mental Processes, Self-Awareness and Interventions*, pp. 281–300. Elsevier Science Publishers BV, North-Holland.

Burke, D. M., Mackay, D., Worthley, J. & Wade, E. (1991). On the tip of the tongue: What causes word finding failures in young and older adults? *Journal of Memory and Language*, **30**, 542–79.

Caine, E. D. (1992). 'Nomenclature and diagnosis of cognitive disorders: a US perspective.' Abstract from Age-related Cognitive Disorders Conference, Nice (Glaxo), June 1992.

Cermak, L. A. (1984). The episodic/semantic distinction in amnesia. In N. Butters & R. L. Squire (eds.) *The Neuropsychology of Memory*, pp. 55–62. Guildford Press, New York.

Chertkow, H. & Bub, D. (1990). Semantic memory loss in dementia of Alzheimer's type. *Brain*, **113**, 397–417.

Chertkow, H., Bub, D. & Seidenberg, M. (1989). Priming and semantic memory loss in Alzheimer's disease. *Brain and Language*, **36**, 420–46.

Christensen, H. & Birrell, P. (1991). Explicit and implicit memory in dementia and normal ageing. *Psychological Research*, **52**, 149–61.

Cockburn, J. & Smith, P. T. (1988). Effects of age and intelligence on everyday memory tasks. In M. M. Gruneberg, P. E. Morris & R. N. Sykes (eds.) *Practical Aspects of Memory: Current Research and Issues*, pp. 132–6. John Wiley and Sons, Chichester.

Cohen, G. & Faulkner, D. (1986). Memory for proper names: age differences in retrieval. *British Journal of Developmental Psychology*, **4**, 187–97.

Colsher, P. L. & Wallace, R. B. (1991a). Epidemiologic considerations in studies of cognitive function in the elderly: methodology and nondementing acquired dysfunction. *Epidemiologic Reviews*, **13**, 1–27.

Colsher, P. L. & Wallace, R. B. (1991b). Longitudinal application of cognitive function measures in a defined population of community-dwelling elders. *Annals of Epidemiology*, **1**, 215–30.

Corkin, S., Growdon, J. H., Nissen, M. J., Huff, F. J., Freed, D. M. & Sagar, H. J. (1984). Recent advances in the neuropsychological study of Alzheimer's disease. In R. J. Wurtman, S. Corkin & J. H. Growdon (eds.) *Alzheimer's Disease: Advances in Basic Research and Therapies*, pp. 375–90. Centre for Brain Sciences and Metabolism Trust, Cambridge, MA.

Cox, B. D., Blaxter, M., Buckle, A. L. J., Fenner, N. P., Golding, J. F., Gore, M., Huppert, F. A., Nickson, J., Roth, M., Stark, J. E., Wadsworth, M. E. J. & Whichelow, M. (1987). *Health and Lifestyle Survey: Preliminary Report of a Nationwide Survey of the Physical and Mental Health, Attitudes and Lifestyle of a Random Sample of 9003 British Adults*. Health Promotion Research Trust, London.

Craik, F. I. M. (1982). Selective changes in encoding as a function of reduced processing capacity. In F. Klix, J. Hoffman & E. van der Meer (eds.) *Cognitive Research in Psychology*, pp. 151–61. North-Holland, Amsterdam.

Craik, F. I. M. (1986). A functional account of age differences in memory. In F. Klix & H. Hagendorf (eds.) *Human Memory and Cognitive Capabilities*, pp. 409–22. North-Holland, Amsterdam.

Craik, F. I. M. & McDowd, J. M. (1987). Age differences in recall and recognition. *Journal of Experimental Psychology: Learning, Memory and Cognition*, **13**, 474–9.

Craik, F. I. M. & Salthouse, T. A. (eds.) (1992). *Handbook of Aging and Cognition*. Lawrence Erlbaum Associates, New Jersey.

Crook, T., Bartus, R. T., Ferris, S. H., Whitehouse, P., Cohen, G. D. & Gershon, S. (1986). Age-associated memory impairment: proposed diagnostic criteria and measures of clinical change – report of a National Institute of Mental Health Work Group. *Developmental Neuropsychology*, **2**, 261–76.

Davis, H. P., Cohen, A., Gandy, M., Colombo, P., Van Dusseldorp, G., Simolke, N. & Romano, J. (1990). Lexical priming deficits as a function of age. *Behavioral Neuroscience*, **104**, 288–97.

Eslinger, P. J. & Damasio, A. R. (1986). Preserved motor learning in Alzheimer's disease. Implications for anatomy and behavior. *Journal of Neuroscience*, **6**, 3006–9.

Folstein, M. F., Folstein, S. E. & McHugh, P. R. (1975). Mini-Mental State Examination. A practical method for grading the cognitive state of patients for the clinician. *Journal of Psychiatric Research*, **12**, 189–98.

Grober, E. & Sliwinski, M. J. (1991). Dual-task performance in demented and nondemented elderly. *Journal of Clinical and Experimental Neuropsychology*, **13**, 667–76.

Grober, E., Buschke, H., Kawas, C. & Fuld, P. (1985). Impaired ranking of semantic attributes in dementia. *Brain and Language*, **26**, 276–86.

Heindel, W. C., Butters, N. & Salmon, D. P. (1989). Impaired learning of a motor skill in patients with Huntington's disease. *Behavioral Neuroscience*, **102**, 141–7.

Hodges, J. R., Salmon, D. P. & Butters, N. (1992). Semantic memory impairment in Alzheimer's disease: failure of access or degraded knowledge? *Neuropsychologia*, **30**, 301–14.

Huff, F. J., Corkin, S. & Growdon, J. H. (1986). Semantic impairment and anomia in Alzheimer's disease. *Brain and Language*, **28**, 235–49.

Hughes, C. P., Berg, L., Danziger, W. L., Coben, L. A. & Martin, R. L. (1982). A new clinical scale for the staging of dementia. *British Journal of Psychiatry*, **140**, 566–72.

Hultsch, D. F., Hammer, M. & Small, B. J. (1993). Age differences in cognitive performance in later life: relationships to self-reported health and activity life style. *Journal of Gerontology, Psychological Sciences*, **48**, 1–11.

Huppert, F. A. (1991a). Neuropsychological assessment of dementia. *Reviews in Clinical Gerontology*, **1**, 159–69.

Huppert, F. A. (1991b). Age-related changes in memory: learning and remembering new information. In F. Boller & J. Grafman (eds.) *Handbook of Neuropsychology*, Vol. 5, pp. 123–47. Elsevier Science Publishers.

Huppert, F. A. & Piercy, M. (1978). Dissociation between learning and remembering in organic amnesia. *Nature*, **275**, 317–18.

Huppert, F. A. & Beardsall, L. (1988). Revealing the concealed: multiple measures of memory in dementia. In M. M. Gruneberg, P. E. Morris & R. N. Sykes (eds.), *Practical Aspects of Memory: Current Research and Issues*, Vol. 2, pp. 34–9. John Wiley and Sons, Chichester.

Huppert, F. A. & Elliott, B. J. (1988). 'The contribution of health and lifestyle variables to cognitive function.' Paper presented at the XXIV International Congress of Psychology, Sydney, August 1988.

Huppert, F. A. & Kopelman, M. D. (1989). Rates of forgetting in normal ageing: a comparison with dementia. *Neuropsychologia*, **27**, 849–60.

Huppert, F. A. & Beardsall, L. (1991). A comparison of clinical, psychometric and behavioural memory tests: findings from a community study of the early detection of dementia. *International Journal of Geriatric Psychiatry*, **6**, 295–306.

Huppert, F. A. & Beardsall, L. (1993). Prospective memory impairment as an early indicator of dementia. *Journal of Clinical and Experimental Neuropsychology*, **15**, 805–21.

Katzman, R., Aronson, M., Fuld, P., Kawas, C., Brown, T., Morgenstern, H., Frishman, W., Gidez, L., Eder, H. & Ooi, W. L. (1989). Development of dementing illnesses in an 80-year-old volunteer cohort. *Annals of Neurology*, **25**, 317–24.

Knopman, D. (1991). Long-term retention of implicitly acquired learning in patients with Alzheimer's disease. *Journal of Clinical and Experimental Neuropsychology*, **13**, 880–94.

Kopelman, M. D. (1985). Rates of forgetting in Alzheimer-type dementia and Korsakoff's syndrome. *Neuropsychologia*, **23**, 623–38.

Kopelman, M. D. (1989). Remote and autobiographical memory, temporal context memory and frontal atrophy in Korsakoff and Alzheimer patients. *Neuropsychologia*, **27**, 437–60.

Light, L. L. & Singh, A. (1987). Implicit and explicit memory in young and older adults. *Journal of Experimental Psychology: Learning, Memory and Cognition*, **13**, 531–41.

Martin, A. & Fedio, P. (1983). Word production and comprehension in Alzheimer's disease: the breakdown of semantic knowledge. *Brain and Language*, **19**, 124–41.

McIntyre, J. S. & Craik, F. I. M. (1987). Age differences in memory for item and source information. *Canadian Journal of Psychology*, **41**, 175–92.

McKhann, G., Drachman, D., Folstein, M., Katzman, R., Price, D. & Stadlan, E. M. (1984). Clinical diagnosis of Alzheimer's disease: report of the NINCDS –ADRDA work group under the auspices of Department of Health and Human Services task force on Alzheimer's disease. *Neurology*, **34**, 939–44.

Miller, E. (1975). Impaired recall and the memory disturbance in presenile dementia. *British Journal of Social and Clinical Psychology*, **14**, 73–9.

Mishkin, M. & Appenzeller, T. (1987). The anatomy of memory. *Scientific American*, **256**, 62–71.

Mishkin, M., Malamut, B. & Bachevalier, J. (1984). Memories and habits: two neural systems. In G. Lynch, J. L. McGaugh & N. M. Weinberger (eds.) *Neurobiology of Learning and Memory*, pp. 65–77. Guildford Press, New York.

Mitchell, D. B. (1989). How many memory systems? Evidence from aging. *Journal of Experimental Psychology: Learning, Memory and Cognition*, **15**, 31–49.

Morris, R. G. (1984). Dementia and the functioning of the articulatory loop system. *Cognitive Neuropsychology*, **1**, 143–57.

Morris, R. G., Gick, M. L. & Craik, F. I. M. (1988). Processing resources and age differences in working memory. *Memory and Cognition*, **16**, 362–6.

Moscovich, M. (1982). A neuropsychological approach to perception and memory in normal and pathological aging. In F. I. M. Craik & S. Trehub (eds.) *Aging and Cognitive Processes*, pp. 55–78. Plenum Press, New York.

Nebes, R. D. (1992). Cognitive dysfunction in Alzheimer's disease. In F. I. M. Craik & T. Salthouse (eds.) *Handbook of Aging and Cognition*, pp. 373–446. Lawrence Erlbaum Associates, New Jersey.

Nebes, R. D. & Brady, C. B. (1988). Integrity of semantic fields in Alzheimer's disease. *Cortex*, **24**, 291–300.

Nebes, R. D. & Brady, C. B. (1990). Preserved organization of semantic attributes in Alzheimer's disease. *Psychology and Aging*, **5**, 574–9.

O'Brien, J. T. & Levy, R. (1992). Age associated memory impairment. *British Medical Journal*, **304**, 5–6.

Partridge, F. M., Knight, R. G. & Feehan, M. (1990). Direct and indirect memory performance in patients with senile dementia. *Psychological Medicine*, **20**, 111–18.

Poon, L. W. (1985). Differences in human memory with aging: nature, causes and clinical implications. In J. E. Birren & K. W. Schiae (eds.) *Handbook of the Psychology of Aging*, 2nd edition, pp. 427–62. Van Nostrand Reinhold, New York.

Poon, L. W., Martin, P., Clayton, Messner, S. A., Noble, C. A. & Johnson, B. M. (1992). The influences of cognitive resources on adaptation and old age. In L. W. Poon (ed.) *The Georgia Centenarian Study. A Special Issue of the International Journal of Aging and Human Development*, pp. 31–46. Baywood Publishing Co. Inc., New York.

Roth, M., Tym, E., Mountjoy, C. Q., Huppert, F. A., Hendrie, H., Verma, S. & Goddard, R. (1986). CAMDEX: a standardised instrument for the diagnosis of mental disorder in the elderly with special reference to the early detection of dementia. *British Journal of Psychiatry*, **149**, 698–709.

Roth, M., Huppert, F. A., Tym, E. & Mountjoy, C. Q. (1988). *CAMDEX: the Cambridge Examination for Mental Disorders of the Elderly*. Cambridge University Press, Cambridge.

Sagar, H. J. (1990). Aging and age-related neurological disease: remote memory. In F. Boller & J. Grafman (eds.) *Handbook of Neuropsychology*, Vol. 4, pp. 311–24. Elsevier Science Publishers, Amsterdam.

Sagar, H. J., Cohen, N. J., Sullivan, E. V., Corkin, S. & Growdon, J. H. (1988). Remote memory function in Alzheimer's disease and Parkinson's disease. *Brain*, **111**, 185–206.

Sagar, H. J., Sullivan, E. & Corkin, S. (1991). Autobiographical memory in normal ageing and dementia. *Behavioural Neurology*, **4**, 235–48.

Salmon, D. P., Shimamura, A. P., Butters, N. & Smith, S. (1988). Lexical and semantic priming deficits in patients with Alzheimer's disease. *Journal of Clinical and Experimental Neuropsychology*, **10**, 477–94.

Salthouse, T. A. (1991). *Theoretical Perspectives on Cognitive Ageing*. Lawrence Erlbaum Associates Inc., New Jersey.

Schacter, D. L., Harbluk, J. L. & McLachlan, D. R. (1984). Retrieval without recollection: An experimental analysis of source amnesia. *Journal of Verbal Learning, Verbal Behaviour*, **23**, 593–611.

Schaie, K. W. (1980). Cognitive development in aging. In L. K. Obler & M. L. Albert (eds.) *Language and Communication in the Elderly*, pp. 7–25. Lexington Books, Massachusetts.

Schaie, K. W. (1983). The Seattle longitudinal study: a 21-year exploration of psychometric intelligence in adulthood. In K. W. Schaie (Ed.) *Longitudinal Studies of Adult Psychological Development*. Guilford Adult Development and Aging Series, vol. 2, pp. 64–135. Guilford Press, New York.

Scherr, P. A., Albert, M. S., Funkenstein, H. H., Cook, N. R., Hennekens, C. H., Branch, L. G., White, L. R., Taylor, J. O. & Evans, D. A. (1988). Correlates of cognitive function in an elderly community population. *American Journal of Epidemiology*, **128**, 1084–101.

Shimamura, A. P., Salmon, D. P., Squire, L. R. & Butters, N. (1987). Memory dysfunction and word priming in dementia and amnesia. *Behavioral Neuroscience*, **101**, 347–51.

Siegler, I. C. (1983). Psychological aspects of the Duke longitudinal studies. In K. W. Schaie (ed.) *Longitudinal Studies of Adult Psychological Development*. Guilford Adult Development and Aging Series, vol. 2, pp. 136–90. Guilford Press, New York.

Siegler, I. C., McCarty, S. M. & Logue, P. E. (1982). Wechsler Memory Scale scores, selective attrition and distance from death. *Journal of Gerontology*, **37**, 176–81.

Storandt, M. & Hill, R. D. (1989). Very mild senile dementia of the Alzheimer type. *Archives of Neurology*, **46**, 383–6.

Tuokko, H., Vernon-Wilkinson, R., Weir, J. & Beattie, B. L. (1991). Cued recall and early identification of dementia. *Journal of Clinical and Experimental Neuropsychology*, **13**, 871–9.

Wechsler, D. A. (1987). *Wechsler Memory Scale – Revised (WMS-R)*. The Psychological Corporation, Harcourt Brace Jovanovich, San Antonio.

Weingartner, H., Grafman, J., Boutelle, W., Kaye, W. & Martin, P. R. (1983). Forms of memory failure. *Science*, **221**, 380–2.

Welsh, K., Butters, N., Hughes, J., Mohs, R. & Heyman, A. (1991). Detection of abnormal memory decline in mild cases of Alzheimer's disease using CERAD neuropsychological measures. *Archives of Neurology*, **48**, 278–81.

Wertheimer, J., Boula, J. G., Brull, J., Gut, A. M., Pierrehumbert, B., Rufini, J., Zinder, M., Brechbuhl, D., El Nadi, A., Mouflin, A. & Montangero, J. (1992). Learning processes in dementia. *International Journal of Geriatric Psychiatry*, **7**, 161–72.

West, R. L. (1988). Prospective memory and aging. In M. M. Gruneberg, P. E. Morris & R. N. Sykes (eds.) *Practical Aspects of Memory: Current Research and Issues*, Vol. 2, pp. 119–25. John Wiley and Sons, Chichester.

Wilson, B., Cockburn, J. & Baddeley, A. D. (1985). *The Rivermead Behavioural Memory Test*. Thames Valley Test Company, Reading.

World Health Organization (1992). *The ICD-10 Classification of Mental and Behavioural Disorders: Clinical Descriptions and Diagnostic Guidelines*. World Health Organization, Division of Mental Health, Geneva.

16

Language in dementia and normal aging

DANIEL KEMPLER AND ELIZABETH M. ZELINSKI

Language is a system of symbolic elements (words), rules for combining these elements into grammatical sentences (syntax), and rules for constructing and using conversations, stories and the like (discourse). Language develops quickly. By the time children are 5 years old, they have a vocabulary of several thousand words and are using all the basic grammatical principles of the language. Until recently it was largely assumed that, barring frank brain injury, language does not change substantially after childhood. However, research in gerontology and psycholinguistics over the past decade has demonstrated subtle but definite changes in language ability across the lifespan (see Kemper (1992) for review). For example, people over the age of 65 years experience word-finding difficulties (Burke et al., 1991) and produce fewer syntactically complex sentences in spontaneous speech and writing (e.g. Kemper, 1992).

Language disorders are among the best-studied symptoms of dementia, and are particularly pronounced in Alzheimer's disease (AD) (for reviews, see Bayles & Kaszniak (1987); Nebes (1989); Kempler (1991)). The incidence of language impairment in dementia is estimated to be between 88% and 95% (Thompson, 1987), and is close to 100% in AD (Cummings et al. 1985). Recent descriptions of language in dementia have confirmed and expanded Alzheimer's original (1907) observation of word-finding deficits, paraphasias (substitutions) and comprehension impairment (e.g. Appell et al., 1982; Bayles, 1982; Obler, 1983). In addition, research has described impairments in the use of discourse which appear early in the disease and impair communication progressively throughout its course (Hutchinson & Jensen, 1980; Ripich & Terrell, 1988; Ulatowska & Chapman, 1991).

Dementia and Normal Aging, eds. F. A. Huppert, C. Brayne & D. W. O'Connor.
© Cambridge University Press 1994.

The purpose of this chapter is to compare the language changes seen in normal aging with those in dementia. In particular, we are interested in determining whether the language deficits observed so easily in dementia are qualitatively different from those seen in normal aging.

Word finding

Knowledge of a particular word encompasses its meaning, pronunciation, its relationship to other words, and its role in sentence structure. For example, we know that the word 'comPUter' is stressed on the second syllable, not the third; and, although the sentence 'The pencil saw the flower' is perfectly grammatical, we know that it does not make sense because there is something about the meaning of the word 'pencil' which precludes it from 'seeing'.

Production and comprehension of words is a more complex task than one might think. Naming an object (called 'confrontation naming') requires visual perception, object recognition, a search for the name among others in a network of object names and concepts, selection of the name, and organization of speech mechanisms for production. Understanding a word involves auditory (or visual) perception and recognition, mapping of the sensory percept to an internal 'dictionary' of words (the lexicon), and accessing knowledge about the concept that the word represents, as well as concepts related to that word. If there is a problem in producing or understanding a word, it can be due to breakdown at any point in these complex sequences.

By about their first birthday, children understand and produce single words reliably. First words are acquired slowly. But around the middle of the second year, there is a surge in vocabulary growth, and children acquire words quickly and easily. By the time a child graduates from high school, she has a vocabulary of about 40000 words (Nagy & Herman, 1987). Therefore we can estimate that children learn approximately 2000–3000 words a year on their way to becoming adult speakers.

Everybody, young and old, demented and not, has at least occasional word-finding difficulty. The question to be considered here is whether or not the naming problems in normal aging and dementia are similar.

Word finding in normal aging

There is little question that normal older adults experience word-finding problems. People over 55 years of age complain about having difficulty remembering names as well as specific words (Zelinski et al., 1980). Burke et al. (1991) studied word finding in a diary study and a laboratory experiment. Comparing younger and older people (over 60 years of age), in both contexts, older people reported more frequent 'tip-of-the-tongue' experiences (a temporary inability to retrieve a word that is recalled eventually) than younger ones. People over 80 years of age also made more errors on confrontation naming than younger people (60 and 70 years of age) (e.g. Borod et al., 1980; Albert et al., 1988). Performance in verbal fluency tasks (generating words within a category such as 'words beginning with F' or 'animals') also declines with age (e.g. Schaie & Parham, 1977; Brown & Mitchell, 1991).

There are two types of explanation for the word-finding problems observed in normal aging. The first is that the structure of lexical knowledge declines with age. The second is that lexical knowledge remains intact, but deficits increase in the ability to retrieve specific words from an intact lexicon. We will consider the argument for a structural decrement with a brief review of the literature (for an extensive review, see Light (1992)).

Generally, it is assumed that knowledge about words is stored in a network of concept nodes, and that the network is organized in terms of strength of relationships among nodes (Anderson, 1983). Network models suggest that, when a concept node is accessed, activation spreads automatically from that concept to related nodes (Neely, 1977). This 'spreading activation' can be observed in the response time to make decisions that letter strings are words ('lexical decision' tasks) or in how quickly a word is read aloud ('naming latency').

In experiments on the structure of lexical knowledge, a semantic priming procedure is often used. In this procedure, word pairs are presented and the subject either names or makes a decision (e.g. 'Is it a word?'; 'Is it alive?') about the second (target) word. It has been found that when a word related to the target word precedes it (e.g. dog-cat), the response to the target is faster than when an unrelated word precedes it (e.g. shoe-cat). The difference between response time (either naming or a lexical decision) for targets following related versus unrelated words is the priming effect, and priming effects are taken to indicate the degree to which the activation has spread through the semantic network (e.g. Foss, 1982).

Semantic priming effects are virtually identical for young and normal older adults. This has been found in an array of manipulations: typical vs. atypical category-exemplar relations (bird-robin vs. bird-duck) (Howard, 1980; Balota & Duchek, 1988); high vs. low associates (animal-cat vs. animal-bull) (Balota & Duchek, 1988); same category members (rain-snow vs. rain-bright), one word describing a property of the other (rain-wet) vs. unrelated word pairs (rain-bright) (Howard et al., 1981); as well as for automatic (unexpected targets, brief delays between presentation of prime and target words) vs. attentional (expected targets, long delays between presentation of prime and target words) (Burke et al., 1987). The constancy of these effects suggests that lexical knowledge is not degraded with age. However, there is new work suggesting that the size of the priming effect may be greater in older than in younger adults, and that it is significant at the level of meta-analysis (Laver & Burke, 1993). This increased priming effect with age has been interpreted to indicate slowing of information transmission across concept nodes (which allows more time for spread of activation), not to a decline in knowledge (see discussion below and Chertkow et al. (1989)). This 'hyperpriming' effect occurs as a main effect of age under different experimental conditions, but does not interact with the kind of priming relationship studied (related vs. unrelated, high vs. low associates), and, therefore, is not related to a loss of a particular type of semantic knowledge, but is rather a general processing change seen with age.

The preservation of the conceptual network between related words, tested indirectly in semantic priming, is also seen in more direct word-production tasks. The words elicited in category generation (Howard, 1980) and word-association tasks (Burke & Peters, 1986) are virtually the same for young and older adults. Additional evidence that word knowledge remains intact in normal aging comes from findings that vocabulary scores do not decline, but often increase with age (Salthouse, 1988). In confrontation naming tasks, older adults are helped by phonological cues more than by semantic cues, as are young adults when they cannot retrieve a word in confrontation naming (Nicholas et al., 1985a). Also, the errors made by older adults are generally circumlocutions ('cutting the wood' for 'sawing') rather than semantically related errors (e.g. calling a 'saw' a 'hammer'), which is common in dementia (see below). This suggests that semantic boundaries between words remain intact.

These data indicate that a disruption of knowledge structures is not the cause of the word-finding problems of older adults. Rather, it is access or retrieval of intact knowledge which is responsible for word-finding deficits in both unimpaired young and older individuals (see Light (1992) for full discussion of this issue).

Word finding in dementia

Alzheimer described a demented woman who 'frequently used perplexing phrases . . . paraphrastic expressions' ('*milk-pourer*' instead of '*cup*') (Alzheimer, 1907, p. 110). Word-finding difficulty is the earliest and most common language symptom of AD (Kempler, 1991). AD patients have difficulty in naming pictures and generating words in conversation. They often substitute semantically related words, or 'place fillers' (e.g. thing, do, it, he).

There have been three primary explanations proposed for word-finding difficulty in dementia, the two discussed above in relation to normal aging (retrieval deficits and loss of lexical knowledge) and visual–perceptual problems which are thought to interfere with the early stages of naming, that is, identifying and recognizing the object to be named. Each of these will be discussed.

There is quite a bit of evidence to support the view that anomia arises from a problem in lexical retrieval for verbal production (the same explanation that was argued for in normal aging). First, as with normal aging, AD patients can often give a related name or circumlocution, suggesting that they know much about the meaning of the word, but cannot find the exact name (e.g. 'cutter' for 'saw'; 'this is for your eyes' for 'glasses') (Bayles & Tomoeda, 1983; Kempler, 1988). Second, AD patients can utilize phonemic (sound) cues to help to retrieve the words, indicating again that the information is there but cannot be retrieved easily (Neils et al., 1988). Third, comprehension of words is generally superior to production of the same words (Kempler, 1988), suggesting that the underlying knowledge can often be accessed in a passive, comprehension task, when the name cannot be generated or retrieved on demand. Last, several researchers have demonstrated that, like normal subjects, AD patients react faster in lexical decision semantic priming tasks (i.e. 'Is it a word?') if the target word (e.g. nurse) is preceded by a related word (e.g. doctor) than if it is preceded by an unrelated word (e.g. shoe), suggesting intact semantic networks (e.g. Nebes et al., 1984).

Another view of word-finding impairments in dementia is that the set of lexical representations (the word knowledge system itself) is disrupted, which results in a permanent degradation of the semantic system. Evidence for this position comes from several sources, demonstrating absent or abnormal priming effects (e.g. Smith et al., 1988; Albert & Milberg, 1989; Nebes et al., 1989). One study (Chertkow et al., 1989) found abnormal priming effects (hyperpriming) associated only with words that were shown to be degraded semantically (i.e. the subjects were not able to answer knowledge probes about the words accurately such as 'Is this a tool or clothing?' and 'Is it sharp or dull?' for the word 'saw'). Other evidence of semantic disruption comes from: semantically related naming errors (e.g. calling a 'dog' a 'cat') (Schwartz et al., 1979); a correspondence between naming and word comprehension errors (Martin & Fedio, 1983; Chertkow et al., 1989; Kempler & Andersen, 1989); and consistency of response across several testing sessions (Huff et al., 1988; Henderson et al., 1990; Kempler, et al., 1994). These findings are consonant with the notion of lexical degeneration, which permanently affects both comprehension and production of specific lexical items.

Although there is a growing consensus that at least some AD patients do exhibit representational impairments, there are only general proposals about the type of disruption which occurs within the lexical representation. For instance, Schwartz et al., (1979, p. 277) discussed the problem as a 'breakdown in the structure of the underlying categories', while Chertkow et al., (1989, p. 430) refer to the 'degraded' semantic representations, and Grober et al. (1985) proposed that the representations are disorganized. In summary, it appears that both lexical retrieval and lexical knowledge are disrupted in AD, making the picture more complicated than that seen for normal aging, where there is only evidence for a deficit in lexical retrieval.

In addition to this evidence supporting both lexical retrieval and representation problems in AD, there are also data suggesting that visual–perceptual problems underlie some of the word-finding difficulty in AD: there is an improvement in naming if the subjects are allowed to have additional sensory cues, such as touching the object (Barker & Lawson, 1968); AD subjects substitute names of visually similar objects in confrontation naming, for instance, calling an 'anchor' a 'hammer' (Rochford, 1971; Logan et al., 1992); and AD subjects are better able to name objects that are very familiar and therefore require less visual recognition (e.g. body parts) than less familiar objects (e.g. a whale) (Rochford, 1971). Kirshner et al. (1984)

showed that perceptual difficulty played a significant role in anomia of AD patients by demonstrating worse naming with progressively degraded visual presentations (actual objects vs. photographs vs. line drawings vs. visually degraded drawings). Convergent evidence for primary visual–perceptual deficits in AD is also provided by reports of degeneration of the retina and optic nerve in AD patients (Sadun & Bassi, 1990; Blanks et al., 1991).

However, visual–perceptual problems account for only a subset of word-finding problems in dementia. For instance, perceptual problems do not explain why AD patients are anomic in spontaneous conversation where no obvious visual–perceptual skills come into play (Kempler et al., 1987). In addition, the perceptual cause is not consistent with the finding that most substitutions in AD are semantically (not visually) related object names (Bayles & Tomoeda, 1983; Huff, 1988; Kempler, 1988). Further evidence against the visual–perceptual argument comes from recent studies showing that some AD patients with significant anomia perform relatively well on independent measures of visual-form discrimination (Huff et al., 1986; Chertkow et al., 1989). So, at best, visual–perceptual deficits only partially explain anomia in AD.

In summary, word-finding problems are among the earliest and most obvious symptoms of AD, but the underlying cause(s) of anomia remain disputed. A review of recent research suggests that the naming in AD is a heterogeneous phenomenon. A straightforward conclusion would be that no single explanation can account for the naming performance in AD. Visual perception, lexical access and deterioration of lexical representations all play a role in anomia of AD. One way to reconcile the variety of results is to acknowledge that AD may affect different components of the lexical processing system in different patients and at different stages of the disease. Some of our work (e.g. Kempler & Andersen, 1989; Henderson et al., 1990; Kempler et al., 1990; 1993) has used variation in consistency of naming errors to address this issue and has found that AD patients differ in the degree to which they suffer from what could be called 'access deficits' – those patients who make inconsistent naming errors and perform poorly on measures of attention – vs. 'linguistic deficits' – demonstrated by consistent naming errors across test sessions. Other researchers have also documented the existence of subgroups of AD patients who present with distinct language performance profiles and may reflect subtypes of the disease (Folstein & Breitner, 1982; Seltzer & Sherwin, 1983; Chui et al., 1985; Knesevich et al., 1985; Chui, 1987). In any discussion of behavioral subgroups, it must be acknowledged that many different behavioral symptoms can be caused, theoretically, by a single mechanism. For instance, Nebes & Brady (1992) propose a single model (i.e. cognitive slowing) to account for a variety of research findings in AD. Although a single mechanism can be posited to explain apparently dissimilar errors, there appears to be evidence for multiple factors causing word-finding problems in AD and no evidence for those same factors in normal aging, setting the two groups apart.

Summary

In examining word-finding problems in normal aging and dementia, both quantitative and qualitative differences between the two groups are found. In normal aging, there is mild word-finding difficulty, attributed to decreased lexical retrieval. In dementia, decreased lexical access also exists, but two differences are apparent. First, the frequency of word-finding problems in itself sets the two groups apart. In normal aging, occasional anomia is observed: in the diary study of tip-of-the-tongue experiences (Burke et al., 1991), the frequency of such problems was about seven times a month for older people and four times a month for young people. By contrast, in dementia, word-finding difficulty can be a prominent symptom, occurring in every utterance. Although there may be quantitative similarity in the number of naming errors made by mild AD subjects and the more anomic normal elderly (e.g. Huff, 1988; Kempler, 1988), in most individual cases and in most group studies, there appears to be little overlap in the frequency of word-finding difficulty, whether tested via confrontation naming or word-list generation (e.g. Cummings et al., 1985; Huff et al., 1986; Kempler, 1988; Bayles et al., 1989). In most cases, the anomia in dementia has a clear effect on communication, but the anomia in normal aging is often unnoticed by all except the speaker. Since anomia creates a functional disability in dementia, but not in normal aging, the quantitative difference between the two has a qualitatively different consequence.

In addition to the marked differences in the level of anomia, the origin of word-finding problems appears to set the two groups apart. In normal aging, intermittent and temporary problems in lexical retrieval appear to explain the anomia; in dementia, multiple factors including perceptual problems, retrieval deficits and loss of conceptual knowledge combine to produce word-finding problems.

Syntax

Knowledge of syntax allows us to tell whether a sentence is grammatical (e.g. 'Boy apple the ate the' may convey some meaning, but it is ungrammatical), and to compute the relationship between words in a sentence. For instance, the sentences 'The boy gave the girl a gift' and 'The girl gave the boy a gift' mean very different things, although the individual words are the same. Syntactic knowledge allows us to determine the different meanings of each by computing the relationships among the words in the sentence.

There is ongoing active debate about the best way to characterize syntactic knowledge and how that knowledge is acquired (Hyams, 1986; MacWhinney, 1987), but the basic patterns of development have been delineated clearly. By the end of the second year (18–24 months), children begin to combine words in novel and flexible ways. Over the following 1–2 years, children master the specific grammatical and morphological constructions of their language (how to ask a question, construct a negative sentence, etc.). There is continued development of grammar at least through early school years, when the more subtle and complex grammatical structures are mastered (Chomsky, 1969; Karmiloff-Smith, 1979). By late childhood, all native speakers of a language produce and comprehend a wide range of grammatical constructions 'automatically', without conscious control, and are able to make uniform judgements about the grammaticality of most sentences.

Normal aging and syntax

Syntactic ability, acquired largely before children go to school, undergoes relatively little change in adulthood. However, Kemper (1992) has reported some subtle changes in production of complex syntactic constructions. In a longitudinal study analyzing the syntactic structures used in diary entries over the adult lifespan, Kemper (1987a) found that by age 70 years, people tended to use less complicated sentences, averaging about 1.4 clauses, whereas in their 20s, their sentences averaged about three clauses. In contrast, the number of words per sentence did not change (about 9.2 at age 70 years, vs. 9.8 at age 20 years). Age did not interact with the relative complexity of particular syntactic constructions; rather, as people aged, they simply produced fewer of all types of constructions. Kynette & Kemper's (1986) analysis of spontaneous speech comparing people in their 50s and 60s with those in their 70s and 80s showed similar patterns of simplification of syntax with age.

Researchers have argued that people are better able to remember what they have understood. On this assumption, many studies report the use of immediate recall paradigms (i.e. imitation) to explore comprehension of various syntactic structures. Kemper (1986) found that adults aged 30–49 years had no difficulty imitating sentences varying in syntactic complexity. People aged 70–89 years had no difficulty imitating sentences with short clauses and those with subordinate clauses at the end of the sentences (sentence-final subordinate clauses: e.g. 'My grandchildren watched what I took out of the oven'). However, the older people had difficulty with subordinate clauses at the beginning of the sentences (sentence-initial subordinate clauses: e.g. 'What I took out of the oven interested my grandchildren'). This interaction of age with syntactic complexity is typical in recall studies (e.g. see: Kemper, 1987b; Norman et al., 1991) as well as studies which require subjects to answer questions about stimuli, relying indirectly on recall (Davis & Ball, 1989; Obler et al., 1991).

Findings such as these have been used to support a hypothesis that stresses the role of memory in sentence comprehension. Sentence comprehension requires coordination of retrieval of information from long-term memory with working memory. Working memory is a limited-capacity system for the simultaneous storage and processing of information (e.g. Baddeley, 1986) and has been implicated in several aspects of sentence comprehension in young normal subjects (e.g. Daneman & Carpenter, 1980; King & Just, 1991; MacDonald et al., 1992). It has also been suggested that working memory capacity is reduced with age (Light et al., 1982). Theories of working memory capacity and its role in sentence processing suggest that sentence-initial subordinate clauses must be stored before being processed as part of the main clause predicate (e.g. Glanzer et al., 1981). Sentence-final subordinate clauses are attached readily to the main clause predicate, which has already been processed. The results of recall studies suggest that older people have difficulty holding sentence-initial subordinate clauses in working memory until they process the main clause. Older people have less difficulty with sentence-final clauses because they are processed subsequent to the main clause. In light of these findings, Kemper (1992) argues that the age-related decrease in production and recall of syntactically complex sentences is due to an age-related reduction in working memory capacity.

However, we note that the decline in recall is only for sentence-initial clauses and it is not a problem of a reduction or loss of knowledge about syntax, but due to a reduction in the efficiency of a cognitive process used to parse sentences. When there is no substantial memory demand, there is no decrease in syntactic ability. Our conclusion is supported by Kynette and Kemper's (1986) observation that, in spontaneous speech, people over 70 years of age showed no increase in the frequency of dysfluencies (e.g. unfinished sentences), incorrect verb tenses, or incorrect grammatical forms, which might be expected if there were a syntactic impairment.

Although it has been suggested here that the origin of apparent deficits in syntactic comprehension is a working memory capacity deficit with age, this explanation does not account for all the data. Stine et al. (1986) examined age differences in recall of sentences equated for the number of words but varying in the number of propositions (ideas). Compare the four-proposition sentence 'The Statue of Liberty was constructed from a framework of steel and a coating of copper' with the 10-proposition sentence 'In many Greek coffee houses, men spend hours reading foreign newspapers or playing backgammon for small stakes'. Although it is assumed that propositionally dense sentences place a greater burden on working memory capacity than sentences with few propositions, because they are harder to recall, age did not interact with density in the Stine et al. study. Note also that the 10-proposition sentence is more syntactically complex. This increase in syntactic complexity did not hamper older peoples' recall differentially, calling into question the working memory deficit hypothesis. Instead, the locus of the problem in sentence recall may not be limited to working memory, but to other, more general aspects of memory (i.e. retrieval of sentence content from long-term memory; see Light et al., 1982; Salthouse, 1991). The written and oral production studies of Kemper and colleagues (Kemper, 1986; Kynette & Kemper, 1986) also may suggest general memory problems as a source of decreasing syntactic complexity because there were no age-related decreases in the spontaneous production of sentence-initial relative to sentence-final subordinate clauses.

Thus, the data suggest that normal older adults are not impaired in syntactic knowledge, but do produce fewer syntactically complex sentences in spontaneous speech and writing, and recall them less well than younger adults. Although the problem is clearly associated with aging, the difficulty is likely to be due to a reduction in working memory capacity or in retrieval of information from long-term memory (see Light (1990)), not due to a syntactic deficit. In fact, although it has been argued that comprehension problems cause memory problems, the opposite appears to be the case: memory deficits in normal older adults affect their comprehension (see also Light (1991)).

Dementia and syntax

Although most anecdotal descriptions of language in AD have observed that syntactic ability appears to be intact, few experimental investigations have addressed this question. Whitaker (1976) described a severely demented patient who spontaneously corrected agrammatic, but not semantically, anomalous sentences in repetition (e.g. 'There are two book on the table' was repeated as 'There are few books on the table' while 'The apple was eaten by a stone' was repeated verbatim). This finding was taken to indicate that grammatical competence was selectively *preserved* in dementia. Schwartz et al. (1979) also examined a single subject in detail, and found that their patient, despite severely impaired lexical (naming) ability, was able to manipulate syntactic structures (e.g. to turn an active into a passive), again supporting the notion that the syntactic processor may in fact be special, and neuropsychologically insulated from the cognitive degeneration seen in dementia. Subsequent attempts to address this issue have found that AD patients produce syntactically complex and well-formed sentences in conversations and narratives. Kempler and colleagues (Kempler, 1984, Kempler et al., 1987) demonstrated that AD patients and age-matched controls did not differ in the range and frequency of syntactic constructions (e.g. relative clauses, questions) used in spontaneous speech and telling a story.

In contrast to the relatively straightforward evidence for preservation of syntactic forms in production, comprehension of syntax is a more complicated story. Schwartz et al. (1979) demonstrated intact comprehension of four syntactic forms (active, passive, preposition and comparative adjectives) by a single demented patient. However, Emery (1988), using the test of syntactic complexity (Emery, 1986) and the Chomsky test of syntax (Chomsky, 1969), documented syntactic comprehension deficits in a sample of 20 AD subjects. These tests evaluate the patient's comprehension of syntax by eliciting verbal responses to grammatically complex stimuli (e.g. 'The dog was bitten by the cat; which animal bit the other and which was bitten?') or gestural responses to complex auditory stimuli (e.g. 'Mickey tells Donald to hop up and down; make him hop'). In contrast to Schwartz et al.'s (1979) findings of preserved comprehension of grammatically complex structures, Emery (1986) found significant impairment in AD patients' ability to process syntactically complex sentences.

The dissociation between intact syntactic production and impaired comprehension in AD may also be explained by memory deficits. Memory and processing demands may affect performance on comprehension tasks more than production tasks, and therefore create an *apparent* comprehension deficit alongside intact production. Emery (1988) argued against this explanation, citing the finding that AD patients were able to *repeat* all the stimuli with good accuracy even though they could not comprehend them, suggesting that the problem is not one of memory, but more likely to be due to deterioration of complex syntactic processing. However, these repetition data do not rule out the possibility that memory problems interfered with performance on her tasks. Commonly, AD patients show intact immediate memory (in repetition), but impaired memory performance with any delay (Buschke & Fuld, 1974; Knopman & Ryberg, 1989). Therefore, any delay between presentation of the sentences and performance of the response task (e.g. acting out the sentence) might be expected to place demands on the memory system not apparent in an imitation task. Even the shift in attention required from listening to the stimulus to acting out the sentence, or the delay between listening to a sentence and then listening to a question about that sentence, may have been sufficient to cause forgetting of the target sentence. In short, although Emery claims to have documented syntactic deficits, the performance patterns she obtained may be better explained by impairments in memory or other nonlinguistic cognitive domains (e.g. attention) that were required to perform her language tasks.

Several studies have now addressed the question of whether sentence comprehension deficits in AD can be attributed to linguistic vs. general nonlinguistic processing demands. Smith (1989) presented a group of 22 AD patients with a picture task to assess comprehension of reciprocals ('The boy and girl are giving gifts to each other') and reflexives ('The boy is spilling paint on himself'), systematically varying elements which contribute to processing difficulty and syntactic complexity (two- vs. four-choice response arrays, and the distance between the reflexive and the referent as in 'The clown is watching the *boy* who is spilling paint on *himself* versus 'The *boy* who is watching the clown is spilling paint on *himself*'). The results demonstrated that both AD patients and controls showed performance decrements as task difficulty increased and both groups showed a similar pattern of errors. These results indicate that comprehension deficits in AD and normal control subjects can be attributed to the same general processing limitations, and not to specifically linguistic deficits.

Waters and colleagues (Waters et al., 1993; Rochon, 1992) have also provided evidence that sentence comprehension impairments in AD may be attributed to 'post-interpretive' demands of the task (e.g. reflection, judgement, storage), rather than to syntactic deficits per se. In their work, these authors make a distinction between two stages in the sentence comprehension process, the first being 'sentence interpretation' (e.g. determining aspects of meaning such as which noun is the agent in a passive sentence), and the second being 'post-interpretive' processing (e.g. matching the literal meaning with real-world knowledge to determine plausibility). This second stage requires more processing resources than the first. Their hypothesis is that AD patients are especially sensitive to increases in difficulty at the post-interpretive rather than the interpretive stage of sentence comprehension, due to their limitation of processing resources. Poorer comprehension performance on sentences with increased number of propositions and correlations between comprehension and working memory are used to support their nonsyntactic 'processing resources' explanation of sentence comprehension deficits.

Thus, in contrast to Emery's results, these more recent findings suggest that sentence comprehension deficits in AD may be attributed at least in part to general processing limitations such as working memory deficits, rather than to a specifically syntactic deficit. That is, syntactic knowledge appears to be intact in AD, but accessing this knowledge in tasks which require other cognitive systems (e.g. memory) causes performance deficits in sentence comprehension.

Summary

Syntactic knowledge appears to be preserved in normal aging and dementia, but both groups' performance is affected by declines in other cognitive capacities – specifically attention and memory. The more severe the memory demands of the task (comprehension > production) and the more severe the memory deficits (AD > normal aging), the more severe the sentence level processing deficits appear to be.

Interestingly, we might conclude from these data that the syntactic deficits in normal aging and dementia appear to be of the same type:

limitations on memory which impair performance on sentence production and comprehension tasks. However, it must be pointed out that this is a general conclusion, and not limited to these populations. The same processing demands also affect young normal subjects' ability to understand sentences. In other words, examination of these two populations has demonstrated that sentences with higher processing demands (more memory) are more difficult to understand (e.g. Stine et al., 1986), and does not provide any evidence for disruption of the syntactic knowledge system in either group.

However, this similarity between the two groups is tempered by two facts. First, the extent (quantity) of the problem is impressively different in the two groups. By definition, the memory deficits seen in dementia are significantly more severe than those seen in normal aging (e.g. McKhann et al., 1984). Therefore, the syntactic deficits resulting from the memory impairment can appear to be more severe as well – particularly in comprehension protocols such as that used by Emery (1985). This different level of impairment in the two groups is highlighted by the manipulations of syntactic complexity which result in performance decrements in the two groups. It is likely that AD patients would show floor effects for recall of multiclause sentences used in the normal aging studies, and that the normal subjects would show near ceiling effects for the stimuli used in the AD studies. Thus, although similar mechanisms are posited for apparent declines, the level of deficit in those mechanisms is much greater in dementia than in normal aging.

Second, despite positing a single mechanism to explain changes in syntactic performance in both groups, the different level of impairment has distinct consequences. Slight deficits in working memory do not impair the normal older person's ability to construct or to understand sentences in daily communication. On the other hand, the severe disruption of memory that is characteristic of dementia does have functional consequences for sentence processing, causing patients to have difficulty in following instructions and conversations. Therefore, while similarities between the two groups can be described as being a quantitative difference, the consequences of these impairments are qualitatively different.

Reference and discourse structure

We join sentences together in order to engage in conversations, tell stories and give lectures. Combining sentences into a coherent and meaningful discourse requires, in addition to lexical and syntactic skills, knowledge of discourse structure and rules for appropriate language use (pragmatics). Much of discourse is governed by general rules – e.g. topics are introduced before details, and, typically, we introduce people into the conversation using proper nouns before we use pronouns (he, she) to refer to them. However, other discourse rules vary from context to context and are determined by, among other things, the relative status, formality, language competence and purpose of the speakers. For instance, rules about when to take a speaking turn and how long a turn to take in conversation are also governed by context-specific criteria: a second of silence is often an indication of a turn boundary in a telephone conversation, while a much longer period of silence and even a direct request to speak may be required before a student takes a turn in a classroom.

The acquisition of discourse structure is distributed widely across childhood. Some aspects (e.g. turn taking) could be considered to arise out of early sound-play and pre-date lexical and syntactic aspects of language. Other more subtle rules of story telling and appropriateness are acquired much later during school years (Bates, 1976; Andersen, 1990).

Because discourse involves many skills (lexical and syntactic ability, integrating concepts within sentences, manipulating references within and between sentences, knowledge about situations and participants, and enough memory to keep track of it all), it is vulnerable to disruption with impairment at any of these levels. In addition, since maintaining a coherent discourse relies more heavily on other cognitive resources (memory in particular) than on lexical or syntactic skills, it might be particularly sensitive, therefore, to deficits in nonlinguistic cognition. Just as discourse is vulnerable to deficits in these areas (lexical, syntactic, cognitive), it is also possible that, due to the many factors that interact to form a discourse, these abilities might be resilient to certain deficits. For example, speakers may be able to compensate for anomia or syntactic deficits and maintain a coherent discourse by reliance on strategies such as paraphrasing, repetition or asking for confirmation.

For the purposes of this chapter, we will focus on two aspects of discourse functioning: pronominal reference and knowledge of discourse macrostructure. Rules of pronoun use govern how and when we use pronouns to refer back to words that were introduced previously in the same sentence, in previous sentences, and even in previous discourses. Knowledge of discourse macrostructures includes, for instance, knowledge of what aspects of a story come first (the introduction comes before the complicating event, which both precede the resolution), and internalized mental scripts for various other verbal activities.

Discourse in normal aging

Cohesive, relevant, appropriate discourse is typical in normal aging. Normal older people are generally able to introduce topics, to build on them, and to refer back to them appropriately throughout a conversation or narrative. However, there have been subtle deficiencies identified in normal older adults' ability to use pronouns in discourse. For instance, older adults are more likely than younger adults to use pronouns that do not specify their referent in spontaneous speech (e.g. Cohen, 1979; Pratt et al., 1989). This problem may be linked to memory deficits where the older speaker has forgotten to establish reference, thought that she already did, or has forgotten the names of characters (see Pratt et al. (1989)).

   In comprehension, subtle deficits in interpreting pronouns have also been documented. Interestingly, there are no observable age differences in terms of pronoun interpretation, as long as information is remembered. However, if memory is required to interpret a discourse accurately, age-related declines appear. For instance, in the pair of sentences (1) and (2) below, research has shown that older adults can use pragmatics, that is, contextualized world knowledge, to assign reference to pronouns accurately:

(1)   Henry spoke at a meeting while John drove to the beach.
(2)   He lectured on the administration.

Light & Capps (1986) found that older adults, like the young, assigned the pronoun 'He' to 'Henry', even though a pronoun such as this is assigned generally to the closest possible antecedent (which would be 'John' in this case). Here, the verbal context biased the reading of the pronoun, and both younger and older adults were able to integrate the contextual information accurately over the two sentences. However, when irrelevant material (about the weather) intervened, placing demands on memory, older people showed reference assignment deficits, that is, assigning the pronoun 'He' to 'John' in the example above, because they could not remember which person was associated with which action. Light and her colleagues (Light, 1992) have also examined pronoun assignments in a variety of conditions and found no age differences. A range of other sentence and text comprehension experiments have similarly found no age differences in interpretation based on contextual bias – that is, older people maintain their ability to use prior context to interpret sentences (e.g. Burke & Harrold, 1988; Zelinski, 1988; Zelinski & Miura, 1988, 1990).

In addition to tracking reference though discourse, each discourse genre has a macrostructure. For instance, conversations involve appropriate turn-taking and stories contain a reliable sequence of elements from the setting to complicating events to the resolution. In contrast to the studies cited above, which documented only subtle, and probably memory-derived, declines in use of pronouns in discourse, studies indicate that there are no age-related difficulties in the use of discourse macrostructures.

One aspect of macrostructure is the ordering of story elements. If sentences from a story are presented in a scrambled order, older people will reorder them spontaneously during recall (Mandel & Johnson, 1984). If a story involves a topic that is familiar to them, older people will include relevant information from what they know about the topic into their memory performance (Hultsch & Dixon, 1983; Light & Anderson, 1983; Zelinski & Miura, 1988).

A few studies have analyzed narratives told by older and younger people about important incidents in their lives – like their first love. In two studies, narratives were produced orally (Kemper et al., 1990; Pratt & Robins, 1991) and, in the third, written extracts from diaries kept over a lifetime were used (Kemper, 1987a). Older adults' stories were rated as appropriate in terms of overall structure: introductions of characters, complex and coherent episodes, and endings that summarized the outcomes of the actions accurately. There was no evidence that the stories told by older people were formed poorly or otherwise reflected a disorganization of knowledge about story macrostructure. In fact, Kemper et al. (1990) reported that English teachers and undergraduate students rated autobiographical stories produced by older people as being better formed than those produced by younger speakers. Similarly, Mergler et al. (1985) found that older people's oral narratives were considered (by undergraduates) to be more interesting and memorable than those produced by younger people.

In summary, studies of discourse do not reveal any deterioration with normal aging. In fact, there may be some increase in discourse skill, at least when describing personally significant autobiographical events. The impression of overall improvement in discourse with age is mitigated by the fact that there are some documented referential problems with respect to pronouns in certain tasks. For instance, Pratt et al. (1989) found about five unspecified referents in narratives produced by people in their 20s and 40s, and an average of eight produced by people in their 70s. While the actual numbers of unspecified referents does increase slightly with age, apparently, the positive ratings of older speakers' narratives suggest that this does not cause an impairment in communicative effectiveness. Thus, we suggest that there are minimal observed deficits in older people's discourse ability and no functional consequences of these impairments. One explanation for this noneffect is that older people may rely on their extensive experience with language to reduce the impact of specific problems with word finding and reference in communication (see also Mackay and Burke (1990) for related arguments on why word-finding problems may not be that frequent). This does not seem to be the case in AD.

Discourse in dementia

Some aspects of discourse are preserved in AD through the mild and moderate stages: AD patients take conversational turns when appropriate and often produce socially ritualized parts of the conversations (greetings, leave takings, small talk, etc.) with appropriate timing and affect. However, there are also discourse problems early on, such as tendency to repeat things unnecessarily ('ideational perseveration'), to be tangential, and to have difficulty with reference, particularly inappropriate use of empty words ('thing', 'do' etc.) and pronouns, creating the impression of empty and incoherent discourse (Nicholas et al., 1985b; Ripich & Terrell, 1988; Ulatowska et al., 1988).

With respect to specific problems in pronominal reference, Kempler and colleagues (Kempler, 1984; Kempler et al., 1987) found that AD patients used significantly more pronouns without clear referents than normal control subjects. Ulatowska et al. (1988) found that decreased informativeness could also be traced back, at least in part, to other related problems with reference, such as the overuse of demonstratives (e.g. *here*, *there*) and exophoric reference (e.g *'this'* without a clear antecedent).

The reason that AD patients have such a difficult time with reference is not clear. AD patients may have simply lost the internalized discourse rule which states that pronouns can be used felicitously only if the referent is clearly indexed within recent discourse. On the other hand, they may have lost the more basic ability to determine what a hearer would need in order to interpret a pronoun (what Ripich & Terrell (1988, p. 14) describe as a loss of the ability to 'take the perspective of the listener'). Or, alternately, the patient may have sufficient memory impairment to have forgotten if or when the referent occurred in previous discourse.

Another obvious source of pronoun overuse is anomia: if a person cannot retrieve a word, she might substitute a pronoun. Nicholas et al. (1985b) investigated the contribution of anomia to discourse incoherence in AD by comparing AD patients' naming ability with elements of empty speech in narrative descriptions of a picture. The authors reported a significant negative correlation between the score of AD patients on the Boston Naming Test (Goodglass & Kaplan, 1983) and the use of indefinite terms (e.g 'thing', 'stuff') as well as a significant positive correlation between the naming scores and the production of 'content elements' (i.e. references to characters and activities in the picture descriptions). However, because many other measures of discourse emptiness (e.g. paraphasias, overuse of pronouns, deictic terms) did not correlate with naming scores, they concluded that the naming deficit did not explain the emptiness of discourse. Of particular interest here is the fact that use of pronouns without antecedents was not correlated with anomia, and therefore suggests that poor pronominal use may be due to other impairments, such as those mentioned above.

In addition to discourse emptiness associated with overuse of pronouns and empty words, another possible source of discourse deficits in AD is the loss of knowledge about discourse structure per se. There is some evidence that AD patients are impaired in this area. Hutchinson & Jensen (1980) analyzed conversations of 10 dementia patients and found several discourse-pragmatic abnormalities including the fact that patients initiated more new topics, often inappropriately. Ripich and colleagues (Ripich & Terrell, 1988; Ripich et al., 1991) also analyzed conversations between AD subjects and normal controls and found that, while the overall conversational structure (genre) was maintained, there were some lower level anomalies, including the fact that the AD subjects spoke in shorter turns and made more attempts to solicit information (e.g. 'Is this coffee?').

Despite the ability to maintain a conversational interchange, analysis of other discourse genres and script knowledge reveals deficits in discourse macrostructure. Ulatowska & Chapman (1991) analyzed normal control and AD subjects' ability to construct a story based on a single picture and a sequence of pictures. Normal subjects included the mandatory story elements of a setting, complicating action and resolution in reasonable proportions to one another. The AD subjects, in contrast, produced more setting information (this component represented the greatest amount of information in the AD narratives), poorly developed action sequences and typically omitted resolutions. Based on these data, the authors conclude that AD subjects 'exhibited impaired narrative superstructure' (Ulatowska & Chapman, 1991, p. 128).

Andersen et al. (1990) evaluated another discourse genre – giving definitions. While this genre is acquired later than conversation or story telling, it is, by adulthood, governed by reliable rules. In their task, which required subjects simply to define several nouns, the authors found that control subjects generated predictably structured definitions, beginning with a superordinate category, and proceeding to specific details regarding functional and perceptual attributes. In contrast, some AD patients produced the correct elements but in an atypical sequence, and others did not produce the 'required' elements at all, often omitting the superordinate category name altogether. Many AD subjects also included personal information (e.g 'My daughter has one') which is not present in the definitions of control subjects. These abnormalities indicate that the knowledge about how to generate this piece of discourse (a definition) is deficient in people with AD.

Discourse genres are structured largely on the basis of internalized scripts – mental representations of the content and sequence of events comprising activities. Recent work has demonstrated that AD patients may also lose the ability to sequence events in familiar scripts – which would also impair their ability to sequence narratives that utilize script knowledge. Harrold et al. (1990) asked AD patients to discriminate and sequence events in three familiar scripts (a wedding, a surprise party and restaurant dining). The patients were required to tell if a particular event belonged in a script at all (e.g 'Is "The bride gives a lecture on English" part of what happens at a wedding?') and then sequence written sentence-pairs accurately (e.g 'Which comes first during a wedding: "The clergyman begins to read the ceremony" or "The bride and groom kiss"'?). AD patients were poor at both the discrimination and sequencing tasks, suggesting that their knowledge base of these mental scripts (including the participants, relations among participants and sequence of events) is impaired.

There are clear discourse problems in AD, and these deficits do not appear to have a single source. Some impairments, such as poor use of pronouns, appear to be secondary to well-documented linguistic problems such as anomia and to cognitive deficits in attention and working memory. There is also evidence that AD patients have pragmatic deficits that limit their ability to take the perspective of the listener and to judge what information is important in a particular discourse. Further, AD appears to impair knowledge of discourse macrostructures that are necessary for, among other things, giving definitions and telling stories.

Summary

Despite evidence for mild word-finding problems and decreases in working memory capacity, older individuals are able to use their considerable expertise with language to structure conversations and stories in a coherent and interesting way. No impairment in functional discourse is seen.

In contrast, discourse produced by AD patients is tangential and incoherent. The impairment is likely to stem from a number of more basic deficits: anomia, severe memory deficits, deficient knowledge of discourse macrostructures, and possibly a difficulty integrating conceptual, grammatical and semantic information – the building blocks of discourse. Unlike normal older people, AD patients are not able to compensate for deficits by relying on areas of preserved function or their years of experience with language. The overall effect is devastating to conversation, and provides convincing evidence that, no matter what similarities might be observed between the two groups in other areas of language, discourse impairments distinguish language in dementia from normal aging.

Summary and conclusions

There are a few similarities between language changes seen in the course of normal aging and those seen in dementia. Specifically, syntactic knowledge appears to be preserved in both groups. This provides evidence that syntactic knowledge is protected from the cognitive and cortical changes seen in both normal and abnormal aging. It is consistent with proposals that certain knowledge systems are modular (or encapsulated) and therefore appear to be independent from certain cognitive operations and dissolutions (Fodor, 1983; 1985; Jorm, 1986;

Kempler et al., 1987). However, there is another part to this story. That is, while syntactic knowledge appears to be preserved, it is clear that syntactic processing of long and propositionally complex sentences can be affected by decreasing memory capacity in both normal aging and dementia. Therefore, while the syntactic knowledge base appears to be uncompromised in both groups, use of that knowledge is sensitive to deficits in other cognitive domains – which are present, although to different degrees, in both groups. Comparison of syntactic ability in normal aging and dementia shows that syntactic knowledge is encapsulated, but the use of that knowledge requires support from other cognitive domains.

Comparisons of lexical abilities in normal aging and dementia illustrate the fact that a superficially similar behavior (i.e word-finding difficulty) can have different causes and that the degree of deficit will predict the impact on communication to a large extent. While normal word-finding problems are due to occasional lexical retrieval deficits, in dementia, word-finding problems probably have several sources (loss of lexical knowledge and perceptual problems complicating the picture), and they are *not* occasional. The differences in source, extent and effect of word-finding problems separate the two groups.

Our comparison of discourse ability in normal aging and dementia drew perhaps the clearest differences between the two populations. Despite the fact that both groups present with word-finding problems and working memory deficits, which might be expected to affect their respective discourse productions, we see very distinct patterns of discourse. Normal older people are able to overcome mild lexical and memory problems and can create coherent, relevant and interesting discourse. Dementia patients, undoubtedly due to the extent of their linguistic and nonlinguistic cognitive problems, produce confusing, incoherent discourse. In discourse, then, we see what perhaps is the most important difference in language abilities of the two groups: in one, subtle language changes occur in an otherwise normal cognitive base; in the other, the cognitive support has deteriorated. In the final analysis, the degree and level of functional impairment requires us to conclude that the differences between language in normal aging and dementia are qualitative.

In reaching the conclusion that the language changes in normal aging and dementia are distinct, we have looked at several types of data. First, we asked whether there was evidence for impairment in particular aspects of language in both groups (e.g. 'Do both groups have word-finding problems?'), and found an affirmative answer. Second, we looked at degree of impairment (e.g. 'Does one group have more frequent word-finding problems than the other'), finding that the degree of impairment distinguished the groups. Third, we asked whether a similar appearing behavior might be due to different underlying causes (e.g. 'Is word-finding difficulty due to retrieval vs. knowledge loss?'), finding evidence for differences between the two groups again. Finally, we wondered whether there were functional consequences of impairments in the two groups (e.g. 'Does word-finding difficulty create misunderstandings in daily communication?'), finding clear differences again.

When all is said and done, we believe the data emphasize differences rather than similarities between the two groups. However, we must acknowledge other explanations for the observations we have made. In fact, there have been recent claims that the two groups differ mainly in degree.

First, an argument can be made that, while studies of selected samples (i.e. most of those reported here) may reveal differences between the two groups, the study of large numbers of individuals from unselected population samples might disclose more notable overlap between normal and demented subjects (e.g. see Chapter 15). That is, individuals with mild dementia may show similar performance patterns to the very old (e.g. over 80 years of age) that are missed in the kind of analyses reported here. Since AD is only diagnosed definitely at post-mortem (McKann et al., 1984), clinical diagnosis necessarily contains some risk of misdiagnosis (e.g. Neary et al., 1986; Sulkava et al., 1983). The effect of misdiagnosis on results will be minimized in a study of groups selected on the basis of clinical investigation, and potentially will be maximized in population studies which will contain many individuals with very mild or borderline cognitive deterioration. AD is a disease that is diagnosed clinically only after it progresses beyond the mildest stages. It is the mildly impaired patients who are most difficult to diagnose, and are therefore the most likely to be confused with normal individuals (i.e. misdiagnosis). It is only at the moderate stages that clinicians become sure of what we are dealing with. In order to increase the likelihood of making veridical comparisons between healthy elderly and AD patients (that is, to compare what we think we are comparing), we believe it is the moderately impaired AD patients who should be compared with the normal population. Although this approach increases the probability of finding group differences, it decreases the prospect of error due to subject misclassification. In addition, in order to limit the chance of subject classification errors and erroneous conclusions further, studies must be extremely careful to control for the effects of all variables that affect performance on cognitive tasks, such as depression and level of education.

Population studies have also concluded that there is more similarity than difference between the normal and demented groups. Nebes and colleagues (Nebes & Madden, 1988; Nebes & Brady, 1992) evaluated a large number of response time (RT) studies performed with young, old and AD subjects (many involving language processing) and suggested that most of the differences between young, old and AD subjects are in quantity rather than in kind (e.g. Nebes, 1992). Their hypothesis is that a single mechanism – generalized cognitive slowing – can account for a wide range of experimental data reviewed in normal aging and AD. They propose specifically that the difference in RT between young and old normal subjects is a constant of about 1.5 (i.e older people take about one and a half times as long as young people to respond), and the difference between young and AD patients is about 2.2 (i.e. AD patients take over twice as long as young people to respond). They propose that criteria for a qualitative difference between groups hinge on significant RT deviation beyond the expected differences outlined above (i.e. disproportionately large RT difference from what their constant would predict for slowing with age and disease).

This position is well argued and elegant, since a single mechanism explains performance on a wide array of tasks. However, there are several issues which mitigate the force of their quantitative explanation for differences that we have described. First, this model is based on RT data, which do not reflect the complexity of the errors discussed in this chapter, errors that highlight the differences between the groups. Although it is likely that cognitive slowing can create distinct error patterns depending on the extent of the deficit, the relationship between cognitive slowing and, for example, types of naming errors or atypical word definitions has yet to be explored and it is unclear how error data fit into an RT theory of impairment. Second, the suggestion that slowing itself causes language difficulties is problematic. This position presumes that slowing is the cause, rather than the result, of deficits in cognitive processes. It might also be argued for instance, that specific lexical retrieval deficits slow down all cognitive processing that involves verbal material. Third, Nebes' position presumes that individual variability in performance represents 'noise' in the data. Since their studies analyze group data, they tend to overlook potentially critical individual factors in performance (see: Folstein & Breitner, 1982; Chui et al., 1985; Kempler et al., 1994). Individual and subgroup data may indicate that performance does not vary on just one dimension (speed), but might reflect different underlying processes. Fourth, recent evidence on normal aging suggests that a general slowing model of performance change is less general than assumed originally, with separate functions needed to explain linguistic compared to nonlinguistic response time phenomena (Lima et al., 1991), and for different chronometric measures of nervous system responses (i.e. cortical evoked potentials vs. manual reaction time) (Bashore et al., 1989). Finally, it is difficult to resolve the apparent conflict between a theory that states that differences between the groups are quantitative in nature with the fact that the real-life consequences of the deficits are so qualitatively different. In order to resolve this conflict, we would have to enhance the theory with a notion of a quantitative threshold that, if crossed, would create qualitative differences. Or in other words, we would conclude that quantity – when there is enough of it – has a quality all its own.

Throughout this chapter, we have emphasized the consequences of language impairments for daily interaction. Even if we demonstrate quantitative parallels, for instance, in the preservation of syntactic knowledge across groups or a continuum of cognitive slowing between young, old normal and AD patients (Nebes & Brady, 1992), these parallels do not capture the obvious differences in the communicative competence of these groups. Young and old nondemented individuals communicate successfully in the entire range of communicative situations (conversations, interviews, telling stories, etc.) with no limitations or special allowances. In contrast, communication with demented individuals is limited severely by their language and cognitive problems. Communication with moderately demented subjects often requires special adjustments such as using shorter sentences, frequent repetitions, slow speech rate, simple vocabulary, and use of other communication modalities (writing, pictures, gestures) to compensate for verbal deficits (Ostuni & Santo Pietro, 1986). Even with these adjustments on the part of the nondemented speaker, it is often impossible to interpret the speech produced by the demented person. This contrast forces us to conclude that the language of normal older and demented individuals is qualitatively different. And it is this qualitative difference that dictates the communicative accommodations necessary for people who want and need to communicate with demented people.

Directions for future research

In closing, it is worth optimistically noting that future research will help to resolve some of the issues that have evolved out of this discussion and to clarify further the nature of the differences between language in normal aging and dementia. Some of our suggestions on how to address these issues further are outlined below.

First, we recommend that experimental research on language should be enhanced by inclusion of measures of functional communication. This will allow us to understand better the relationship between experimentally measurable deficits and the effects of these deficits on daily communication and activities.

Second, the literature reviewed here makes it difficult to compare older normal and demented individuals because methods used to evaluate the two groups are often not comparable (see, for example, the stimuli used in syntactic experiments for normal aging vs. AD), and few studies include all three groups (young, old and demented) necessary for the comparison. Therefore, we recommend the use of both young and older normal controls in research on dementia and the use of comparable materials and tasks with these three groups to allow more valid group comparisons.

Third, we have suggested at several points that memory interacts with the language decline in both normal aging and dementia. However, the precise relationship between specific aspects of memory (working vs. long-term) and specific language tasks is not well understood. To clarify this relationship further, two methodological suggestions can be made:

(1) Independent measures of memory function could be included in studies of language processing to afford direct comparisons between particular aspects of memory and language processing (for example, see Rochon (1992) as well as Small et al. (1991) for prototypes of this type of inquiry)

(2) On-line methods such as those used to study language processing in normal young and aphasic patients (e.g. Tyler, 1992) could be utilized to evaluate the moment-by-moment components of language processing which would minimize the reliance on memory for task performance.

These methodologies hold promise to illuminate the mechanisms underlying language breakdown, which will supplement our discussion of deficits in the 'end product' (i.e. errors) of language processing.

Finally, future research will also need to explore individual and subgroup differences, investigating, for example, the performance differences in the normal populations between the old and very old and the differences between subgroups of dementia subjects, such as: those with early vs. late onset (Seltzer & Sherwin, 1983; Filley et al., 1986; Faber-Langendoen et al., 1988; Selnes et al., 1988); particular patterns of language impairment (Becker et al., 1988; Kempler et al., 1994); familial vs. nonfamilial disease (Knesevich et al., 1985); and distinct patterns of brain damage (Foster et al., 1983; Chase et al., 1984).

References

Albert, M. & Milberg, W. (1989). Semantic processing in patients with Alzheimer's disease. *Brain and Language*, **37**, 163–71.
Albert, M. S., Heller, H. S. & Milberg, W. (1988). Changes in naming ability with age. *Psychology and Aging*, **3**, 173–8.
Alzheimer, A. (1907). Of a particular disease of the cerebral cortex. *Zentralblatt vur Nervenheilkunde und Psychiatrie*, **30**, 177–9. (Translation and commentary by Wilkins, R. H. & Brody, I. A. (1969) Alzheimer's disease, *Archives of Neurology*, **21**, 109–10.)
Andersen, E. S. (1990). *Speaking with Style: the Sociolinguistic Skills of Children*. Routledge, New York.
Andersen, E. S., Clancy, P. & White, E. (1990). 'The disruption of discourse organization in Alzheimer's disease.' Paper presented at the International Pragmatics Association, Barcelona, July 1990.
Anderson, J. R. (1983). A spreading activation theory of memory. *Journal of Verbal Learning and Verbal Behavior*, **22**, 261–95.
Appell, J., Kertesz, A. & Fisman, M. (1982). A study of language functioning in Alzheimer patients. *Brain and Language*, **17**, 73–91.
Baddeley, A. (1986). *Working memory*. Clarendon, Oxford.
Balota, D. A. & Duchek, J. M. (1988). Age-related differences in lexical access, spreading activation, and simple pronunciation. *Psychology and Aging*, **3**, 84–93.
Barker, M. G. & Lawson, J. S. (1968). Nominal aphasia in dementia. *British Journal of Psychiatry*, **114**, 1351–6.
Bashore, T. R., Osman, A. & Heffley, E. F. (1989). Mental slowing in elderly persons: a cognitive psychophysiological analysis. *Psychology and Aging*, **4**, 235–44.
Bates, E. (1976). *Language and Context: the Acquisition of Pragmatics*. Academic Press, New York.
Bayles, K. A. (1982). Language function in senile dementia. *Brain and Language*, **16**, 265–80.
Bayles, K. A. & Tomoeda, C. K. (1983). Confrontation naming impairment in dementia. *Brain and Language*, **19**, 98–114.

Bayles, K. A. & Kaszniak, A. W. (1987). *Communication and Cognition in Normal Aging and Dementia*. Little, Brown and Co., Boston.

Bayles, K. A., Boone, D. R., Tomoeda, C. K., Slauson, T. J. & Kaszniak, A. W. (1989). Differentiating Alzheimer's patients from the normal elderly and stroke patients with aphasia. *Journal of Speech and Hearing Research*, **54**, 74–87.

Becker, J. T., Huff, F. J., Nebes, R. D., Holland, A. & Boller, F. (1988). Neuropsychological function in Alzheimer's disease. *Archives of Neurology*, **45**, 263–8.

Blanks, J. C., Torigoe, Y., Hinton, D. R. & Blanks, R. H. (1991). Retinal degeneration in the macula of patients with Alzheimer's disease. *Annals of the New York Academy of Sciences*, **640**, 44–6.

Borod, J. C., Goodglass, H. & Kaplan, E. (1980). Normative data on the Boston Diagnostic Aphasia Examination, Parietal Lobe Battery, and the Boston Naming Test. *Journal of Clinical Neuropsychology*, **2**, 209–15.

Brown, A. S. & Mitchell, D. B. (1991). Age differences in retrieval consistency and response dominance. *Journal of Gerontology: Psychological Sciences*, **46**, P332–9.

Burke, D. M. & Peters, L. (1986). Word associations in old age: evidence for consistency in semantic encoding during adulthood. *Psychology and Aging*, **1**, 283–92.

Burke, D. M. & Harrold, R. M. (1988). Automatic and effortful semantic processes in old age: Experimental and naturalistic approaches. In L. L. Light & D. M. Burke (eds.) *Language, Memory, and Aging*, pp. 100–16. Cambridge University Press, New York.

Burke, D. M., White, H. & Diaz, D. L. (1987). Semantic priming in young and older adults: evidence for age-constancy in automatic and attentional processes. *Journal of Experimental Psychology: Human Perception and Performance*, **13**, 79–88.

Burke, D. M., Mackay, D. G., Worthley, J. A. & Wade, E. (1991). On the tip of the tongue: what causes word finding failures in young and older adults? *Journal of Memory and Language*, **30**, 542–79.

Buschke, H. & Fuld, P. A. (1974). Evaluating storage, retention, and retrieval in disordered memory and learning. *Neurology*, **24**, 1019–25.

Chase, T. N., Foster, N. L., Fedio, P., Brooks, R., Mansi, L. & DiChiro, G. (1984). Regional cortical dysfunction in Alzheimer's disease as determined by positron emission tomography. *Annals of Neurology*, **15**, 170–4.

Chertkow, H., Bub, D. & Seidenberg, M. (1989). Priming and semantic memory loss in Alzheimer's disease. *Brain and Language*, **36**, 420–46.

Chomsky, C. (1969). *The Acquisition of Syntax in Children from 5–10*. MIT Press, Cambridge, Mass.

Chui, H. C. (1987). The significance of clinically defined subgroups of Alzheimer's disease. *Journal of Neural Transmission*, (supplement), **24**, 57–68.

Chui, H. C., Teng, E. L., Henderson, V. W. & Moy, A. C. (1985). Clinical subtypes of dementia of the Alzheimer type. *Neurology*, **35**, 1544–50.

Cohen, G. (1979). Language comprehension in old age. *Cognitive Psychology*, **11**, 412–29.

Cummings, J. L., Benson, D. F., Hill, M. A. & Read, S. (1985). Aphasia in dementia of the Alzheimer type. *Neurology*, **29**, 315–23.

Daneman, M. & Carpenter, P. (1980). Individual differences in working memory and reading. *Journal of Verbal Learning and Verbal Behavior*, **19**, 450–66.

Davis, G. A. & Ball, H. E. (1989). Effects of age on comprehension of complex sentences in adulthood. *Journal of Speech and Hearing Research*, **32**, 143–50.

Emery, O. B. (1985). Language and aging. *Experimental Aging Research*, **11**, 3–60.

Emery, O. B. (1986). Test for Syntactic Complexity. *Language and Communication*, **6**, 63–4.

Emery, O. B. (1988). Language and memory processing in senile dementia Alzheimer's type. In L. L. Light & D. M. Burke (eds.) *Language, Memory and Aging*, pp. 221–43. Cambridge University Press, New York.

Faber-Langendoen, K., Morris, J. C., Knesevich, J. W., LaBarge, E., Miller, J. P. & Berg, L. (1988). Aphasia in senile dementia of the Alzheimer type. *Annals of Neurology*, **23**, 365–70.

Filley, C. M., Kelly, J. & Heaton, R. K. (1986). Neuropsychologic features of early- and late-onset Alzheimer's disease. *Archives of Neurology*, **43**, 574–6.

Fodor, J. (1983). *The Modularity of Mind, an Essay on Faculty Psychology*. MIT Press, Cambridge, Mass.

Fodor, J. (1985). Precis of the modularity of mind. *The Behavioral and Brain Sciences*, **8**, 1–42.

Folstein, M. F. & Breitner, J. C. S. (1982). Language disorder predicts familial Alzheimer's disease. In S. Corkin (ed.) *Alzheimer's Disease: a Report of Progress (Aging, vol 19)*, pp. 197–200. Raven Press, New York.

Foss, D. J. (1982). A discourse on semantic priming. *Cognitive Psychology*, **14**, 590–607.

Foster, N. L., Chase, T. N., Fedio, P., Patronas, N. J., Brookes, R. A. & DiChiro, G. (1983). Alzheimer's disease: focal cortical changes shown by positron emission tomography. *Neurology*, **33**, 961–5.

Glanzer, M., Dorfman, D. & Kaplan, B. (1981). Short-term storage in the processing of text. *Journal of Verbal Learning and Verbal Behavior*, **20**, 656–70.

Goodglass, H. & Kaplan, E. (1983). *The Boston Naming Test*. Lee and Febiger, Philadelphia.

Grober, H., Buschke, H., Kawas, C. & Fuld, P. (1985). Impaired ranking of semantic attributes in dementia. *Brain and Language*, **26**, 276–86.

Harrold, R. M., Andersen, E. S., Clancy, P. & Kempler, D. (1990). Script knowledge deficits in Alzheimer's disease. Paper presented at the International Neuropsychological Society, July, Innsbrück. *Journal of Clinical and Experimental Neuropsychology*, **12**, 397.

Henderson, V., Mack, W., Freed, D., Kempler, D. & Andersen, E. (1990). Naming consistency in Alzheimer's disease. *Brain and Language*, **39**, 530–8.

Howard, D. V. (1980). Category norms: a comparison of the Battig and Montague (1969) norms with the responses of adults between the ages of 20 and 80. *Journal of Gerontology*, **35**, 225–31.

Howard, D. V., McAndrews, M. P. & Lasaga, M. I. (1981). Semantic priming of lexical decisions in young and old adults. *Journal of Gerontology*, **36**, 707–14.

Huff, F. J. (1988). The disorder of naming in Alzheimer's disease. In L. L. Light & D. M. Burke (eds.) *Language, Memory and Aging*, pp. 209–20. Cambridge University Press, New York.

Huff, F. J., Corkin, S. & Growdon, H. J. (1986). Semantic impairment and anomia in Alzheimer's disease. *Brain and Language*, **28**, 235–49.

Huff, F. J., Mack, L., Mahlmann, J. & Greenberg, S. (1988). A comparison of lexical–semantic impairments in left hemisphere stroke and Alzheimer's disease. *Brain and Language*, **34**, 262–78.

Hultsch, D. F. & Dixon, R. A. (1983). The role of pre-experimental knowledge in text processing and adulthood. *Experimental Aging Research*, **9**, 17–22.

Hutchinson, J. M. & Jensen, M. (1980). A pragmatic evaluation of discourse communication in normal and senile elderly in a nursing home. In L. Obler & M. Albert (eds.) *Language and Communication in the Elderly*, pp. 59–74. D. C. Heath and Company, Lexington, Mass.

Hyams, N. M. (1986). *Language Acquisition and the Theory of Parameters*. D. Reidel Co., Boston.

Jorm, A. F. (1986). Controlled and automatic information processing in senile dementia: a review. *Psychological Medicine*, **16**, 77–88.

Karmiloff-Smith, A. (1979). Language development after five. In P. Fletcher & M. Garman (eds.) *Language Acquisition*. Cambridge University Press, Cambridge.

Kemper, S. (1986). Imitation of complex syntactic constructions by elderly adults. *Applied Psycholinguistics*, **7**, 277–88.

Kemper, S. (1987a). Life-span changes in syntactic complexity. *Journal of Gerontology*, **42**, 323–8.

Kemper, S. (1987b). Syntactic complexity and elderly adults' prose recall. *Experimental Aging Research*, **13**, 47–52.

Kemper, S. (1992). Language and aging. In F. I. M. Craik & T. A. Salthouse (eds.) *The Handbook of Aging and Cognition*, pp. 213–72. Erlbaum, Hillsdale, NJ.

Kemper, S., Rash, S. R., Kynette, D. & Norman, S. (1990). Telling stories: the structure of adults' narratives. *European Journal of Cognitive Psychology*, **2**, 205–28.

Kempler, D. (1984). 'Syntactic and symbolic abilities in Alzheimer's disease.' Ph.D. dissertation, UCLA.

Kempler, D. (1988). Lexical and pantomime abilities in Alzheimer's disease. *Aphasiology*, **2**, 147–59.

Kempler, D. (1991). Language changes in dementia of the Alzheimer type. In R. Lubinski (ed.) *Dementia and Communication*, pp. 98–114. B. C. Decker, Inc., Philadelphia.

Kempler, D. & Andersen, E. (1989). Language subgroups in Alzheimer's disease. Paper presented at the Gerontological Society of America. Minneapolis, November. *Gerontologist*, **29**, p. 140A.

Kempler, D., Curtiss, S. & Jackson, C. (1987). Syntactic preservation in Alzheimer's disease. *Journal of Speech and Hearing Research*, **30**, 343–50.

Kempler, D., Andersen, E., Hunt, M. & Henderson, V. W. (1990). Linguistic and attentional contributions to anomia in Alzheimer's disease. Paper presented at the International Neuropsychological Society, July, Innsbruck. *Journal of Clinical and Experimental Neuropsychology*, **12**, 398.

Kempler, D., Andersen, E. S. & Henderson, V. W. (1994). Linguistic and attentional contributions to anomia in Alzheimer's disease. *Journal of Cognitive Neuroscience*, in press.

King, J. & Just, M. A. (1991). Individual differences in syntactic processing: the role of working memory. *Journal of Memory and Language*, **30**, 580–602.

Kirshner, H. S., Webb, W. G. & Kelly, M. P. (1984). The naming disorder of dementia. *Neuropsychologia*, **22**, 23–30.

Knesevich, J. W., Toro, F. R., Morris, J. C. & LaBarge. (1985). Aphasia, family history, and the longitudinal course of senile dementia of the Alzheimer type. *Psychiatry Research*, **14**, 255–63.

Knopman, D. S. & Ryberg, S. (1989). A verbal memory test with high predictive accuracy for dementia of the Alzheimer type. *Archives of Neurology*, **46**, 141–5.

Kynette, D. & Kemper, S. (1986). Aging and the loss of grammatical forms: a cross-sectional study of language performance. *Language & Communication*, **6**, 43–9.

Laver, G. D. & Burke, D. M. (1993). Why do semantic priming effects increase in old age? A meta-analysis. *Psychology and Aging*, **8**, 34–43.

Light, L. L. (1990). Interactions between memory and language in old age. In J. E. Birren & K. W. Schaie (eds.), *Handbook of the Psychology of Aging*, pp. 275–90. Academic Press, New York.

Light, L. L. (1991). Memory and aging: four hypotheses in search of data. *Annual Review of Psychology*, **42**, 333–76.

Light, L. L. (1992). The organization of memory in old age. In F. I. M. Craik & T. A. Salthouse (eds.) *The Handbook of Aging and Cognition*, pp. 111–66. Erlbaum, Hillsdale, NJ.

Light, L. L. & Anderson, P. A. (1983). Memory for scripts in young and older adults. *Memory and Cognition*, **11**, 435–44.

Light, L. L. & Capps, J. L. (1986). Comprehension of pronouns in young and older adults. *Developmental Psychology*, **22**, 580–5.

Light, L. L., Zelinski, E. M. & Moore, M. (1982). Adult age differences in reasoning from new information. *Journal of Experimental Psychology: Learning, Memory, and Cognition*, **8**, 435–47.

Lima, S. D., Hale, S. & Myerson, J. (1991). How general is general slowing? Evidence from the lexical domain. *Psychology and Aging*, **6**, 416–25.

Logan, C. G., Buckwalter, J. G. & Henderson, V. W. (1992). Boston Naming Test Error Analysis in Alzheimer's disease. *Society for Neuroscience Abstracts*, **18**, 736.

MacDonald, M. C., Just, M. A. & Carpenter, P. (1992). Working memory constraints on the processing of syntactic ambiguity. *Cognitive Psychology*, **24**, 469–92.

Mackay, D. G. & Burke, D. M. (1990). Cognition and aging: a theory of new learning and the use of old connections. In T. M. Hess (ed.) *Aging and Cognition: Knowledge Organization and Utilization*, pp. 213–63. Elsevier, North-Holland.

MacWhinney, B. (ed.) (1987). *Mechanisms of Language Learning*. Lawrence Erlbaum, Hillsdale, NJ.

Mandel, R. G. & Johnson, N. S. (1984). A developmental analysis of story recall and comprehension in adulthood. *Journal of Verbal Learning and Verbal Behavior*, **23**, 643–59.

Martin, A. & Fedio, P. (1983). Word production and comprehension in Alzheimer's disease: the breakdown of semantic knowledge. *Brain and Language*, **19**, 124–41.

McKhann, G., Drachman, D., Folstein, M., Katzman, R., Price, D. & Stadian, E. M. (1984). Clinical diagnosis of Alzheimer's disease: report of the NINCDS –ADRDA work group unde the auspices of Department of Health and Human Services Task Force on Alzheimer's Disease. *Neurology*, **34**, 939–44.

Mergler, N., Faust, M. & Goldstein, M. (1985). Storytelling as an age-dependent skill. *International Journal of Aging and Human Development*, **20**, 205–28.

Nagy, W. E. & Herman, P. A. (1987). Breadth and depth of vocabulary knowledge: implications for acquisition and instruction. In M. G. McKeown & M. E. Curtis (eds.) *The Nature of Vocabulary Acquisition*, pp. 19–35. Lawrence Erlbaum, Hillsdale, NJ.

Neary, D., Snowden, J. S., Mann, D. M., Bowen, D. M., Sims, N. R., Northern, B., Yates, P. D. & Davison, A. N. (1986). Alzheimer's disease: a correlative study. *Journal of Neurology, Neurosurgery and Psychiatry*, **49**, 229–37.

Nebes, R. D. (1989). Semantic memory in Alzhcimer's disease. *Psychological Bulletin*, **106**, 377–94.

Nebes, R. D. (1992). Cognitive dysfunction in Alzheimer's disease. In F. I. M. Craik & T. A. Salthouse (eds.) *The Handbook of Aging and Cognition*, pp. 373–448. Erlbaum, Hillsdale, NJ.

Nebes, R. D. & Madden, D. J. (1988). Different patterns of cognitive slowing produced by Alzheimer's disease and normal aging. *Psychology and Aging*, **3**, 102–4.

Nebes, R. D. & Brady, C. B. (1992). Generalized cognitive slowing and severity of dementia in Alzheimer's disease: implications for the interpretation of response-time data. *Journal of Clinical and Experimental Neuropsychology*, **14**, 317–26.

Nebes, R. D., Martin, D. C. & Horn, L. C. (1984). Sparing of semantic memory in Alzheimer's disease. *Journal of Abnormal Psychology*, **93**, 321–30.

Nebes, R. D., Brady, C. G. & Huff, F. J. (1989). Automatic and attentional mechanisms of semantic priming in Alzheimer's disease. *Journal of Clinical and Experimental Neuropsychology*, **11**, 219–30.

Neely, J. H. (1977). Semantic priming and retrieval from lexical memory: roles of inhibitless spreading activation and limited capacity attention. *Journal of Experimental Psychology, General*, **106**, 226–54.

Neils, J., Brennan, M. M., Cole, M., Boller, F. & Gerdeman, B. (1988). The use of phonemic cueing with Alzheimer's disease patients. *Neuropsychologia*, **26**, 351–4.

Nicholas, M., Obler, L., Albert, M. & Goodglass, H. (1985a). Lexical retrieval in healthy aging. *Cortex*, **21**, 595–606.

Nicholas, M., Obler, L., Albert, M. & Helm-Estabrooks, N. (1985b). Empty speech in Alzheimer's disease and fluent aphasia. *Journal of Speech and Hearing Research*, **28**, 405–10.

Norman, S., Kemper, S., Kynette, D., Cheung, H. & Anagnopoulos, C. (1991). Syntactic complexity and adults' running memory span. *Journal of Gerontology: Psychological Sciences*, **46**, P346–51.

Obler, L. K. (1983). Language and brain dysfunction in dementia. In S. Segalowitz (ed.) *Language Functions and Brain Organization*, pp. 267–82. Academic Press, New York.

Obler, L. K., Fein, D., Nicholas, M. & Albert, M. L. (1991). Auditory comprehension and aging: decline in syntactic processing. *Applied Psycholinguistics*, **12**, 433–52.

Ostuni, M. J. & Santo-Pietro, E. (1986). *Getting Through: Communicating when Someone You Know has Alzheimer's Disease*. The Speech Bin, Princeton.

Pratt, M. W. & Robins, S. W. (1991). That's the way it was: age differences in the structure and quality of adults' personal narratives. *Discourse Processes*, **14**, 73–85.

Pratt, M. W., Boyes, C., Robins, S. & Manchester, J. (1989). Telling tales: aging, working memory, and the narrative cohesion of storytellers. *Developmental Psychology*, **25**, 628–35.

Ripich, D. N. & Terrell, B. Y. (1988). Cohesion and coherence in Alzheimer's disease. *Journal of Speech and Hearing Disorders*, **53**, 8–14.

Ripich, D. N., Vertes, D., Whitehouse, P., Fulton, S. & Ekelman, B. (1991). Turn-taking and speech act patterns in the discourse of senile dementia of the Alzheimer's type patients. *Brain and Language*, **40**, 330–43.

Rochford, G. (1971). A study of naming errors in dysphasic and in demented patients. *Neuropsychologia*, **9**, 437–43.

Rochon, E. (1992). 'The Nature and Determinants of Sentence Comprehension Impairments in Patients with Alzheimer's Disease.' August 1992. Ph.D. The School of Human Communication Disorders, McGill University.

Sadun, A. A. & Bassi, C. J. (1990). Optic nerve damage in Alzheimer's disease. *Ophthamology*, **97**, 9–17.

Salthouse, T. A. (1988). Effects of aging on verbal abilities: examination of the psychometric literature. In L. L. Light & D. M. Burke (eds.) *Language, Memory, and Aging*, pp. 17–35. Cambridge University Press, Cambridge.

Salthouse, T. A. (1991). *Theoretical perspectives on cognitive aging*. Erlbaum, Hillsdale, NJ.

Schaie, K. W. & Parham, I. A. (1977). Cohort-sequential analyses of adult intellectual development. *Developmental Psychology*, **13**, 649–53.

Schwartz, M., Marin, O. & Saffran, E. (1979). Dissociations of language function in dementia: a case study. *Brain and Language*, **7**, 277–306.

Selnes, O. A., Carson, K., Rovner, B. & Gordon, B. (1988). Language dysfunction in early- and late-onset possible Alzheimer's disease. *Neurology*, **38**, 1053–6.

Seltzer, B. & Sherwin, I. (1983). A comparison of clinical features in early- and late-onset primary degenerative dementia. *Archives of Neurology*, **40**, 143–6.

Small, J. A., Kempler, D. & Andersen, E. S. (1991). Syntactic comprehension and attention in Alzheimer's disease. Paper presented at the Gerontological Society of America, October, San Francisco. *The Gerontologist*, **31**, (Special Issue II) 86.

Smith, S. (1989). 'Syntactic comprehension in Alzheimer's disease.' Paper presented at the Academy of Aphasia. Santa Fe, October 1989.

Smith, S., Butters, N. & Granholm, E. (1988). Activation of semantic relations in Alzheimer's and Huntington's disease. In H. Whitaker (ed.) *Neuropsychological Studies of Nonfocal Brain Damage*, pp. 265–85. Springer-Verlag, New York.

Stine, E. A. L., Wingfield, A. & Poon, L. W. (1986). How much and how fast: rapid processing of spoken language in later adulthood. *Psychology and Aging*, **1**, 303–11.

Sulkava, R., Haltia, M., Paetau, A., Wikstroem, J. & Palo, J. (1983). Accuracy of clinical diagnosis in primary degenerative dementia: correlation with neuropathological findings. *Journal of Neurology, Neurosurgery and Psychiatry*, **46**, 9–13.

Thompson, I. M. (1987). Language in dementia. *International Journal of Geriatric Psychiatry*, **2**, 145–61.

Tyler, L. K. (1992). *Spoken Language Comprehension: an Experimental Approach to Normal and Disordered Processing*. MIT Press, Cambridge, Mass.

Ulatowska, H. K. & Chapman, S. B. (1991). Discourse Studies. In R. Lubinski (ed.) *Dementia and Communication*, pp. 115–32. BD Decker, Inc., Philadelphia.

Ulatowska, H., Allard, L., Donnell, A., Bristow, J., Haynes, S. M., Flower, A. & North, A. J. (1988). Discourse performance in subjects with dementia of the Alzheimer type. In. H. Whitaker (ed.) *Neuropsychological Studies in Nonfocal Brain Damage*, pp. 108–31. Springer-Verlag, New York.

Waters, G. S., Caplan, D., Rochon, E. & Waters, G. (1993). Two stages of sentence comprehension and their impairment in patients with Alzheimer's disease. Submitted.

Whitaker, H. (1976). A case of the isolation of the language function. In H. Whitaker & H. Whitaker (eds.) *Studies in Neurolinguistics*, vol 2, pp. 1–58. Academic Press, New York.

Zelinski, E. M. (1988). Integrating information from discourse: do older adults show deficits? In L. L. Light & D. M. Burke (eds.) *Language and Memory in Old Age*, pp. 117–32. Cambridge University Press, Cambridge.

Zelinski, E. M. & Miura, S. A. (1988). Effects of thematic information on script memory in young and old adults. *Psychology and Aging*, **3**, 292–9.

Zelinski, E. M. & Miura, S. A. (1990). Anaphor comprehension in young and older adults. *International Journal of Aging and Human Development*, **31**, 111–34.

Zelinski, E. M., Gilewski, M. J. & Thompson, L. W. (1980). Do laboratory tasks relate to self-assessment of memory in the young and old? In L. W. Poon. J. L. Fozard, L. S. Cermak, D. Arenberg & L. W. Thompson (eds.) *New Directions in Memory and Aging: Proceedings of the George Talland Memorial Conference*, pp. 519–44. Lawrence Erlbaum Associates, Hillsdale, NJ.

17

Visuospatial dysfunction in dementia and normal aging

J. VINCENT FILOTEO, DEAN C. DELIS, PAUL J. MASSMAN AND
NELSON BUTTERS

Whereas much attention has been given to the study of memory deficits in Alzheimer's disease (AD) and normal aging, relatively few studies have investigated visuospatial dysfunction in these populations. This is surprising, given that visuospatial dysfunction is one of the most common sequelae of Alzheimer's disease (Cogan, 1985; Mendez et al., 1990b), and that visuospatial abilities tend to decline with normal aging (Albert & Kaplan, 1980; Kaplan, 1980). Several reasons may underlie this disparity. Research on memory dysfunction has been guided by strong theoretical frameworks that posit distinct *components* of memory (e.g. encoding versus retrieval; Butters et al., 1985). Such theoretical frameworks have generated numerous investigations of the spared and impaired components of memory following focal and diffuse brain damage. In contrast, visuospatial dysfunction has resisted fractionation into meaningful spared and impaired components (Newcombe, 1985). Typically, impaired performance on tasks of visuospatial abilities are combined into one category and are labeled as 'visuospatial dysfunction', 'constructional apraxia', or 'constructional difficulties'. This 'lumping' of visuospatial deficits has masked the presence of possible visuospatial syndromes of spared and impaired component processes (Delis & Bihrle, 1989).

A second problem in this area is that AD patients often display heterogeneous cognitive profiles. Specifically, subgroups of AD patients have been found to show primarily verbal or visuospatial deficits on clinical tests (Naugle et al., 1985; Martin et al., 1986). These differential patterns of impairment are associated with hemispheric asymmetries in glucose hypometabolism (Koss et al., 1985; Grady et al., 1990). In light of these findings, Martin and colleagues (Martin et al., 1986; Martin, 1990) have cautioned against averaging data across

Dementia and Normal Aging, eds. F. A. Huppert, C. Brayne & D. W. O'Connor.
© Cambridge University Press 1994.

individual AD patients, and have stressed the importance of studying subgroups of AD patients.

A third problem concerns the verbal/spatial distinction itself. The common subdivision of AD patients according to their relative strengths in verbal (left hemisphere) functions or spatial (right hemisphere) functions may characterize the nature of their spatial deficits inaccurately. Past studies of unilateral brain-damaged patients suggest that damage to *either* hemisphere can produce spatial dysfunction, and different components of spatial analysis are impaired depending upon the side of the cerebral insult. Thus, the question arises as to whether or not dissociations in visuospatial processing can also occur in AD, a more diffuse disease process that often presents with asymmetrical hemispheric involvement.

A fourth problem is related to the methodology used in studying visuospatial deficits in AD and normal aging. As indicated elsewhere in this volume, past studies of cognitive impairment in AD have utilized age- and education-matched controls who may not be entirely representative of the general population of elderly people. The use of such highly selective control samples in past studies makes it difficult to investigate continuum and categorical models of the cognitive impairments in AD and normal aging. Clearly, more population studies must be conducted in order to address this issue adequately.

In this chapter, we review past studies of visuospatial dysfunction in AD patients and normal elderly and discuss their strengths and limitations. We also describe a series of studies from our laboratory which investigated the spared and impaired components of visuospatial processing in subgroups of AD patients and matched elderly controls. Finally, we discuss the results of past studies in terms of continuum versus categorical models of dementia and normal aging.

Throughout this chapter, we make extensive use of the phrase 'normal elderly'; therefore, it is important to clarify what we mean by this terminology. In general, the criteria for specifying normal elderly across the investigations that we review were based on either informal or structured interviews of subjects that elicited self-reports of past neurological, psychiatric or medical disorders that could have an impact on brain functioning. Potentially some of these studies may be confounded because they fail to rule out these conditions using extensive medical screens. Nevertheless, when referring to normal elderly in this chapter, we mean those individuals who did not report a medical history that would have precluded their participating in the various studies reviewed.

Past studies of visuospatial dysfunction in Alzheimer's disease

Using standardized clinical tests and other visuoconstructional tasks, past studies have reported that patients with AD exhibit deficits beyond that observed in normal aging (Cummings & Benson, 1983; Mendez et al., 1990b). Relative to highly selective groups of age-matched controls, AD patients have been found to demonstrate constructional deficits on the Block Design subtest of the WAIS (Whitehead, 1973) and WAIS-R (Mohr et al., 1990). AD patients also demonstrate impairments in drawing to command and in copying common two-dimensional and three-dimensional objects (e.g. clocks, daisies, faces, and houses; Brouwers et al., 1984; Cogan, 1985; Mohr et al., 1990; Ober et al., 1991). For example, Rouleau et al., (1992) found that, when asked to produce drawings of clocks, AD patients tended to commit more errors which violated the overall configuration and symmetry of the clock (e.g. they drew the numbers outside the clock's boundary).

In a recent study, Ober et al. (1991) examined AD patients' visuo-constructional abilities and found that their performance was related significantly to glucose metabolic activity in temporal–parietal cortices. Specifically, AD patients' impaired scores on scales which measured constructional abilities in terms of overall recognizability, attention to detail, accuracy of detail, accuracy of configuration, and neglect and symmetry, were all highly associated with glucose metabolism in temporal–parietal regions. It has been well documented that these cortical regions play an important role in visuospatial processing (de Renzi, 1982; Newcombe, 1985). The results of the Ober et al. (1991) study suggest that the visuoconstructional deficits exhibited by AD patients are due in large part to temporal–parietal lobe involvement, which is a typical neuropathological characteristic of AD (Friedland et al., 1985).

Patients with AD have been found to exhibit deficits on a host of other visuospatial tasks that do not have a constructional component, including

(1) Identifying common objects and faces (Eslinger & Benton, 1983; Cogan, 1985; Mendez et al., 1990a)
(2) Synthesizing visual information (Mendez et al., 1990a; Mohr et al., 1990)
(3) Perceiving figure–ground discriminations (Capitani et al., 1988; Mendez et al., 1990a)

(4) Discriminating between two or more complex visual forms (Brouwers et al., 1984; Mendez et al., 1990a)
(5) Judging line orientations (Eslinger & Benton, 1983; Eslinger et al., 1985; Ska et al., 1990)

The deficits exhibited by AD patients on these visuospatial tasks are also consistent with the temporal–parietal lobe involvement often observed in this disease.

Most studies of visuospatial dysfunction in dementia and normal aging have used clinical tests (e.g. WAIS-R Block Design subtest) and other complex tasks that tap multiple cognitive domains. These tasks place significant demands on novel-problem solving and manipulo-motor abilities in addition to visuospatial functions (Ryan & Butters, 1986). It is unclear to what extent the performances of AD patients and the normal elderly on these complex tests are related to deficits in their other areas of function. Therefore, the use of elementary perceptual tasks that place minimal demands on other cognitive skills is important for investigating visuospatial dysfunction in dementia and in normal aging.

Another limitation of most past studies is that visuospatial dysfunction was regarded as being a unitary disorder, and no attempt was made to isolate spared and impaired component processing. However, a few studies have investigated component processes of visuospatial abilities in AD on backward visual masking tasks. In these tasks, subjects are asked to identify a visual target after the presentation of a visual mask. The target stimuli are typically letters or digits and the mask is either a patterned mask composed of similar physical characteristics to the target stimuli (e.g. letter fragments), or a homo-geneous mask composed of different physical characteristics (e.g. a flash of light).

Past studies have indicated that the degree to which the mask inter-feres with subjects' ability to identify target stimuli is dependent on the physical characteristics of the mask (Turvey, 1973). Specifically, research with young normal subjects indicates that the homogeneous mask interferes with peripheral processes (e.g. perceptual extraction of physical characteristics such as contrast) which occur at an earlier processing stage, whereas the patterned mask interferes with central processes (e.g. perceptual integration of the physical features) which occur at a later processing stage. It has been suggested that the pat-terned mask interferes with central processes by 'interrupting' the per-ceptual processing of the target stimuli. This interruption leads to decreased target recognition (Turvey, 1973).

In an earlier study, Miller (1977) found that AD patients were more susceptible to backward masking than were normal elderly controls. Subsequent studies compared AD patients' performances on backward masking tasks which used both a homogeneous mask and a patterned mask (Schlotterer et al., 1983; Coyne et al., 1984). It was found that AD patients' perception of target stimuli was affected more by a patterned mask than a homogeneous mask, relative to normal elderly. This finding led the authors to suggest that central visual processes are more impaired than peripheral processes in AD. Studies such as these are important for two reasons: (1) they use tasks which minimize the demands placed on other cognitive abilities, and (2) they attempt to identify the spared and impaired component processes of visuospatial abilities in AD.

In a series of studies in our laboratory, we attempted to characterize spared and impaired visuospatial components better following unilateral brain-damage. A key feature of our investigations was the use of hierarchical stimuli that consist of a large (global) form made up of numerous smaller (local) forms (see Figure 17.1). These hierarchical stimuli are methodologically superior to common clinical stimuli such as faces and block designs because

(1) The two levels of the stimuli provide a clear distinction between 'parts' and 'wholes'
(2) Forms at the two levels can be from the same stimulus category (e.g. letters, numbers, or nonlinguistic shapes)
(3) Stimuli at the two levels can be the same (e.g. the number '1'

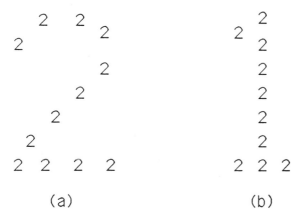

(a)   (b)

Figure 17.1. Examples of global–local stimuli: (a) consistent stimuli;
(b) inconsistent stimuli (Massman et al., 1993).

at both levels), or different (e.g. the number '1' at one level and the number '2' at the other), which allows for an analysis of the possible interference effects between two perceptual levels

Results from our studies indicate that pronounced dissociations in global–local processing occur in patients with unilateral brain-damage. Specifically, we found that patients with damage to the right hemisphere are impaired selectively in perceiving, copying, recalling, and recognizing global forms relative to local forms, whereas patients with damage to the left hemisphere display the opposite pattern (Delis et al., 1986, 1988a; Robertson & Delis, 1986; see also Delis et al., 1988b). These studies demonstrated that specific components of visuo-spatial functioning can be impaired selectively following focal injury to the brain. The results from these studies invited the question of whether or not dissociations in visuospatial functioning could also occur in patient groups with more diffuse but asymmetric neuropathol-ogy such as found in AD.

In a recent study (Massman et al., 1993), we investigated whether subgroups of AD patients exhibit dissociations in visuospatial analysis of global–local stimuli on a task of directed attention that had minimal manipulo-motor and memory components. In this study, AD patients were divided into subgroups on the basis of their standard scores on the Boston Naming Test (BNT; Kaplan et al., 1983) and the WISC-R Block Design subtest (BD; Wechsler, 1974). The standard scores for the AD patients were derived from a normative sample who were matched for age and education with the patient group. AD patients who performed at least one standard deviation higher on the BNT than on the BD were assigned to the high verbal subgroup. Those patients who performed at least one standard deviation higher on the BD than on the BNT were assigned to the high spatial subgroup. A third subgroup attained equivalent standard scores on the BNT and BD and was labeled the equal subgroup.

Four global–local stimuli were used in this experiment:

A large '1' composed of smaller '1s' (consistent condition)

A large '1' composed of smaller '2s' (inconsistent condition)

A large '2' composed of smaller '2s' (consistent condition)

A large '2' composed of smaller '1s' (inconsistent condition)

The stimuli were presented individually on a computer screen in two randomized blocks of 64 trials. On the first block, subjects were asked to attend to either the large numbers only or the small numbers only (thus, subjects were asked to 'direct' their attention). On the second block, subjects were asked to attend to the other level only. The word 'large' or 'small' was displayed on a sign in front of the monitor to assist the subjects in remembering and maintaining set during each block of trials. Subjects were asked simply to press one key if they saw a '1' and another key if they saw a '2'. Accuracy data were analyzed for the inconsistent stimuli, because the accuracy rate for about half the AD patients in the two asymmetric subgroups fell below 75%, thereby precluding analysis of reaction time data due to problems in speed/accuracy tradeoffs.

The results indicated that, as predicted, the high spatial patients made significantly more errors when making perceptual judgments at the local level, whereas the high verbal patients made significantly more errors when making perceptual judgments at the global level. The equal subgroup (i.e. patients with equivalent levels of impairment on traditional verbal and visuospatial tests) exhibited similar error rates when responding either to the global or local levels. In the consistent condition, the cross-over effect between the high verbal and high spatial subgroups was attenuated but still significantly different (see Figure 17.2).

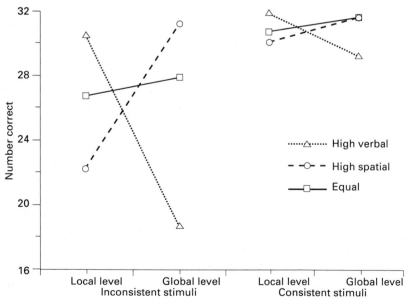

Figure 17.2. Mean local and global accuracy scores in the inconsistent and consistent stimulus conditions in the three Alzheimer's disease subgroups (Massman et al., 1993).

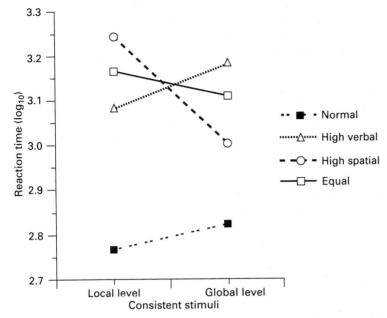

Figure 17.3. Local and global median reaction times ($\log_{10}$ units) in the consistent stimulus condition in the three Alzheimer's disease subgroups and the normal controls (Massman et al., 1993).

A control experiment using single large or small '1s' and '2s' indicated that the global–local dissociations found in the subgroups of AD patients were not due to differences in the absolute size of the global and local forms, but to their hierarchical spatial relationship. The global–local dissociations found in this study are consistent with our findings from another study which required subjects to recall and to draw global–local stimuli following a brief presentation (Delis et al., 1992).

The AD patients' accuracy rates in the consistent stimulus condition were above 75%; therefore, the reaction time (RT) performances of the normal controls and the AD patients were analysed. The RT results in the consistent condition paralleled the results obtained from the error analysis. As can be seen in Figure 17.3, the high spatial subgroup had a higher (i.e. more impaired) mean RT when responding to the local level, whereas the high verbal subgroup had a higher mean RT when responding to the global level. Furthermore, the mean difference in RT when responding to the global level versus the local level for the high spatial subgroup was significantly different from the mean RT difference for the high verbal subgroup. That is, the high spatial subgroup was relatively quicker when responding to the global level compared to the local level, whereas the high verbal subgroup was relatively quicker when responding to the local level compared to the global level.

Three implications can be drawn from these findings. First, subgroups of AD patients exhibited pronounced global–local dissociations on a spatial task that has minimal manipulo-motor or memory components. This finding suggests that AD patients exhibit a primary perceptual deficit independent of other impairments (e.g. in motor manipulation). Second, correct responding in the inconsistent condition required subjects to inhibit responding to discordant information at the nondirected hierarchical level. The pronounced impairments exhibited by AD patients with asymmetric hemispheric involvement in this condition suggest that AD patients are impaired severely in inhibiting responses to their 'strong' level when directing attention to their 'weak' level. Third, asymmetric patients displayed mild global–local dissociations even when interference was absent (i.e. in the consistent condition), suggesting that fundamental perceptual mechanisms are also affected in AD.

Past studies of visuospatial dysfunction in the normal elderly

Investigation of cognitive changes associated with aging have indicated that visuospatial abilities decline markedly with age. On standardized measures of intelligence, for example, scores on subtests that depend heavily upon visuospatial abilities tend to decline significantly with age compared to scores on subtests that measure verbal abilities (Meudell & Greenhalgh, 1987; Koss et al., 1991). These results have led some authors to suggest that the right hemisphere ages more rapidly than the left (Goldstein & Shelly, 1981; Meudell & Greenhalgh, 1987).

Relative to younger controls, normal elderly tend to perform worse on constructional tasks such as assembling blocks (Ardila & Rosselli, 1989; Koss et al., 1991), and drawing to command and copying two-dimensional designs and three-dimensional objects (Plude et al., 1986; Ardila & Rosselli, 1989). In addition, age-associated decline has been found on other perceptual tasks that do not have a construction component, including facial matching (Benton et al., 1981; Eslinger & Benton, 1983), visual synthesis (Fozard et al., 1977), and figure–ground discrimination (Capitani et al., 1988). Two studies have indicated that normal elderly are impaired at judging line orientations

(Benton et al., 1981; Eslinger & Benton, 1983); however, in a recent study, Ska et al. (1990) did not find an age effect on this task.

Normal elderly perform worse than younger controls on backward visual masking tasks when either a homogeneous mask or a patterned mask is used (Walsh et al., 1979; Till & Franklin, 1981; Schlotterer et al., 1983). However, a striking dissociation between AD patients and normal elderly occurs across masking types. Although both AD patients and normal elderly perform worse than young controls on both patterned and homogeneous masks, AD patients are dispro-portionately more impaired on patterned masks (Schlotterer et al., 1983; Coyne et al., 1984). These results indicate that both peripheral and central processing decline with old age; however, AD affects central processing to a greater extent than would be expected in nor-mal aging. The central processing deficits of AD patients are not sur-prising given that this disease is characterized by the involvement of temporal–parietal cortices (Friedland et al., 1985).

In the consistent condition in our global–local attention experiment (Massman et al., 1993), the mean global–local RT difference score for the normal elderly did not differ significantly from that of the high verbal AD subgroup: both groups demonstrated a *local* RT advantage (see Figure 17.2). In contrast, the mean difference score of the normal elderly differed significantly from that of the high spatial subgroup with AD. Thus, the RT performance of the elderly controls was similar to that of the high verbal subgroup with AD and different from that of the high spatial subgroup with AD. The local processing advantage found with the older subjects in this study is similar to the local pro-cessing advantage found with patients with right-hemisphere damage reported in past studies (Delis et al., 1986, 1988a).

These results appear to support the notion that the right hemisphere ages more rapidly than the left, as other authors have suggested pre-viously (Goldstein & Shelly, 1981; Meudell & Greenhalgh, 1987). However, in another experiment which investigated global–local pro-cessing in the elderly, we found that subjects demonstrated a *global* processing advantage on a visual memory task (Akshoomoff-Haist et al., 1989). The global processing advantage exhibited by these sub-jects became more pronounced with increasing age. These findings, which are difficult to explain, suggest that the type of task may influ-ence whether normal subjects exhibit a global or local processing advantage.

The majority of studies reporting a decline in visuospatial func-tioning with age have used a cross-sectional approach. However, the use of cross-sectional methods in studying age effects on cognitive functions has been controversial, and it is now widely believed that longitudinal studies provide a better estimate of such effects (Schaie, 1988). One reason for the shift towards longitudinal methodology in aging research is that cross-sectional data do not account for possible cohort effects. That is, when cross-sectional data obtained from one age-group is compared to data from another age-group, it is difficult to assess other variables that may lead to cohort differences, such as environmental influences, educational factors and state of health (Benton & Sivan, 1984). Several studies have demonstrated the importance of assessing the effects of cohort differences on various cognitive tasks (Schaie & Hertzog, 1983; Hertzog & Schaie, 1988). In a recent study, Schaie (1989) found that, in contrast to longitudinal data, cross-sectional data underestimated the effects of aging on a test of visuoperceptual speed. Because most previous studies that have investigated the effects of age on visuospatial processing have used primarily cross-sectional designs, it is unknown whether or not the age-related decrements reported in these studies are attenuated or overestimated. Thus, in order to determine better the true effects of age on visuospatial functioning, both longitudinal and cross-sectional methods should be employed.

Implications of past research findings on continuum versus categorical models of dementia and normal aging

The experimental results reviewed in this chapter suggest that AD patients are more impaired on tests of visuospatial functioning in comparison to normal elderly. However, most of the past studies contrasting the performances of AD patients and normal elderly have used highly selective groups of control subjects. In most of these studies, potential control subjects were excluded on the basis of memory and other cognitive complaints. This selection bias may tend to underrepresent those normal elderly who have experienced a general cognitive decline associated with advanced age. Thus, based solely on these past studies, it is difficult to ascertain whether the impairments observed in AD patients and normal elderly exist on a continuum or are the result of categorically distinct processes. In order to address this issue, future research investigating visuospatial functioning in these groups should use large population samples and should not exclude subjects based on cognitive criteria (e.g. a history of memory problems).

Despite the fact that these past studies do not address the continuum versus categorical debate directly, they do provide some clues relating to this important topic and provide some direction for future research.

Past studies of visuospatial dysfunction in AD and normal aging have attempted to identify quantitative differences between these groups on traditional measures (e.g. WISC Block Design). A number of these studies have indicated that decrements in visuospatial functioning are associated with *both* dementia and aging. That is, on traditional tests of visuospatial abilities, AD patients are impaired relative to normal elderly controls and also the latter are impaired relative to younger controls. Since both demented and normal aging exhibit deficits on these tasks, this suggests that AD patients' impairments are perhaps an exaggeration of those seen in normal aging. Thus, the results of past studies that have used *traditional* measures of visuospatial functioning suggest that the decrements observed in AD and normal aging are not categorically distinct; rather, they appear to fall along a continuum of impairment.

In contrast, an analysis of qualitative differences between the performances of AD patients and normal elderly on visuospatial tasks may reveal categorically different deficits that are masked in traditional tests. The results from our recent studies indicate that component processes of visuospatial abilities can be impaired differentially in both AD patients and normal elderly. Our results also indicate that the pattern of deficits observed in subgroups of AD patients and normal elderly can in fact be qualitatively different. Although our results do not necessarily refute the continuum hypothesis, they do suggest that future research should investigate the differential impairment of component processes in these groups on visuospatial tasks. It may be that subgroups of normal elderly people also display differential processing of global and local stimuli. Thus, applying this process-oriented approach to population studies may help to elucidate the relationship between AD and normal aging and will provide further insight into the debate between categorical and continuum models of cognitive decline.

Acknowledgments   The preparation of this chapter was supported in part by funds from the Medical Service of the Department of Veterans Affairs, and by National Institute of Aging Grant AG-05131 and AG-08204 to the University of California, San Diego, USA.

References

Akshoomoff-Haist, N., Delis, D. C. & Costanza, C. (1989). Age-related changes in memory for visual hierarchical stimuli. *Journal of Clinical and Experimental Neuropsychology*, **11**, 68.

Albert, M. S. & Kaplan, E. (1980). Organic implications of neuropsychological deficits in the elderly. In L. W. Poon, J. L. Fozard, L. S. Cermak, D. Arenberg & L. W. Thompson (eds.) *New Directions in Memory and Aging*, pp. 403–42. LEA, Hillsdale.

Ardila, A. & Rosselli, M. (1989). Neuropsychological characteristics of normal aging. *Developmental Neuropsychology*, **5**, 307–20.

Benton, A. L. & Sivan, A. B. (1984). Problems and conceptual issues in neuropsychological research in aging and dementia. *Journal of Clinical Neuropsychology*, **6**, 57–63.

Benton, A. L., Eslinger, P. J. & Damasio, A. R. (1981). Normative observations on neuropsychological test performances in old age. *Journal of Clinical Neuropsychology*, **3**, 33–42.

Brouwers, P., Cox, C., Martin, A., Chase, T. & Fedio, P. (1984). Differential perceptual–spatial impairment in Huntington's and Alzheimer's dementia. *Archives of Neurology*, **41**, 1073–6.

Butters, N., Wolfe, J., Martone, E., Granholm, E. & Cermak, L. S. (1985). Memory disorders associated with Huntington's disease: verbal recall, verbal recognition, and procedural memory. *Neuropsychologia*, **6**, 729–44.

Capitani, E., Della Salla, S., Lucchelli, F., Soave, P. & Spinnler, H. (1988). Perceptual attention in aging and dementia measured by Gottschaldt's Hidden Figure Test. *Journal of Gerontology*, **41**, 157–63.

Cogan, D. G. (1985). Visual disturbances with focal progressive dementing disease. *American Journal of Ophthalmology*, **100**, 68–72.

Coyne, A. C., Liss, L. & Geckler, C. (1984). The relationship between cognitive status and visual information processing. *Journal of Gerontology*, **39**, 711–17.

Cummings, J. L. & Benson, D. F. (1983). *Dementia: a Clinical Approach.* Butterworth Publishers, Stoneham.

Delis, D. C. & Bihrle, A. M. (1989). Fractionation of spatial cognition following focal and diffuse brain damage. In A. Ardila & F. Ostrosky-Solis (eds.) *Brain Organization of Language and Cognitive Processes*. Plenum Press, New York.

Delis, D. C., Robertson, L. C. & Efron, R. (1986). Hemispheric specialization of memory for hierarchical stimuli. *Neuropsychologia*, **24**, 205–14.

Delis, D. C., Kiefner, M. & Fridlund, A. J. (1988a). Visuospatial dysfunction following unilateral brain damage: dissociations in hierarchical and hemispatial analysis. *Journal of Clinical and Experimental Neuropsychology*, **10**, 421–31.

Delis, D. C., Kramer, J. H. & Kiefner, M. (1988b). Visuospatial functioning before and after commissurotomy: disconnections in hierarchical processing. *Archives of Neurology*, **45**, 462–5.

Delis, D. C., Massman, P. J., Butters, N., Salmon, D. P., Shear, P. K., Demadura, T. L. & Filoteo, J. V. (1992). Spatial cognition in Alzheimer's disease: Subtypes of global-local impairment. *Journal of Clinical and Experimental Neuropsychology*, **14**, 463–77.

de Renzi, E. (1982). *Disorders of Space Exploration and Cognition*. Wiley, New York.

Eslinger, P. J. & Benton, A. L. (1983). Visuoperceptual performances in aging and dementia: clinical and theoretical implications. *Journal of Clinical Neuropsychology*, **5**, 213–20.

Eslinger, P. J., Damasio, A. R., Benton, A. L. & Van Allen, M. (1985). Neuropsychologic detection of abnormal mental decline in older persons. *Journal of the American Medical Association*, **253**, 670–4.

Fozard, J., Wolf, E., Bell, B., McFarland, R. A. & Podolsky, S. (1977). Visual perception and communication. In J. E. Birren & K. W. Schaie (eds.) *Handbook of the Psychology of Aging*, pp. 497–34. Van Nostrand, New York.

Friedland, R. P., Budinger, T. F., Koss, E. & Ober, B. A. (1985). Alzheimer's disease: anterior–posterior and lateral hemispheric alterations in cortical glucose utilization. *Neuroscience Letters*, **53**, 235–40.

Goldstein, G. & Shelley, C. (1981). Does the right hemisphere age more rapidly than the left? *Journal of Clinical Neuropsychology*, **3**, 65–78.

Grady, C. L., Haxby, J. V., Schapiro, M. B., Gonzales-Aviles, A., Kumar, A., Ball, M. J., Heston, L. & Rapoport, S. (1990). Subgroups in dementia of the Alzheimer type identified by using positron emission tomography. *Journal of Neuropsychiatry and Clinical Neurosciences*, **2**, 373–84.

Hertzog, C. & Schaie, K. W. (1988). Stability and change in adult intelligence: 2. Simultaneous analysis of longitudinal means and covariance structures. *Psychology and Aging*, **3**, 122–30.

Kaplan, E. (1980). Changes in cognitive style with aging. In L. K. Obler & M. L. Albert (eds.) *Language and Communication in the Elderly*, pp. 121–32. Lexington Books, Lexington.

Kaplan, E., Goodglass, H. & Weintraub, S. (1983). *Boston Naming Test*. Lea and Febiger, Philadelphia.

Koss, E., Friedland, R. P., Ober, B. A. & Jagust, W. J. (1985). Differences in lateral hemispheric asymmetrics of glucose utilization between early- and late-onset Alzheimer-type dementia. *American Journal of Psychiatry*, **142**, 638–40.

Koss, E., Haxby, J. V., DeCarli, C., Schapiro, M. B., Friedland, R. P. & Rapoport, S. I. (1991). Patterns of performance preservation and loss in healthy aging. *Developmental Neuropsychology*, **7**, 99 113.

Martin, A. (1990). Neuropsychology of Alzheimer's disease: the case for subgroups. In M. F. Schwartz (ed.) *Modular Deficits in Alzheimer-Type Dementia*. MIT Press, Cambridge, Mass.

Martin, A., Brouwers, P., Lalonde, F., Cox, C., Teleska, P., Fedio, P., Foster, N. L. & Chase, T. N. (1986). Towards a behavioral typology of Alzheimer's patients. *Journal of Clinical and Experimental Neuropsycholgoy*, **8**, 594–610.

Massman, P. J., Delis, D. C., Filoteo, J. V., Butters, N., Salmon, D. P. & Demadura, T. L. (1993). Mechanisms of spatial impairment in Alzheimer's disease subgroups: differential breakdown of directed attention to global–local stimuli. *Neuropsychology*, **7**, 172–81.

Mendez, M. F., Mendez, J. A., Martin, R., Smyth, K. A. & Whitehouse, P. J.

(1990a). Complex visual disturbances in Alzheimer's disease. *Neurology*, **40**, 439–43.

Mendez, M. F., Tomsak, R. L. & Remler, B. (1990b). Disorders of the visual system in Alzheimer's disease. *Journal of Clinical Neuro-opthalmology*, **100**, 62–9.

Meudell, P. R. & Greenhalgh, M. (1987). Age related differences in left and right hand skill and in visuo-spatial performance: their possible relationships to the hypothesis that the right hemisphere ages more rapidly than the left. *Cortex*, **23**, 431–45.

Miller, E. (1977). A note on visual information processing in presenile dementia: a preliminary report. *British Journal of Social and Clinical Psychology*, **16**, 99–100.

Mohr, E., Litvan, I., Williams, J., Fedio, P. & Chase, T. N. (1990). Selective deficits in Alzheimer and Parkinsonian dementia: visuospatial function. *The Canadian Journal of Neurological Sciences*, **17**, 292–7.

Naugle, R. I., Cullum, C. M., Bigler, E. D. & Massman, P. J. (1985). Neuropsychological and computerized axial tomography volume characteristics of empirically derived dementia subgroups. *Journal of Nervous and Mental Disease*, **173**, 596–604.

Newcombe, F. (1985). Neuropsychology qua interface. *Journal of Clinical and Experimental Neuropsychology*, **7**, 663–81.

Ober, B. A., Jagust, W. J., Koss, E., Delis, D. C. & Friedland, R. P. (1991). Visuoconstructive performances and regional cerebral metabolism in Alzheimer's disease. *Journal of Clinical and Experimental Neuropsychology*, **13**, 752–72.

Plude, D. J., Milberg, W. P., & Cerella, J. (1986). Age differences in depicting and perceiving tridimensionality in simple line drawing. *Experimental Aging Research*, **12**, 221–5.

Robertson, L. C. & Delis, D. C. (1986). 'Part–whole' processing in unilateral brain damaged patients: dysfunction of hierarchical organization. *Neuropsychologia*, **24**, 363–70.

Rouleau, I., Salmon, D. P., Butters, N., Kennedy, C. & McGuire, K. (1992). Quantitative and qualitative analyses of clock drawings in Alzheimer's and Huntington's disease. *Brain and Cognition*, **18**, 70–87.

Ryan, C. & Butters, N. (1986). The neuropsychology of alcoholism. In D. Wedding, A. M. Horton & J. Webster (eds.) *The Neuropsychology Handbook: Behavioral and Clinical Perspectives*. Springer, New York.

Schaie, K. W. (1988). Ageism in psychological research. *American Psychologist*, **43**, 179–83.

Schaie, K. W. (1989). Perceptual speed in adulthood: cross-sectional and longitudinal studies. *Psychology and Aging*, **4**, 443–53.

Schaie, K. W. & Hertzog, C. (1983). Fourteen-year cohort-sequential analyses of adult intellectual development. *Developmental Psychology*, **19**, 531–43.

Schlotterer, B., Moscovitch, M. & Crapper-McLachlan, D. (1983). Visual processing deficits as assessed by spatial frequency contrast sensitivity and backward masking in normal ageing and Alzheimer's disease. *Brain*, **107**, 309–25.

Ska, B., Poissant, A. & Yves, J. (1990). Line orientation judgment in normal elderly and subjects with dementia of Alzheimer's type. *Journal of Clinical and Experimental Neuropsychology*, **12**, 695–702.

Till, R. E. & Franklin, D. L. (1981). On the locus of age differences in visual information processing. *Journal of Gerontology*, **36**, 200–10.

Turvey, M. T. (1973). On peripheral and central processes in vision: interference from an information-processing analysis with patterned stimuli. *Psychological Review*, **80**, 1–52.

Walsh, D. A., Williams, M. V. & Hertzog, C. K. (1979). Age-related differences in two stages of central perceptual processes: the effects of short duration targets and criterion differences. *Journal of Gerontology*, **34**, 234–41.

Wechsler, D. (1974). *Wechsler Intelligence Scale for Children – Revised*. The Psychological Corporation, New York.

Whitehead, A. (1973). The pattern of WAIS performance in elderly psychiatric patients. *British Journal of Social and Clinical Psychology*, **12**, 435–6.

PART VI

Neurobiology of dementia and normal aging

18

Dementia and normal aging: neuropathology

MARGARET M. ESIRI

Common experience leads us to believe that to some extent mental decline is a universal consequence of old age. Almost all perceptive elderly people are subjectively aware that their mental function is not as good as it was when they were young or middle-aged. Yet most such people are not clinically demented, the rate of their mental decline is very slow and they are well able to continue to live independent lives in the community. They are sometimes referred to as suffering from the benign forgetfulness of old age. Clinical dementia refers, in most cases, to a different order of magnitude of decline. It progresses more noticeably, results in dependency and decreases life expectancy. Neuropathologists who search in the brain for the substratum of dementia have to bear in mind that they are likely to stumble on the structural basis of the more common, perhaps universal, 'benign forgetfulness', and need to try to distinguish this from the pathology of clinical dementia.

Systematic examination of changes in the human brain with aging has taken place only relatively recently. There are a number of different reasons why this should be so. The brain can be examined effectively only at autopsy, and autopsies on the very elderly have always tended to be carried out less frequently than on young subjects. The changes that occur with age are subtle and varied and, in order to be seen, some require special stains for microscopy. The difficulties of assessing the numbers of cells in brain nuclei, or over widely dispersed volumes such as the cerebral cortex, are formidable, and results are still often controversial. Often, insufficient attention has been paid to changes in volume of a region and efforts have been directed mainly at estimating cell densities (Pakkenberg & Gundersen, 1988). Large numbers of brains need to be examined when studying age- or

Dementia and Normal Aging, eds. F. A. Huppert, C. Brayne & D. W. O'Connor.
© Cambridge University Press 1994.

disease-specific alterations in neuron populations because of the high degree of variability among normal controls. Finally, there are difficulties in extrapolating from observations on more readily accessible, but generally short-lived, animal brains to those of humans. Despite these difficulties, there is now a considerable body of evidence about changes that occur in the human brain with aging and dementia. These are discussed below with an emphasis on whether or not each can best be considered to form a continuum with 'normality' at one end and 'dementia' at the other.

The ideal starting position for a neuropathologist setting out to investigate this question might be to have available for unlimited study the whole brains from a large number (hundreds at least) of subjects who had had their mental powers comprehensively analysed shortly before death. No such opportunity can present itself, if only because techniques used for some forms of study preclude the use of the same tissue for other purposes. Therefore, we need to assemble the limited evidence available from a number of studies of different aspects of change in relatively small numbers of brains from subjects whose pre-mortem mental state has been assessed more or less adequately. In order to keep this chapter to a reasonable length, only changes most commonly associated with dementia, those of Alzheimer's disease (AD), will be considered here.

Changes in brain weight and volume associated with aging and dementia

Many of the early autopsy studies of brain weight and volume changes with age included unselected hospital cases from which cases of AD were not excluded specifically. Only studies of prospectively assessed subjects can ensure that cases of dementia have been eliminated from a group of elderly subjects. There have been no large autopsy studies of the brains of prospectively assessed, cognitively well preserved, elderly subjects. Those studies that have sought information retrospectively about the pre-mortem social and intellectual function of their subjects provide the best evidence available at present.

Normal aging

There is evidence that the weight and volume of the brain diminish modestly, gradually and unremittingly in healthy old age. Most of this evidence comes from autopsies, but evidence on brain volume changes also comes from computerized tomography scans (not reviewed here). Conclusions from several autopsy studies are summarized in Table 18.1. An increase in the size of the brains of *young* subjects during the course of this century needs to be taken into consideration in comparing old and young subjects' brains for evidence of shrinkage in old age and the study by Miller et al. (1980), for example, takes this change into account. Comparisons of cranial capacity and brain volume to derive a ratio of skull capacity to brain volume also get around this variable, since cranial capacity does not vary with age (Davis & Wright, 1977). The findings of these two studies are in close agreement that brain weight and volume remain more or less constant up to about 50 years of age. Thereafter there is a constant loss of about 2–3% per decade over the next four decades.

On inspection, the most noticeable change with aging in the brain is a slight narrowing of the cerebral cortical gyri and widening of the sulci. The hippocampus and amygdala also participate in this atrophic process. The volume of the ventricular system and subarachnoid space enlarges progressively as the brain shrinks (Hubbard & Anderson, 1981a, b), and the leptomeninges show a mild thickening due to collagen deposition. The overall reductions in weight and volume of the brain with normal aging mask regional variations which need to be taken into account before attempting to reach conclusions regarding the inevitability of loss of brain substance with aging. The volume loss of white matter after age 70 years is greater than that of grey matter (Anderson et al., 1983). For example, Anderson et al. (1983) found a volume loss in cerebral neocortex of only 2–3% between the ages of 70 and 85 years, but a reduction of 8% in the basal ganglia (which contain more white matter) and of 11% in cerebral white matter over the same period. However, atrophy in the subiculum of the hippocampus was greater and amounted to 28%.

Dementia

In dementia due to AD, brain weights often fall within the 95% confidence limits for normal elderly subjects, but a few lie outside the lower limit. Some studies, though not all, have found reduced mean weights in AD of some 7–15% compared with age-matched controls (Table 18.2). Because of the wide range in weight of normal brains these differences are not always statistically significant. Brain weights are

Table 18.1. *Volumetric and weight changes in the brain with aging*

No. of cases studied[a] (age range in years)	Nature of study[b]	Information on pre-mortem mental state	Site	Main findings	Reference
1090 (20–80)	Measurement of fresh brain wt.	None	Whole brain	Redn. of 8.6% in males and 10.6% in females between ages 20–30 and 70–80 yrs	Pakkenberg & Voigt (1964)
28 (65–92)	Measurement of brain wt.	Retro.; undem.	Whole brain	No signif. change in wt. over age range studied	Tomlinson et al. (1968)
1670 (20–89)	Measurement of fresh brain wt.	None	Whole brain	Redn. of 7% in males and 7.1% in females between ages 20–30 and 70–80 yrs	Chrzanowska & Beben (1973)
100 (55–94)	Measurement of brain vol., and cranial cavity vol.	87 retro. normal, no retro. dem.	Whole brain	Brain vol. loss of 10% over age range studied	Davis & Wright (1977)
4736 (birth–86+)	Measurement of fresh brain wt.	None	Whole brain	Redn. of 11% in males and 11.2% in females between ages 19–21 and over 86 yrs	Dekaban & Sadowsky (1978)

No. of cases (age range)	Method	Design	Region	Findings	Reference
1261 (25–80)	Measurement of fresh brain wt.	None	Whole brain	Redn. of wt. of approx. 2 g per yr between ages 30–80 yrs and approx. 5 g per yr after 80 yrs	Ho et al. (1980)
24–38 (19–85+)	S.-auto. measurement of capillary density	Retro.; undem.	Cortex, putamen, CWM	No change in vol. of cerebral cortex with age. Marked redn. of vol. of putamen and CWM after age 65 yrs	Meier-Ruge et al. (1980)
130 (20–90)	Auto. morphom. of total vol. and grey and white matter vols.	Retro.; undem.	One or both hemis.	Vol. redn. of 2% per decade after 50 yrs	Miller et al. (1980)
18 (68–95)	Point counting morphom. and comparison of brain vol. and cranial capacity	Retro.; undem.	Whole brain and mult. regions	5% loss of brain vol. in advanced old age	Hubbard & Anderson (1981a)
26 (23–95)	Measurement of cerebral ventric. vol.	Retro.; undem.	Whole brain	Signif. but modest rise in ventric. vol. with age	Hubbard & Anderson (1981b)

Table 18.1. *Contd*

No. of cases studied[a] (age range in years)	Nature of study[b]	Information on pre-mortem mental state	Site	Main findings	Reference
19 (69–95)	S.-auto. morphom. of vol. and measurement of brain vol. and cranial capacity and brain wt.	Retro.; undem.	Whole brain and cortex/hippo. vols.	Reduced vol. and wt. of approx. 11.4% over age range studied. Insignif. change in cortex vol. except in hippo. where redn. of 28% was found	Anderson et al. (1983)
76 (29–90)	Point counts for macroscopic evaluation. S. auto. for neuron density	Retro.; undem.	Cortical areas 6,7,11,17, basal ganglia, thalamus, etc.	6% redn. in total brain vol. by late 70s. Deep grey nuclei more affected than cortex. Redn. in cortex vol. seen only in front.	Haug et al. (1983)
25 (not given)	Measurement of wt. and vol. displacement	Retro.; undem.	Hemi.	Wt. reduced in those over 80 yrs by 9% cf. those less than 80 yrs. Similar redn. in vol.	Mountjoy et al. (1983)

No. (age range)	Method	Study type	Region	Findings	Reference
12 (37–86)	Point counting of cerebral cortex vol. and surface area	Retro.; undem.	Hemi.	Relative vol. of front. showed insig. decline with age. Signif. redn. in surface area of front. with age	Eggers et al. (1984)
24000 (not given)	Measurement of brain wt.	None	Whole brain	6% redn. in brain wt. at 75 yrs compared with 25 yrs	Haug (1985)
67 (10–97)	Measurement of cortical thickness/area	Retro.; undem.	Temp. cortex (22) and hippo.	No signif. redn. in temp. cortex thickness with age; signif. redn. in hippo. area with age	Mann et al. (1985)
81 (45–54) and 386 (70–9)	Measurement of brain wt. and ventric. size	Retro.; undem. (most) and dem., the 2 gps. being analysed together	Whole brain wt. and lateral ventric. size	Signif. redn. of approx. 7 g per yr in women aged 70–9 yrs, and insignif. redn. in men. Similar slight incr. in size of lateral ventrics. Brain wt. correlated signif. with body wt.	Skullerud (1985)

Table 18.1. *Contd*

No. of cases studied[a] (age range in years)	Nature of study[b]	Information on pre-mortem mental state	Site	Main findings	Reference
51 (24–100)	S.-auto. morphom. for cortical width; measurement of brain wt., and cerebral hemi. wt.	Retro.; undem. some (more elderly) prosp. undem.	Whole brain and hemi. wts.; cortex width and laminar widths in three areas (9/10/46, 38 and 39/40)	Signif. redn. of 18% in whole brain wt. and 21% in hemi. wt. between those aged 20–49 yrs and those aged over 70 yrs. Redn. occurred mainly after 55 yrs. Signif. redn. in cortical thickness in front and temp. cortex of 15% and 10% respectively.	Terry et al. (1987)

| 38 (50–100) | S.-auto. morphom. for cortical width; measurement of brain wt. (as hemi.-brain wt. ×2) | Retro.; undem. | Whole brain wt.; cortex width in three areas | Brain wt. of those aged 70–100 yrs, 8% less than those aged 50–65 yrs, 7–8% redn. in cortical thickness in sup. temp. and inf. par. between those aged 50–65 and 80–100 yrs | Hansen et al. (1988) |

aIncludes studies with 12 or more cases.

bAll studies were made at autopsy unless otherwise stated.

AD, Alzheimer's disease; AMC, age-matched controls; auto., automatic; capill., capillary; cing., cingulate; clin., clinical/clinically; CWM, cerebral white matter; decr. decrease; dem., dementia/demented; diff(s)., difference(s); front., frontal lobe (Brodmann area); gp(s)., group(s); hemi(s)., cerebral hemisphere(s); hippo., hippocampus; incr., increase; inf., inferior; insig., insignificant; LGB, lateral geniculate body; loc. cer., locus coeruleus; mamm. bods., mammillary bodies; morphom., morphometry; mult., multiple; nuc. bas., nucleus basalis; occ., occipital cortex; P, argyrophilic plaques; par., parietal lobe (Brodmann area); pathol., pathology; prosp., prospectively tested; redn(s)., reduction(s); retro., retrospective analysis of notes or other information available; S.-auto., semiautomatic (includes automatic measurements with manual editing); s.-quant., semi-quantitative; signif., significant; sup., superior; NFT, neurofibrillary tangles; temp., temporal lobe (Brodmann area); undem., undemented; ventric(s)., ventricle(s)/ ventricular.

Table 18.2. *Volumetric and weight changes in the brain in Alzheimer's disease*

No. of cases studied[a]	Nature of study[b]	Information on pre-mortem mental state	Site	Main findings	Reference
50	Measurement of brain wt.	Clin. diagnosis of dem. with scores given prospectively	Whole brain	No signif. diff. from AMC, though trend to lower wt.	Tomlinson et al. (1970)
13	Auto. morphom. of total vol. and grey and white matter vols.	Clin. diagnosis of dem.	Hemi.	Total vol. 18% lower than for AMC	Miller et al. (1980)
15	Point counting morphom. and comparison of brain vol. with cranial capacity	Clin. diagnosis of dem.	Whole brain and mult. regions	Those less than 80 yrs showed excess loss of brain vol. compared with AMC, up to 18%, mean 12.7%. In those over 80 yrs no signif. redn. compared with AMC. Cerebral cortex vol. redn. up to 25% in those less than 80 yrs, insig. redn. in those over 80 yrs. Regional vol. loss greatest for temp.	Hubbard & Anderson (1981a)

n	Method	Basis of diagnosis	Measure	Results	Reference
23	Measurement of brain vol. by displacement and vol. proportion of ventrics. by point counting	Clin. diagnosis of dem.	Cerebral ventric. vol.	57% had ventric. vol. above upper limit of normal	Hubbard & Anderson (1981b)
14	Measurement of brain wt.	Clin. diagnosis of dem.	Whole brain	Brain wt. redn. of 8% compared with 10 AMC	Terry et al. (1981)
25	Measurement of hemi. wt. and vol. by water displacement	Clin. diagnosis of dem.	Hemi.	15% redn. in hemi. wt. in those less than 80 yrs and 13% redn. in whole gp. compared with AMC. Vol. of hemi. signif. reduced compared with AMC in whole gp. and in those less than 80 yrs but not in those more than 80 yrs	Mountjoy et al. (1983)
32	Measurement of cortical thickness and point counting morphom. for hippo. area in cross section; measurement of brain wt.	Clin. diagnosis of dem.	Whole brain; cortical thickness in temp.; hippo. area	Signif. redn. in brain wt. of 5% compared with AMC; signif. redn. of 28% in temp. cortex thickness and of 12% in hippo. area compared with AMC	Mann et al. (1985)

Table 18.2. *Contd*

No. of cases studied[a]	Nature of study[b]	Information on pre-mortem mental state	Site	Main findings	Reference
113	Measurement of brain wt. as twice fixed hemi. wt. S.-auto. morphom. for measurement of cortical width	Clin. diagnosis of AD, some with prosp. assessment	Hemi. wts.; cortical width in mult. areas	Brain wts. signif. reduced compared with AMC by 13% in cases less than 66 yrs and by 7% in those over 69 yrs. Cortex width reduced by 9–26% compared with AMC; greatest redn. in inf. par. cortex	Hansen et al. (1988)
150	Measurement of hemi. wts.	Clin. diagnosis of AD	Hemi.	Wts. of hemis. from 15% of men and 11% of women fell outside 95% confidence limits for their age gp.	Joachim et al. (1988)

| 16 | Measurement of brain wt. and ventric. vol. S.-auto. morphom. for cortex, CWM and subcortical grey areas | Clin. diagnosis of AD | Hemi. and mult. areas | Brain wt. signif. lower by 9% than for AMC. Ventric. vol. 40% greater than for AMC. Cortex area reduced 13–24% and CWM by 3–19%. No signif. redn. in vol. of subcortical nuclei except amygdala (reduced by 24%). Hippo. cross-sectional area at LGB reduced 10% | de la Monte et al. (1989) |

See Table 18.1 for abbreviations and key.

reduced more in younger subjects than older ones with AD, when comparisons are made with age-matched controls (Hansen et al., 1988).

Changes in volume of varying extent in different parts of the brain in AD have been described in recent studies. For example, de la Monte (1989) found cortical atrophy to be more striking at the level of the amygdala than in anterior frontal cortex, and white matter area reductions were also greatest at the level of the amygdala. Hansen et al. (1988) found cortical width reductions that were greater in temporal and parietal regions than in the frontal cortex. Subcortical nuclei were not reduced in area compared with age-matched controls in the study by de la Monte (1989), apart from the amygdala which, however, showed marked mean atrophy of 24%. The hippocampal area at the level of the lateral geniculate body was reduced by a mean of 10%. Hubbard & Anderson (1981a) found a more significant reduction in brain volume in those less than 80 years of age at death compared with those over 80 years. In the latter group the only region with significantly reduced volume was the temporal lobe cortex, which was reduced by 20% compared with age-matched controls.

Summary

In summary, there is a slight reduction in brain size in old age, maintained into the ninth decade. It is more noticeable in white than grey matter and the changes in grey matter are not uniform in different parts of the brain. In AD, brain weights and volumes may fall within the normal range, but some are lower, particularly among the younger patients. To try to explain these gross findings on aging, we need to examine the changes found at the microscopic level.

Microscopic changes in the brain associated with aging and dementia

A number of different microscopic changes need to be considered, starting with alterations in number and size of nerve cells.

Changes in nerve cell numbers and size

Many different techniques have been used to estimate numbers of nerve cells. Some have involved counting using the eye and an eye-piece grid, for example, to count neurons in strips from the outer to the innermost boundaries of the cortex or vice versa. Others have made use of semiautomatic or automatic cell counting devices. Initially, the difficulties of automatic cell counting were under-estimated generally, but now they are appreciated better and are over-come by manual editing. Alterations in cell volume complicate automatic cell counting, because, in changing from one size category to another, cells may be interpreted erroneously as being lost.

Normal aging   Data from several recent studies are summarized in Tables 18.3 and 18.4. Of the nerve cell populations investigated so far, alterations with normal aging are still controversial, with wide variations in results from different studies, which are not readily accounted for. There seems to be no doubt that nerve cell populations are heterogeneous, with some showing cell loss and cell shrinkage, others showing shrinkage without significant loss, and yet others show-ing neither shrinkage nor loss. Some studies show a trend towards neuron loss which fails to reach significance possibly because the number of brains examined was relatively small. Several studies that show significant neuron loss found differing degrees of loss in different cell populations, again emphasizing the selectivity of change from one population to another. Neuron loss, when present, is generally slight in extent: for example, about 1% per year after the age of 70 years in neocortex and medial hippocampus in the study by Anderson et al. (1983); 10–15% loss in neocortex from 24 to 100 years in the study by Terry et al. (1987); and 6–25% in neocortex in those aged 80 to 100 years compared with those aged 50 to 65 years in the study by Hansen et al. (1988). Large cortical neurons, principally pyramidal neurons, show the greatest losses in most studies, but this is at least partly accounted for by shrinkage. Thus, in the study by Terry et al. (1987), the loss of cortical neurons in the large neuron class was largely offset by an increase in neurons in the small neuron class. One study (Braak & Braak, 1986) found a much greater loss (47%) of non-pyramidal than of pyramidal cells in the brains of non-demented elderly people. There are a number of subcortical nuclei in which no age-specific neuron loss has been found: inferior olives (Moatamed, 1966); deep cerebellar nuclei (Heidary & Tomasch, 1969); the seventh

Table 18.3. *Changes in nerve cell numbers in normal aging*

No. of cases studied[a] (age range in years)	Nature of study[b]	Information on pre-mortem mental state	Site	Main findings	Reference
28 (0–75)	Manual counts	None	Seventh nerve nucleus	No change in nerve cell nos. after age 1 yr	van Buskirk (1945)
20 (newborn–95)	Manual counts	None	Pre- and post-central gyrus, sup. and inf. temp. gyri, striate cortex	Approx. 50% of neurons in sup. temp. gyrus and slightly fewer in other areas lost by age 90 yrs	Brody (1955)
18 (41–87)	Manual counts	Retro.; undem.	Sup. front gyrus	8% annual decrement of neurons over age range studied	Brody (1970)
23 (newborn–90)	Manual counts	None	Ventral cochlear nucleus	No signif. loss of neurons over age range studied	Konigsmark & Murphy (1970)
90 (0–100+)	Manual counts	Retro.; no neurological or organic psychiatric disorder	Cerebellar Purkinje cells	Mean redn. of 2.5% of cells per decade. Total counts 6–8% higher in males than females	Hall et al. (1975)

No. (age range)	Method	Material	Region	Findings	Reference
18 (47–89)	S.-auto.	Retro.; undem.	Hippo.	Approx. 27% loss of pyramidal neurons between ages 45 and 95 yrs	Ball (1977)
24 (14–87)	Manual counts	Retro.; undem.	Loc. cer. and subcoeruleus	40% redn. in cell no. after 63 yrs	Vijayashankar & Brody (1977)
29 (21–91)	Manual counts	Retro.; undem.	Hippo.	20% redn. after age 68 yrs	Mouritzen Dam (1979)
23 (20–87)	Ultrasound disruptions of fixed tissue and counts of suspended stained cells in a counting chamber	Retro.; no neurological disease	Striate cortex (macular projection area)	At least 50% loss of neurons by age 80 yrs	Devaney & Johnson (1980)
64 (18–95)	Auto.	All cases aged over 65 yrs retro. undem. Many had had prosp. assessment, showing undem.	Pre- and post-central, sup. temp., and inf. temp. gyri, gyrus rectus	Approx 35% loss of small neurons and 50% loss of large neurons between 20 and 90 yrs. Little diff. in extent of loss between different areas	Henderson et al. (1980)
38 (19–94)	Auto. measurement of capill. parameters	Retro.; undem.	Pre-central cortex, putamen	Approx. 60% incr. in capill. fraction in putamen with age, but no change in cortex	Meier-Ruge et al. (1980)

Table 18.3. *Contd*

No. of cases studied[a] (age range in years)	Nature of study[b]	Information on pre-mortem mental state	Site	Main findings	Reference
25 (32–93)	Normal	Retro.; undem.	Loc. cer.	60–70% redn. in neuron no. by eighth and ninth decades	Tomlinson et al. (1981)
20 (70–85)	Auto.	Retro.; undem.	Cortex (11,22,24) and subiculum	15–16% loss of neurons between ages studied at annual rate of 1%	Anderson et al. (1983)
25	S.-auto.	Retro.; undem.	Mult. cortical area (8,9,20–2,24,7,17)	Trivial diffs. between those aged less than 80 and over 80 yrs except in inf. temp. and par. cortex where cell counts in columns in those aged over 80 yrs were reduced by 19% and 15% respectively	Mountjoy et al. (1983)

No. (age range)	Method	Type	Region	Findings	Reference
30 (40–88)	Manual counts	Retro.; undem.	Mid portion of nuc. bas.	No signif. diff. in neuron counts between those younger and older than 65 yrs	Whitehouse et al. (1983)
17 (25–87)	Manual counts	Retro.; many alcoholic	Nuc. bas.	No correlation between no. of neurons and age	Chiu et al. (1984)
86 (15–96)	Auto.	Retro.; undem.	Hippo.	Loss of 3.6% of pyramidal neurons per decade over age range studied	Miller et al. (1984)
20–50+ (20–100+)	Auto.	Retro.; undem.	Cortex (6,11,17,20)	No neuron loss with age over age range studied	Haug (1985)
67 (50–90)	Manual counts	Retro.; undem.	Temp. cortex (22), hippo.	7.5% redn. in pyramidal neurons in temp. cortex and 6.2% redn. in pyramidal neurons in hippo. in each decade over age range studied	Mann et al. (1985); (see also Mann et al. (1984))
28 (10–93)	Auto. on sections showing oxytocin and vasopressin immunoreactivity	Retro.; undem.	Supraoptic and paraventricular nuclei	No loss of neurons with age	Fliers et al. (1985)

Table 18.3. *Contd*

No. of cases studied[a] (age range in years)	Nature of study[b]	Information on pre-mortem mental state	Site	Main findings	Reference
28 (10–93)	Auto. on sections showing vasopressin immuno-reactivity	Retro.; undem.	Suprachiasmic nucleus	After 80 yrs, vasopressin and total neurons reduced by 54% compared with those aged between 61–80 yrs	Swaab et al. (1985)
18 (28–96)	Manual counts	Retro.; no neurological disorder	Cortex (11)	'Fairly constant' number of pyramidal neurons even in extreme old age. Non-pyramidal neurons showed loss of 47% with age	Braak & Braak (1986)
51 (24–100)	S.-auto.	Retro.; undem.	Mult. cortical areas (9/10/46, 38,39/40)	10–15% loss of neurons over age range studied. Inf. par. cortex least affected and mid-front. most affected	Terry et al. (1987)

| 48 (50–100) | S.-auto. | Retro.; undem. | Mult. cortical areas (9/10/46, 39,39/40) | Large neurons reduced by 23–39% in those aged 80–100 yrs compared with those aged 50–65 yrs. Total neurons reduced by 6–25% between those age gps. Larger redns. in sup. temp. and inf. par. than in mid front. cortex | Hansen et al. (1988) |

See Table 18.1 for abbreviations and key.

Table 18.4. *Changes in nerve cell volume in normal aging*

No. of cases studied[a] (age range in years)	Nature of study[b]	Information on pre-mortem mental state	Site	Main findings	Reference
13 (19–95)	S.-auto.	Retro.; undem.	Cortex	No redn. in nerve cell vol. until 85 yrs; signif. slight redn. between 85 and 94 yrs	Meier-Ruge et al. (1980)
20 (70–85)	Auto.	Retro.; undem.	Cortex (11) gyrus rectus, sup. temp. gyrus (22), cing. gyrus (24)	Neuronal vol. reduced 7–20% between 70 and 85 yrs	Anderson et al. (1983)
76 (20–100+)	S.-auto.	Retro.; undem.	Cortical areas 6,11 and 17	Mean neuronal shrinkage by 80 yrs of 30% in area 6, 20% in area 11 and 10% or less in areas 7 and 17	Haug (1985)

28 (10–93)	Auto. cf immunocyto-chemically stained vasopressin and oxytocin neurons	Paraventricular and supraoptic nuclei	Retro.; undem.	No change in oxytocin cell size with age. Vasopressin cells showed slight decrease to sixth decade, then increase	Fliers et al. (1985)
51 (24–100)	S.-auto.	Mult. cortical areas (9/10/46, 38,39/40)	Retro.; undem.	'Salient change was shrinkage of large neurons reflected in redn. in no. of large neurons and increase in no. of small neurons over age range studied'	Terry et al. (1987)

See Table 18.1 for abbreviations and key.

nerve nucleus (van Buskirk, 1945); the ventral cochlear nucleus (Konigsmark & Murphy, 1970); and the nucleus basalis of Meynert (Whitehouse et al., 1983; Chiu et al., 1984).

Cell shrinkage is more common than cell loss in some studies of normal brain aging (Table 18.4), but again it does not occur in all types of nerve cell, and in some studies is confined to those aged over 85 years (Meier-Ruge, 1988). Large cortical neurons are those reported most regularly to show shrinkage with age (Haug, 1985; Terry et al., 1987). There is no evidence to suggest that nerve cell shrinkage or loss are either accelerated or reduced in extreme old age.

Dementia   There is general agreement that substantially more nerve cells are lost from the brain in AD than in normal aging, but there are variable reports of the extent of the loss (Table 18.5). Nerve cell loss is recognized to be an important component of the disease, some studies finding higher correlations of mental impairment with cortical nerve cell loss than with plaques and tangles (discussed below) (Neary et al., 1986; Hubbard et al., 1990). Furthermore, nerve cell loss is irreversible and any therapeutic strategy that aims to restore mental function to AD sufferers must take account of it. Total neuron losses varying from 40% to 50% in the hippocampus (Ball, 1977; Mann et al., 1985), up to 79% in the nucleus basalis, (Whitehouse et al., 1982), and from 15% to 58% in the cortex (Hansen et al., 1988) have been described in AD. Temporal cortex generally shows more severe neuron loss than frontal cortex. Large neurons, principally pyramidal neurons, are more affected than small ones. Younger patients with AD tend to show more neuron loss than older ones. For example, neuron loss was not significant in AD patients aged over 80 years, but was significant in those aged under 80 years in the study by Mountjoy et al. (1983). On the other hand, in the study by Hansen et al. (1988) neuron loss was not significantly greater in the younger than in the older cases of AD.

Reductions in nerve cell volume are also more marked in AD than in normal aging. For example, reductions in volume of 48% to 55% in nerve cells of frontal, temporal and pre-central cortex are described by Meier-Ruge et al. (1985).

Summary   There is probably definite, but not very severe, nerve cell loss in the brain in normal aging and rather more shrinkage of nerve cells. These changes continue, apparently steadily, into extreme old age but do not occur in all nerve cell populations. In AD, nerve cell loss is substantial, probably clinically important and often accompanied by severe shrinkage of remaining neurons. Nerve cell loss occurs in many of the same populations of cells affected by mild loss and shrinkage in normal aging, such as cortical and hippocampal pyramidal neurons, but some additional populations are affected as well. Moreover, the greater magnitude of the AD changes, and the fact that the cell loss is more marked in the younger cases, supports the view that AD is a disease and not a manifestation of normal aging.

Other changes in normal brain constituents associated with normal aging and dementia

Normal aging   The accumulation of lipofuscin increases progressively with age in some neurons (Mann et al., 1978; Brizzee & Ordy, 1981), but this is not obviously related to a drop-out of cells from the affected populations (Mann et al., 1978; Swaab, 1991). Lipofuscin-rich nuclei include the inferior olives, lateral geniculate bodies and certain other thalamic nuclei. Some cortical pyramidal cells also accumulate lipofuscin.

A reduction in nucleolar volume has been documented in some neurons, including cortical pyramidal cells, in old age (Mann et al., 1981). This is thought to reflect reduced protein synthetic capability.

Golgi studies of cortical pyramidal neurons have shown a reduction in length and number of dendrites and a loss of dendritic spines in old age (Scheibel et al., 1975; Scheibel, 1981; Nakamura et al., 1985). However, other studies indicate that there are extensions to some dendritic trees, possibly indicative of attempts at regeneration to compensate for loss of other dendrites (Buell & Coleman, 1981; Coleman & Flood, 1986). It has been suggested that such regenerative change in the cerebral cortex may explain why the volume of cortex is reduced to less than that of white matter in normal aging (Anderson et al., 1983).

Measures of synaptic terminations using immunolabelling for synaptophysin, a protein localized to synapses, show a 15–20% reduction in synapses in frontal cortex between the ages of 16 and 98 years (Masliah et al., 1993). Electron microscopic studies show a similar 14–20% reduction in synaptic density in the frontal cortex during aging (Huttenlocher, 1979; Gibson, 1983).

Dementia   Lipofuscin accumulation in nerve cells has not been shown to be excessive in AD. Reduction in nucleolar volume is greater in

Table 18.5. *Changes in nerve cell numbers in Alzheimer's disease*

No. of cases studied[a]	Nature of study[b]	Information on pre-mortem mental state	Site	Main findings	Reference
21	S.-auto.	Clin. diagnosis of senile dem.	Cortex (mid-front., pre-central, post-central sup. temp., occ.)	No signif. redn. in neuron counts compared with AMC	Terry et al. (1977)
18	S.-auto.	Clin. diagnosis of senile dem.	Front., temp. and pre-central cortex	40% decr. in large neurons in front and 46% in temp. cortex compared with AMC. No correlation of cell counts with plaque nos. in adjacent sections	Terry et al. (1981)
15	Manual counts	Clin. diagnosis of AD with psychological testing	Loc. cer.	56% redn. in pigmented cells compared with AMC	Tomlinson et al. (1981)
25	S.-auto.	Clin. diagnosis of dem.	Mult. cortical areas (8,9,20–22,24,7,17)	Signif. redn. of 18% in neurons per mm^2 in inf. front. and sup. temp. gyri. Signif.	Mountjoy et al. (1983)

				redn. of 22–31% in neurons in four cortical columns in all areas except 7 and 17, compared with AMC. Neuron counts correlated weakly with P and strongly with NFT in the same control areas	
21	Auto.	Clin. diagnosis of dem.	Gyrus rectus, temp. cortex (22), hippo.	Vol. of cortex occupied by large neurons reduced by 26% in front, and 37% in temp. compared with AMC. Redn. only signif. in those aged less than 80 yrs. Signif. neuron loss in subiculum and of neuropil in all areas at all ages	Hubbard & Anderson (1985)

Table 18.5. *Contd*

No. of cases studied[a]	Nature of study[b]	Information on pre-mortem mental state	Site	Main findings	Reference
32	Manual counts	Clin. diagnosis of AD	Temp. cortex and hippo.	Redn. of pyramidal nerve cells per unit vol. of 60% in temp. cortex and 40% in hippo. compared with AMC. Loss of neurons greater in younger cases	Mann et al. (1985) (see also Mann et al. (1984))
20	Auto.	Clin. diagnosis of dem.	Loc. cer.	Redn. of 55% in pigmented neurons compared with AMC	Bondareff & Mountjoy (1986)
32	Manual counts	Clin. diagnosis of AD	Temp. cortex, hippo., nucl. bas., loc. cer.	Neuron loss of approx. 58% in temp. cortex, 47% in hippo., 48% in nucl. bas. and 64% in loc. cer. compared with AMC	Mann et al. (1986)

17	Manual counts	Clin. diagnosis of pre-senile dem. with biopsy diagnosis of AD	Mid-temp., gyrus, cortex (biopsy)	No. of pyramidal neurons reduced by 60% in layer III and 56% in layer V compared with AMC. Nuclear vol. of some cells reduced by 38% and 36%, nucleolar vol. by 27% and 34% and RNA content by 22% and 25% respectively	Neary et al. (1986)
15	Manual counts	Clin. diagnosis of dem.	Ventral tegmental area and substantia nigra	40–60% loss of neurons in ventral tegmental area and 15% loss in substantia nigra compared with AMC	Mann et al. (1987b)
113	S.-auto.	Clin. diagnosis of dem.	Mult. cortical areas (9/10/46, 38,39/40)	Total no. of neurons reduced signif. by 15–36% compared with AMC. Large neurons showed even greater redns. Most severe loss was in inf. par. cortex	Hansen et al. (1988)

Table 18.5. *Contd*

No. of cases studied[a]	Nature of study[b]	Information on pre-mortem mental state	Site	Main findings	Reference
13	Manual counts	Clin. diagnosis of AD	Loc. cer., nuc. bas., dorsal raphe nucleus	Redn. of 39% for large neurons in nuc. bas., of 64% for pigmented cells in loc. cer. and 66% for neurons in dorsal raphe nucleus compared with AMC	Wilcock et al. (1988)
22	Manual counts	Clin. diagnosis of AD, prosp.	Loc. cer., dorsal raphe and central sup. raphe nuclei	Redn. to 30%, 19% and 33% of AMC for rostral, mid and caudal loc. cer. respectively. Redn. to 64% of AMC for caudal dorsal raphe nucleus. No loss in other regions	Zweig et al. (1988)
22	Manual counts	Clin. diagnosis of AD	Substantia nigra, ventral tegmental area	No significant loss of neurons compared with AMC	Gibb et al. (1989)

See Table 18.1 for abbreviations and key.

cortical neurons in AD than in age-matched controls. In a biopsy study, reduction in nucleolar volume correlated well with the extent of neuropsychological deficit (Neary et al., 1986). The loss of dendrites and dendritic spines is exaggerated in AD in comparison with age-matched controls (Scheibel et al., 1975; Scheibel, 1981) and does not appear to be compensated for by regenerative changes (Buell & Coleman, 1981; Coleman & Flood, 1986).

In AD the degree of synaptic loss in frontal cortex exceeds that found in normal aging and shows a strong correlation with cognitive deficit (DeKosky & Scheff, 1990; Terry et al., 1991). Decreases of 45% in the synaptic markers synaptophysin and spectrin have been recorded in frontal cortex with lesser decreases in visual and entorhinal cortex and hippocampus (Masliah et al., 1989, 1991; Weiler et al. 1990). Quantitative electron microscopy on frontal cortex in biopsy and autopsy samples have likewise shown a 27–42% loss of synapses (Davies et al., 1987; Scheff et al., 1990).

Summary   In two of the four features considered here – reduction in nucleolar volume and loss of dendrites and dendritic spines – the changes seen in AD are qualitatively similar but quantitatively greater than those seen in normal aging. In this respect, the changes may be considered to fit the 'continuum model' for aging and AD. However, this is not true for the other two features considered, for lipofuscin accumulation is not apparently excessive in AD and regenerative changes in dendritic arborizations are not seen in AD.

Development of plaques and tangles in aging and dementia

Plaques and tangles are the two main pathological hallmarks of AD (Tomlinson & Corsellis, 1984). They are also found to a lesser extent in normal aging, although they are not found in normal young and middle-aged people. Plaques are abnormal focal groups of argyrophilic degenerate neuritic processes centred around extracellular deposits of fibrillary proteinaceous, argyrophilic amyloid (see below), with some admixed astrocytic and microglial cell processes. Tangles are accumulations of argyrophilic fibrillary material composed ultrastructurally of paired, helically wound filaments in the cell bodies of neurons. In AD, plaque and tangle densities are correlated with each other and with the degree of cognitive impairment and extent of biochemical change in the brain (see, for example, the review by Mountjoy, 1988). Tangle densities also correlate with neuronal loss in AD in cerebral cortex and hippocampus, although not in the locus coeruleus and nucleus basalis (Bondareff et al., 1989).

Normal aging　Numerous studies have compared plaque and tangle counts in AD with those of age-matched control cases. However, the latter groups have, in general, had less systematic prospective assessment than the demented groups, so that the data for the numbers and distribution of plaques and tangles in so-called normal aging is less secure than for AD. For example, when the brains were examined in a general hospital series and notes and relatives were consulted in unusual detail retrospectively, 5.7% of the cases had clinical and pathological evidence of AD and another 8.6% had pathological changes suggestive of pre-clinical AD that distinguished them from the remainder (Hubbard et al., 1990). Therefore, without prospective assessment, one must expect autopsy series from acute hospital populations to include a small proportion of AD cases. Evidence from some studies on the occurrence of plaques and tangles in normal aging is summarized in Table 18.6. The occurrence of tangles in hippocampus and neocortex needs to be considered separately because it has been recognized that the hippocampus is much more vulnerable to tangle formation than the neocortex. This is clear from Table 18.6, from which it can be seen that the majority of cases aged over 60 years had some tangles (usually only a few) in the hippocampus, although very few cases had any tangles in the neocortex. Plaques were distributed more evenly between these two sites and were found commonly in small numbers. Those in the subiculum tended to increase in numbers with age in the study by Hubbard & Anderson (1981a).

Dementia　Semiquantitative and quantitative data for plaques and tangles in hippocampus and neocortex in AD are given in Table 18.7. Plaques were generally numerous at both these sites and in most studies were significantly more numerous than in age-matched, non-demented controls. Tangles were almost invariably numerous in the hippocampus, significantly more numerous than in age-matched controls, and in cortex were almost invariably present even if not numerous. The difference in densities between AD and controls is generally more striking for tangles than for plaques, and correlations with severity of dementia are more marked for tangles than plaques (Wilcock Esiri, 1982; Mountjoy et al., 1983). In the study by Hubbard & Anderson (1981a) the number of plaques in the subiculum tended to increase with age, whereas the number of tangles at the same site was not related to age in the demented subjects. In the study by Hansen et al. (1988), younger cases of AD had significantly more tangles than older cases, and Mann et al. (1985) found more tangles and plaques in younger cases.

Summary These studies show that in normal aging the numbers of brains containing plaques and tangles increases progressively from 60 to 90 years of age, but the numbers studied in the tenth decade are limited and the results at this age may therefore not be reliable. In the study that included the largest number of brains by Miller et al. (1984), 9% of brains of those aged under 55 years and 90% of brains of those aged over 85 years contained tangles, and the corresponding figures for plaques were zero and 72%. All cases of AD, by definition, contain both plaques and tangles. The crucial difference between the brains of normal elderly people and those with AD lies in the much *larger numbers* of plaques and, particularly, tangles found in AD. In AD, there is also a tendency for densities of plaques and tangles to be higher in younger patients (Mann et al., 1985). It seems, therefore, that the *numbers* of plaques and tangles in AD and normal aging do not form a continuum, but show a bimodal distribution (Tomlinson, 1982; Mountjoy, 1988; Köster et al., 1989; Hubbard et al., 1990). The *distribution* of tangles is also much more widespread in AD than in normal aging. A further point of distinction between normal aging and AD is that, whereas the density of tangles and plaques tends to increase with age in the hippocampus in undemented individuals, in AD, tangle densities tend to be higher in the younger cases.

In AD, nerve cell populations that develop tangles also show substantial drop-out of nerve cells. Published studies do not examine directly whether the same is true of nerve cell populations in normal aging. However, it is noteworthy that the hippocampus, which is among the most severely affected region with regard to nerve cell loss in normal aging, is also the region most vulnerable to tangle formation (Ball, 1977; Ulrich, 1985; Mann et al., 1987a; Hubbard et al., 1990).

Development of Hirano bodies, granulovacuolar degeneration and vascular and parenchymal amyloid deposits in aging and dementia

Hirano bodies and granulovacuolar degeneration Hirano bodies and granulovacuolar degeneration are pathological changes that occur in

Table 18.6. Occurrence of brain plaques and tangles in normal aging

No. of cases studied[a] (age range in years)	Nature of study[b]	Information on pre-mortem mental state	Site	Main findings	Reference
28 (65–92)	Manual counts of P and NFT	Retro.; undem.	Cerebral cortex and hippo.	P: none in 6 cases; <5 per field in 14 cases; >5 per field in 8 cases. NFT: none in 11 cases; some in hippo. in 14 cases; some in hippo., few in cortex in 1 case. The 8 cases with most numerous NFT in hippo. had higher P counts than the overall mean.	Tomlinson et al. (1968)
75 (30–98)	Manual counts of P and NFT	Retro.; undem.	Frontal cortex, hippo.	Nos. of cases with P and NFT correlated with age >60 yrs, but nos. of P and NFT per case were not correlated with age	Dayan (1970a)
55 (50–89)	Manual counts of P and NFT	Retro.; undem.	Hippo.	Rise in prevalence and quantity of P and NFT with age	Morimatsu et al. (1975)

19 (47–89)	S.-auto. counts of NFT	Retro.; undem.	Hippo.	Very slight, regular, rise in NFT nos. with age from sixth to ninth decades	Ball (1976)
617 (30–80+)	Manual counts of P and NFT	Retro.; undem.	Medial temp. cortex, hippo., front. and par. cortex	Linear incr. in prevalence of NFT with age (found in 50% at 50–9 yrs, >80% at 60–9 yrs and almost 100% at over 70 yrs). Also, a regular incr. in density of NFT in medial temp. lobe up to 89 yrs. P much less prevalent than NFT but also showed rise with age	Matsuyama & Nakamura (1978)
18 (68–95)	Point counting of area occupied by P; manual count of NFT as % of nucleated neurons	Retro.; undem.	Subiculum	Slight incr. in area occupied by P with increasing age. % of neurons with NFT not related to age	Hubbard & Anderson (1981a)

Table 18.6. *Contd*

No. of cases studied[a] (age range in years)	Nature of study[b]	Information on pre-mortem mental state	Site	Main findings	Reference
14 (65–102)	Manual counts of P and NFT	Prosp. tested and shown undem.	Cortex of all main lobes and hippo.	Low to moderate nos. of P in neocortex and hippo.; very low NFT counts in neocortex and hippo.	Wilcock & Esiri (1982)
199 (49 cases <55; 150 cases >64)	Manual s.-quant. assessment of P and NFT	Retro.; undem.	Cerebral cortex and hippo.	Presence of P and NFT correlated and both present at rate that incr. steadily after 70 yrs	Miller et al. (1984)
67 (10–97)	Manual counts of P and NFT	Retro.; undem.	Temp. cortex (22) and hippo.	In those aged >65 yrs, P and NFT incr. with age. Mean nos. of P: 0.5 in temp. cortex and 1.3 in hippo. Mean nos. of NFT: 0.8 in temp. cortex and 6.6 in hippo.	Mann et al. (1985)
60 (6–84)	Manual s.-quant. assessment of P and NFT	Retro.; undem.	Front temp., amygdala, hippo., nuc. bas.	32 cases (30 cases <65) had no P or NFT; 15 cases (14 over 60 yrs) had some P and NFT (NFT mainly in hippo.); 11	Mann et al. (1987a)

22 (60–90)	Manual counts of P and NFT	Prosp. tested and shown undem. (some also included in Wilcock & Esiri, 1982)	Coronal section of hippo. at level of LGB	cases had NFT only (mainly in hippo.); 1 case had P only (mainly in amygdala) No P in 15 cases; <80 P in 4 cases; >80 P in 12 cases; no NFT in 7 cases; <50 NFT in 7 cases; >50 NFT in 3 cases	Köster et al. (1989)
66 (60–95)	Manual counts of NFT	Retro., including interview with relative; undem.	Front (6), temp. (22), hippo., nuc. bas.	No NFT in cortex in 60 cases; few NFT in cortex in 6 cases; no NFT in hippo in 25 cases; <10 NFT in hippo. in 16 cases; no NFT in nuc. bas. in 11 of 61 examined; all but 4 of remainder contained <50 NFT in nuc. bas.	Hubbard et al. (1990)

See Table 18.1 for abbreviations and key.

Table 18.7. *Occurrence of brain plaques and tangles in Alzheimer's disease*

No. of cases studied[a]	Nature of study[b]	Information on pre-mortem mental state	Site	Main findings	Reference
48	Manual counts of P and NFT	Clin. diagnosis of dem.	Mult. cortical areas, mamm. bods., amygdala and hippo.	Highest counts of P and NFT found in amygdala; counts of P and NFT in each area were correlated	Jamada & Mehraein (1968)
40	Manual counts of P and NFT	Clin. diagnosis of dem.	Front. cortex, hippo.	All except one case had NFT in hippo; there were signif. more NFT in hippo. than in AMC. This was not so for P	Dayan (1970b)
50	Manual counts of P and NFT	Clin. diagnosis of dem. and prosp. dem. scores given	Cerebral cortex, hippo.	P in cortex signif. more numerous than in AMC; NFT in hippo. signif. more numerous than in AMC; NFT also found in cortex (not found in AMC)	Tomlinson et al. (1970)

61	Manual counts of P and NFT	Clin. diagnosis of dem.	Hippo.	Signif. more P and NFT than in AMC. No correlation between nos. of P and NFT and severity of dem.	Morimatsu et al. (1975)
15	Point counting of area occupied by P. Manual count of % of nucleolated neurons with NFT	Clin. diagnosis of dem.	Subiculum, cortex	Area occupied by P increased with age; % of neurons with NFT not related to age	Hubbard & Anderson (1981a)
35	Manual counts of P and NFT	Clin. diagnosis of dem. with dem. scores given prosp.	Cerebral cortex of all main lobes, hippo.	High correlation between severity of dem. and no. of NFT; weaker correlation with no. of P.	Wilcock & Esiri (1982)
32	Manual counts of P and NFT	Clin. diagnosis of dem.	Temp. cortex (22) and hippo.	P and NFT signif. more numerous in younger cases in temp. cortex but not in hippo.	Mann et al. (1985)
17	Manual counts of P and NFT	Clin. diagnosis of pre-senile dem. with biopsy confirmation of AD	Mid temp. gyrus biopsy	P and NFT counts were correlated. NFT counts were signif. correlated with pyramidal neuron loss	Neary et al. (1986)

Table 18.7. *Contd*

No. of cases studied[a]	Nature of study[b]	Information on pre-mortem mental state	Site	Main findings	Reference
13	Manual counts of P and NFT	Clin. diagnosis of dem. with prosp. assessment	Front. cortex and hippo.	All but 1 case had many cortical P and all but 4 had many hippo. P; all but 4 had cortical NFT and all but 1 had hippo. NFT	Crystal et al. (1988)
113	Manual counts of P and NFT	Clin. diagnosis of dem.	Three areas of cerebral cortex (9/10/46, 38,39/40)	Signif. more NFT in those aged under 65 yrs than those aged over 70 yrs	Hansen et al. (1988)
150	Manual counts of P and NFT	Clin. diagnosis of dem.	Cerebral cortex	131 cases fulfilled Khatchaturian (1985) criteria for diagnosis of AD. 103 cases had moderately high or high nos. of cortical NFT. 28 cases had small nos. of cortical NFT in cortex	Joachim et al. (1988)

16	Manual counts of P and NFT	Clin. diagnosis of dem. with prosp. assessment	Hippo.	All cases had >50 NFT and >20 P per coronal section of hippo.	Köster et al. (1989)
21	Manual counts of P and NFT	Clin. diagnosis of dem. with prosp. assessment	Front., temp. cortex, hippo.	P most numerous in cortex; NFT most numerous in hippo. All cases had P and NFT, and these were ten-fold higher than in AMC	Zubenko et al. (1989)
12	Manual counts of NFT	Clin. diagnosis of dem.	Cerebral cortex, (front., temp.), hippo., nuc. bas.	All cases had >80 NFT per coronal section of hippo. All had at least a few NFT in cortex	Hubbard et al. (1990)

See Table 18.1 for abbreviations and key.

the hippocampus in AD. Like plaques and tangles, they can also be found to a slight extent in normal aging (Woodard, 1962; Tomlinson & Kitchener, 1972; Ball & Lo, 1977; Ball, 1983). Again, like plaques and tangles, they are much more abundant in AD than in normal aging, with an apparent bimodal density distribution in these two states.

Vascular and parenchymal amyloid deposits

Vascular amyloid deposits in AD are abnormal fibrillary deposits in the walls of leptomeningeal and cortical blood vessels of a protein termed A4 or β protein. Identical deposits of β/A4 amyloid also occur at the centres of argyrophilic plaques and more diffusely in cerebral cortex and other areas, but not in tangles. β/A4 protein is composed of a polypeptide sequence derived by proteolytic cleavage from part of a much larger protein, the amyloid precursor protein (APP), which forms a constituent of cell membranes, including nerve cell membranes, and whose function is unknown (Kang et al., 1987). It is thought likely that abnormal processing and degradation of APP is responsible for its deposition in blood vessel walls, plaques and elsewhere. These deposits are found not only in AD but also in normal aging. The vessels containing amyloid may leak and occasionally give rise to slight or more extensive subarachnoid or intracerebral haemorrhage.

Normal aging   The proportion of undemented subjects in which some cerebrovascular amyloid can be detected rises steadily with age from 60 to 97 years, according to the studies by Mountjoy et al. (1982) and Vinters & Gilbert (1983), although Esiri & Wilcock (1986) found no such increase in prevalence with age over 70 years and reported a more constant prevalence of slightly over 30% in elderly subjects without AD. Vascular amyloid in normal aging is usually mild in degree and is accompanied almost invariably by some cortical plaques, although the density of each is not correlated closely. Recent studies have investigated the prevalence, density and distribution of A4 or β amyloid using antisera or monoclonal antibodies to the polypeptide (Tagliavini et al., 1988; Yamaguchi et al., 1988; Braak et al., 1989; Bugiani et al., 1989; Ikeda et al., 1989; Ogomori et al., 1989). Using this method of detection, which is claimed to be more sensitive than traditional staining, 60% of non-demented control brains from people aged 50–98 years were found to contain β/A4 amyloid deposits either in vessels or in grey matter parenchyma in the form of argyrophilic plaques, or in smaller or more diffuse non-argyrophilic deposits ('pre-amyloid') (Ogomori et al., 1989). There was some evidence that the prevalence of β/A4 protein deposits increased with age. The prevalence of vascular β/A4 amyloid actually appears to have been no higher in this study than in earlier studies using traditional stains. Parenchymal deposits of β/A4 protein were shown by Davies et al. (1988) to be present in 45% of 110 unselected coronets autopsies on cases over 50 years of age. The prevalence of β/A4 deposits rose from 19% in the sixth decade to 79% in the ninth decade.

Dementia Almost all cases of AD show some degree of vascular amyloid deposition detectable using traditional amyloid or silver stains (Glenner, 1983; Joachim et al., 1988). The extent of vascular deposits is variable and does not correlate closely with plaque or tangle counts, or with age or severity of cognitive impairment. Immunostaining for β/A4 protein in AD shows more widespread parenchymal deposits of this protein than are seen with silver and traditional amyloid stains. Vascular deposits of β/A4 protein are found in 100% of cases of AD using this method (Ogomori et al., 1989). Some of the parenchymal deposits occur at sites that are largely devoid of conventional plaques, most noticeably in cerebellar cortex, but also in many deep grey nuclei of basal ganglia, thalamus, and brain stem and even, in some cases, in the spinal cord (Bugiani et al., 1989; Ogomori et al., 1989).

Summary Vascular amyloid deposits show a similar relationship to normal aging and AD as do plaques, but their extent is harder to quantify. In consequence, few attempts have been made to correlate the extent of vascular amyloid deposition to the other variables in AD, such as biochemical alterations and severity of cognitive impairment. Detection of the β/A4 protein in amyloid deposits using immunostaining shows a steady increase in its appearance with normal aging but, as with plaques and tangles, there is substantially more of it in AD such as to suggest that AD is a manifestation of clearly abnormal β/A4 metabolism.

Discussion and conclusions

Many of the changes that occur in the brain in normal aging resemble qualitatively those found in AD: reduced volume and weight of the brain, number and size of neurons, development of plaques, tangles, granulovacuolar degeneration, Hirano bodies and vascular and parenchymal β/A4 amyloid deposits. However, there is a profound difference in the *abundance* of all these changes between normal aging and AD. If AD were an exaggeration of normal aging one might expect the abundance of these changes to be moderate in most elderly people, low in the exceptionally cognitively well-preserved and high in those with AD. Despite the shortcomings of some of the evidence it is clear that this is *not* what is found. Most healthy elderly people, including the exceptionally well-preserved, have very mild degrees of change (perhaps sufficient to explain 'benign forgetfulness'?) or none, and the minority, those with AD, have relatively severe degrees of change (Skullerud, 1985). It seems, therefore, that people are susceptible to either a mild or a severe form of Alzheimer-type change as they age. The severe form may be further subdivisible if it is accepted that early onset AD is more severe than late onset AD (Mountjoy et al., 1983; Hansen et al., 1988). Similarly, people may be susceptible to mild or severe forms of other neurodegenerative changes, for example, of the type seen in Parkinson's disease. We do not know what factors determine susceptibility to AD, except in the few cases in which genetic factors are clearly involved, in familial AD or AD occurring in Down's syndrome. In other cases there may be different mechanisms involved, not all of which are necessarily determined wholly by heredity. For example, one recent line of investigation has shown that patients with a number of degenerative neurological diseases, including AD, have an impaired capacity to metabolize sulphur-containing compounds (Steventon et al., 1990). Such a genetically determined impairment might be expected to reduce the capacity to detoxify common endogenous and exogenous sulphur-containing compounds, rendering those affected liable to intoxication if subjected to a lifetime dose of pro-toxin or toxin above a threshold level. It is easy to propose ways in which genetic and environmental factors of this sort might interact to produce a disease of late life such as AD.

The literature on aging and the brain includes contributions from many different disciplines. It is noticeable that those who favour the view that aging and AD, or dementia, form a continuum are chiefly to be found among researchers who deal with living people – geriatricians, psychiatrists and psychologists. Biochemists and neuropathologists who study the brain tend to take the opposite view. The clinicians evaluate the net performance of the brain, which must represent the outcome of many different influences. Biochemists and neuropathologists tend to examine individual items – chemical or structural – and see a different pattern. How can the two differing views be reconciled? Perhaps the effects of two or more discontinuous processes become merged, and appear as one when the sum total of brain performance is examined in the clinical setting. Thus, in the very old, in whom the pathology of AD, if it develops, tends to be mild, the deficits produced may appear to fall on a continuum with normal aging, and indeed much of the cell loss present in very elderly sufferers from AD can be ascribed to an aging effect rather than to AD. But this continuum has no place for younger, severer, AD sufferers, and that should make us pause and search for mechanisms for this disease other than time alone. Greater understanding of such mechanisms may show that even the mild changes in the brains of normal elderly people are not an inevitable consequence of aging.

References

Anderson, J. M., Hubbard, B. M., Coghill, G. R. & Slidders, W. (1983). The effect of advanced old age on the neurone content of the cerebral cortex. *Journal of the Neurological Sciences*, **58**, 233–44.

Ball, M. (1976). Neurofibrillary tangles and the pathogenesis of dementia: a quantitative study. *Neuropathology and Applied Neurobiology*, **2**, 395–410.

Ball, M. (1977). Neuronal loss, neurofibrillary tangles and granulovacuolar degeneration in the hippocampus with ageing and dementia: a quantitative study. *Acta Neuropathologica*, **37**, 111–18.

Ball, M. (1983). Granulovacuolar degeneration. In B. Reisberg (ed.) *Alzheimer's Disease – the Standard Reference*, pp. 62–8. Free-Press MacMillan, NY.

Ball, M. J. & Lo, P. (1977). Granulovacuolar degeneration in the ageing brain and in dementia. *Journal of Neuropathology and Experimental Neurology*, **36**, 474–87.

Bondareff, W. & Mountjoy, C. Q. (1986). Numbers of neurons in nucleus locus ceruleus in demented and non-demented patients: rapid estimation and correlated parameters. *Neurobiology of Aging*, **7**, 297–300.

Bondareff, W., Mountjoy, C. Q., Roth, M. & Hauser, D. C. (1989). Neurofibrillary degeneration and neuronal loss in Alzheimer's disease. *Neurobiology of Aging*, **10**, 709–15.

Braak, H. & Braak, E. (1986). Ratio of pyramidal cells versus non-pyramidal cells in the human frontal isocortex and changes in ratio with ageing and Alzheimer's disease. *Progress in Brain Research*, **70**, 185–212.

Braak, H., Braak, E., Ohm, T. & Bohl, J. (1989). Alzheimer's disease: mismatch between amyloid plaques and neuritic plaques. *Neuroscience Letters*, **103**, 24–8.

Brizzee, K. R. & Ordy, J. M. (1981). Age pigments, cell loss and functional implications in the brain. In R. S. Sohal (ed.) *Age Pigments*, pp. 317–24. Elsevier, Amsterdam.

Brody, H. (1955). Organisation of the cerebral cortex III. A study of ageing in the human cerebral cortex. *Journal of Comparative Neurology*, **102**, 511–56.

Brody, H. (1970). Structural changes in the aging nervous system. *Interdisciplinary Topics in Gerontology*, **7**, 9–21.

Buell, S. J. & Coleman, P. D. (1981). Quantitative evidence for selective dendritic growth in normal ageing but not in senile dementia. *Brain Research*, **214**, 23–41.

Bugiani, O., Giaccone, G., Frangione, B., Ghetti, B. & Tagliavini, F. (1989). Alzheimer patients: preamyloid deposits are more widely distributed than senile plaques throughout the central nervous system. *Neuroscience Letters*, **103**, 263–8.

Chiu, H. C., Bondareff, W., Zarow, C. & Slager, U. (1984). Stability of neuronal number in human nucleus basalis of Meynert with age. *Neurobiology of Aging*, **5**, 83–8.

Chrzanowska, G. & Beben, A. (1973). Weight of the brain and body height in man between the ages of 20 and 89 years. *Folia Morphologica (Warszawa)*, **32**, 391–406.

Coleman, P. D. & Flood, D. G. (1986). Dendritic proliferation in the ageing brain as a compensatory repair mechanism. *Progress in Brain Research*, **70**, 227–37.

Crystal, H., Dickson, D., Fuld, P., Masur, P., Scott, R., Mehler, M., Masden, J., Kawar, C., Aronson, M. & Wolfson, L. (1988). Clinicopathological studies in dementia: nondemented subjects with pathologically confirmed Alzheimer's disease. *Neurology*, **38**, 1682–7.

Davies, C. A., Mann, D. M. A., Sumpter, P. Q. & Yates, P. O. (1987). A quantitative morphometric analysis of the neuronal and synaptic content of the frontal and temporal cortex in patients with Alzheimer's disease. *Journal of the Neurological Sciences*, **78**, 151–64.

Davies, L., Wolska, B., Hilbich, C., Multhaus, G., Martins, R., Simms, G., Beyreuther, K. & Masters, C. L. (1988). A4 amyloid protein deposition and the diagnosis of Alzheimer's disease. *Neurology*, **38**, 1688–93.

Davis, P. J. M. & Wright, E. A. (1977). A new method for measuring cranial cavity volume and its application to the assessment of cerebral atrophy at autopsy. *Neuropathology and Applied Neurobiology*, **3**, 341–58.

Dayan, A. D. (1970a). Quantitative histological studies on the aged human brain. I. Senile plaques and neurofibrillary tangles in normal patients. *Acta Neuropathologica*, **16**, 85–94.

Dayan, A. D. (1970b). Quantitative histological studies on the aged human brain. II. Senile plaques and neurofibrillary tangles in senile dementia. *Acta Neuropathologica*, **16**, 95–102.

Dekaban, A. S. & Sadowsky, D. (1978). Changes in brain weights during the span of human life: relation of brain weights to body heights and body weights. *Annals of Neurology*, **4**, 345–56.

DeKosky, S. T. & Scheff, S. W. (1990). Synapse loss in frontal cortex biopsies in Alzheimer's disease: correlation with cognitive severity. *Annals of Neurology*, **27**, 457–64.

de la Monte, S. M. (1989). Quantitation of cerebral atrophy in preclinical and end-stage Alzheimer's disease. *Annals of Neurology*, **25**, 450–9.

Devaney, K. O. & Johnson, H. A. (1980). Neuron loss in the ageing visual cortex of man. *Journal of Gerontology*, **35**, 836–41.

Eggers, R., Haug, H. & Fisher, D. (1984). Preliminary report on macroscopic age changes in the human prosencephalon. A stereologic investigation. *Journal für Hirnforschung*, **25**, 129–39.

Esiri, M. M., Wilcock, G. K. (1986). Cerebral amyloid angiopathy in dementia and old age. *Journal of Neurology, Neurosurgery and Psychiatry*, **49**, 1221–6.

Fliers, E., Swaab, D. F., Pool, C. W. & Verwer, R. W. H. (1985). The vasopressin and oxytocin neurons in the human supraoptic and paraventricular nucleus: changes with aging and in senile dementia. *Brain Research*, **342**, 45–53.

Gibb, W. R. G., Mountjoy, C. Q., Mann, D. M. A. & Lees, A. J. (1989). The substantia nigra and ventral tegmental areas in Alzheimer's disease and Down's syndrome. *Journal of Neurology, Neurosurgery and Psychiatry*, **52**, 193–203.

Gibson, P. H. (1983). EM study of the number of cortical synapses in the brains of ageing people and people with Alzheimer-type dementia. *Acta Neuropathologica*, **62**, 127–33.

Glenner, G. G. (1983). Alzheimer's disease: multiple cerebral amyloidosis. In Banbury Report 15: Cold Spring Harbour Symposium on *Biological Aspects of Alzheimer's Disease*, pp. 137–44. Cold Spring Harbour, New York.

Hall, T. C., Miller, A. K. H., Corsellis, J. A. N. (1975). Variations in the human Purkinje cell population according to age and sex. *Neuropathology and Applied Neurobiology*, **1**, 267–92.

Hansen, L. A., De Teresa, R., Davies, P. & Terry, R. D. (1988). Neocortical morphometry, lesion counts, and choline acetyltransferase levels in the age spectrum of Alzheimer's disease. *Neurology*, **38**, 48–54.

Haug, H. (1985). Are neurons of the human cerebral cortex really lost during ageing? A morphometric examination. In J. Traber & W. H. Gispen (eds) *Senile dementia of the Alzheimer type*, pp. 150–63. Springer, Berlin.

Haug, H., Barmwater, U., Eggers, R., Fischer, D., Kühl, S. & Sass, N. L. (1983). Anatomical changes in ageing brain. *Aging*, **21**, 1–12.

Heidary, H. & Tomasch, J. (1969). Neuron numbers and perikaryon areas in the human cerebellar nuclei. *Acta Anatomica*, **74**, 290–6.

Henderson, G., Tomlinson, B. E. & Gibson, P. H. (1980). Counts in human cerebral cortex in normal adults throughout life using an image analysing computer. *Journal of the Neurological Sciences*, **46**, 113–36.

Ho, K-C., Roessmann, U., Straumfjord, J. V. & Monroe, G. (1980). Analysis of brain weight. *Archives of Pathology and Laboratory Medicine*, **104**, 635–9.

Hubbard, B. M. & Anderson, J. M. (1981a). A quantitative study of cerebral atrophy in old age and senile dementia. *Journal of the Neurological Sciences*, **50**, 135–45.

Hubbard, B. M. & Anderson, J. M. (1981b). Age, senile dementia and ventricular enlargement. *Journal of Neurology, Neurosurgery and Psychiatry*, **44**, 631–5.

Hubbard, B. M. & Anderson, J. M. (1985). Age-related variations in the neuron content of the cerebral cortex in senile dementia of Alzheimer type. *Neuropathology and Applied Neurobiology*, **11**, 369–82.

Hubbard, B. M., Featon, G. W. & Anderson, J. M. (1990). A quantitative histological study of early clinical and preclinical Alzheimer's disease. *Neuropathology and Applied Neurobiology*, **16**, 111–21.

Huttenlocher, P. R. (1979). Synaptic density in human frontal cortex – developmental changes and effects of aging. *Brain Research*, **163**, 195–205.

Ikeda, S., Allsop, D. & Glenner, G. G. (1989). Morphology and distribution of plaque and related deposits in the brains of Alzheimer's disease and control cases. An immunohistochemical study using amyloid β-protein antibody. *Laboratory Investigation*, **60**, 113–22.

Jamada, M. & Mehraein, P. (1968). Verteilungsmuster der senilen veränderungen im Gehirn. Die Beteiligung des limbischen Systems bei hirnatrophischen Prozessen des Seriums und bei Morbus Alzheimer. *Zeitgeist für Neurologie und Psychiatrie*, **211**, 308–24.

Joachim, C. L., Morris, J. H. & Selkoe, D. J. (1988). Clinically diagnosed Alzheimer's disease: autopsy results in 150 cases. *Annals of Neurology*, **24**, 50–6.

Kang, J., Lemaire, H. G., Unterbeck, A., Salbaum, J. M., Masters, C. L., Grzeschik, K. H., Multhaup, G., Beyreuther, K. & Müller-Hill, B. (1987). The precursor of Alzheimer's disease amyloid A4 protein resembles a cell-surface receptor. *Nature*, **325**, 733–6.

Khachaturian, Z. S. (1985). Diagnosis of Alzheimer's disease. *Archives of Neurology*, **42**, 1097–104.

Konigsmark, B. W. & Murphy, E. A. (1970). Neuronal populations in the human brain. *Nature*, **228**, 1335–6.

Köster, R., Esiri, M. M. & Wilcock, G. K. (1989). Pathologic diagnosis of Alzheimers. *Neurology*, **39**, 1268.

Mann, D. M. A., Yates, P. O. & Stamp, J. E. (1978). The relationship between lipofuscin pigment and ageing in the human nervous system. *Journal of the Neurological Sciences*, **37**, 83–93.

Mann, D. M. A., Neary, D., Yates, P. O., Lincoln, J., Snowden, J. S. & Stanworth, P. (1981). Neurofibrillary pathology and protein synthetic capability in nerve cells in Alzheimer's disease. *Neuropathology and Applied Neurobiology*, **7**, 37–47.

Mann, D. M. A., Yates, P. O. & Marcyniuk, B. (1984). Monoaminergic neurotransmitter systems in presenile Alzheimer's disease and in senile dementia of Alzheimer type. *Clinical Neuropathology*, **3**, 199–205.

Mann, D. M. A., Yates, P. O. & Marcyniuk, B. (1985). Some morphometric observations on the cerebral cortex and in hippocampus in Alzheimer's presenile dementia, senile dementia of Alzheimer type and Down's syndrome in middle age. *Journal of the Neurological Sciences*, **69**, 139–59.

Mann, D. M. A., Yates, P. O. & Marcyniuk, B. (1986). A comparison of nerve cell loss in cortical and subcortical structures in Alzheimer's disease. *Journal of Neurology, Neurosurgery and Psychiatry*, **49**, 310–12.

Mann, D. M. A., Tucker, C. M., Yates, P. O. (1987a). The topographic distribution of senile plaques and neurofibrillary tangles in the brains of non-demented persons of different ages. *Neuropathology and Applied Neurobiology*, **13**, 123–39.

Mann, D. M. A., Yates, P. O. & Marcyniuk, B. (1987b). Dopaminergic neurotransmitter systems in Alzheimer's disease and in Down's syndrome at middle age. *Journal of Neurology, Neurosurgery and Psychiatry*, **50**, 341–4.

Masliah, E., Terry, R. D., De Teresa, R. M. & Hansen, L. A. (1989). Immunohisto-chemical quantification of the synapse-related protein synaptophysin in Alzheimer's disease. *Neuroscience Letters*, **103**, 234–9.

Masliah, E., Terry, R. D., Alford, M., De Teresa, R. M. & Hansen, L. A. (1991). Cortical and subcortical patterns of synaptophysin-like immuno-reactivity in Alzheimer's disease. *American Journal of Pathology*, **138**, 235–46.

Masliah, E., Mallory, M., Hansen, L., De Teresa, R. & Terry, R. D. (1993). Quantitative synaptic alterations in the human neocortex during normal aging. *Neurology*, **43**, 192–7.

Matsuyama, H. & Nakamura, S. (1978). Senile changes in the brain in the Japanese: incidence of Alzheimer's neurofibrillary change and senile plaques. In R. Katzman & R. D. Terry (eds.) *Alzheimer's Disease and Related Disorders (Aging*, vol. 7), pp. 287–97. Raven Press, New York.

Meier-Ruge, W. (1988). Morphometric methods and their potential value for gerontological brain research. In J. Ulrich (ed.) *Histology and Histopathology of the Ageing Brain. Interdisciplinary Topics in Gerontology*, vol. 25, pp. 90–100. Karger, Basel.

Meier-Ruge, W., Hurziker, O., Schulz, U., Tobler, H. J. & Schweizer, A. (1980). Stereologic changes in the capillary network and nerve cells of the ageing human brain. *Mechanisms and Ageing and Development*, **14**, 233–43.

Meier-Ruge, W., Ulrich, J. & Stähelin, H. B. (1985). Morphometric investigation of nerve cells, neuropil and senile plaques in senile dementia of the Alzheimer type. *Archives of Gerontology and Geriatrics*, **4**, 219–29.

Miller, A. K. H., Alston, R. L. & Corsellis, J. A. N. (1980). Variation with age in the volumes of grey and white matter in the cerebral hemispheres of man. Measurements with an image analyser. *Neuropathology and Applied Neurobiology*, **6**, 119–32.

Miller, F. de W., Hicks, S. P., D'Amato, C. J. & Landis, J. R. (1984). A descriptive study of neuritic plaques and neurofibrillary tangles in an autopsy population. *American Journal of Epidemiology*, **120**, 331–41.

Moatamed, F. (1966). Cell frequencies in the human olivary complex. *Journal of Comparative Neurology*, **128**, 109–16.

Morimatsu, M., Hirai, S., Muramatsu, A. & Yoshikawa, M. (1975). Senile degenerative brain lesions and dementia. *Journal of the American Geriatrics Society*, **23**, 390–406.

Mountjoy, C. Q. (1988). Number of plaques and tangles, loss of neurons: their correlation with deficient neuro-transmitter synthesis and the degree of dementia. In J. Ulrich (ed.) *Histology and Histopathology of the Ageing Brain. Interdisciplinary Topics in Gerontology*, vol. 25, pp. 74–89. Karger, Basel.

Mountjoy, C. Q., Tomlinson, B. E. & Gibson, P. H. (1982). Amyloid and senile plaques and cerebral blood vessels. *Journal of the Neurological Sciences*, **57**, 89–103.

Mountjoy, C. Q., Roth, M., Evans, N. J. R. & Evans, H. (1983). Cortical neuronal counts in normal elderly controls and demented patients. *Neurobiology of Aging*, **4**, 1–11.

Mouritzen Dam, A. (1979). The density of neurons in the human hippocampus. *Neuropathology and Applied Neurobiology*, **5**, 249–64.

Nakamura, S., Akiguclin, J., Kameyama, M. & Mizuno, N. (1985). Age-related changes of pyramidal cell basal dendrites in layers III and V of human motor cortex. A quantitative Golgi study. *Acta Neuropathologica*, **65**, 281–4.

Neary, D., Snowden, J. S., Mann, D. M. A., Bowen, D. M., Sims, N. R., Nathen, B., Yates, P. O. & Davison, A. N. (1986). Alzheimer's disease: a correlative study. *Journal of Neurology, Neurosurgery and Psychiatry*, **49**, 229–37.

Ogomori, K., Kitamoto, T., Tateishi, J., Sato, Y., Suetsugu, M. & Abe, M. (1989). β-protein amyloid is widely distributed in the central nervous system of patients with Alzheimer's disease. *American Journal of Pathology*, **134**, 243–51.

Pakkenberg, B. & Gundersen, H. J. G. (1988). Total number of neurons and glial cells in human brain nuclei estimated by the disector and the fractionator. *Journal of Microscopy*, **150**, 1–20.

Pakkenberg, H. & Voigt, J. (1964). Brain weight of the Danes, a forensic material. *Acta Anatomica*, **56**, 297–307.

Scheff, S. W., DeKosky, S. T., Price, D. A. (1990). Quantitative assessment of cortical synaptic density in Alzheimer's disease. *Neurobiology of Aging*, **11**, 29–37.

Scheibel, A. B. (1981). The gerohistology of the ageing human forebrain: some structuro-functional considerations. In S. J. Enna, T. Samorajski & B. Beer (eds.) *Aging*, vol. 17, pp. 31–42. Raven Press, NY.

Scheibel, M. E., Lindsay, R. D., Tomiyasu, U. & Scheibel, A. B. (1975). Progressive dendritic changes in ageing human cortex. *Experimental Neurology*, **47**, 392–403.

Skullerud, K. (1985). Variations in the size of the human brain. *Acta Neurologica Scandinavica*, **71**, (supplement 102), 1–95.

Steventon, G. B., Heathfield, M. T. E., Sturman, S., Waring, R. H. & Williams, A. C. (1990). Xenobiotic metabolism in Alzheimer's disease. *Neurology*, **40**, 1095–8.

Swaab, D. F. (1991). Brain aging and Alzheimer's disease, 'wear and tear' versus 'use it or lose it'. *Aging*, **12**, 317–24.

Swaab, D. F., Fliers, E. & Partiman, T. S. (1985). The suprachiasmatic nucleus of the human brain in relation to sex, age and senile dementia. *Brain Research*, **342**, 37–44.

Tagliavini, F., Giaccone, G., Frangione, B. & Bugiani, O. (1988). Preamyloid deposits in the cerebral cortex of patients with Alzheimer's disease and nondemented individuals. *Neuroscience Letters*, **93**, 191–6.

Terry, R. D., Fitzgerald, C., Peck, A., Millner, J. & Farmer, P. (1977). Cortical cell counts in senile dementia. *Journal of Neuropathology and Experimental Neurology*, **36**, 633.

Terry, R. D., Perk, A., De Teresa, R. & Schecter, R. (1981). Some morphometric aspects of the brain in senile dementia of the Alzheimer type. *Annals of Neurology*, **10**, 184–92.

Terry, R. D., De Teresa, R. & Hansen, L. A. (1987). Neocortical cell counts in normal human adult aging. *Annals of Neurology*, **21**, 530–9.

Terry, R. D., Masliah, E., Salmon, D. P., Butters, N., De Teresa, R., Hill, R., Hansen, L. A. & Katzman, R. (1991). Physical basis of cognitive alterations in Alzheimer disease: synapse loss is major correlate of cognitive impairment. *Annals of Neurology*, **30**, 572–80.

Tomlinson, B. E. (1982). Plaques, tangles and Alzheimer's disease. *Psychological Medicine*, **12**, 449–59.

Tomlinson, B. E. & Corsellis, J. A. N. (1984). Ageing and the dementias. In J. H. Adams, J. A. N. Corsellis & L. W. Duchen (eds.) *Greenfield's Neuropathology*, 4th edition, pp. 951–1025. Arnold, London.

Tomlinson, B. E. & Kitchener, D. (1972). Granulovacuolar degeneration of the hippocampal pyramidal cells. *Journal of Pathology*, **106**, 165–85.

Tomlinson, B. E., Blessed, G. & Roth, M. (1968). Observations on the brain of non-demented old people. *Journal of the Neurological Sciences*, **7**, 331–56.

Tomlinson, B. E., Blessed, G. & Roth, M. (1970). Observations on the brains of demented old people. *Journal of the Neurological Sciences*, **11**, 205–42.

Tomlinson, B. E., Irving, D. & Blessed, G. (1981). Cell loss in the locus coeruleus in senile dementia of Alzheimer type. *Journal of the Neurological Sciences*, **49**, 419–28.

Ulrich, J. (1985). Alzheimer changes in nondemented patients younger than sixty five: possible early stages of Alzheimer's disease and senile dementia of Alzheimer type. *Annals of Neurology*, **17**, 273–7.

van Buskirk, C. (1945). The seventh nerve complex. *Journal of Comparative Neurology*, **82**, 303–34.

Vijayashankar, N. & Brody, H. (1977). A quantitative study of the pigmented neurons in the nuclei locus coeruleus and subcoeruleus in man as related to aging. *Journal of Neuropathology and Experimental Neurology*, **38**, 490–7.

Vinters, H. V. & Gilbert, J. J. (1983). Cerebral amyloid angiopathy: incidence and complications in the aging brain 2. The distribution of amyloid vascular changes. *Stroke*, **14**, 924–8.

Weiler, R., Lassmann, H., Fischer, P., Jellinger, K. & Winkler, H. (1990). A high ratio of chromogranin A to synaptin/synaptophysin is a common feature of brains in Alzheimer and Pick disease. *FEBS Letters*, **263**, 337–9.

Whitehouse, P. J., Price, D. L., Struble, R. G., Clark, A. W., Coyle, J. T. & Delong, M. R. (1982). Alzheimer's disease and senile dementia: loss of neurons in the basal forebrain. *Science*, **215**, 1237–9.

Whitehouse, P. J., Parhad, I. M., Iledreen, J. C., Clark, A. W., White, C. L. III, Struble, R. G. & Price, D. L. (1983). Integrity of the nucleus basalis of Meynert in normal aging. *Neurology Supplement*, **33**, 159.

Wilcock, G. K. & Esiri, M. M. (1982). Plaques, tangles and dementia: a quantitative study. *Journal of the Neurological Sciences*, **56**, 343–56.

Wilcock, G. K., Esiri, M. M., Bowen, D. M. & Hughes, A. O. (1988). The differential involvement of subcortical nuclei in senile dementia of Alzheimer type. *Journal of Neurology, Neurosurgery and Psychiatry*, **51**, 842–9.

Woodard, J. S. (1962). Clinico-pathological significance of granulovacuolar degeneration in Alzheimer's disease. *Journal of Neuropathology and Experimental Neurology*, **21**, 85–91.

Yamaguchi, H., Hirai, S., Morimatsu, M., Shoji, M. & Ihara, Y. (1988). A variety of cerebral amyloid deposits in the brains of the Alzheimer-type dementia demonstrated by beta-protein immunostaining. *Acta Neuropathologica*, **76**, 541–9.

Zubenko, G. S., Moossy, J., Martinez, J., Rao, G. R., Kopp, U. & Hanin, I. (1989). A brain regional analysis of morphologic and cholinergic abnormalities in Alzheimer's disease. *Archives of Neurology*, **46**, 634–8.

Zweig, R. M., Ross, C. A., Hedreen, J. C., Steele, C., Cardillo, J. E., Whitehouse, P. J., Folstein, M. F. & Price, D. L. (1988). The neuropathology of aminergic nuclei in Alzheimer's disease. *Annals of Neurology*, **24**, 233–42.

19

Cholinergic component of dementia and aging

E. K. PERRY, J. A. COURT, M. A. PIGGOTT & R. H. PERRY

> Everyone complains of his memory, but no one complains of his judgement.
>
> *(Les Maximes 89, de la Rochefoucauld)*

Compared with other species, the human brain is not only the most sophisticated in terms of information processing, but also the most susceptible to the appearance with time of specific lesions such as senile plaques. Neuritic, A4-positive plaques occur primarily in areas of greatest 'plasticity' and the vulnerability of regions such as entorhinal cortex and hippocampus may be linked directly to their role in the storage of new information. If there is some kind of theoretical limit to the programming capacity of the normal brain then functional abnormalities in, for example, memory may be, to a greater or lesser extent, an inevitable consequence of aging. Arguments as to whether normal cerebral aging and Alzheimer's disease are part of the same fundamental process, distinguished only by degree (see for example Perry & Perry, 1988; Storandt, 1988) are not just academic. If they are similar, then increasing life expectancy by whatever means will only further increase the prevalence of Alzheimer's disease and the prospects for prevention appear to be remote. However, if the pathogenesis of Alzheimer's disease and normal brain aging do share a common mechanism, analysis of aging itself may provide new insights into the disease process at its earliest stages and in itself may generate successful therapeutic strategies. The present chapter subscribes to the view that some forms of dementia, notably Alzheimer's disease, are neurochemically contiguous with the aging process and that, in terms of devising appropriate therapeutic strategies, investigation of the aging brain may be one of the best approaches to the problem of Alzheimer's disease itself. In other forms of dementia, notably that of the Lewy body type, which is second in prevalence to Alzheimer's

Dementia and Normal Aging, eds. F. A. Huppert, C. Brayne & D. W. O'Connor. © Cambridge University Press 1994.

disease in the elderly demented population and appears to be distinct from normal aging at least pathologically (R. H. Perry et al., 1989, 1990a), prevention may be a more realistic long-term objective.

This chapter on neurochemistry is focused on the transmitter acetylcholine, since a robust framework exists for examining alterations in this particular system in the context of age-related memory impairments and the more severe cognitive deficits in dementia. The 'cholinergic hypothesis' (reviewed in Perry (1986, 1988)) continues to survive despite various theories. These theories include: the key role of amyloidoisis or abnormal neurofilament formation in cerebral dysfunction; and the role of multiple transmitter pathology in mental symptoms such as memory loss. The hypothesis has not attempted, however, to encompass aetiopathological aspects nor does it explain all aspects of functional change in the aging brain or demented individual. It suggests rather that the principal basis of the confusion (impaired working memory and visuospatial deficits, for example) is the declining function of the neocortical cholinergic system which originates in the basal forebrain. This conclusion is apparent, to a modest degree, in some normal elderly individuals and evident, to a devastating extent, in dementing disorders such as Alzheimer's disease.

Methods of investigation

Parameters

Numerous cholinergic 'markers' delineating the structure, chemistry and function of basal forebrain cholinergic neurons are applicable to investigations of aging and, to a lesser extent, dementia. Morphologically, the numbers and size of the cholinergic neuronal perikarya which extend, rostrally, from the septal nuclei and caudally to the nucleus of Meynert, can be assessed together with the presence (in the human but not other aging species) of such disease-related histopathological features as neurofibrillary tangles and Lewy bodies. The extent and normality of the axonal arborization of the neurons can be monitored in the fibre tracts emanating from the basal forebrain and in terminal processes situated in target areas such as the cortex, hippocampus and amygdala, by using appropriate cytochemical markers such as choline acetyltransferase, the receptor for nerve growth factor (NGF), and in some instances acetylcholinesterase. Neurochemically, these enzyme and receptor activities provide, in regions of neuronal perikarya or cortical target areas, indices of the extent and activity of the basal forebrain cholinergic system. Other neurochemical markers include high affinity choline uptake (hemicholinium binding), the vesicular acetylcholine transporter (vesamicol binding) and a variety of cholinergic receptors, both muscarinic and nicotinic which further exist as structurally and pharmacologically different subtypes situated both presynaptically and postsynaptically. All these cholinergic-related proteins can be either quantified in dispersed tissue or visualized at the microanatomic or cellular level using immunocytochemical or autoradiographic techniques. In many instances, probes are available for the respective mRNA species, although the relatively short half life of the latter, and discrepancies between message and protein levels, suggest that information on RNA alone may be insufficient to gauge neuronal activity. Functional measures of the cholinergic system, generally only applicable to experimental animal or human biopsy tissue in vitro, include: the rate of acetylcholine synthesis; basal and stimulated transmitter release; high affinity choline uptake; responses to acetylcholine – both electrophysiological and neurochemical, receptor activated second messenger production – and release of acetylcholinesterase. Compensatory receptor responses to cholinergic drugs administered in vivo provide a biological measure of the integrity of the system in the living brain. Psychopharmacologically, a range of agonist and antagonist drugs are available to manipulate the cholinergic system in vivo, although, since these are not specific to basal forebrain neurons nor even to the central as opposed to peripheral nervous system, interpretation of the behavioural or mental response is difficult.

A new dimension has been added recently to the pathophysiological studies of basal forebrain cholinergic neurons with the discovery that these cells interact specifically with NGF (reviewed by Whittemore & Seigel, 1987; Ebendal, 1989). Not only NGF but also closely related molecules including brain derived neurotrophic factor (BDNF) and neurotrophin-3 (Maisonpierre et al., 1990), appear to be synthesized most actively in the hippocampus and other target areas of this cholinergic system, notably the cerebral cortex. The existence of high affinity receptors for NGF (and probably other growth factors, see Rodriguez-Tébar et al., (1990)) on cholinergic basal forebrain neurons provides mechanisms whereby these neurons can – through retrograde axonal transport and nuclear interaction – respond to trophic factors (increasing axonal arborization and the level of choline acetyltransferase, for example). At the morphological level, NGF receptor provides another useful 'marker' of these neurons (see above), although whether the receptor localization is cholinergic specific is not yet clear. Certainly, low affinity receptors exist on other neuronal populations (Richardson et al., 1986; Buck et al., 1988). Any contemporary analysis of the basal forebrain cholinergic system in aging and dementia does need, however, to include the levels (both protein and mRNA) of NGF and related molecules, the NGF receptor and, where appropriate, more dynamic aspects such as the response to NGF. This is a research area in aging and neurodegenerative disease where exploration is only in its infancy.

Pitfalls

Biological studies of aging and dementia in human and laboratory animals are complicated by a variety of problems which can be difficult to resolve:

(1) Species and strain differences undoubtedly exist with respect to the onset and extent of normal aging (see Table 19.1)

(2) Aging may be a heterogeneous process involving individual variability within a normal population (see, for example, Fischer et al., 1989)

(3) Heterogeneity of the aging process may be due to factors unrelated to normal aging, such as superimposed disease. In human studies for example, the normal aged population may include preclinical cases of Alzheimer's disease

(4) Discrepancies may arise in the conclusions reached from different studies of aging as a result of the precise brain area, number of individuals and age range that are selected

(5) The question of whether age- or disease-related changes are sufficiently extensive to be functionally significant depends on the degree of redundancy or compensation in neuronal circuitry

(6) Neurodegenerative changes in aging and disease may be obscured by compensatory mechanisms such as axonal sprouting, changes in transmitter release or receptor number, affinity and cellular responses

(7) Functional disturbances may reflect changes in subtle neurophysiological mechanisms which, unlike relatively crude measures of neuron numbers, transmitter, enzyme or receptor levels, cannot be investigated readily

Table 19.1. *Influence of aging on cholinergic activities in mammalian brain*[a]

Activity	Parameter	Observation	Species	References
Basal forebrain perikarya	Number	25% loss from 60–90 years, affecting minority of individuals	Human	Bigl et al., 1987; Perry & Perry, 1988
		23% loss from 0–90 years 20% loss in septum and diagonal band	Human	Lowes-Hummel et al., 1989
			Rat	Fischer et al., 1989; Nunzi et al., 1989
	Size	Shrinkage	Mouse	Mesulam et al., 1987
		Decrease in cross section in memory impaired aged group	Rat	Fischer et al., 1989; Altavista et al., 1990
	Acetylcholinesterase	Decrease (30%) in number of positive neurons	Rat	Altavista et al., 1990
	NGF receptor	Shrinkage and vacuolation in subpopulation of aged	Rat	Koh & Loy, 1988; Koh et al., 1989
	Firing	Alterations in septohippocampal neurons in subgroup with impaired performance	Rat	Lamour et al., 1989
Acetylcholine	Level	Increased	Rat	Takei et al., 1989
		Unchanged, together with choline	Mouse	Yavin et al., 1989

Table 19.1. *Contd*

Activity	Parameter	Observation	Species	References
	Release	Extracellular release from cortex decreased 50%	Rat	Wu et al., 1988
		Slice release on electrical stimulation decreased 50%	Rat	Giovannelli et al., 1988
		Reduction on K+ evoked release	Rat	Vannucchi & Pepeu, 1987; Takei et al., 1989; Araujo et al., 1990
		Nucleus basalis stimulated release unchanged	Rat	Kurosawa et al., 1989
High affinity choline uptake		Decrease (offset by acetylcarnitine)	Rat	Curti et al., 1989
		Reduction in cortex	Rat	Williams & Rylett, 1990
Choline acetyltransferase	Enzyme activity	Decline in forebrain, best predictor spatial learning deficits	Rat	Gallagher et al., 1990
		Cortical reduction in Fisher, but not Wistar, strain	Rat	Michalek et al., 1989
		Cortical reduction correlated with declining memory and paradoxical sleep	Rat	Stone et al., 1989

	Decrease in hippocampus, forebrain, amygdaloid nucleus	Rat	Springer et al., 1989; Araujo et al., 1990; Goudsmit et al., 1990 Hiramatsu et al., 1989
	Hippocampal decline (offset by Chinese herbal drug)	Rat	
	No change in cortex and hippocampus (Wistar strain)	Rat	Sirvio et al., 1988a,b; Schwarz et al., 1990
	Decline in hippocampus and cortex from 60–100 years	Human	Perry & Perry, 1988
Immunohistochemistry	Enlarged processes and clusters (as in Alzheimer's disease)	Rat	Armstrong et al., 1988
Modulation	Increase after learning in young but not old (impaired learning)	Rat	Nakamura & Ishihara, 1989
Acetylcholinesterase Enzyme activity	Reduction in hippocampus and cortex	Rat	Springer et al., 1989; Haba et al., 1988; Pintor et al., 1988; Sirvio et al., 1988a,b, 1989a; Nakamura & Ishihara, 1989
Modulation	Increase in young but not old after training	Rat	Nakamura & Ishihara, 1989
Histochemistry	Abnormal neurites increased (preceding βA4 deposits)	Monkey	Cork et al., 1990

Table 19.1. *Contd*

Activity	Parameter	Observation	Species	References
		Modest loss of neurites in entorhinal and temporal cortex	Human	Geula & Mesulam, 1989
	Solubility	Proportion of detergent soluble enzyme decreased	Rat	Sirvio et al., 1989b
Muscarinic receptor	Ligand binding site number	Decline in cortex and hippocampus	Rat	Popova & Petkov, 1989; Araujo et al., 1990; Schwartz et al., 1990
		M_1 and M_2 reduction in cortex	Rat	Biegon et al., 1989
		Decrease in temporal cortex (autoradiography) preceding memory deficit	Monkey	Wagster et al., 1990
		Reduction in several areas, including cortex correlates with working memory impairment	Rat	Kadar et al., 1990
		Reduction in substantia innominata, cortex and hippocampus	Human	Cortes et al., 1987; Rinne, 1987

Affinity	Increase in K_d	Rat	Sirvio et al., 1988a,b; Peitrzak et al., 1989
PI response	Unchanged	Rat	Surichamorn et al., 1989
	Increase after septohippocampal lesion retained	Rat	Court et al., 1990
CAMP formation	Inhibition unchanged in hippocampus	Rat	Abdallah et al., 1990
DFP modulation	Normal receptor down regulation absent in some aged individuals	Rat	Pintor et al., 1988
	Recovery after down regulation delayed	Rat	Pintor et al., 1990
Ethanol modulation	Increase in young (50%) absent in aged	Rat	Peitrzak et al., 1989
Scopolamine modulation	Changes in induced young but not aged	Mouse	Pilch and Muller, 1988a,b
	Similar in young and aged	Rat	Peitrzak et al., 1989
	Induced EEG changed decreased	Rat	Buzsaki et al., 1988
Arecoline modulation	Induced increase in glucose utilization unchanged	Rat	Soncrant et al., 1989
Nicotinic receptor			
Ligand binding site number	Dramatic loss from 1–14 months	Rat	Zhang et al., 1990

Table 19.1. *Contd*

Activity	Parameter	Observation	Species	References
		Decrease in temporal cortex precedes memory deficit	Monkey	Wagster et al., 1990
		Reduction in hippocampus and cortex	Rat	Araujo et al., 1990
		Reduction in hippocampus 40–90 years	Human	E. K. Perry et al., 1987
		Steady decline in frontal cortex from maturity to tenth decade	Human	Court et al., 1993
	Immunohistochemistry	Positive neurons in cortex decreased 50% from middle to old age	Human	Schröder et al., 1991
Trophic	NFG binding	Decrease in hippocampus and basal forebrain (offset by acetylcarnitine)	Rat	Angelucci et al., 1988
	NGF receptor/ Immunohistochemistry	Decline in number of positive neurons in diagonal band in subpopulation, correlated closely with spatial learning	Rat	Koh & Loy, 1988; Koh et al., 1989
		Reduction in terminal and fibre reactivity in hippocampus (30–90 years)	Human	Kerwin et al., 1991

	Description	Species	Reference
	Decreased basal forebrain neuronal and absent dendritic reactivity	Rat	Gomez-Pinilla et al., 1989
	Decreased number and size of reactive neurons in septum	Rat	Markram & Segal, 1990
NGF	Decreased in forebrain	Rat	Larkfors et al., 1988
	Decline in hippocampus, postnatally	Monkey	Hayashi et al., 1990
	Unchanged in hippocampus, increased in cortex, no relation to memory impairment	Rat	Hellwig et al., 1990
NGF mRNA	Decreased in Fisher but not Sprague Dawley strain	Rat	Larkfors et al., 1987
NGF effect	Ameliorates spatial deficits in old, impaired, individuals	Rat	Fischer et al., 1987
	Stimulation of choline acetyltransferase and high affinity uptake to same extent in young and old	Rat	Williams & Rylett, 1990

[a]Based on reports from 1987 to 1991 on postmaturity aging effects on basal forebrain cholinergic neurons and target areas (unless otherwise stated).

Abbreviations: CAMP, cyclic adenosine monophosphate; DFP, di-isopropylfluorophosphate; EEG, electroencepholograph; K_d, dissociation constant; K^+, potassium; M_1 and M_2, subtypes of the muscarinic receptors; PI, phosphoinositide (hydrolytic response).

(8) Disease studies (especially in postmortem human brain) include end-stage abnormalities; primary pathological events may be obscured or even obliterated

(9) In comparisons between control and diseased human populations, it is often impossible to match for certain variables (drug effects or agonal status in degenerative dementia, for example)

In spite of these caveats, the current literature on the role of the cholinergic system provides an overwhelming body of evidence suggesting a critical involvement of this transmitter in both aging and dementia.

Aging

The seminal work of Drachman & Leavitt (1974) on the effects of the anticholinergic drug scopolamine in human volunteers originally drew attention to the role of the cholinergic system in the aging human brain. Normal young volunteers so treated experienced memory deficits similar to those observed in elderly subjects. Together with clinical observations that the elderly are generally much more susceptible than younger adults to the side effects of anticholinergic medication (Hicks & Davis, 1980) – an increased vulnerability to atropine 'psychosis' which includes acute confusion and delirium – the experimental work suggested strongly that there was an age-related decline in cholinergic activity in the human brain. Over 15 years later, studies on laboratory animals from a number of research groups, notably those of Fischer et al. (1987, 1989) have revealed that amongst aging rodents a subpopulation of animals with severe memory impairment exists with degenerative changes in basal forebrain cholinergic neurons (Table 19.1). The inconsistencies in the literature in the intervening period, regarding both human and laboratory animal central nervous system (CNS) cholinergic activity as a function of aging, no doubt reflect, at least partly, problems associated with some of the factors outlined above.

The conclusions of Michael Decker, reviewing the subject in 1987, were as follows:

> The oft-stated generalization that normal aging is characterized by disruption of cholinergic input to the hippocampus and cortex is not

entirely correct. Instead it appears that age-related changes are not consistently found on measures such as the activity of ChAT [choline acetyltransferase] or the content of ACh [acetylcholine] in these regions, basal levels of ACh release in cortex, and the number of cholinergic neurons in the basal forebrain. The responsivity of the cholinergic system, however, is altered during normal aging. ACh synthesis and stimulation-induced release of ACh are diminished in aged animals. Further, the electrophysiological response of postsynaptic neurons to ACh is reduced during aging.

A fresh appraisal of the subject based on numerous studies reported since then – to the beginning of 1991 (see Table 19.1) is that if proper account is taken of species and regional variations and attention given to the possible existence of behaviourally impaired subgroups within the aged population, then the 'oft-stated generalization' is more than amply justified with respect to most aspects of the cholinergic system.

All the cholinergic parameters so far measured (Table 19.1) undergo age-related changes in most of, if not all, the reported studies. The enzyme choline acetyltransferase which synthesizes acetylcholine and was considered previously to be an 'inconsistent' measure of aging is reported as being decreased in eight of 10 independent investigations (Table 19.1). Negative findings may well relate to species differences, since, according to Michalek et al. (1989), the enzyme declines in Fisher (which may experience accelerated aging) but not Wistar or Sprague Dawley rat strains. The cholinergic enzyme loss in the aged animals reported in one study (Gallagher et al., 1990) was, amongst 15 neurochemical parameters investigated, the most accurate predictor of spatial learning deficits. Also of particular interest are the findings of Nakamura & Ishihara (1989) that young, but not old animals, experience an increase in choline acetyltransferase as a result of learning, and of Hiramatsu et al., (1989) that the Chinese herbal medicine, sho-saiko-to-go-keishi-ka-shakuyaku-to, offsets the hippocampal age-related enzyme loss. A further striking correlation between cholinergic neurochemical activity and memory decline in the aged rodent is provided by Koh and Loy (1988), who reported a correlation coefficient in excess of 0.7 for the atrophy of NGF receptor positive basal forebrain neurons related to the extent of spatial learning. The decline in cortical and forebrain NGF binding evident in aged rats is reportedly offset by acetylcarnitine (Angelucci et al., 1988) and other drug effects included prevention in the age-related decline in cortical muscarinic receptor binding by piracetam (Pilch & Muller, 1988a,b).

Although the numbers of muscarinic receptors are reported consistently to decline with age, alterations in linked second messenger activities (such as phosphoinositide turnover) are not apparent (Table 19.1). Age-related changes in receptor responses, for example those induced by drugs (Table 19.1), would thus seem to reflect primarily a decline in the number of molecules present – although changes in muscarinic

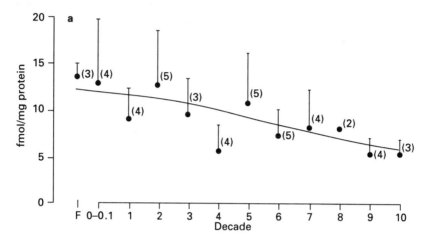

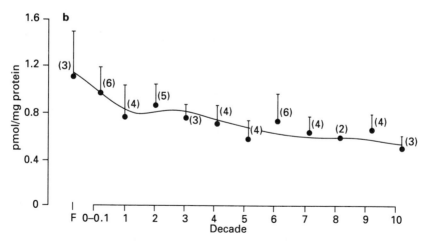

Figure 19.1. Loss of (a) nicotinic (nicotine) binding and (b) glutamate N-methyl-D-aspartate (MK801) binding in the normal human frontal cortex (Brodmann area 9) as a function of age. Points and bars represent mean values ± standard deviation (numbers of individuals in parentheses). On the 'Decades' scale, F refers to fetal cases and 0–0.1 refers to neonates and those under 1 year. Correlation coefficients were, respectively, 0.470 (p<0.001) and 0.596 (p<0.001) for the nicotine and (^{3}H) MK801-binding versus age.

receptor affinity have also been reported (Sirvio et al., 1988a; Peitrzak et al., 1989). In addition to muscarinic receptor binding, the nicotinic receptor undergoes an even more extensive age-related decline which may occur at an earlier stage (before or at maturity, see Figure 19.1 and Table 19.1). Such a trend, linking the developmental and aging period, raises the question of whether the two stages can be considered separately. A continuum may exist, for example, between neuronal elimination during development and postmaturity. Interestingly, the number of nicotinic, but not muscarinic, receptors declines further in Alzheimer's disease, being lower than in age-matched (elderly) controls (Table 19.2).

Very few of the recent published reports on the cholinergic system of the aging mammalian brain have included man. Explanations may include the difficulty of obtaining clinically and pathologically assessed normal tissue over a span of up to 10 decades. Moreover, Decker's (1987) review pinpointed a high degree of controversy amongst the various reports on human brain published previously, with equal numbers of authors claiming a significant decrease or no change in choline acetyltransferase in the neocortex or hippocampus.

An investigation of 66 individuals, each screened carefully for the absence of neurological or psychiatric disease (and, in the older cases, for the absence of significant neuropathological abnormality) and aged between 28 weeks gestation to 93 years has indicated clearcut area-specific changes in the enzyme choline acetyltransferase (see the published reports in Table 19.1). These are evident (Figure 19.2) most strikingly in the hippocampus – an area which, despite variations in the size and cortical convolutions of individual human brains, can be dissected consistently. The decline in activity postmaturity is evident in this area in middle age (from 30 to 40 years) onwards and occurs later in the adjacent entorhinal cortex. Interestingly, in the cerebellum there is no obvious decline postmaturity but, in contrast, a dramatic loss occurs perinatally. The latter may reflect the less 'plastic' nature of the adult compared with the developing cerebellum or the postnatal development of other neuronal systems. The contrast in age-related trends in cholinergic enzyme activity in human brain between archicortical areas, such as the hippocampus, and the cerebellum is of further interest in view of the susceptibility of the former, but not the latter, to neuritic plaque formation. Thus, although amyloid or βA4-amyloid reactive deposits are evident throughout the human nervous system with increasing age, neuritic plaques involving degenerating or reactive, proliferating neuronal processes are confined generally

Table 19.2. *Comparison of cholinergic activities in aging, Alzheimer's and Lewy body disease[a]*

Activity	Parameter	Aging[b]	Alzheimer's disease	Lewy body dementia[c]
Basal forebrain perikarya	Neuron number	Modest reduction	Loss varies from minimal to extensive	Extensive reduction in demented Parkinson cases
	Neuron size	Shrinkage	Shrinkage	nd
Transmitter synthesis	High affinity choline uptake	Decreased	Decreased	nd
	Choline acetyltransferase	Enzyme activity decreased / Immunocytochemical abnormalities	Decrease in enzyme activity correlated with degree dementia / Immunocytochemical abnormalities	Decreased, extensively in hallucinating cases / nd
Transmitter storage/and release	Evoked release	Diminished	nd	nd
	Vesamicol binding	nd	Increased	nd
Transmitter degradation	Acetylcholinesterase	Activity decreased, neuritic abnormalities	Decreased, including loss of histochemically reactive neurites	Decreased
Receptors	Muscarinic	Decrease in number of ligand binding sites/ increase in affinity	Number decreased or unchanged	Increased number

Nicotinic	Decrease in number of ligand binding and immunoreactive sites	Decreased	Decreased
Trophic NGF NGF mRNA	Decreased/normal Decreased	nd Normal in cortex and hippocampus	nd
NGF receptor	Immunohistochemical loss (neuronal and neurite)	Reduction in positive neurons and possibly neurites	Immunoreactive neurons reduced by 90% (demented Parkinson's cases)
	mRNA decreased (?)	Overall level unchanged, increased mRNA in surviving neurons	nd

[a] Activities in Alzheimer's and Lewy body disease are compared with age-matched (i.e. elderly) controls. For references on cholinergic neurochemistry in Alzheimer's disease, see reviews by Perry (1986, 1988), Cummings & Benson (1987), Giacobini et al. (1989) and including nerve growth factor (NGF) (Perry, 1990a,b). Other original papers include those on vesamicol binding (Ruberg et al., 1990), the nicotinic receptor (E. K. Perry et al., 1990d; Sugaya et al., 1990) and NGF (Enfors et al., 1990; Kerwin et al., 1991); original references on the cholinergic system in Lewy body dementia include Dickson et al. (1987) and E. K. Perry et al. (1990a,b,c); and on NGF in Parkinson's disease (Mufson et al., 1991).

[b] Changes in aging are an amalgamation of human and animal data (see Table 19.1).

[c] The term Lewy body dementia used here is inclusive of dementia in Parkinson's disease.

nd, Data not available.

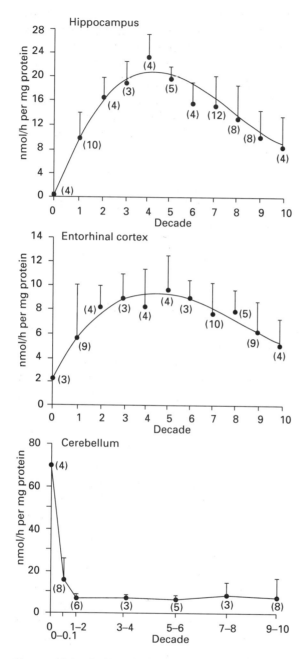

Figure 19.2. Choline acetyltransferase as a function of age in the normal human brain. Points and bars represent mean values ± standard deviation (number of individuals in parentheses). On the 'Decades' scale, zero refers to fetal cases and 0–0.1 refers to neonates and those under 1 year.

to the cortex, being particularly dense in the archicortex. These are very occasionally apparent in fifth and sixth decades and become progressively more common until, in the tenth decade, it is rare for an individual not to be affected to some degree (R. H. Perry et al., 1990b). From this scenario, it is apparent that neurochemical changes are evident in transmitter systems such as the cholinergic at a stage before neuritic plaque formation occurs, a conclusion also reached by Cork et al. (1990) in their study of acetylcholinesterase in the cerebral cortex of the rhesus monkey (Table 19.1). Neuritic, as opposed to non-neuritic βA4 reactive, plaques may reflect neurodegenerative events, therefore, and not just the deposition of amyloid.

The age-related decline in choline acetyltransferase in the human hippocampus (60% in the tenth compared with the third decade) is more extensive than that evident in the aging rodent brain. This species difference is consistent with previous investigations which include, for example, a loss of over half the substantia nigra neurons in the human brain (third to tenth decade) compared with a loss of less than 20% in rodents (reviewed by Cotman & Peterson (1989)). The reasons for such a difference are not clear but could include the greatly extended lifespan of man and perhaps the inadvertent inclusion of preclinical cases of CNS disease in amongst the older normal individuals.

The latter explanation for the extensive cholinergic enzyme loss in the cortex becomes more likely if the view is upheld that all individuals progress, to a greater or lesser extent with increasing age, towards Alzheimer's disease. A further unresolved issue is the functional significance of the loss of cholinergic activity in the normal aging human hippocampus. None of the individuals included suffered from dementia, an aspect which was closely investigated through contact with clinical and nursing staff or relatives at the time of autopsy and which indicated that mental ability and, in the adults, the capacity for self care were not in doubt. However, the group was not assessed for the presence or absence of milder forms of cognitive impairment – a daunting task given the great variation in, for example, learning between individuals and the need to repeat assessments at regular intervals. Therefore, it can be only a matter for speculation that the extensive (over 50%) decline in hippocampal cholinergic activity may relate to moderate deficits in working memory experienced by many elderly people. Such deficits include information processing in general and the period required for learning and recall, especially in tasks requiring division of attention (Crook et al., 1986). However, from the quantitative viewpoint it can be stated with certainty, that symptoms of dementia are not evident until the neurochemical deficit exceeds 60% – a reduction which is close to the 70% apparent in the older cases of Alzheimer's disease compared with young controls (Figure 19.3).

Of great interest to the theme of the present chapter is the finding that in a parallel series of clinically and pathologically established cases of Alzheimer's disease (E. K. Perry et al., 1990d; R. H. Perry et al., 1990a), an opposite trend was apparent with increasing age (Figure 19.3). The younger cases of the disease demonstrated a more extensive cholinergic enzyme loss than the older cases – an observation not in itself new – and in the hippocampus the normal and diseased groups were much less clearly distinguished in the ninth decade (no cases with Alzheimer's disease were available for study in the tenth decade). These trends are discussed more fully in the following section.

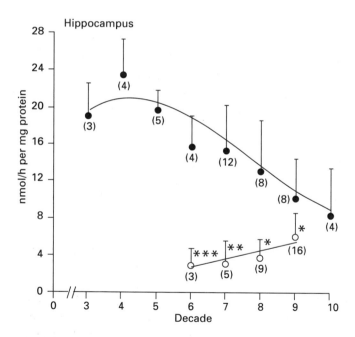

Figure 19.3. Choline acetyltransferase in Alzheimer's disease (open circles) compared with normal (filled circles; see also Figure 19.1) cases as a function of age. Points and bars represent mean ± standard deviation (number of individuals in parentheses). Differences between the normal group and the group with Alzheimer's disease were significant (*p<0.05, **p<0.02 and ***p<0.001).

Dementia

It is not clear whether the trend whereby the incidence of dementia rises steeply from 5% to 20% of the population, as age increases from the eighth to ninth decade, persists into the tenth decade. If the incidence does continue to rise exponentially with increasing age then, given the current absence of any effective treatment, the problems arising from substantially extending the human lifespan beyond the proverbial three score years and ten would seem to be insuperable. Whether effective treatment is likely to emerge depends on the nature of the disorder and, in the elderly, dementia can be due to a wide variety of diseases. These have been classified previously into two broad categories according to whether the disease shares the manifestations of normal aging or is associated with its own unique pathological features (Perry & Perry, 1988). In the one category, no pathological feature is specific to the disease process; each is apparent to a lesser extent in the brains of many normal old people. The two principal examples of this category of disease, which account for the majority of demented old people, are dementia of the Alzheimer and cerebrovascular types. The classical neuropathological features of these – plaques, tangles and ischaemia, for example – are evident to a limited extent in the majority of the normal elderly population (Tomlinson et al., 1968) and also in other related diseases such as Parkinson's (R. H. Perry et al., 1990a). In the other category, the neuropathological features are not evident in the normal aging human brain and tend to distinguish the disease from all others. Included in this category are much rarer diseases such as Pick's, Creutzfeldt–Jakob's, Gerstmann–Straussler, Binswanger's, Hallervorden–Spatz and Huntington's disease, together with a range of conditions associated with dementia arising from traumatic, neoplastic, infectious, dietary or toxic (e.g. alcoholic) events. It is not yet entirely clear to which of these categories Parkinson's disease, which is sometimes associated with dementia, and Lewy body dementia (variously described as diffuse Lewy body disease, senile dementia of the Lewy body type, Lewy body variant of Alzheimer's disease) belong. It has been argued recently that Lewy bodies (unlike plaques) are not associated with the normal aging process, being present in under 3% of normal individuals over the age of 70 years, and that their presence in the brain denotes specifically the existence of Lewy body disease, which includes a spectrum of psychiatric and neurological disorders (E. K. Perry et al., 1990b). Thus, Lewy body dementia would appear to belong to the second disease category. The increased occurrence of Alzheimer-type pathology in Lewy body dementia and Parkinson's disease, together with many of the category 2 diseases (Perry & Perry, 1989) should not incidentally confuse the issue of classification, since a wide variety of insults may, as a secondary feature, lead to accelerated aging.

The implications of this basic classification scheme are that the aetiology of diseases such as Alzheimer's is, like individual aging, complex, involving a variety of interacting genetic and environmental factors and that prevention will, in the majority of cases, be extremely difficult. In contrast, those diseases with a specific pathology may be due to a single aetiopathological factor which can be more readily identified and controlled. Whatever the ultimate merits of this classification system, it is worth comparing the neurochemistry of diseases in both categories with that of normal aging. Alzheimer's disease and Lewy body dementia provide common examples of each type in which the cholinergic system has been examined in some detail.

A comparison of various cholinergic parameters in normal aging, Alzheimer and Lewy body type of dementia is provided in Table 19.2. The proposal that Alzheimer's disease represents an extension of the normal aging process is supported clearly by the data on cell counts, choline acetyltransferase, acetylcholinesterase and the nicotinic receptor. The original data illustrated in Figure 19.3 provide further convincing evidence that, regarding choline acetyltransferase in at least the hippocampus, the normal group and the group with Alzheimer's disease tend to converge with increasing age. In those over 80 years of age, the overlap between the two groups is extensive and, as with the prevalence of plaque formation in archicortical areas, it is often difficult to allocate an individual case to the correct clinical category (normal or demented) on the basis of a section of the hippocampus. Such a degree of convergence is not evident in neocortical areas, but that it is so obvious in the archicortex supports the notion that aging and Alzheimer's disease are distinguishable only by degree – both in quantitative and regional anatomical terms.

The situation is less clear regarding the muscarinic receptor which, in contrast to normal aging, is not reported consistently to be further reduced in the disease compared with age-matched controls (Table 19.2). Alterations in vesamicol binding, a measure of acetylcholine storage in, and release from, synaptic vesicles, are also difficult to interpret, since this parameter does not change in the experimentally cholinergic-lesioned animal brain and increases in the disease may reflect compensatory mechanisms in surviving neurites (Ruberg et al.,

1990). Further evidence that Alzheimer's disease may not be an exaggeration of aging is to be found in reports that NGF mRNA is unchanged, compared with age-matched controls, in the disease, despite being reduced in aging (Tables 19.1 and 19.2). Since reports on NGF in aging are controversial, however, and since this molecule is thought to be synthesized by pyramidal neurons which in, for example, the hippocampus, undergo degenerative changes in Alzheimer's disease, the data need to be interpreted cautiously at this stage.

The proposal that Alzheimer and Lewy body type of dementia involve fundamentally different mechanisms, the latter also differing from normal aging, does not immediately receive substantial support from the investigations of the cholinergic system so far conducted (Table 19.2). Thus, although neuronal loss and (in the majority of Lewy body dementia cases suffering from visual hallucinations (E. K. Perry et al., 1990a)) reductions in choline acetyltransferase are more extensive than in cases with Alzheimer's disease, these differences appear to be quantitative. Strong correlations between neuronal loss and the cortical cholinergic enzyme evident in Parkinson's, but not Alzheimer's, disease (Perry et al., 1985) do indicate, however, that qualitative differences may exist. Whereas, as in Alzheimer's disease and, to a lesser extent, aging, degeneration of the basal forebrain cholinergic system appears to be retrograde, in Parkinson's disease and perhaps also Lewy body dementia the pathology may be primarily subcortical in origin.

A clearcut qualitative difference between Alzheimer and Lewy body types of dementia is evident in the behaviour of the muscarinic receptor (Table 19.2). The increase in binding sites (primarily M_1 subtype) reported consistently in Parkinson's disease and also apparent in Lewy body dementia (E. K. Perry et al., 1990a) is not generally apparent in Alzheimer's disease. Previously, it has been argued that this difference may reflect the presence of tangles in cholinoceptive neurons in Alzheimer's disease which interferes with the normal supersensitive response to denervation (E. K. Perry et al., 1990d). Whether or not this is so, the alteration in Lewy body disease is the opposite to that seen in normal aging and as such provides at least one firm line of evidence that this type of dementia is distinct from the aging process.

Whatever the theoretical considerations, a practical aspect of the increased muscarinic receptor binding in Lewy body but not Alzheimer type dementia is the implication for therapy. Thus, if cholinoceptive neurons are demonstrating their functional integrity by expressing increased numbers of receptors, potential cholinergic therapy such as anticholinesterase drugs aimed at increasing synaptic acetylcholine may be more effective in Lewy body compared with Alzheimer-type dementia. The same conclusion is reached on the basis of the greatly increased number of cortical neurofibrillary tangles in the latter compared with the former. One further consideration regarding drug treatment of the cholinergic deficit in dementia is the increasing evidence of a loss of nicotinic receptor sites. As investigations become progressively more refined with respect to receptor subtypes, cellular localization (immunohistochemistry) and autoradiographic analysis, it is clear that the receptor loss may be more extensive (>75%) than reported previously (Whitehouse et al., 1988; Sugaya et al., 1990; Schröder et al., 1991, Perry et al., unpublished observations). Thus, cholinergic therapeutic strategies may need to include attempts to raise the level of the receptor by co-administering nicotine, for example. Administration of nicotine itself or in tobacco is associated with an increase in receptor numbers (Wonnacott, 1987) and, since the receptor declines so inexorably during aging (Figure 19.1) any attempts to offset this trend might well be beneficial. Most interestingly, it has been claimed recently that, in familial Alzheimer's disease, onset of dementia is delayed by an average of six years in members of the family who use tobacco (van Duijn & Hofman, 1991). Unfortunately, smoking is not itself renowned for prolonging human life, although nicotine administered orally or transdermally may, with appropriate dosage, be relatively free of untoward side effects. No doubt the nicotinic receptor will receive greater attention from the viewpoint of therapy in dementia over the next decade.

Emerging concepts

It remains to be determined whether the division of dementing disorders into categories according to the relation they bear to the normal aging process is justified. An extensive body of information, both histopathological and neurochemical, undoubtedly supports the concept of a continuum between aging and Alzheimer's disease – at least with respect to the majority of parameters and brain regions. Amongst the theoretical implications of such a connection (mentioned in the first section), one important outcome in relation to future research strategies is that examining the normal aging process in such areas as the human hippocampus may provide a valuable 'model' – perhaps one of the best available – for the earliest stages of Alzheimer's disease. The present findings in the aging human hippocampus for example suggest that functional or degenerative changes in the cholinergic input may precede the formation of neuritic plaques, and that amyloid deposition does not necessarily initiate the pathological cascade. It may well be that disturbances in the metabolism of the amyloid precursor protein precede both events.

The postulate that diseases such as Parkinson's disease and Lewy body dementia are distinct from the normal aging process gains some support from the present analysis but would benefit from further neuropathological and neurochemical data – not only on the cholinergic but also on other transmitter systems which are affected. The nigrostriatal system degenerates in both diseases to a greater or lesser extent (for comparisons, see E. K. Perry et al., 1990c) and it would be interesting to determine whether a similar convergence (as seen in the hippocampus) between aging normal and diseased subjects occurs in this pathway.

The recently discovered role of trophic factors in the nervous system has opened up major new avenues in neurodegenerative disease and aging research. In terms of the programmed cell death which occurs during development and aging, trophic factor interaction constitutes a most likely candidate as a key controlling mechanism. Whether such degeneration is due to decreased trophic factor production by the target tissue or receptor interaction and consequential events within the neuron is unclear. The evidence so far obtained on the cholinergic system in both aging and Alzheimer's disease (Tables 19.1 and 19.2) tends to suggest that the synthesis and production of NGF may be unimpaired, that the receptor is still present on surviving neurons (perhaps even at increased levels, by way of compensation), but that neurons lose their responsiveness progressively. This is supported by the presence of neuritic abnormalities and cholinergic enzyme deficits generally in excess of the actual loss of neurons. Some, as yet undetermined, factor must be responsible for the retrograde degeneration, suggested by extensive reductions in terminal cholinergic enzyme but only modest loss of the basal forebrain neurons. Degeneration could relate to impaired axonal transport of NGF and/or its receptor complex, the response of the neuron to NGF at the level of gene transcription, or perhaps an involvement not of NGF but of one of the other closely related trophic factors such as BDNF.

Whilst the basal forebrain cholinergic system may be especially vulnerable to aging and CNS disease (perhaps for the same reason that it plays a role in memory – its very 'plasticity' or adaptability – see E. K. Perry et al. (1990c), there is no doubt that many of the other neurotransmitter systems are also affected. Thus, changes in the aging human brain such as impaired vision and hearing together with alterations in mood and sleep patterns and perhaps even positive aspects, such as wisdom and in some instances increased creativity, are likely to have a biological counterpart in age-related changes of other neuronal populations. There is no doubt a need to consider these different systems not only individually but also in conjunction with each other. In relation to transmitter interactions, for example, the incidence of visual hallucinations in Lewy body dementia appears to be related to a monoaminergic : cholinergic imbalance in the cortex (E. K. Perry et al., 1990a). Interestingly, hallucinatory experiences decline from childhood to adulthood and rapid eye movement sleep (which parallels hallucinoid imagery during dreaming) decreases progressively from infancy to old age (see Leonard (1992), pp. 14–17). Such age-related trends may reflect the earlier development and decline of monoaminergic (for example serotonergic) compared with cholinergic activity in the human brain with increasing age. The prospects for future research on the aging human brain, particularly conducted in conjunction with cognitive assessments, clearly extend beyond the investigation of age-related disease to an understanding of some of the great mysteries of the mind itself.

Acknowledgement   Very many thanks to Mrs M. Middlemist for preparation of this manuscript and especially the tables.

References

Abdallah, E. A. M., Pou, W. S. & el-Fakahanay, E. E. (1990). Aging does not alter muscarinic receptor mediated inhibitor of cyclic AMP formation in the striatum and hippocampus. *Brain Research*, **534**, 234–6.

Altavista, M. C., Rossi, P., Bentivoglio, A. R., Crociani, P. & Albanese, A. (1990). Aging is associated with a diffuse impairment of forebrain cholinergic neurons. *Brain Research*, **508**, 51–9.

Angelucci, L., Ramacci, M. T., Taglialatela, G., Hulsebosch, C., Morgan, B., Werrbach-Perez, K. & Perez-Polo, R. (1988). Nerve growth factor binding in aged rat central nervous system: effect of acetyl-L-carnitine. *Journal of Neuroscience Research*, **20**, 491–6.

Araujo, D. M., Lapchak, P. A., Meaney, M. J., Collier, B. & Quirion, R. (1990). Effects of aging on nicotinic and muscarinic autoreceptor function in the rat brain: relationship to presynaptic cholinergic markers and binding sites. *Journal of Neuroscience*, **10**, 3069–78.

Armstrong, D. M., Hersh, L. B. & Gage, F. H. (1988). Morphologic alterations of cholinergic processes in the neocortex of aged rats. *Neurobiology of Aging*, **9**, 199–205.

Biegon, A., Hanau, M., Greenberger, V. & Segal, M. (1989). Aging and brain cholinergic muscarinic receptor subtypes: an autoradiographic study in the rat. *Neurobiology of Aging*, **10**, 305–10.

Bigl, V., Arendt, T., Fischer, S., Werner, M. & Arendt, A. (1987). The cholinergic system in aging. *Gerontology*, **33**, 172–80.

Buck, C. R., Martinez, H. J., Chao, M. V. & Black, L. B. (1988). Differential expression of the nerve growth factor receptor gene in multiple brain areas. *Developmental Brain Research*, **44**, 259–68.

Buzsaki, G., Bickford, R. G., Armstrong, D. M., Ponomareff, G., Chen, K. S., Ruiz, R., Thal, L. J. & Gage, F. H. (1988). Electric activity in the neocortex of freely moving young and aged rats. *Neuroscience*, **26**, 735–44.

Cork, L. C., Masters, C., Beyreuther, K. & Price, D. L. (1990). Development of senile plaques. Relationships of neuronal abnormalities and amyloid deposits. *American Journal of Pathology*, **137**, 1383–92.

Cortes, R., Probst, A. & Palacios, J. M. (1987). Quantitative light microscopic autoradiographic localization of cholinergic muscarinic receptors in the human brain: forebrain. *Neuroscience*, **20**, 65–107.

Cotman, C. W. & Peterson, C. (1989). Aging in the nervous system. In G. J. Siegel (ed.) *Basic Neurochemistry*, pp. 523–40. Raven Press, New York.

Court, J. A., Keith, A. B., Kerwin, J. M. & Perry, E. K. (1990). Fimbria-fornix lesions in aged rats cause increased carbachol-stimulated phosphoinositide hydrolysis in the hippocampus but no change in muscarinic receptor binding. *Brain Research*, **532**, 333–5.

Court, J. A., Piggott, M. A., Perry, E. K., Barlow, R. B. & Perry, R. H. (1992). Age associated decline in high affinity nicotine binding in human brain frontal cortex does not correlate with changes in choline acetyltransferase. *Neuroscience Research Communications*, **10**, 125–33.

Crook, T., Bartus, R. T., Ferris, S. H., Whitehouse, P., Cohen, G. D. & Gershon, S. (1986). Age associated memory impairment. Proposed diagnostic criteria and measure of clinical change: report of a National Institute of Mental Health work group. *Developmental Neuropathology*, **2**, 261–76.

Cummings, J. L. & Benson, D. F. (1987). The role of the nucleus basalis of Meynert and dementia: review and reconsideration. *Alzheimer Disease and Associated Disorders*, **1**, 128–45.

Curti, D., Dagani, F., Galmozzi, M. R. & Marzatico, F. (1989). Effect of aging and acetyl-L-carnitine on energetic and cholinergic metabolism in rat brain regions. *Mechanisms of Ageing and Development*, **47**, 39–45.

Decker, M. W. (1987). The effects of aging on hippocampal and cortical projections of the forebrain cholinergic system. *Brain Research Reviews*, **12**, 423–38.

Dickson, D. W., Davies, P. & Mayeur, P. (1987). Diffuse Lewy body disease: neuropathological and biochemical studies of six patients. *Acta Neuropathologica*, **75**, 8–15.

Drachman, D. A. & Leavitt, J. (1974). Human memory and the cholinergic system, a relationship to aging? *Archives of Neurology*, **30**, 113–21.

Ebendal, T. (1989). NGF in CNS: experimental data and clinical implications. *Progress in Growth Research*, **1**, 143–59.

Enfors, P., Lindefors, N., Chan-Palay, V. & Persson, H. (1990). Cholinergic neurons of the nucleus basalis express elevated levels of nerve growth factor receptor mRNA in senile dementia of the Alzheimer type. *Dementia*, **1**, 125–37.

Fischer, W., Wictorin, K., Bjorklund, A., Williams, L. R., Varon, S. & Gage, F. H. (1987). Amelioration of cholinergic neuron atrophy and spatial memory impairment in aged rats by nerve growth factor. *Nature*, **329**, 65–8.

Fischer, W., Gage, F. H. & Bjorklund, A. (1989). Degenerative changes in forebrain cholinergic nuclei correlate with cognitive impairments in aged rats. *European Journal of Neuroscience*, **1**, 34–45.

Gallagher, M., Burwell, R. D., Kodsi, M. H., McKinney, M., Southerland, S., Vella-Rountree, L. & Lewis, M. H. (1990). Markers for biogenic amines in the aged rat brain: relationship to decline in spatial learning ability. *Neurobiology of Aging*, **11**, 507–14.

Geula, C. & Mesulam, M. M. (1989). Cortical cholinergic fibres in aging and Alzheimer's disease. *Neuroscience*, **33**, 469–81.

Giacobini, E., DeSarno, P., Clark, B. & McIlhany, M. (1989). The cholinergic receptor system in the human brain: neurochemical and pharmacological aspects in aging and Alzheimer's disease. *Progress in Brain Research*, **29**, 335–43.

Giovannelli, L., Giovannini, M. G., Pedata, F. & Pepeu, G. (1988). Purinergic modulation of cortical acetylcholine release is decreased in aging rats. *Experimental Gerontology*, **23**, 175–81.

Gomez-Pinilla, F., Cotman, C. W. & Nieto-Sampedro, M. (1989). NGF receptor immunoreactivity in aged rat brain. *Brain Research*, **479**, 255–62.

Goudsmit, E., Luine, V. N. & Swaab, D. F. (1990). Testosterone locally increases vasopressin content but fails to restore choline acetyltransferase activity in other regions in the senescent male rat brain. *Neuroscience Letters*, **112**, 290–6.

Haba, K., Ogawa, N., Kawata, M. & Mori, A. (1988). A method for parallel determination of choline acetyltransferase and muscarinic cholinergic receptors: application in aged-rat brain. *Neurochemical Research*, **13**, 951–5.

Hayashi, M., Yamashita, A. & Shimizu, K. (1990). Nerve growth factor in the primate central nervous system: regional distribution and ontogeny. *Neuroscience*, **36**, 683–9.

Hellwig, R., Fischer, W., Hock, C., Gage, F. H., Bjorklund, A. & Thoenen, H. (1990). Nerve growth factor levels and choline acetyltransferase activity in the brain of aged rats with spatial memory impairments. *Brain Research*, **537**, 123–30.

Hicks, R. & Davis, J. M. (1980). Pharmacokinetics in geriatric psychopharmacology. In: C. Eisdorfer & W. F. Fann (eds.) *Psychopharmacology of Aging*, pp. 169–212. MTP Press Ltd., England.

Hiramatsu, M., Haba, K., Edamatsu, R., Hamada, H. & Mori, A. (1989). Increased choline acetyltransferase activity by Chinese herbal medicine Sho-saiko-to-go-keishi-ka-shakuyaku-to in aged rat brain. *Neurochemical Research*, **14**, 249–51.

Kadar, R., Silbermann, M., Weissman, B. A. & Levy, A. (1990). Age related

changes in the cholinergic components within the central nervous system.
II. Working memory impairment and its relation to hippocampal muscarinic
receptors. *Mechanisms of Ageing and Development*, **55**, 139–49.

Kerwin, J. M., Morris, C. M., Perry, R. H. & Perry, E. K. (1991). Nerve
growth factor receptor immunoreactivity in the human hippocampus.
Neuroscience Letters, **121**, 178–82.

Koh, S., Chang, P., Collier, T. J. & Loy, R. (1989). Loss of NGF receptor
immunoreactivity in basal forebrain neurons of aged rats: correlation with
spatial memory impairment. *Brain Research*, **498**, 397–404.

Koh, S. & Loy, R. (1988). Age-related loss of nerve growth factor sensitivity
in rat basal forebrain neurons. *Brain Research*, **440**, 396–401.

Kurosawa, M., Sato, A. & Sato, Y. (1989). Well-maintained responses of
acetylcholine release and blood flow in the cerebral cortex to focal electrical
stimulation of the nucleus basalis of Meynert in aged rats. *Neuroscience
Letters*, **100**, 198–202.

Lamour, Y., Bassant, M. H., Robert, A. & Joly, M. (1989). Septo-hippocampal
neurons in the aged rat: relation between their electrophysiological and
pharmacological properties and behavioural performances. *Neurobiology of
Aging*, **10**, 181–6.

Larkfors, L., Ebendal, T., Whittemore, S. R., Persson, H., Hoffer, B. &
Olson, L. (1987). Decreased level of nerve growth factor (NGF) and its
messenger RNA in the aged rat brain. *Progress in Brain Research*, **3**, 55–60.

Larkfors, L., Ebendal, T., Whittemore, S. R., Persson, H., Hoffer, B. &
Olson, L. (1988). Developmental appearance of nerve growth factor in the rat
brain: significant deficits in the aged forebrain. *Progress in Brain Research*,
78, 27–31.

Leonard, B. E. (1992). *Fundamentals of Psychopharmacology*. John Wiley and
Sons, Chichester.

Lowes-Hummel, P., Gertz, H. J., Ferszt, R. & Cervos Navarro, J. (1989). The
basal nucleus of Meynert revised: the nerve cell number decreases with age.
Archives of Gerontology and Geriatrics, **8**, 21–7.

Maisonpierre, P. C., Belluscio, L., Friedman, B., Alderson, R. F., Wigand,
S. J., Furth, M. E., Lindsay, R. M. & Yancopoulos, G. D. (1990). NT-3,
BDNF, and NGF in the developing rat nervous system: parallel as well as
reciprocal patterns of expression. *Neuron*, **5**, 501–9.

Markram, H. & Segal, M. (1990). Regional changes in NGF receptor
immunohistochemical labelling in the septum of the aged rat. *Neurobiology of
Aging*, **11**, 481–4.

Mesulam, M.-M., Mufson, E. J. & Rogers, J. (1987). Age related shrinkage
of cortically projecting cholinergic neurons: a selective effect. *Annals of
Neurology*, **22**, 31–6.

Michalek, H., Fortuna, S. & Pintor, A. (1989). Age-related differences in brain
choline acetyltransferase, cholinesterases and muscarinic receptor sites in two
strains of rats. *Neurobiology of Aging*, **10**, 143–8.

Mufson, E. J., Presley, L. N. & Kordower, J. H. (1991). Nerve growth factor
receptor immunoreactivity within the nucleus basalis (Ch4) in Parkinson's
disease: reduced cell numbers and co-localization with cholinergic neurons.
Brain Research, **539**, 19–30.

Nakamura, S. & Ishihara, T. (1989). Region selective increase in activities of

CNS cholinergic marker enzymes during learning of memory tasks in aged rats. *Pharmacology, Biochemistry and Behavior*, **34**, 805–10.

Nunzi, M. G., Milan, F., Guidolin, D., Polato, P. & Toffano, G. (1989). Effects of phosphatidylserine administration of age-related structural changes in the rat hippocampus and septal complex. *Pharmacopsychiatry*, **22**, (supplement 2), 125–8.

Peitrzak, E. R., Wilce, P. A. & Shanley, B. C. (1989). Plasticity of brain muscarinic receptors in aging rats: the adaptive response to scopolamine and ethanol treatment. *Neuroscience Letters*, **104**, 331–5.

Perry, E. K. (1986). The cholinergic hypothesis – ten years on. *British Medical Bulletin*, **42**, 63–9.

Perry, E. K. (1988). Annotation: Alzheimer's disease and acetylcholine. *British Journal of Psychiatry*, **152**, 737–40.

Perry, E. K. (1990a). Hypothesis linking plasticity, vulnerability and nerve growth factor to basal forebrain cholinergic neurons. *International Journal of Geriatric Psychiatry*, **5**, 223–32.

Perry, E. K. (1990b). Nerve growth factor and the basal forebrain cholinergic system: a link in the aetiopathology of neurodegenerative dementias? *Alzheimer Disease and Associated Disorders*, **4**, 1–13.

Perry, E. K. & Perry, R. H. (1988). Aging and dementia: neurochemical and neuropathological comparisons. In A. S. Henderson & J. H. Henderson (eds.) *Etiology of dementia of Alzheimer's type*, pp. 213–30. John Wiley and Sons, Chichester.

Perry, E. K. & Perry, R. H. (1989). Amyloid and Alzheimer's disease: a question of specificity. *Neurobiology of Aging*, **10**, 473–4.

Perry, E. K., Curtis, M., Dick, D. J., Candy, J. M., Atack, J. R., Bloxham, C. A., Blessed, G., Fairbairn, A., Tomlinson, B. E. & Perry, R. H. (1985). Cholinergic correlates of cognitive impairment in Parkinson's disease: comparisons with Alzheimer's disease. *Journal of Neurology, Neurosurgery and Psychiatry*, **48**, 413–21.

Perry, E. K., Perry, R. H., Smith, C. J., Dick, D. J., Fairbairn, A., Blessed, G., Candy, J. M., Johnson, M. & Edwardson, J. A. (1987). Nicotinic receptor abnormalities in Alzheimer's and Parkinson's disease. *Journal of Neurology, Neurosurgery and Psychiatry*, **50**, 806–9.

Perry, E. K., Kerwin, J., Perry, R. H., Irving, D., Blessed, G. & Fairbairn, A. F. (1990a). Cerebral cholinergic activity is related to the incidence of visual hallucinations in senile dementia of Lewy body type. *Dementia*, **1**, 2–4.

Perry, E. K., Marshall, E., Kerwin, J., Smith, C. J., Jabeen, S., Cheng, A. V. & Perry, R. H. (1990b). Evidence of a monoaminergic-cholinergic imbalance related to visual hallucinations in Lewy body dementia. *Journal of Neurochemistry*, **55**, 1454–6.

Perry, E. K., Marshall, E., Smith, C. J., Perry, R. H., Irving, D., Blessed, G. & Fairbairn, A. F. (1990c). Cholinergic and dopaminergic activities in senile dementia of Lewy body type. *Alzheimer Disease and Associated Disorders*, **4**, 87–95.

Perry, E. K., Smith, C. J., Court, J. A. & Perry, R. H. (1990d). Cholinergic nicotinic and muscarinic receptors in dementia of Alzheimer, Parkinson and Lewy body types. *Journal of Neural Transmission*, **2**, 149–58.

Perry, R. H., Irving, D., Blessed, G., Perry, E. K. & Fairbairn, A. F. (1989). Clinically and neuropathologically distinct form of dementia in the elderly. *Lancet*, **i**, 166.

Perry, R. H., Irving, D., Blessed, G., Fairbairn, A. F. & Perry, E. K. (1990a). Senile dementia of Lewy body type: a clinically and pathologically distinct form of Lewy body dementia. *Journal of the Neurological Sciences*, **95**, 119–35.

Perry, R. H., Irving, D. & Tomlinson, B. E. (1990b). Lewy body prevalence in the aging brain: relationship to neuropsychiatric disorders, Alzheimer-type pathology and catecholaminergic nuclei. *Journal of the Neurological Sciences*, **100**, 223–33.

Pilch, H. & Muller, W. E. (1988a). Piracetam elevates muscarinic cholinergic receptor density in the frontal cortex of aged but not of young mice. *Psychopharmacology*, **94**, 74–8.

Pilch, H. & Muller, W. E. (1988b). Chronic treatment with choline or scopolamine indicates the presence of muscarinic cholinergic receptor plasticity in the frontal cortex of young but not of aged mice. *Journal of Neural Transmission*, **71**, 39–43.

Pintor, A., Fortuna, S., Volpe, M. T. & Michalek, H. (1988). Muscarinic receptor plasticity in the brain of senescent rats; down-regulation after repeated administration of diisopropyl fluorophosphate. *Life Sciences*, **42**, 2113–21.

Pintor, A., Fortuna, S., DeAngelis, S. & Michalek, H. (1990). Impaired recovery of brain muscarinic receptor sites following an adaptive down-regulation induced by repeated administration of diisopropyl fluorophosphate in aged rats. *Life Sciences*, **46**, 1027–36.

Popova, J. S. & Petkov, V. D. (1989). Age-related changes in rat brain muscarinic receptors and betadrenoreceptors. *General Pharmacology*, **20**, 581–4.

Richardson, P. H., Verge Issa, V. M. K. & Riopelle, R. J. (1986). Distribution of neuronal receptors for nerve growth factor in the rat. *Journal of Neuroscience*, **6**, 2312–21.

Rinne, J. D. (1987). Muscarinic and dopaminergic receptors in aging human brain. *Brain Research*, **404**, 162–8.

Rodriguez-Tébar, A., Dechant, G. & Barde, Y.-A. (1990). Binding of brain derived neurotrophic factor to the nerve growth factor receptor. *Neuron*, **4**, 487–52.

Ruberg, M., Mayo, W., Brice, A., Duyckarts, C., Hauw, J. J., Simon, H., LeMoal, M. & Agid, Y. (1990). Choline acetyltransferase activity and (^{3}H)vesamicol binding in the temporal cortex of patients with Alzheimer's disease, Parkinson's disease and rats with basal forebrain lesions. *Neuroscience*, **35**, 327–32.

Schröder, H., Giacobini, E., Struble, R. G., Zilles, K. & Maelicke, A. (1991). Nicotinic cholinoceptive neurons of the frontal cortex are reduced in Alzheimer's disease. *Neurobiology of Aging*, **12**, 259–62.

Schwarz, R. D., Bernabei, A. A., Spencer, C. J. & Pugsley, T. A. (1990). Loss of muscarinic M1 receptors with aging in the cerebral cortex of Fisher 344 rats. *Pharmacology, Biochemistry and Behavior*, **35**, 589–93.

Sirvio, J., Hervonen, A. & Riekkinen, P. J. (1988a). Cholinergic binding in the hippocampus of the aging male rat. *Comparative Biochemistry and Physiology*, **90**, 161–3.

Sirvio, J., Valjakka, A., Jolkkonen, J., Hervonen, A. & Riekkinen, P. J. (1988b). Cholinergic enzyme activities and muscarinic binding in the cerebral cortex of rats of different age and sex. *Comparative Biochemistry and Physiology*, **90**, 245–8.

Sirvio, J., Pitkanen, A., Paakkonen, A., Partanen, J. & Riekkinen, P. J. (1989a). Brain cholinergic enzymes and cortical EEG activity in young and old rats. *Comparative Biochemistry and Physiology*, **94**, 277–83.

Sirvio, J., Riekkinen, P. J. & Hervonen, A. (1989b). Age-dependence of the solubility fractions of acetylcholinesterase in the cerebral cortex and cerebellum of the rat. *Neuroscience Letters*, **96**, 218–22.

Soncrant, T. T., Holloway, H. W., Greig, N. H. & Rapoport, S. I. (1989). Regional brain metabolic responsivity to the muscarinic cholinergic agonist arecoline is similar in young and Fischer-344 rats. *Brain Research*, **487**, 255–66.

Springer, J. E., Tayrien, M. W. & Loy, R. (1989). Regional analysis of age-related changes in the cholinergic system of the hippocampal formation and basal forebrain of the rat. *Brain Research*, **407**, 180–4.

Stone, W. S., Altman, H. J., Berman, R. F., Caldwell, D. F. & Kilbey, M. M. (1989). Association of sleep parameters and memory in intact old rats and young rats with lesions in the nucleus basalis magnocellularis. *Behavioral Neuroscience*, **103**, 755–64.

Storandt, M. (1988). Relationship of normal aging and dementing diseases in later life. In A. S. Henderson & J. H. Henderson (eds.) *Etiology of dementia of Alzheimer's type*, pp. 231–40. John Wiley and Sons, Chichester.

Sugaya, K., Giacobini, E. & Chiappinelli, V. A. (1990). Nicotinic acetylcholine receptor subtypes in human frontal cortex: changes in Alzheimer's disease. *Journal of Neuroscience*, **27**, 349–59.

Surichamorn, W., Abdallah, E. A. & el-Fakahanay, E. E. (1989). Aging does not alter brain muscarinic receptor-mediated phosphoinositide hydrolysis and its inhibition by phorbol esters, tetrodotoxin and receptor desensitization. *Journal of Pharmacology and Experimental Therapeutics*, **251**, 543–9.

Takei, N., Nihonmatsu, L. & Kawamura, H. (1989). Age-related decline of acetylcholine release evoked by depolarizing stimulation. *Neuroscience Letters*, **101**, 182–6.

Tomlinson, B. E., Blessed, G. & Roth, M. (1968). Observations on the brains of non-demented old people. *Journal of the Neurological Sciences*, **7**, 331–56.

van Duijn, C. & Hofman, A. (1991). Relation between nicotine intake and Alzheimer's disease. *British Medical Journal*, **302**, 1491–4.

Vannucchi, M. G. & Pepeu, G. (1987). Effect of phosphatidylserine on acetylcholine release and content in cortical slices from aging rats. *Neurobiology of Aging*, **8**, 403–7.

Wagster, M. V., Whitehouse, P. J., Walker, L. C., Kellar, K. J. & Price, D. L. (1990). Laminar organization and age-related loss of cholinergic receptors in temporal neocortex of rhesus monkey. *Journal of Neuroscience*, **10**, 2879–85.

Whitehouse, P. J., Martino, A. M., Wagster, M. V., Price, D. L., Mayeux, R., Atack, J. R. & Kellar, K. J. (1988). Reductions in (^{3}H)nicotine acetylcholine binding in Alzheimer's disease and Parkinson's disease – an autoradiographic study. *Neurology*, **38**, 720–3.

Whittemore, S. R. & Seigel, A. (1987). The expression localization and functional significance of β-nerve growth factor in the central nervous system. *Brain Research Reviews*, **12**, 439–64.

Williams, L. R. & Rylett, R. J. (1990). Exogenous nerve growth factor increases the activity of high-affinity choline uptake and choline acetyltransferase in brain of Fisher 344 male rats. *Journal of Neurochemistry*, **55**, 1042–9.

Wonnacott, S. (1987). Brain nicotine binding sites. *Human Toxicology*, **6**, 343–53.

Wu, C. F., Bertorelli, R., Sacconi, M., Pepeu, G. & Consolo, S. (1988). Decrease of brain acetylcholine release in aging freely-moving rats detected by microdialysis. *Neurobiology of Aging*, **9**, 357–61.

Yavin, E., Tanaka, Y. & Ando, S. (1989). Phospholipid-derived choline intermediates and acetylcholine synthesis in mouse brain synaptosomes. *Journal of Neuroscience Research*, **24**, 241–6.

Zhang, X., Wahlstrom, G. & Nordberg, A. (1990). Influence of development and ageing on nicotinic receptor subtypes in rodent brain. *International Journal of Developmental Neuroscience*, **8**, 715–21.

20

Molecular characterization of the neurodegenerative changes which distinguish normal aging from Alzheimer's disease

CLAUDE M. WISCHIK, CHARLES R. HARRINGTON AND
ELIZABETA B. MUKAETOVA-LADINSKA

It is now 100 years since the discovery of the 'senile plaque' by Blocq & Marinesco (1892). And yet the clinical syndrome of dementia occurring in late adult life, in which these lesions appear, did not become known by the names of the discoverers of the plaque, but by the name of the discoverer of the neurofibrillary tangle (both lesions are shown in Figure 20.1). The reason that Alzheimer, and those who followed him, felt the neurofibrillary tangle provided a better neuropathological correlate of the clinical syndrome he also described in his initial report (Alzheimer, 1907) was that the 'senile plaque', as the name suggests, is a common neuropathological feature of normal aging. To his way of thinking, such a change could not be the cause of the clinical syndrome of dementia he described, since such changes were also observed in the brains of those who reached old age with their mental faculties intact.

Some schools of thought give prominence to the plaque as the lesion by which Alzheimer's disease should be diagnosed (Khachaturian, 1985), and maintain that the abnormal protein deposits found in the plaque (β-amyloid protein derived from the amyloid precursor protein, APP) hold the key to the understanding of the molecular pathogenesis of the disease (Hardy & Allsop, 1991). One could be forgiven, therefore, for wondering whether the name had not enshrined a historical error of judgement.

The issues which arise in considering the aptness or otherwise of the name of the disease go directly to the heart of the problem which the present volume seeks to address. This dilemma was first articulated

Dementia and Normal Aging, eds. F. A. Huppert, C. Brayne & D. W. O'Connor.
© Cambridge University Press 1994.

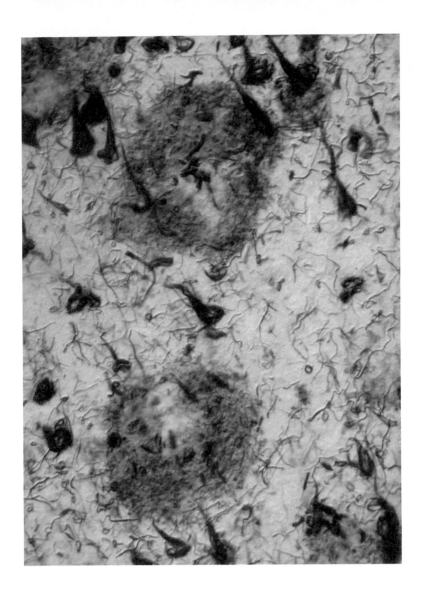

Figure 20.1. Alzheimer's disease neuropathology visualized by immunohistochemistry using a (paired helical filament) PHF-specific tau monoclonal antibody (mAb) 423. This section shows labelling of neurofibrillary tangles, neuritic plaques and dystrophic neurites throughout the neuropil in the frontal cortex. Photograph provided by R. Mena.

FACING PAGE 470

by Kraepelin (1910): 'The clinical significance of Alzheimer's disease is at present unclear. While the anatomic findings suggest that this condition deals with an especially severe from of senile dementia, some circumstances speak to a certain extent against this, namely the fact that the disease may arise even at the end of the fifth decade. One would describe such cases at least in terms of "senium praecox", if not more preferably that this disease is more or less independent of age'. This ambiguous statement remains strangely appropriate, after almost a century of research on the subject.

At the biological/molecular level, the question which can be put most usefully is: what are the changes which occur in the brains of those who become demented which distinguish them from those which are seen in the course of normal aging? This apparently simple formulation of the question avoids the philosophical difficulty raised by Kraepelin: can one have 'Alzheimer's disease' in the senium, or is this a contradiction in terms? However, this attempt to formulate a pragmatic biological question runs into another philosophical problem concerning the nature of biological causation.

In defining the biological changes which distinguish normal from demented old age, one is automatically speaking of the biological cause of the pathological changes which are characteristic of Alzheimer's disease. It has been claimed recently that paint mutations which lead to changes in the processing of APP are linked with dementia in certain rare kindreds with an autosomal dominant form of this disorder (Goate et al., 1991; Murrell et al., 1991). Therefore, it has been argued that all cases of Alzheimer's disease, whether genetic or sporadic, must be caused by abnormal processing of APP (Hardy & Allsop, 1991). However, abnormal processing of APP, giving rise to 'senile plaques', is actually a widespread phenomenon in the normal aging population (Barcikowska et al., 1989; Delaère et al., 1990). Nevertheless, such is the force which has been attributed by some to the genetic argument that the changes which best distinguish normal from pathological aging of the brain, i.e. neurofibrillary pathology (Wilcock & Esiri, 1982; Tierney et al., 1988; Delaère et al., 1989; Duyckaerts et al., 1990; Braak & Braak, 1991; Arriagada et al., 1992), are in danger of coming to be regarded as being mere epiphenomena.

Having outlined some of the philosophical difficulties inherent in any approach to this problem, the present chapter focuses on the question: what distinguishes normal from pathological aging of the brain? In doing so, we examine first the results obtained from the molecular characterization and measurement of the neurofibrillary pathology of Alzheimer's disease. These changes are then considered in relation to the changes associated with abnormal processing of APP and the force of the genetic evidence as it stands.

Molecular characterization of the neurofibrillary pathology of Alzheimer's disease

The two hallmark lesions of Alzheimer's disease are shown in Figure 20.1. They are the neurofibrillary tangle and the neuritic plaque. In addition, the figure shows extensive abnormal dystrophic neurites in the neuropil. All these structures have been visualized by means of a single monoclonal antibody (mAb 423). That is, there is at least one antigenically distinct species which is common to all the lesions seen.

The monoclonal antibody used to produce this picture has the property of recognizing a molecular species which is present in the paired helical filament (PHF). Thus, all the deposits seen in Figure 20.1 are sites of accumulation of PHFs. The PHF was described initially by Kidd (1963) as the main fibrous constituent of the neurofibrillary tangle. As also noted by Kidd in his initial report, PHFs are found more easily by electron microscopy in the neuropil and in plaques than in neurofibrillary tangles. This can be seen in Figure 20.1 as the abundance of labelled dystrophic neurites. That such neurites are predominantly dendritic in character and contain PHFs has been confirmed in a recent ultrastructural study (Braak & Braak, 1988).

The PHF is a polymer made up of a repeating C-shaped subunit which has an approximate molecular mass of 100 kDa, and is surrounded by a fuzzy coat which accounts for a further 20 kDa per subunit (Wischik, 1989). One can distinguish between the regular core and the fuzzy coat of the PHF by the relatively greater susceptibility to protease digestion of the fuzzy coat. Thus, after digestion with a broad spectrum protease, PHFs have some 20% less mass as measured by scanning-transmission electron microscopy (Wischik et al., 1988a). The monoclonal antibody used in Figure 20.1 has the property of recognizing both the protease-resistant core PHF and also fuzzy PHFs, although a higher antibody concentration is required if the fuzzy coat is left intact (Figure 20.2).

The mAb 423 used in Figure 20.1 also has the property of recognizing a 12 kDa protein fragment which can be released in an essentially pure form from highly enriched bulk preparations of protease-resistant acid-treated core PHFs from Alzheimer's disease brain tissues (Wis-

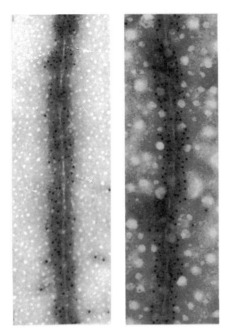

Figure 20.2. Paired helical filaments decorated with mAb 423 visualized by immunoelectronmicroscopy.

chik et al., 1988b). This fragment is derived from a specific functional segment of a longer protein, known as the microtubule-associated protein tau. The 12 kDa fragment corresponds to the region of tau which contains three tandem repeats of 31 amino acid residues each, and is thought to function as the microtubule binding domain of tau (Figure 20.3).

Normal function and distribution of tau protein

Tau protein is one of a family of proteins which copurify with preparations of microtubules. A strategy used in the purification of microtubules is their propensity to disassemble into their constituent proteins at temperatures of less than 10°C. The main constituents are a pair of proteins known as α- and β-tubulin. These constituents can also be made to reassemble into the characteristic cylindrical microtubule polymer. Proteins which copurify with microtubules during the course of disassembly and reassembly are known as microtubule-associated proteins. They have been found to have the property of facilitating microtubule

Microtubule

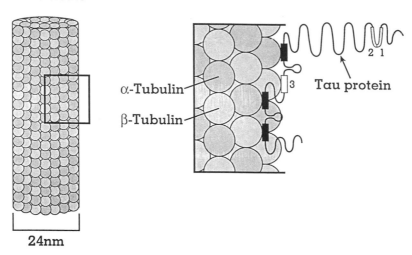

α-Tubulin

β-Tubulin

Tau protein

24nm

Figure 20.3. Microtubules consist of protofilaments composed of α- and β-tubulin subunits. Tau protein is involved in the assembly of axonal microtubules. Six different isoforms of tau protein exist which arise by alternative splicing. The largest isoform contains three inserted segments. The third insert occurs in the middle of a three tandem repeat region each of which acts as a microtubule binding domain. Reproduced from Harrington & Wischik (1994).

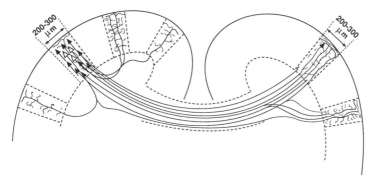

Figure 20.4. Cortico-cortical association fibres in the cortex. These fibres are the axons of pyramidal cells which are particularly vulnerable to neurofibrillary pathology of the Alzheimer type. These fibres mediate the bulk of associative processing in the cortex. In Alzheimer's disease, tau protein, which ought to be in the axons, is sequestered with paired helical filaments which accumulate in the somatodendritic compartment. It is hypothesized that this leads to functional disconnection in the cortex, which manifests itself as dementia.

assembly by copolymerizing on the surface of the polymer as it forms. Indeed, the tandem repeat region of tau and other related microtubule-associated proteins functions as the microtubule binding domain (Figure 20.3).

Tau protein is specifically an axonal microtubule-associated protein. That is, it functions to stabilize microtubules, particularly in the cortico-cortical association circuits of the neocortex (Figure 20.4). These microtubules are required for rapid transport of synaptic vesicles, mitochondria and other cellular components between the cell body, where they are produced, to the synaptic terminals, where they are required for interneuronal communication. As it happens, the neurofibrillary changes described by Alzheimer affect particularly the pyramidal cells which mediate cortico-cortical connectivity in the neocortex.

Measurement of changes in tau protein in Alzheimer's disease

The mAb 423 used to demonstrate the pathology of Alzheimer's disease in Figure 20.1 has been used as the basis for an immunochemical assay for PHF–tau protein complex in brain homogenate (Harrington et al., 1990, 1991). This antibody has the property of recognizing only the 12 kDa tau fragment released from the core PHF (Novak et al., 1991). There is no recognition of normal tau protein, either in immunoblots or in the conditions of the immunoassay on which quantification depends.

The properties of mAb 423 can be contrasted with those of mAb 7.51, which also recognizes the repeat region of tau, but is not selective for PHF–tau (Novak et al., 1991). Indeed mAb 7.51 does not recognize the tau in the PHF core so long as this remains bound within the PHF, but does recognize the 12 kDa fragment following release from the PHF. Thus, mAb 7.51 can be used in two ways. In the absence of an acid extraction step, mAb 7.51 measures only the normal, soluble tau protein which is found in brain tissues. In the PHF fraction, mAb 7.51 can be used after an acid extraction step to provide a second, independent measure of tau released from the PHF core. Thus, the measurements obtained by using mAb 423 for PHF–tau can be confirmed independently by using mAb 7.51 (Harrington et al., 1991).

These assays for normal tau and PHF–tau have been used in a study in which tissue has been dissected into grey and white matter for several regions from the association neocortex and medial temporal lobe of patients with Alzheimer's disease and control cases (Mukaetova-Ladinska et al., 1992a). The regional distribution of normal soluble tau protein is shown in Figure 20.5a. The highest levels of normal tau are found in frontal, temporal and parietal cortices in adult controls. The white matter predominance expected for an axonal protein is seen only in frontal cortex. The high grey matter levels can be attributed to the axonal contribution to grey matter. There is a major loss of normal tau in the Alzheimer's disease cases. The levels are uniformly low in all brain regions, but the greatest decrease is found in frontal and temporal neocortex.

The results of measuring PHF–tau by either of the two methods described above are also shown in Figure 20.5b. Substantial PHF accumulation is not observed in control brain tissues. The regions of greatest PHF accumulation in Alzheimer's disease differ somewhat from those expected from histological studies. Generally, it is thought that neurofibrillary tangles are most abundant in the hippocampus. This is not, however, the region of highest PHF accumulation relative to wet weight of tissue. This suggests that there is a discrepancy between the severity of pathology detected by histological and biochemical methods.

The reason for this discrepancy can be understood when the biochemical measures of PHF content are compared with quantitative histological measures of neurofibrillary tangles, plaques and dystrophic neuropil threads. Two distinct measures of plaques were made: counts

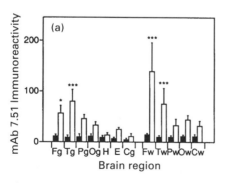 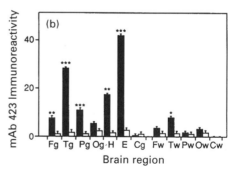

Figure 20.5. Biochemical measurements of (a) normal soluble tau and (b) PHF–tau (paired helical filament) in post-mortem brain tissue described from 10 cases with Alzheimer's disease (shaded) and 10 controls (unshaded). F, frontal; T, temporal; P, parietal; O, occipital lobes; H, hippocampus; E, entorhinal cortex; C, cerebellum; for grey (g) and white (w) matter. Significant differences between the two groups of cases is shown (*p<0.05; **p<0.01; ***p<0.001). Reproduced from Wischik et al., in CIBA Foundation Symposium No. 169: *Aluminium in Biology and Medicine*, Wiley, Chichester, 1992.

Table 20.1. *Correlation between PHF accumulation in grey matter and neuropathological lesions in Alzheimer's disease*

Lesion	mAb 423	mAb 7.51
Total plaques	ns	ns
Diffuse plaques	ns	ns
Neuritic plaques	<0.0001	<0.0001
Dystrophic neurites	<0.0001	<0.001
Intracellular tangles	<0.02	ns
Extracellular tangles	ns	ns

The level of significance is indicated for p <0.05; ns, not significant.

of plaques detected with an anti-tau antibody and counts of plaques detected with an anti-β-amyloid antibody. Table 20.1 shows that the histological variable which corresponds most closely to the biochemical PHF content is the extent of dystrophic neurite pathology, followed by neuritic plaques. Tangles are relatively poor indicators of total PHF content.

This is shown with greatest clarity in a subset of cases found to have high PHF levels overall and particularly in the occipital cortex (Mukaetova-Ladinska et al., 1992a). In these cases, neither the number of neurofibrillary tangles nor the number of neuritic plaques could be used to distinguish between cases with high or low PHF levels in the occipital cortex. The only histological indicator of high PHF content in these cases was the amount of dystrophic neurite pathology.

These observations have a direct bearing on the controversial question of diagnosing Alzheimer's disease in the absence of neurofibrillary tangles. Terry et al. (1987) have pointed out that a substantial proportion of cases in whom a clinico-pathological diagnosis of Alzheimer's disease could be made had no neurofibrillary tangles in the neocortex. For this reason, emphasis has been placed on plaque counts (Khachaturian, 1985), and indeed on β-amyloid plaque counts (Price et al., 1991), in the neuropathological diagnosis of Alzheimer's disease. However, the findings based on biochemical measurement of PHF content in brain tissues suggest that this is the wrong approach to the problem. The issue is not whether tangles are, or are not, required for diagnosing Alzheimer's disease, but whether a diagnosis can be made in the absence of extensive PHF accumulation, regardless of the histological form that these accumulations take.

PHF accumulation as the process which mediates destruction of nerve cells in Alzheimer's disease

It has been possible to distinguish immunohistochemically between intracellular and extracellular neurofibrillary tangles (Bondareff et al., 1990). An intracellular tangle is one which is contained within a pyramidal cell. An extracellular tangle is a swollen, dispersed, tangle-like structure left behind in the extracellular space after the death of the pyramidal cell. These latter structures are sometimes called 'tombstone' tangles. In a recent study of neurofibrillary pathology in the CA1 region of hippocampus, it was found that cases with high extracellular tangle counts had low surviving neuron counts (Bondareff et al., 1993). Indeed, a significant negative correlation was found between the surviving neuron count and either the total tangle count ($r = -0.77$, $p < 0.001$) or the extracellular tangle count ($r = -0.72$, $p < 0.001$). These findings demonstrate that it is neurofibrillary pathology which is actually responsible for neuronal destruction. If some other process were destroying cells, the predicted link between cell loss and neurofibrillary tangle count would be random.

This matter has been taken further in a recent study of PHF levels in cases divided on the basis of high or low extracellular tangle counts in the neocortex (Mukaetova-Ladinska et al., 1992b). Cases with high extracellular tangle counts have very much higher levels of PHFs than cases with low extracellular tangle counts. Again, these findings suggest that there is a close link between accumulation of PHFs and eventual destruction of nerve cells. If PHF accumulation were an epiphenomenon, one would predict that cases with lower surviving neuron counts ought to have lower PHF levels, since there would be fewer cells in which this presumed ancillary process might occur.

Tau protein changes in normal and pathological aging

In the results described earlier, all control cases were grouped together. When the control cases were divided into those older or younger than 65 years of age, PHF accumulation could not be used to discriminate between older and younger controls. As seen in Figure 20.6, PHF accumulation is a feature of Alzheimer's disease, not of aging.

This situation contrasts with that found in relation to normal tau levels. As shown in Figure 20.6a, younger controls have higher levels of normal soluble tau protein than do older controls. Cases with Alz-

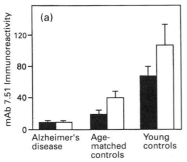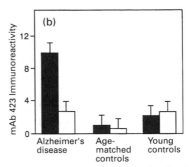

Figure 20.6. Distribution of (a) normal soluble tau and (b) PHF–tau (paired helical filament) as a function of aging and Alzheimer's disease. Grey (shaded) and white (unshaded) matter was dissected from six regions (excluding cerebellum) of all cases described in Figure 20.5. Normal aging is associated with a decline in normal tau content that is accentuated in Alzheimer's disease. PHF accumulation can be used to discriminate Alzheimer's disease cases from controls, but is not a feature of normal aging. PHFs accumulate predominantly in the grey matter. Reproduced from Wischik et al. in CIBA Foundation Symposium No. 169: *Aluminium in Biology and Medicine*, Wiley, Chichester, 1992.

heimer's disease have even lower levels than do aged controls. There is a significant inverse correlation between age and level of soluble tau ($r = -0.82$, $p < 0.01$). The age-related loss of tau cannot be explained by accumulation into a PHF-like insoluble compartment (Mukaetova-Ladinska et al., 1992a).

Chronological age is also used conventionally in the differentiation between pre-senile and senile dementia of the Alzheimer's type. When PHF levels were compared in Alzheimer's disease cases below and above the age 65 years, no significant difference was found between those dying before and after this age. However, when the dividing age was shifted to 80 years, there was a significant difference in both PHF content and counts of neuritic plaques and in dystrophic neuritic pathology, but not in counts of neurofibrillary tangles (Mukaetova-Ladinska et al., 1992b). This suggests that the more severe variant of Alzheimer's disease is equally common before and after the age of 65 years. It is only after the age of 80 years that it becomes possible at death to discern the separation of a group with less severe pathology.

These findings have a direct bearing on the concept of 'senium praecox', and the notion that Alzheimer's disease represents an exaggeration of the changes of normal aging. Firstly, in regard to PHF accumulation, a clear distinction can be drawn between aging with and without dementia. Secondly, in those who become demented, the relationship with aging is inverted. That is, the more severe pathology is observed in those who die younger, the less severe pathology in those who are more elderly. These considerations do not apply to levels of soluble tau protein. A decrease in the amount of soluble tau protein is a feature of normal aging. Loss of soluble tau, however, does not by itself provide an indication of transition into a state in which high levels of PHFs are observed.

A very similar pattern has emerged from the study of a larger sample of 18 cases of Alzheimer's disease (mean age: 77.7 ± 10.7 years) and 15 controls representative of the adult life span (mean age: 57.1 ± 19.0 years) (Mukaetova-Ladinska et al., 1993). Further prospective studies on community populations are under way which would include a wider range of neuropsychologically assessed subjects. This would allow both the age-related and the pathological cognitive and behavioural changes to be examined as a step toward understanding the pathophysiology that leads to their development.

Changes in processing of the amyloid precursor protein in aging and in Alzheimer's disease

APP is thought to be a cell surface protein whose functions are not known. Unlike tau protein, which is specific for the central nervous system, only certain forms of APP, designated by mRNA length, are brain specific (Neve et al., 1988). Studies at the level of mRNA have failed to support the hypothesis that Alzheimer's disease is characterized by any change in the absolute quantity or ratio of APP subtypes (Johnson et al., 1988; Tanaka et al., 1988; Koo et al., 1990; Oyama et al., 1991). Attempts to express various portions of APP in transgenic animals, although heralded as providing the first animal model of Alzheimer's disease pathology (Kawabata et al., 1991), have failed to produce neurofibrillary pathology, and the relevant claims have now been withdrawn. Thus, there is at present no support for the hypothesis that simple over-expression of APP causes β-amyloid pathology, nor for the suggestion that it causes neurofibrillary pathology of the type described by Alzheimer.

More sophisticated theories of the origin of β-amyloid deposits in the brain have attempted to take account of the emerging complexity of post-translational processing of APP. In certain cell types, the large N-terminal domain of the APP molecule (Figure 20.7) is released in a secreted form by cleavage at or near residue 612, corresponding to

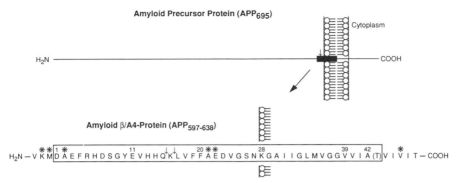

Figure 20.7. Schematic representation of the shortest form of the amyloid precursor protein (APP$_{695}$). Larger isoforms (APP$_{751}$ and APP$_{770}$) are produced by alternative splicing to include a Kunitz type II serine protease inhibitor domain (KPI). The segment of the molecule which is now known to accumulate as β-amyloid deposits in Alzheimer's disease corresponds to the short stretch which spans the outer part of the cell membrane and extends into the extracellular space. Normal secretory cleavage, which releases the long N-terminal portion of APP, occurs in the N-terminal half of β/A4 (indicated by arrows), and within a portion of the molecule regarded as being critical for the polymerization of β/A4 fibrils. Mutations so far observed in APP are indicated by asterisks. Three separate mutations, C-terminal to the β/A4 domain (isoleucine substituted with valine, phenylalanine or glycine) occur in a small number of familial Alzheimer's disease cases (Chartier-Harlin et al., 1991; Goate et al., 1991; Murrell et al., 1991). Probable Alzheimer's disease in two related Swedish pedigrees is associated with a double mutation that results in the substitution of lysine and methionine residues, adjacent to the N-terminus of β/A4, with asparagine and leucine (Mullan et al., 1992). Mutations linked with cerebral haemorrhage in a limited number of families have been observed within the extracellular portion of the β/A4 domain (residues 2, 21 and 22; with asterisks) (Levy et al., 1990; Hendricks et al., 1992; Peacock et al., 1993). Cases with the mutation at residue 21 are also affected with dementia (Hendricks et al., 1992).

residue 16 of the 42-residue segment of APP, termed 'β/A4', found in histological β-amyloid deposits in Alzheimer's disease. Cleavage at this site would be within the minimal 13 amino acid residue segment required for polymerization of β/A4 fibrils in vitro. Thus, it is proposed that normal secretory processing of APP would preclude deposition of β/A4 fibrils in the extracellular space, which is the characteristic feature of β-amyloid pathology. From this, it is proposed that deposition of β/A4 is the consequence of aberrant processing, which results in cleavage of APP at or near residue 638, which would have to occur in the transmembrane segment of the molecule (Selkoe, 1991).

There is increasing evidence that abnormal processing of APP occurs in the course of normal aging. Although β-amyloid deposits were thought initially to be associated only with the classical plaques and cerebrovascular amyloid of Alzheimer's disease (Masters et al., 1985; Wong et al., 1985; Allsop et al., 1986), a much more extensive distribution has been found using anti-β-amyloid antibodies. These take the form of 'diffuse plaques' (Yamaguchi et al., 1988). Ultrastructurally, these deposits consist of small bundles of amyloid fibrils interspersed with amorphous material located in the extracellular space between astrocytic processes (Yamaguchi et al., 1991). These deposits are very widespread, occurring in brain areas that appear to be largely unaffected clinically in Alzheimer's disease and in tissues other than the brain (Joachim et al., 1989; Ogomori et al., 1989).

The failure of PHF accumulation to correlate with β-amyloid deposits (Table 20.1) confirms the same result obtained by histological methods. Thus, the regional distribution of diffuse amyloid deposits does not correlate with neurofibrillary pathology (Delaère et al., 1989; Tabaton et al., 1989; Wisniewski et al., 1989; Akiyama et al., 1990), and cannot be used to distinguish between normal aging and Alzheimer's disease (Barcikowska et al., 1989; Delaère et al., 1990). All the available quantitative studies point to the conclusion that the processes leading to β-amyloid deposits and neurofibrillary pathology are independent of each other even in the same brain region (Armstrong, 1991; Armstrong et al., 1991). Although the bulk of β-amyloid deposits do not appear to be associated with clinical deficit, neurofibrillary pathology, or even loss of synapses (Terry et al., 1991), there have been attempts recently to prove that β-amyloid deposits are neurotoxic in brain tissues (Yankner et al., 1989; Frautschy et al., 1991; Kowall et al., 1991) and in tissue culture (Roher et al., 1991). The toxicity that is observed in cultured cells appears to be related more closely to the formation of gelatinous aggregates around neurons, and this, in turn, depends on the propensity of β/A4 peptides to self-aggregate in vitro. The relevance of these phenomena to those which occur in vivo is open to question.

β/A4 deposits and aging pigments

Another site of β/A4 accumulation which has become apparent recently is within so-called lipofuscin granules (Grundke-Iqbal et al., 1989). Lipofuscin has been defined as a 'membrane-bound lysosmal organelle, which contains lipoidal moieties, exhibits yellow to brown coloration, emits yellow to greenish autofluorescence under ultraviolet light, and accumulates progressively with age under normal physiological conditions' (Sohal & Wolfe, 1986, pp. 171–2). The ceroid-lipofuscinoses are a group of inherited storage diseases of children, characterized by brain and retinal atrophy and accumulation of fluorescent lipopigment in neurons and in a wide variety of other cells. The biochemical basis of these diseases has not been defined.

Analysis of this lipopigment from a number of tissue sources has shown that two-thirds of the lipopigment mass is proteinaceous, and Palmer et al. (1989) have shown that subunit 9 of the mitochondrial ATP synthetase enzyme complex accounts for 73% of the protein present in ovine ceroid-lipofuscinosis. Recently, we have identified the same protein in the lipofuscin deposits found in aged brain tissues, along with several other mitochondrial proteins (C. M. Wischik, unpublished). There appears, therefore, to be an abnormality of lysosomal processing, which particularly affects the turnover of mitochondria by autophagic vacuoles, which occurs with aging. There is evidence for a link between abnormal processing of APP and lipofuscin deposits not only in normal aging but also in juvenile ceroid-lipofuscinosis (Wisniewski et al., 1990).

β/A4 deposits and neurofibrillary pathology

Several groups have reported labelling of neurofibrillary tangles by antibodies raised against β/A4 peptides (Hyman et al., 1989; Bondareff et al., 1990; Tabaton et al., 1991). Such colocalization of tau and apparent β/A4 epitopes is of great potential theoretical interest, since it would provide a means of linking the two major forms of pathology of Alzheimer's disease. Labelling of some extracellular neurofibrillary tangles with antisera raised against preparations of β/A4 isolated from brain tissues from a patient with Alzheimer's disease and with antisera raised against synthetic β/A4 peptides has been subject to two different interpretations: exposure of intrinsic PHF–core epitopes in the course of extracellular degradation of tangles (Hyman et al., 1989; Tabaton et al., 1991), or secondary deposition of β-amyloid within extracellular tangles (Yamaguchi et al., 1991). We have reported that cases that had labelling of extracellular tangles in the CA1 region of the hippocampus by classical anti-β-amyloid antibodies tended to have more β-amyloid pathology, more extracellular tangles and a younger age of onset than cases without β-amyloid immunoreactivity in extracellular tangles (Bondareff et al., 1993). This would be more consistent with the secondary deposition argument.

Genetics of APP and Alzheimer's disease

A causal link between abnormal processing of APP and the neurofibrillary pathology of Alzheimer's disease rests largely on inferences drawn from certain cases of familial dementia with a point mutation resulting in the substitution of valine for isoleucine, as indicated in Figure 20.7. This is a conservative substitution, and has been identified in several kindreds with familial dementia (Goate et al., 1991). Further cases have been identified in which mutations result in substitution of amino acids near the N- or C-terminus of the β/A4 domain (Figure 20.7). The neuropathological characterization of these cases is far from clear, and appears to be variable. It has been claimed that some cases have the typical pathology of Alzheimer's disease. Others have been shown to have cortical Lewy bodies, but not cortical neurofibrillary pathology (Hardy et al., 1991). Furthermore, a mutation identified at residue 22 of β/A4 (indicated in Figure 20.7) is associated not with Alzheimer's disease, but with a condition of cerebrovascular amyloidosis, which causes dementia through multiple infarctions (Levy et al., 1990). Finally, an additional mutation, adjacent to this, results in dementia but tangles are absent (Hendricks et al., 1992).

The force of the genetic argument is at present far from clear. Mutations in APP are associated with the appearance of β-amyloid deposits in brain tissues, but not necessarily with the appearance of the neurofibrillary pathology required for a diagnosis of Alzheimer's disease. That is to say, these mutations do appear to be causal of neurological disease, but not necessarily of Alzheimer's disease. This situation is in no way different from that of normal aging. Abnormal processing of APP which is a common feature of aging appears to be a pre-condition which favours the appearance of neurofibrillary degeneration. However, it need not be a direct cause. There are other factors, for example environmental, or other genetic factors which may be more stringent determinants of classical Alzheimer's disease pathology. Abnormal processing of APP need not be, either epidemiologically or aetiologically, the most important factor predisposing to dementia of the Alzheimer type.

Summary

The molecular changes which distinguish brain tissues taken from persons who have died from advanced dementia from those taken from persons who have died with relatively normal mental function have been reviewed briefly in the present chapter. The question raised at the beginning, whether Alzheimer's disease had been named correctly after the discoverer of neurofibrillary pathology, appears to be answerable in the affirmative. The biochemical, rather than simply histological, measurement of Alzheimer's disease pathology has tended to confirm, albeit with reservations, Alzheimer's fundamental intuition that the degenerative 'neurofibrillary' change within cells that he discovered is, indeed, the trademark of a process which distinguishes between normal aging and clinical dementia.

Molecular studies have shown that the appearance of neurofibrillary pathology which is visible in the light microscope is associated with a major redistribution of a protein essential for maintaining the function of microtubules within the cortico-cortical association circuits of the neocortex. Normal tau protein is reduced to levels substantially below those found in the course of normal aging, and there is a major accumulation of an altered form of tau protein within protease-resistant, non-functional polymers (PHFs) in the somatodendritic compartment of cortical pyramidal cells. Since these changes are linked directly to the process which destroys pyramidal cells throughout the brain, it seems reasonable to infer that these changes are also directly responsible for the functional impairment seen clinically as dementia.

These changes are not part of the normal aging process. From the results presented here, it is clear that biochemical measurement of PHF accumulation could be used diagnostically to distinguish between normal aging of the brain and the incipient changes which could be expected to lead to neurofibrillary degeneration. Normal aging is characterized most clearly in the present context as one of the conditions in which significant accumulation of PHFs does not occur.

The arguments which have been advanced on the basis of the presence of neurofibrillary tangles in the hippocampus in the course of normal aging, and their absence in the neocortex in certain cases with undoubted dementia, are essentially without foundation when the biochemical tools are available to look beyond histological appearances. The occasional neurofibrillary tangles seen in the hippocampus in the course of normal aging do not predict a PHF content which differs statistically from that found in the brains of young control patients.

For reasons which are unclear, neurofibrillary tangles that appear in
the hippocampus are associated with lower PHF levels than are found
in other brain regions. At the other end of the scale, for example in
occipital cortex, it is possible to have very extensive PHF accumulation
in the absence of neurofibrillary tangles. Thus, the question is not
whether tangles are, or are not, specific to Alzheimer's disease, but
whether it is possible to diagnose Alzheimer's disease in the absence
of extensive PHF accumulation.

References

Akiyama, H., Tago, H., Itagaki, S. & McGeer, P. L. (1990). Occurrence of
diffuse amyloid deposits in the presubicular parvopyramidal layer in
Alzheimer's disease. *Acta Neuropathologica*, **79**, 537–44.

Allsop, D., Landon, M., Kidd, M., Lowe, J. S., Reynolds, G. P. & Gardner,
A. (1986) Monoclonal antibodies raised against a subsequence of senile plaque
core protein react with plaque cores, plaque periphery and cerebrovascular
amyloid in Alzheimer's disease. *Neuroscience Letters*, **68**, 252–6.

Alzheimer A. (1907), Über eine eigenartige Erkrankung der Hirnrinde.
Allegemeine Zeitschrif für Psychiatrie und Psychisch Gerichtiche Medizine, **64**,
146–8.

Armstrong, R. A. (1991) The relationship between senile plaques,
neurofibrillary tangles and amyloid (A4) deposits in Alzheimer's disease: a
principal components analysis. *Neuroscience Research Communications*, **9**,
91–7.

Armstrong, R. A., Myers, D., Smith, C. U. M., Cairns, N. & Luthert, P. J.
(1991). Alzheimer's disease: the relationship between the density of senile
plaques, neurofibrillary tangles and A4 protein in human patients.
Neuroscience Letters, **123**, 141–3.

Arriagada, P. V., Growdon, J. H., Hedley-White, E. T. & Hyman, B. T. (1992)
Neurofibrillary tangles but not senile plaques parallel duration and severity of
Alzheimer's disease. *Neurology*, **42**, 631–9.

Barcikowska, M., Wisniewski, H. M., Bancher, C. & Grundke-Iqbal, I. (1989)
About the presence of paired helical filaments in dystrophic neurites
participating in the plaque formation. *Acta Neuropathologica*, **78**, 225–31.

Blocq, P. & Marinesco G. (1892) Sur les lésions et la pathogénie de l'épilepsie
des dite essentielle. *Semaine Médicale*, **12**, 445–6.

Bondareff, W., Wischik, C. M., Novak, M., Amos, W. B., Klug, A. & Roth,
M. (1990) Molecular analysis of neurofibrillary degeneration in Alzheimer's
disease: an immunohistochemical study. *American Journal of Pathology*, **137**,
711–23.

Bondareff, W, Mountjoy, C. Q., Wischik, C. M., Hauser, D. L., LaBree, L. D.
& Roth, M. (1993) Evidence for subtypes of Alzheimer's disease and
implications for etiology. *Archive of General Psychiatry*, **50**, 350–6.

Braak, H. & Braak, E. (1988). Neuropil threads occur in dendrites of
tangle-bearing nerve cells. *Neuropathology and Applied Neurology*, **14**, 39–44.

Braak, H. & Braak, E. (1991). Neuropathological stageing of Alzheimer-related changes. *Acta Neuropathologica*, **82**, 239–59.

Chartier-Harlin, M.-C., Crawford, F., Houlden, H., Warren, A., Hughes, D., Fidani, L., Goate, A., Rossor, M., Roques, P., Hardy, J. & Mullan, M. (1991). Early-onset Alzheimer's disease caused by mutations at codon 717 of the β-amyloid precursor protein gene. *Nature*, **353**, 844–6.

Delaère, P., Duyckaerts, C., Brion, J. P., Poulain, V. & Hauw J.-J. (1989), Tau, paired helical filaments and amyloid in the neocortex: a morphometric study of 15 cases with graded intellectual status in aging and senile dementia of the Alzheimer type. *Acta Neuropathologica*, **77**, 645–53.

Delaère, P., Duyckaerts, C., Masters, C., Beyreuther, K., Piette, F. & Hauw J.-J. (1990). Large amounts of neocortical βA4 deposits without neuritic plaques nor tangles in a psychometrically assessed, non-demented person. *Neuroscience Letters*, **116**, 87–93.

Duyckaerts, C., Delaère, P., Hauw, J.-J., Abbamondi-Pinto, A. L., Sorbi, S., Allen, I., Brion, J.-P., Flament-Durant, J., Duchen, L., Kauss, J., Schlote, W., Lowe, J., Probst, A., Ravid, R., Swaab, D. F., Renkawek, K. & Tomlinson, B. (1990). Rating of the lesions in senile dementia of the Alzheimer type: concordance between laboratories. A European multicenter study under the auspices of EURAGE. *Journal of the Neurological Sciences*, **97**, 295–323.

Frautschy, S. A., Baird, A. & Cole, G. M. (1991). Effects of injected Alzheimer β-amyloid cores in rat brain. *Proceedings of the National Academy of Sciences, USA*, **88**, 8362–6.

Goate, A., Chartier-Harlin, M.-C., Mullan, M., Brown, J., Crawford, F., Fidani, L., Giuffra, L., Haynes, A., Irving, N., James, L., Mant, R., Newton, P., Rooke, K., Roques, P., Talbot, C., Pericak-Vance, M., Roses, A., Williamson, R., Rossor, M., Owen, M. & Hardy, J. (1991). Segregation of a missense mutation in the amyloid precursor protein gene with familial Alzheimer's disease. *Nature*, **349**, 704–6.

Grundke-Iqbal, I., Iqbal, K., George, L., Tung, Y.-C., Kim, K. S. & Wisniewski, H. M. (1989). Amyloid protein and neurofibrillary tangles coexist in the same neuron in Alzheimer disease. *Proceedings of the National Academy of Sciences, USA*, **86**, 2853–7.

Hardy, J. & Allsop, D. (1991). Amyloid depositions as the central event in the aetiology of Alzheimer's disease. *Trends in Pharmacological Sciences*, **12**, 383–8.

Hardy, J., Mullan, M., Chartier-Harlin, M.-C., Brown, J., Goate, A., Rossor, M., Collinge, J., Roberts, G., Luthert, P., Lantos, P., Naruse, S., Janeko, K., Tsuji, S., Miyatake, T., Shimizu, T., Kojima, T., Nakano, I., Yoshioka, K., Sakaki, Y., Miki, T., Katsuya, T., Ogihara, T., Roses, A., Pericak-Vance, M., Haan, J., Roos, R., Lucotte, G. & David, F. (1991). Molecular classification of Alzheimer's disease. *Lancet*, **337**, 1342–3.

Harrington, C. R., Edwards, P. C. & Wischik C. M. (1990). Competitive ELISA for measurement of tau proteins in Alzheimer's disease. *Journal of Immunological Methods*, **134**, 261–71.

Harrington, C. R., Mukaetova-Ladinska, E. B., Hills, R., Edwards, P. C., Montejo de Garcini, E., Novak, M. & Wischik, C. M. (1991). Measurement of distinct immunochemical presentations of tau protein in Alzheimer disease. *Proceedings of the National Academy of Sciences, USA*, **88**, 5842–6.

Harrington, C. R., & Wischik, C. M. (1994). Molecular pathobiology of Alzheimer's disease. In A. Burns & R. Levy (eds.). *Dementia*, pp. 209–38. Chapman and Hall, London.

Hendricks, L., Van Duijn, C. M., Cras, P., Cruts, M., Van Hul, W., van, Harskamp F., Warren, A., McInnis, M. G., Antonarakis, S. E., Martin, J.-J., Hofman, A. & van Broeckhoven, C. (1992). Presenile dementia and cerebral haemorrhage linked to a mutation at codon 692 of the β-amyloid precursor protein gene. *Nature Genetics*, **1**, 218–21.

Hyman, B. T., Van Hoesen, G. W., Beyreuther, K. & Masters, C. L. (1989). A4 amyloid protein immunoreactivity is present in Alzheimer's disease neurofibrillary tangles. *Neuroscience Letters*, **101**, 352–5.

Joachim, C. L., Mori, H. & Selkoe, D. J. (1989) Amyloid β-protein deposition in tissues other than brain in Alzheimer's disease. *Nature*, **341**, 226–30.

Johnson, S. A., Pasinetti, G. M., May, P. C., Ponte, P. A., Cordell, B. & Finch, C. E. (1988). Selective reduction of mRNA for the β-amyloid precursor protein that lacks a Kunitz-type protease inhibitor motif in cortex from Alzheimer brains. *Experimental Neurology*, **102**, 264–8.

Kawabata, S., Higgins, G. A. & Gordon J. W. (1991). Amyloid plaques, neurofibrillary tangles and neuronal loss in brains of transgenic mice overexpressing a C-terminal fragment of human amyloid precursor protein. *Nature*, **354**, 476–8.

Khachaturian, Z. S. (1985). Diagnosis of Alzheimer's disease. *Archives of Neurology*, **42**, 1097–105.

Kidd, M. (1963). Paired helical filaments in electron microscopy in Alzheimer's disease. *Nature*, **197**, 192–3.

Koo, E. H., Sisodia, S. S., Archer, D. R., Martin, L. J., Weidemann, A., Beyreuther, K., Fischer, P., Masters, C. L. & Price, D. L. (1990). Precursor of amyloid protein in Alzheimer disease undergoes fast anterograde axonal transport. *Proceedings of the National Academy of Sciences, USA*, **87**, 1561–5.

Kowall, N. W., Beal, M. F., Busciglia, J., Duffy, L. K. & Yankner, B. A. (1991). An in vivo model for the neurodegenerative effects of β amyloid and protection by substance P. *Proceedings of the National Academy of Sciences, USA*, **88**, 7247–51.

Kraepelin, E. (1910). *Psychiatrie*, 8th edition, vol. 2, pp. 616–32. Barth, Leipzig.

Levy, E., Carman, M. D., Fernandez-Madrid, I. J., Power, M. B., Lieberburg, I., van Duinen, S. G., Bots, G. T. A. M., Luyendijk W. & Frangione B. (1990). Mutation of the Alzheimer's disease amyloid gene in hereditary cerebral haemorrhage, Dutch type. *Science*, **248**, 1124–6.

Masters, C. L., Multhaup, G., Simms, G., Pottgiesser, J., Martins, R. N. Beyreuther, K. (1985). Neuronal origin of a cerebral amyloid: neurofibrillary tangles of Alzheimer's disease contain the same protein as the amyloid of plaque cores and blood vessels. *EMBO Journal*, **4**, 2757–63.

Mukaetova-Ladinska, E. B., Harrington, C. R., Hills, R., O'Sullivan, A., Roth, M. & Wischik, C. M. (1992a). Regional distribution of paired helical filaments and normal tau proteins in aging and in Alzheimer's disease with and without occipital lobe involvement. *Dementia* **3**, 61–9.

Mukaetova-Ladinska, E. B., Harrington, C. R., Xuereb, J. H. & Wischik, C. M. (1992b). Molecular and neuropathological heterogeneity in Alzheimer's disease. *Neuropathology and Applied Neurobiology*, **18**, 634–5.

Mukaetova-Ladinska, E. B., Harrington, C. R., Roth, M. & Wischik, C. M. (1993) Biochemical and anatomical redistribution of tau protein in Alzheimer's disease. *American Journal of Pathology*, **143**, 565–78.

Mullan, M., Crawford, F., Axelman, K., Houlden, H., Lilius, L., Winblad, B. & Lannfelt, L. (1992). A pathogenic mutation for probable Alzheimer's disease in the APP gene at the N-terminus of β-amyloid. *Nature Genetics*, **1**, 345–7.

Murrell, J., Farlow, M., Ghetti, B. & Benson, M. D. (1991). A mutation in the amyloid precursor protein associated with hereditary Alzheimer's disease. *Science*, **253**, 97–8.

Neve, R. L., Finch, E. A. & Dawes, L. R. (1988). Expression of the Alzheimer amyloid precursor gene transcripts in the human brain. *Neuron*, **1**, 669–77.

Novak, M., Jakes, R., Edwards, P. C., Milstein, C. & Wischik, C. M. (1991). Difference between the tau protein of Alzheimer paired helical filament core and normal tau revealed by epitope analysis of mAbs 423 and 7.51. *Proceedings of the National Academy of Sciences, USA*, **88**, 5837–41.

Ogomori, K., Kitamoto, T., Tateishi, J., Sato, Y., Suetsugu, M. & Abe, M. (1989). β-protein amyloid is widely distributed in the central nervous system of patients with Alzheimer's disease. *American Journal of Pathology*, **134**, 243–51.

Oyama, F., Shimada, H., Oyama, R., Titani, K. & Ihara, Y. (1991). Differential expression of β amyloid protein precursor (APP) and tau mRNA in the aged human brain: individual variability and correlation between APP-751 and four-repeat tau. *Journal of Neuropathology and Experimental Neurology*, **50**, 560–78.

Palmer, D. N., Martinus, R. D., Cooper, S. M., Midwinter, G. G., Reid, J. C. & Jolly, R. D. (1989). Ovine ceroid lipofuscinosis. The major lipopigment protein and the lipid-binding subunit of mitochondrial ATP synthase have the same NH$_2$-terminal sequence. *Journal of Biological Chemistry*, **264**, 5736–40.

Peacock, M. L., Warren, J. T., Roses, A. D. & Fink, J. K. (1993). Novel polymorphism in the region of the amyloid precursor protein gene. *Neurology*, **43**, 1254–6.

Price, J. L., Davis, P. B., Morris, J. C. & White, D. L. (1991). The distribution of tangles, plaques and related immunohistochemical markers in healthy aging and Alzheimer's disease. *Neurobiology of Aging*, **12**, 295–312.

Roher, A. E., Ball, M. J., Bhave, S. V. & Wakade, A. R. (1991). β-amyloid from Alzheimer disease brains inhibits sprouting and survival of sympathetic neurons. *Biochemical and Biophysical Research Communications*, **174**, 572–9.

Selkoe, D. J. (1991). The molecular pathology of Alzheimer's disease. *Neuron*, **6**, 487–98.

Sohal, R. S. & Wolfe L. S. (1986). Lipofuscin: characteristics and significance. *Progress in Brain Research*, **70**, 171–83.

Tabaton, M., Mandybur, T. I., Perry, G., Onorato, M., Autilio-Gambetti, L. & Gambetti, P. (1989). The widespread alteration of neurites in Alzheimer's disease may be unrelated to amyloid deposition. *Annals of Neurology*, **26**, 771–8.

Tabaton, M., Cammarata, S., Mancardi, G., Manetto, V., Autilio-Gambetti, L., Perry, G. & Gambetti, P. (1991). Ultrastructural localization of β-amyloid, τ, and ubiquitin epitopes in extracellular neurofibrillary tangles. *Proceedings of the National Academy of Sciences, USA*, **88**, 2098–102.

Tanaka, S., Nakamura, S., Ueda, K., Kameyama, M., Shiojiri, S., Takahashi, Y., Kitaguchi, N. & Ito, H. (1988). Three types of amyloid protein precursor mRNA in human brain: their differential expression in Alzheimer's disease. *Biochemical and Biophysical Research Communications*, **157**, 472–9.

Terry, R. D., Hansen, L. A., DeTeresa, R., Davies, P., Tobias, H. & Katzman, R. (1987). Senile dementia of the Alzheimer type without neocortical neurofibrillary tangles. *Journal of Neuropathology and Experimental Neurology*, **46**, 262–8.

Terry, R. D., Masliah, E., Salmon, D. P., Butters, N., DeTeresa, R., Hill, R., Hansen, L. A. & Katzman, R. (1991). Physical basis of cognitive alterations in Alzheimer's disease: synapse loss is the major correlate of cognitive impairment. *Annals of Neurology*, **30**, 572–80.

Tierney, M. C., Fisher, R. H., Lewis, A. J., Zorzitto, M. L., Snow, W. G., Reid, D. W. & Nieuwstraten, P. (1988). The NINCDS–ADRDA work group criteria for the clinical diagnosis of probable Alzheimer's disease: a clinicopathologic study of 57 cases. *Neurology*, **38**, 359–64.

Wilcock, G. K. & Esiri, M. M. (1982). Plaques, tangles and dementia: a quantitative study. *Journal of the Neurological Sciences*, **56**, 407–17.

Wischik C. M. (1989). Cell biology of the Alzheimer tangle. *Current Opinion in Cell Biology*, **1**, 115–22.

Wischik, C. M., Novak, M., Edwards, P. C., Klug, A., Tichelaar, W. & Crowther, R. A. (1988a). Structural characterization of the core of the paired helical filament of Alzheimer disease. *Proceedings of the National Academy of Sciences, USA*, **85**, 4884–8.

Wischik, C. M., Novak, M., Thogersen, H. C., Edwards, P. C., Runswick, M. J., Jakes, R., Walker, J. E., Milstein, C., Roth, M. & Klug A. (1988b). Isolation of a fragment of tau derived from the core of the paired helical filament of Alzheimer's disease. *Proceedings of the National Academy of Sciences, USA*, **85**, 4506–10.

Wischik, C. M., Harrington, C. R., Mukaetova-Ladinska, E. M., Novak, M., Edwards, P. C. & McArthur, F. K. (1992) Molecular characterization and measurement of Alzheimer's disease pathology: implications for genetic and environmental aetiology. In CIBA Foundation Symposium No. 169: *Aluminium in Biology and Medicine*, pp. 268–302. Wiley, Chichester.

Wisniewski, H. M., Bancher, C., Barcikowska, M., Wen, G. Y. & Currie, J. (1989). Spectrum of morphological appearance of amyloid deposits in Alzheimer's disease. *Acta Neuropathologica*, **78**, 337–47.

Wisniewski, K. E., Maslinska, D., Kitaguchi, T., Kim, K. S., Goebel, H. H. & Haltia, M. (1990). Topographic heterogeneity of amyloid β-protein epitopes in brains with various forms of neuronal ceroid lipofuscinoses suggesting defective processing of amyloid precursor protein. *Acta Neuropathologica*, **80**, 26–34.

Wong, C. W., Quaranta, V. & Glenner, G. G. (1985). Neuritic plaques and cerebrovascular amyloid in Alzheimer disease are antigenically related *Proceedings of the National Academy of Sciences, USA*, **82**, 8729–32.

Yamaguchi, H., Hirai, S., Morimatsu, M., Shoji, M. & Ihara, Y. (1988). A variety of cerebral amyloid in the brains of the Alzheimer-type dementia by β-protein immunostaining. *Acta Neuropathologica*, **76**, 541–9.

Yamaguchi, H., Nakazato, Y., Shoji, M., Okamoto, K., Ihara, Y., Morimatsu, M & Hirai, S. (1991). Secondary deposition of beta amyloid within extracellular neurofibrillary tangles in Alzheimer-type dementia. *American Journal of Pathology*, **138**, 699–705.

Yankner, B. A., Dawes, L. R., Fisher, S., Villa-Komaroff, L., Oster-Granite, M. L. & Neve, R. L. (1989). Neurotoxicity of a fragment of the amyloid precursor associated with Alzheimer's disease. *Science*, **245**, 417–20.

21

Genetic linkage in Alzheimer's disease

S.-J. RICHARDS AND C. VAN BROECKHOVEN

It will be obvious to the reader of this volume that Alzheimer's disease (AD) has devastating consequences for the carers and relatives of the affected person as well as for the sufferers. Furthermore, it will be understood that attempts to fathom the underlying aetiology are diverse, ranging from determining precise cognitive deficits to investigating the pathological events. However, problems with accurate diagnosis whilst the patient is alive have been further compounded by a lack of global uniformity in evaluating post-mortem tissues. Stemming from these frustrations, the way was paved for optimism in the power of linkage studies to isolate the gene responsible for AD. Genetic linkage studies for AD are now several years down the road, and, although commanding much press interest and financial resources, one must ask whether they are in reality suffering from the same problems which have impeded other areas of AD research over the years? This chapter will outline the requirements of linkage studies and assess how close the field of AD research is to fulfilling these prerequisites.

An introduction to genetic linkage

When the Austrian monk, Gregor Mendel, in the nineteenth century observed how inherited characteristics of the garden pea were passed down from generation to generation, he could hardly have foreseen the implications that his conclusions would have for human genetics. Genetic linkage is based on the laws of Mendelian inheritance and, while few would dispute the value of this approach to locating and isolating disease-associated genes, the implications for the human species of the prospect of isolating and manipulating genes regulating intelligence, emotion and behaviour are more controversial.

In brief, Mendelian law claims that: (1) inherited characteristics are

Dementia and Normal Aging, eds. F. A. Huppert, C. Brayne & D. W. O'Connor. © Cambridge University Press 1994.

determined by pairs of genes; (2) the two members of a single pair of genes (alleles) pass to different gametes during reproduction; and (3) different gene pairs assort to different gametes independently of each other. Based on these assumptions of Mendel and his contemporaries, linkage of disease genes to DNA markers of known chromosomal origin was pioneered. One of the first genetic diseases to be studied using recombinant DNA techniques was Duchenne muscular dystrophy. Although this disorder had been assigned previously to the X chromosome at the region Xp21 on the basis of a number of apparently balanced translocations in females (Lindenbaum et al. 1979; Zatz et al., 1981), Murray et al. (1982) established loose linkage ($\tau = 0.15$ approx.) for Duchenne muscular dystrophy using an X chromosome DNA probe. Since then, this approach has been used to claim chromosomal locations for many other diseases including Huntington's chorea, Charcot Marie tooth disease, schizophrenia and cystic fibrosis, to name but a few.

Epidemiological studies have indicated that there is good evidence to attribute a proportion of AD to the inheritance of an autosomal dominant gene defect thus rendering the disorder appropriate for a molecular genetics approach to locating and isolating the gene(s) responsible (Davies, 1986). The incidence of familial AD (FAD) is disputed, with conservative estimates suggesting that 5% of total AD cases are inherited whereas more extreme estimates suggest that the figure is nearer to 95% (Breitner et al., 1988).

Within an autosomal dominant disorder such as AD (i.e. the disease gene needs only to be on one of the pair of chromosomes for the disease to be observed), the affected parent will have the FAD gene on one chromosome and the normal copy of the gene on the homologous chromosome. Thus, any child with one affected parent will have a 50% chance of inheriting the chromosome bearing the disease gene. Genetic linkage exploits the tendency for alleles at nearby loci to segregate together during meiosis. Loci demonstrating genetic linkage are termed 'genetically linked'.

In order to introduce variation to the species, recombination occurs during meiosis which may alter the relationship between alleles at the disease and marker loci. Approximately 52 crossovers occur at male meiosis (this number is greater for females) which represents between one and six crossovers per chromosome – depending on the length of the chromosome (McKusick & Ruddle, 1977). It has been suggested further that these crossover events occur more frequently at the ends of the chromosome (telomeric) than near the centromere (Laurie et al., 1982). Such exchanges of genetic material produce recombinant gametes and a 'recombination fraction' may be deduced from the number of such recombinant gametes expressed as a proportion of the total number of gametes or offspring. The recombination fraction is denoted by the Greek letter τ.

The closer the disease and marker loci are situated to one another on the chromosome, the less likelihood there is of crossing over between the two loci, hence the number of recombinant gametes will be small. Thus, when two loci are situated very closely the recombination fraction is considered to be zero (tight linkage). Conversely, the further apart the loci are, the greater the likelihood of crossovers occurring and of subsequent increase in the number of recombinant gametes. In turn, this produces a greater recombination fraction and when this is equal to 50%, independent assortment has occurred. Where disease and marker loci are spaced widely on the same chromosome, recombination events can give rise to four equally likely outcomes. Since some regions of chromosomes are more susceptible to recombination than others, the recombination fraction is only able to reflect 'genetic distance'. It does not measure the physical distance between two loci.

The primary way of establishing genetic linkage between a disease and marker loci is the demonstration that the recombination fraction is significantly less than 50%. Several methods have been devised for this analysis, the most widely used of which is the lod score calculation (logarithm of the odds ratio) (Conneally & Rivas, 1980; Ott, 1985). The first steps in undertaking a genetic linkage analysis of an autosomal dominant disorder such as AD involve ascertaining the pattern of inheritance of a polymorphic DNA marker within affected and non-affected family members. An example of this may be seen in Figure 21.1 in which a single copy DNA marker with three alleles A,B and C has been used to screen genomic DNA obtained from each family member across three generations. The affected male (1) is homozygous

Family 1

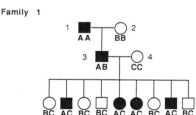

Figure 21.1. Linkage analysis of this pedigree demonstrates that the disease locus segregates with allele A (Family 1).

for allele A, while his unaffected wife (2) is homozygous for allele B. The couple's affected son (3) has inherited one copy of each of the alleles A and B. The son's unaffected wife (4) is homozygous for the third allelic position, C. Scores obtained from the third generation reveal that the disease locus segregates with allele A. Thus, marker and disease loci are genetically linked, since all four affected offspring are A, while the five unaffected offspring are B (all individuals have inherited allele C from their unaffected mother) making a total of nine non-recombinants.

If the FAD gene and the DNA marker being investigated for linkage have their loci on different chromosomes, then by chance each child in the family who receives the chromosome with the marker may receive the chromosome with the FAD gene locus. This becomes less likely as more offspring are included in the investigation. A measure of the statistical significance of the departure from that expected by chance alone is given by the lod score of observing such a departure by independent assortment. A lod score of 3 or greater is the accepted criterion to demonstrate linkage at a statistically significant level.

To return to Family 1, if the FAD gene and DNA marker loci are not linked, the probability of a departure from independent assortment occurring by chance is the same as calling heads or tails correctly for nine consecutive tosses of a coin (i.e. $(0.5)^9 = 0.002$). However, if these loci are linked with a recombination fraction of 0.1, the likelihood of the FAD gene segregating with allele A or the normal gene with allele B is 0.9 for each child. The probability of not observing a recombination event in any of the nine children is $(0.9)^9$ (i.e. 0.4). Thus, recombination at 0.1 is a more likely explanation than no linkage; in fact, it is 200 times more likely to be correct $(0.4/0.002 = 200)$. Similarly, if the recombination fraction is truly zero for this family, a recombination event cannot occur, the probability of the observed outcome is 1, resulting in a likelihood ratio of 1/0.002 (i.e. 500). To calculate the lod scores for the various recombination fractions within this hypothetical family, the logarithms (base of 10) need to be determined for the likelihood ratios. Thus, for a recombination fraction of 0.1, the lod score is 2.3 ($\log_{10} 200$), and when the recombination fraction is 0 the lod score is 2.7 ($\log_{10} 500$).

Within our hypothetical Family 2 (Figure 21.2), the youngest son (unaffected) possesses alleles A and C. This indicates one of two possibilities – either a recombination event has occurred between the FAD gene and the marker within this individual, or allele A is not segregating with the disease. This latter possibility is less likely but cannot be

Family 2

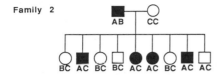

Figure 21.2. A recombination event between the disease locus and the marker at allele C is the likely explanation of the youngest son being 'unaffected' (Family 2).

excluded, since there is no information about the previous generation. Thus, regardless of which situation is correct, a zero recombination fraction has to be rejected, since it has a probability of zero, i.e. a lod score of minus infinity ($-\infty$).

Invariably, genetic linkage studies require pooled data from more than one family. This involves calculating the lod scores for the recombination value at several points (e.g at 0.1 intervals from 0.0 to 0.4) and then combining these values (Table 21.1). The highest lod score value obtained is the one assessed for statistical significance, and linkage is accepted when a lod score of 3 or greater is obtained. When applied to an autosomal dominant disorder with complete penetrance (i.e. the disease appears in each generation) such as AD, the chance of false identification of linkage with a particular probe is less than one in a thousand. However, typically many different probes are used for screening for linkage, so that the chances of a false positive result increases accordingly. Indeed, Rao et al. (1978) consider that false linkages are obtained in up to 2% of cases. While negative lod scores indicate the absence of linkage, scores between 2 and 3 are considered to be ambiguous. To overcome an inconclusive result, more families may be added to the study, or more informative markers can be used to analyse segregation in existing family members (van Broeckhoven

Table 21.1. *Cumulative lod scores for Families 1 and 2*

	Recombination fraction				
	0.00	0.10	0.20	0.30	0.40
Family 1	2.7	2.3	1.8	1.3	0.7
Family 2	−0.0	1.0	0.9	0.6	0.3
Combined	−0.0	3.3	2.7	1.9	1.0

Taken from Yates & Connor (1986).

et al., 1988). Similarly, multi-point analysis (analysis of multiple pair-wise lod scores) may be used, which involves mapping the disease locus in relation to a number of marker loci in the region.

Lod scores may be calculated directly (Ott, 1985), by tables (Race & Sanger, 1975) or by computer programs, i.e. two-point or multi-point analysis. Two-point analysis appropriately handles data where information about recombinant meiosis is available across three generations (as demonstrated in Family 1), or in two-generation pedigrees where the recombinant meioses are unknown.

Of course, the possibility of such linkage analyses is totally dependent upon the availability of informative DNA probes. DNA restriction fragment length polymorphisms (RFLPs) are detected as a consequence of DNA base changes, insertions or deletions (of a single base or of a longer sequence) which subsequently remove, insert or rearrange restriction enzyme sites (Botstein et al., 1980). Such variations have been shown to occur in the normal population once in every 100–200 hundred base pairs around the β-globin locus (Jeffreys, 1979) and may be detected using random DNA probes (Wyman & White, 1980). The Mendelian inheritance of these RFLPs has proved to be valuable as genetic markers. DNA probes used within linkage studies have invariably comprised single-copy DNA sequences representing two allele systems. Depending on the presence of a restriction enzyme site, these markers have yielded RFLPs at the same locus (Botstein et al., 1980). The more polymorphic the marker, the greater the likelihood of the marker being informative. The discovery of markers containing a variable number of tandem repeats (VNTRs) producing multiple alleles has increased the possibility of extracting information about allelic segregation with the disease gene (Nakamura et al., 1987). To date, most VNTRs have been mapped to the telomeres of chromosomes, which may be exploited for telomerically situated disease genes (such as Huntington's disease), but may be of little advantage to isolating the more centromeric FAD gene.

Hunting the gene for familial Alzheimer's disease

In the majority of linkage studies, tracking the disease locus has involved screening pedigrees with DNA markers located throughout the genome, i.e. markers representing the various chromosomes. This can be expensive, labour intensive and time consuming. Indeed, it has often taken several years of such analyses to establish the presence of a disease locus on a particular chromosome. However, the nets didn't have to be cast so far afield in ascertaining with which chromosome to start the search for the FAD gene. Indeed, one of the landmarks in genetic disease history yielded a clue. In 1959, Lejeune et al. discovered the first human chromosomal disease – trisomy 21 (Down syndrome). Subsequently, it was discovered that Down syndrome individuals develop the neuropathological characteristics of AD if they survive to middle life (Burger & Vogel, 1973; Oliver & Holland, 1986; Mann et al., 1989). Thus, chromosome 21 was the obvious autosome to start screening for the FAD gene.

Further evidence supporting chromosome 21 as the autosome carrying the FAD locus came from mapping the β/A4 protein gene to the region 21q11–q22 of chromosome 21 (Goldgaber et al., 1987; Kang et al., 1987; Robakis et al., 1987; Tanzi et al., 1987). The β/A4 protein is intrinsic to the neuropathological plaque core and cerebral vasculature depositions observed in both AD and Down syndrome cases over the age of 30 years (Mann et al., 1987). The youngest trisomy 21 case with amyloid deposits so far identified was 13 years old and immunocytochemical studies have shown that amyloid is deposited in the brains of trisomy 21 individuals approximately 50 years before that observed in the normal aging population (Rumble et al., 1989).

In 1987, St George Hyslop and colleagues reported preliminary data indicating the presence of a disease locus on the long arm of chromosome 21, in the region of the anonymous DNA markers, D21S1/S11 and D21S16. These markers implicated a region closer to the centromere (21q11.2–21q21) than the region (21q22) associated with Down syndrome. The data were collected from four extended AD pedigrees (Table 21.2) in which AD segregated as an autosomal dominant disorder. However, since the lod scores for D21S16 and D21S1/S11 did not exceed the criterion score of 3.0 (2.32 ($\tau = 0.00$) and 2.37 ($\tau = 0.08$) respectively), positive linkage could not be confirmed in these pedigrees by two-point lod scores but could be supported by multipoint analysis.

In the same year, Tanzi et al. (1987) published data suggesting that the FAD locus segregated close to the amyloid gene locus within AD pedigrees. To investigate the possibility of the amyloid gene as a candidate for the FAD gene, van Broeckhoven et al. (1987) used an RFLP for the β/A4 gene, to examine its segregation within two extended, Belgian pedigrees with early-onset AD ($\approx$35 years) and five UK families with late-onset AD ($\approx$65 years). Linkage analysis within these families revealed crossover events had occurred within one Belgian

Table 21.2. *Characterization of FAD pedigrees*

Family no.	Mean age of onset (yrs)	No. of generations	No. of AD cases described	No. of AD cases confirmed post-mortem
FAD 1	52.0±6.23	8	54	7
FAD 2	48.7±5.73	6	20	3
FAD 3	49.8±4.84	6	23	9
FAD 4	39.9±7.18	8	48	6

AD, Alzheimer's disease; FAD, familial Alzheimer's disease.

early-onset, and one UK late-onset pedigree, indicating a recombination between the amyloid gene and the FAD locus. This suggested strongly that these two loci are genetically distinct unless the recombination event occurred within the amyloid gene locus. Furthermore, the linkage data obtained from this analysis placed the amyloid gene closer to the Down syndrome region (21q22) than was reported previously.

Since these early studies, many research groups have actively sought families in which AD segregates as an autosomal dominant disorder and, to date, well over a hundred pedigrees have been evaluated using a recombinant DNA approach. Data analysis from individual groups has yielded variable results. Subsequent to the previous report supporting genetic linkage of AD with the chromosome 21 markers D21S1/S11 and D21S16 loci (St George Hyslop et al., 1987), van Broeckhoven et al. (1988, 1990a) have obtained positive lod scores within the two extended Belgian pedigrees with the chromosome 21 marker D21S13 (peak lod score = +1.02, $\tau=0.12$) but have failed to detect linkage by two-point analyses with any of these chromosome 21 markers. In a small, cumulative study (inclusive of the St George Hyslop et al. (1990) data), linkage for D21S16 by two-point analysis has been demonstrated (Goate et al., 1989). Within the same study, the cumulative values obtained could not support linkage for D21S1/S11. In a further two unrelated AD pedigrees, including the Volga-German pedigree, linkage for the D21S1/S11 loci could not be established (Pericak-Vance et al., 1988; Schellenberg et al., 1989).

In an attempt to discern whether this failure to confirm linkage reflected a true non-replication or rather aetiological heterogeneity, or differences in data sampling, etc., a corporate analysis was undertaken on 48 described AD pedigrees. From these families 153 affected family members were typed with the five anonymous DNA markers (D21S13, D21S16, D21S52, D21S1 and D21S11), representing three genetic loci (van Broeckhoven et al., 1988). At a recombination fraction of 0.20, pooled data indicated a lod score of 3.26 for D21S13/S16 and 3.22 for D21S1/S11 (Table 21.3) (St George Hyslop et al., 1990).

To investigate 'age of onset' as a determining factor for linkage of AD to chromosome 21, the same data were subjected to further cumulative analysis. Pedigrees were assigned to one of two groups according to whether their mean age of onset for AD was earlier, or later, than 65 years. Table 21.4 reveals linkage for the markers D21S13/S16 and D21S1/S11 within the group whose age of onset for AD was under 65 years, but there was a failure to confirm linkage with any of the markers investigated within the group whose age of onset was over 65 years. These observations suggest that more than one mechanism contribute to dementia in AD.

The apparent linkage for early age of onset pedigrees within which AD is represented as an autosomal dominant trait would confirm the generally held view that AD is caused by a genetic defect on chromosome 21. However, some researchers do not find this linkage data alone so convincing and a scepticism for chromosome 21 may not be ill founded (Roses, 1989). Evidence for additional FAD loci may exist on chromosomes 19 and 14 (Schellenberg et al., 1992). Additional evidence supporting the involvement of chromosome 21 may be derived from: (1) the incidence of AD-like neuropathologies in trisomy 21 (Down syndrome) individuals; and (2) animal models implicating genes which in humans are associated with chromosome 21. However, neither of these lines of evidence can link the dementia to the neuropathological hallmarks of the disease conclusively and directly.

To date, the lack of comprehensive investigations concerning chromosomally karyotyped trisomy 21 and unbalanced translocations of the 'obligate region' of chromosome 21 Down syndrome cases in relation to their potential for developing AD-type dementia make it impossible to state categorically that all trisomy 21 individuals will suffer from AD. Similarly, it cannot be claimed that all Down syndrome cases karyotypically determined as having only the region of chromosome 21 below the FAD region in excess will escape the disorder. Frustratingly, the field of psychiatric/psychological testing lacks the diagnostic procedures to assess moderately or severely mentally handicapped people for AD-associated dementia. However, there is

Table 21.3. *Two-point lod scores for chromosome 21 markers*

	D21S13/S16						D21S52						D21S1/S11					
Lod score recombination fraction (θ)	0.00	0.05	0.10	0.20	0.30	0.40	0.00	0.05	0.10	0.20	0.30	0.40	0.00	0.05	0.10	0.20	0.30	0.40
Total lod scores	−∞	−3.04	1.11	3.26	2.48	0.91	−∞	−9.72	−4.40	−0.24	0.78	0.45	−∞	−3.54	1.04	3.22	2.47	0.92

From St George Hyslop et al. (1990).

Table 21.4. *Cumulative lod scores for pedigrees according to age of onset*

Locus	Age of onset (years)	Cumulative lod score at recombination fraction (θ)						Peak lod score (Z at θ)
		0.00	0.05	0.10	0.20	0.30	0.40	
D21S13/S16	≤65	−∞	−0.97	2.17	3.51	2.49	0.90	3.60 at 0.17
	>65	−∞	−2.07	−1.06	−0.25	−0.02	0.02	0.02 at 0.40
D21S52	≤65	−∞	−3.86	−0.13	2.09	1.93	0.85	2.22 at 0.24
	>65	−11.3	−5.86	−4.27	−2.33	−1.15	−0.40	—
D21S1/S11	≤65	−∞	1.14	3.81	4.28	2.82	1.00	4.50 at 0.17
	>65	−16.5	−4.68	−2.77	−1.06	−0.35	−0.08	—

Z, lod scores; — minus scores.
From St George Hyslop et al. (1990).

little disagreement that a gradual regression occurs in the cognitive ability of Down syndrome individuals from the age of 19 years onward. Whether this reflects a cessation of the close supervision provided by special education to handicapped children in the UK, cortical cell loss, or both, is unknown. Oliver & Holland (1986) are undertaking a comprehensive psychiatric analysis of Down syndrome individuals in an attempt to clarify whether trisomy 21 individuals living to middle age will experience AD dementia.

A more definitive statement is that most Down syndrome cases will develop amyloid plaques and, later, neurofibrillary tangles in numbers that are sufficient to fulfil the criteria for a post-mortem confirmation of AD (Mann et al., 1987, 1989; Davies et al., 1988; Rumble et al., 1989). It remains to be established whether all trisomy 21 individuals fulfil this criteria while unbalanced, translocation Down syndrome cases which do not have the FAD region in excess lack elevated numbers of these neuropathological features. Indeed, as more antibodies are raised against different epitopes of the pathological proteins involved in AD, the tighter the comparison will become between the plaques and tangles observed in Down syndrome and AD cases (Mann et al., 1989).

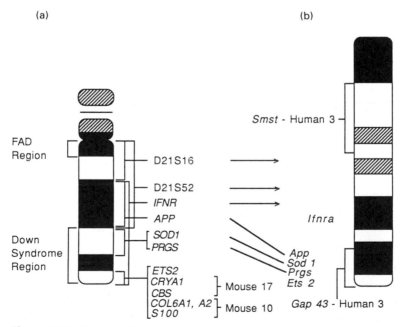

Figure 21.3. Synteny between (a) mouse chromosome 16 and (b) human chromosome 21 for the region spanning the FAD locus.

Further evidence supporting the implication of a chromosome 21 gene defect for the aetiology of the neuropathology observed in both AD and Down syndrome comes from an animal model derived from the trisomy 16 mouse. Murine chromosome 16 is syntenic to human chromosome 21 for the FAD region (Reeves et al., 1987), so that the trisomy 16 mouse may mirror the AD association with human trisomy 21 (Figure 21.3). Disappointingly, this aneuploidy is lethal at approximately 16–18 days of gestation. In order to prolong the life of cortical tissues, a neural transplantation system has been used in which trisomy 16 cortical tissues are implanted into a cortical site in young normal mouse recipients. These trisomic grafts accumulate proteins associated with human AD, and this neuropathology develops with age (Richards et al., 1991). Within this model neither Hirano nor Lewy bodies have been observed. However, since mouse chromosome 16 is larger than human 21, and there exist genes on this chromosome which are represented on human chromosomes other than 21 (Figure 21.3), it is conceivable that the neuropathological consequences for trisomy 16 may be influenced by genes located on the region of mouse chromosome 16 which is not syntenic to human 21.

Alzheimer's disease revisited

The data reviewed within this chapter attempt to explain the disparity in the chromosome 21 linkage data obtained by different research groups for the various pedigrees. Heterogeneity by the age of onset of AD dementia is used to accommodate the entire rag, tag and bobtail of aetiologies – from monogenic or polygenic genetic effects through to environmental influences, or even a mixture of the two. But how does this truly explain the conflicting and perplexing dimensions of the disease?

The fundamental problem in understanding this disease is that not one aspect of AD is as yet defined or characterized unambiguously. Psychological, psychiatric and neurological diagnostic procedures are hard pressed to distinguish between multi-infarct dementia, Lewy body dementia and AD dementia, especially in cases where the dementia is in its early stages. For research purposes, clinical diagnosis must be supplemented by post-mortem confirmation, yet little consensus is forthcoming even from this branch of science. This is demonstrated in a recent study in which brains from six AD patients were distributed for analysis to eleven established neuropathology centres throughout

Europe (Duyckaerts et al., 1990). The variable results reflect the divergent histological staining techniques used within the different laboratories. Moreover, while consensus existed between laboratories for the most severely demented cases, this was not so for the moderately or mildly demented individuals. Thus, as in clinical diagnosis, the confirmation of AD was most accurate within the severely demented cases. Clearly, a reliable marker for AD dementia is needed and developments in this area are being pursued keenly (Navaratnam et al., 1991).

Genetic linkage studies are dependent upon accurate diagnosis. For example, in a recent case, a mutation in the APP gene (a gene associated with AD neuropathology) has led Goate et al. (1991) to conclude that the valine to isoleucine change observed may be the aetiology of AD in this and other AD cases. However, although the authors claim that autopsy confirmation on one affected member had been undertaken, it appears that this brain manifested cortical and brainstem Lewy bodies in addition to amyloid angiopathy. Since there is little, if any, evidence to suggest that patients with AD are predisposed to develop Lewy bodies as a secondary phenomenon in the brain, nor that Lewy bodies co-exist with amyloid plaques and neurofibrillary tangles in Down syndrome (Gibb et al., 1989), this case is clearly atypical. Furthermore, it is circular to include a pedigree in which a mutation occurs within a known chromosome 21 gene to establish linkage to chromosome 21. In particular, the use of this case or any other families with a similar mutation to contribute to the cumulative genetic linkage data scores is dubious (Family 26 in the St George Hyslop (1990) study and Family 2 in the Goate et al. (1989) study). Indeed, when Family 26 is removed from this most recent and largest international linkage analysis (St George Hyslop et al., 1990) the total peak lod score derived by two-point analysis (Z at τ) is 1.94, not 3.26, for D21S13/S16 at 0.20 recombination fraction, and 1.90 not 3.22 for D21S1/S11 (see Table 21.3).

The Val–Ile mutation at position 717 of the amyloid precursor protein (APP) gene has been detected in a further three early-onset, Japanese FAD kindreds (Naruse et al., 1991; Yoshioka et al., 1991) and in an American pedigree. An APP, Phe-Val substitution has also been detected at position 717 (Murrell et al., 1991) and it is possible that further cases with different substitutions will be revealed as more families are screened for these mutations. However, the Val–Ile mutation has not been detected in any of 55 Italian pedigrees or in 100 early-onset, familial and sporadic Belgian AD cases (van Duijn et al., 1991). This suggests that if a mutation within the amyloid gene is the underlying cause of AD in these pedigrees, it is not the underlying aetiology of the disease in the majority of early-onset, familial cases. While misdiagnosis for AD has been estimated at around 30% (Khatchaturian, 1985), a diagnostic error is likely to be detected in an early-onset, autosomal dominant disorder. Moreover, it is difficult to explain the absence of the mutation in the majority of early-onset familial cases as resulting from lack of paternity (where the child is illegitimate, of a previous marriage or adopted), laboratory errors or environmental influences. However, it will be essential to determine whether these rare cases present with an atypical neuropathology, especially in view of the association between point mutations within the APP and neuropathological amyloid depositions within human hereditary cerebral haemorrhage with amyloidosis (Dutch type) (Levy et al., 1990; van Broeckhoven et al., 1990b) and familial amyloid polyneuropathy (Benson, 1989). Several different mutations have been detected within the APP within Creutzfeldt–Jacob disease and Gerstmann–Straussler disease (Brown et al., 1991).

Needless to say, research groups involved actively in a genetic linkage approach to AD will be screening their familial and sporadic AD cases for mutations and, in time, a clearer picture will emerge regarding the incidence in early- vs. late-onset cases, and familial vs. sporadic cases and whether they occur in the normal population. For example, if three out of 200 screened cases of AD were found to carry the mutation then at least 1800 normal, unrelated people would have to be negative to justify the conclusion that the chances of a mutation occurring in AD cases was higher than that in the normal population (at a chance level of one in a thousand, which is equivalent to a lod score of 3.0). Similarly, if four cases were positive out of 200 screened, then approximately 600 normal, unrelated individuals would have to be judged to be negative. The number of control cases screened so far is clearly inadequate to conclude that the identified cases of a mutation within the APP gene are other than a chance occurrence.

The identification of mutations in the APP have raised a number of interesting questions about the contribution of amyloid to the disease process. Firstly, have sufficient controls been examined to exclude the possibility that these mutations are rare recombination events unrelated to AD? Secondly, if these mutations (and others N-terminal to the existing mutations) do contribute to the early age of onset of the disease in these pedigrees, at what level are they exerting their effects? Finally, in the event of dementia being the outcome of cortical cell death, what are the implications for cell viability of mutations in a rapidly transported transmembrane protein? To address this latter point, many studies have explored the toxicity of synthetic β/A4 peptides in vivo and in vitro. However, as is frequently the case for AD research, the results of these studies are variable and conflicting (Price et al., 1992).

Amyloid is a rapidly transported, axonal protein which, if prevented from being transported, results in accumulations of the protein occurring within the cell cytoplasm. Eventually, such accumulations would result in the breakdown of intracellular processing and degeneration implicating a range of cytoskeletal proteins such as tau, ubiquitin and others. Events leading to failure of appropriate axonal transport could be numerous and diverse ranging from loss of pre-synaptic or post-synaptic regulation and transmembrane transport through to the performance of proteolytic enzymes involved in normal intracellular processing. Indeed, within normal aging, synaptic contacts are lost and the more synapses a cell loses the greater the risk of accumulating amyloid intracellularly. Thus, early-onset AD pedigrees demonstrating a transmembrane domain mutation may be at increased risk of cortical cell death by virtue of the mutation increasing the instability of the cell membrane (inappropriate processing of the post-cleavage domain from the membrane) leading to a failure of appropriate intracellular processing and eventual cell death (Haass et al., 1992a,b). Similarly, within trisomy 21 cases not only are synaptic contacts lost prematurely but also expression of the additional copy of the chromosome 21 amyloid gene may result in a greater amount of amyloid protein requiring axonal transport. Thus, it is plausible that any event causing axonal degeneration or abnormal processing within an amyloid-producing cell type could result in the formation of neuropathological amyloid deposits.

An exciting development in understanding the sequence of pathological events and the processes involved in AD has been reported recently by Caputo et al. (1991) in which intracellular β/A4 amyloid binds tau. The speculation being that complexes of these two proteins give rise to the paired helical filaments observed at post-mortem. An excellent review outlining current thinking on the contribution of amyloid to the neuropathology of AD has been prepared by Yanker & Mesulam (1991) and includes an update on the neuropathologies induced in mice transgenic for different regions of the APP gene.

Meanwhile, the APP mutations have highlighted the growing awareness of neuropathologists to the dilemma of interpreting an extended

AD phenotype e.g. Lewy bodies, amyloid angiopathy, core and diffuse amyloid plaques and neurofibrillary tangles. On this subject, Kosaka (1990) has subdivided diffuse Lewy body dementia (DLBD) into *common* and *pure* types. Thus, Lewy bodies co-existing with moderate/ severe numbers of plaques and tangles are considered to be *common* DLBD, while cortical Lewy bodies without plaques and tangles are deemed to be *pure* DLBD. The presence of the pure form of DLBD in many cases suggests that cortical Lewy bodies alone can cause cortical dementia, therefore it is difficult to discern the relative roles of Lewy bodies, plaques and tangles in the dementia within the British APP mutation pedigree. The long-awaited report concerning the neuro-pathological comparisons of the AD mutation and non-mutation AD cases has still to be published.

Similarly, in an impressive study undertaken in Newcastle by Perry et al. (1990a,b), an association was identified between AD-type pathology and Lewy body disorders. In particular, a proportion of patients with Lewy body disorders develop more cortical senile plaques and neurofibrillary tangles than would be expected within the general population. However, the consensus of both investigators for determining a diagnosis in favour of AD appears to reflect elevated numbers of plaques (of the *core* as opposed to the *diffuse* type) and tangles in proportion to the number of Lewy bodies. Ironically, the neuropathological procedures for detecting cortical Lewy bodies are also criticized for poor consensus between laboratories – a problem shared by AD pathology.

In reviewing the available data on 88 'described' AD pedigrees, St George Hyslop et al. (1989) considered that only twenty-six families contained sufficient numbers of AD individuals in multiple generations to support the argument for an autosomal dominant trait for specific, individual pedigrees. Further doubts concerning the integrity of AD families to fulfil diagnostic criteria is illustrated in another international linkage report by the same author (St George Hyslop et al., 1990). Dismally few families had any neuropathological confirmation and of the 20 British families which contributed to the analysis, 50% comprised one generation only, and in only six of the 20 families had AD been confirmed neuropathologically.

The problems of overlapping clinical definitions of AD-like dementias, and the lack of consistency between laboratories to identify with sufficient accuracy the number of plaques and tangles (with or without Lewy bodies), outline the ease with which pedigrees may be misdiagnosed as being AD, yet may be contributing to cumulative genetic linkage studies. While this chapter has focused on the problems presented by inadequate diagnosis to linkage investigations, other difficulties also exist. AD linkage studies are hampered by the majority of cases falling into the late-onset category. The difficulty being that there are rarely two affected generations who are simultaneously available for sampling, and often a family member dies of unrelated causes before reaching the age of onset for AD. Therefore, information is lost as to whether the individual was affected or unaffected. The extent to which data derived from AD linkage studies has been contaminated by misdiagnosis, sporadic AD cases, lack of penetrance and non-paternity has as yet to be realized. However, perhaps the most devastating prospect for genetic linkage is heterogeneity with the resulting likelihood that pedigrees sampled may represent more than one aetiology. A more general problem for genetic linkage studies today is the application of a statistically based level of analysis which was developed for inherited diseases where the diagnosis of the disorder was unambiguous. The application of these analyses to disorders where diagnostic ambiguities exist (particularly within the field of mental health), has led to a number of spurious linkage reports being published and suggests that a lod score of 3.0 is insufficiently stringent.

The future of molecular genetics for AD is dependent upon increasing the numbers of carefully scrutinized pedigrees and, within these families, establishing convincing lod scores with a range of probes mapped to the vicinity of the FAD locus, regardless of whether the locus is on chromosome 21, 19 or 14. A genetic linkage approach to AD will be reliable only with extended AD pedigrees, early and consistent ages of onset, several generations clinically and neuropathologically defined (by the same neuropathology laboratory – if possible), the identification of a reliable marker for AD and in parallel the development of diagnostic assays. If this seems difficult to achieve, it should be remembered that a genetic linkage approach to schizophrenia or manic depression is a minefield by comparison!

The debate continues as to whether AD should be perceived as a continuum of normal aging within which everyone would suffer from the dementia should they live long enough, or alternatively whether changes leading to AD dementia are distinct from those associated with normal aging and the issues central to the debate are well addressed within this volume. The extent to which genetic linkage clarifies the position is in itself debatable. If the mutations identified in the APP are confirmed as being causative of the dementia in the very few early-onset AD families the argument would swing in favour of a distinct defect – an all or nothing event. However, the fact that the dementia takes a minimum of 35–40 years to become manifest suggests a more complex interaction which may be age-factor dependent. Furthermore, strong evidence is emerging for a heterogeneous aetiology for the neuropathology in the majority of AD cases in which amyloid itself is not the key agent. This points towards abnormal cellular processing (Haass et al., 1992a,b; Schellenberg et al., 1992) of which the precise mechanisms involved have yet to be defined. However, these are likely to be influenced by a range of events – environmental, genetic, head trauma, normal aging and others – but with cell death being the outcome. Whatever the causes of cell death, AD dementia appears to be associated closely with the loss of cells located within specific cortical areas. The 'threshold' hypothesis (outlined in Chapter 10) in which a baseline level of a particular neuronal population is required for normal cognition suggests that to fall below this number – due to any of the events discussed previously – impairs cognition and, subsequently, the manifestation of AD symptoms. Frustratingly, it may be simply the number of hippocampal cells derived during gestation and in the early neonatal period that will determine vulnerability to the dementia. Thus, a boxer born with high numbers of hippocampal neurons can afford to lose more neurons through head injury than a Down syndrome individual who starts life with far fewer. Indeed, while a mutation may be the aetiology of neuronal cell death within some pedigrees, FAD may be no more than the inherited predisposition for deriving fewer numbers of cortical neurons during gestation. Clearly, this would bring into the field of AD research those developmental neurobiologists investigating the mechanisms underlying cell division, differentiation, target recognition and programmed cell death.

The application of genetic linkage to inherited disorders aims to identify the disease gene and, having achieved this, the challenge remains to develop a therapeutic intervention. If mutations in the amyloid gene do prove to be causative of AD dementia in rare families, then blood samples for DNA testing should reveal accurately whether an individual carries the mutation. Of course, even a negative test result for the known APP mutations does not rule out the possibility of the individual being at risk from some other contributing factor.

Clearly, it is the ambition of most pharmaceutical companies with an AD research interest to develop a drug therapy or diagnostic assay system for the disease. Yet, increased understanding of the disease brings with it the dilemma – is it in the individual's best interest to know whether at the age of 35, 65 or 85 years he/she will develop a chronically debilitating disease for which there is currently no cure, no therapeutic intervention and no hope of spontaneous recovery? To what extent will individuals who undergo genetic screening be obliged to reveal their results to insurance agencies? Furthermore, is AD a disorder we should consider screening for prenatally? Obviously, these questions have been raised in response to the availability of prenatal diagnosis for many of the disabling diseases such as Huntington's chorea and cystic fibrosis, and the issues raised are the subject of extensive moral, political and personal debate. However, surely pregnancy termination of positively screened fetuses cannot be contemplated seriously for a disease that is not manifested, in the majority of cases, until after the sixth decade. With anxiety mounting in administrators of health care programmes and social services agencies because of the ever increasing numbers of the elderly population in need of long-term medical care, it is disappointing that governments are not investing more into research programmes aimed at identifying ways of protecting the brain from the cellular degeneration that occurs in AD.

Acknowledgements   Sincere thanks to Dr S. B. Dunnett, Dr B. J. Sahakian and Dr J. R. W. Yates (University of Cambridge, UK), Dr W. R. G. Gibb (Institute of Psychiatry, London, UK), Dr D. M. A. Mann (University of Manchester, UK), Dr N. Quinn (Institute of Neurology, London, UK) and Dr R. H. Perry (Newcastle General Hospital, Newcastle upon Tyne, UK) for their helpful discussions.

Glossary

Alleles: alternative forms of a gene at the same chromosomal locus

Aneuploidy: any chromosome number that is not an exact multiple of the haploid number

Autosome: any chromosome other than the sex chromosomes (X and Y)

Autosomal dominant mutation: a mutation that exerts its full effect on the individual's phenotype despite the presence of another, normal allele of the gene on the paired chromosome. The mutation may be located on any chromosome other than the X or Y chromosome

Centromere: the site on the chromosome that provides the attachment for the chromosome to the spindle during mitosis

Crossovers: exchanges of genetic material between homologous chromosomes during meiosis

Heterogeneity: different genetic backgrounds producing the same observable characteristics

Homozygous: carrying two identical alleles at a particular locus, one on each of a pair of chromosomes

Karyotype: the assessed chromosomal complement of the individual or of a cell

Linkage: the location of two or more genes or markers on the same chromosome

Locus/loci: the specific location of gene(s) on a chromosome

Lod: logarithm of the odds ratio – a statistically based analysis employed in genetic linkage

Marker: a detectable allelic difference

Meiosis: cell division which occurs during gamete production

Obligate region: the chromosomal region considered to be necessary for the manifestation of a particular phenotype

Penetrance: the frequency of which the genotype is expressed

Phenotype: the physical manifestation of a genetic trait

Polymorphic: demonstrating genetic variation

Polymorphism: any characteristic that shows genetic variation within a population

Probe: a DNA fragment which is used to identify a complementary sequence. Invariably the fragment is visualized by the incorporation of a radioisotope or a fluorescent marker

Recombinant: where the marker and disease locus have segregated during meiosis

Restriction fragment length polymorphisms (RFLPs): a difference in a DNA sequence revealed by changes in restriction enzyme recognition sites

Segregation: the separation of allelic genes during meiosis

Syntenic: the same loci are located on the same chromosome

Telomere/telomeric: the tip of a chromosome

Translocation: a chromosomal rearrangement in which two different chromosomes are broken and reattached incorrectly to each other. In a *balanced* translocation the same amount of chromosomal material is inherited, whereas in an *unbalanced* translocation chromosomal material is either gained or lost

Trisomy: three copies of a particular chromosome per cell being inherited rather than the normal two, i.e. instead of one copy from each parent, two copies are received from one parent and a single copy of the same chromosome is received from the other parent

References

Benson, M. D. (1989). Familial amyloidotic polyneuropathy. *Trends in Neuroscience*, **12**, 88–92.

Botstein, D., White, R., Skolnik, M. & Davies, R. (1980). Construction of a genetic linkage map in man using restriction fragment length polymorphisms. *American Journal of Human Genetics*, **32**, 314–31.

Breitner, J. C. S., Silverman, J. S., Mohs, R. C. & David, K. L. (1988). Familial aggregation in Alzheimer's disease: comparison of risk among relatives of early- and late-onset cases and among male and female relatives in successive generations. *Neurology*, **38**, 207–12.

Brown, P., Goldfarb, L. G. & Gajdusek, D. C. (1991). The new biology of spongioform encephalopathy: infectious amyloidoses with a genetic twist. *Lancet*, **337**, 1019–22.

Burger, P. C. & Vogel, F. S. (1973). The development of the pathologic changes of Alzheimer's disease and senile dementia in patients with Down syndrome. *American Journal of Pathology*, **73**, 457–76.

Caputo, C. B., Wischik, C., Sobel, I. R. E., Kirschner, D. A., Fraser, P. E. & Brunner, W. F. (1991). Possible contribution of the C-terminus of β-amyloid protein precursor (APP) to Alzheimer paired helical filaments (PHF's). *Neuroscience Abstracts*, **17**, 573.6.

Conneally, P. M. & Rivas, M. L. (1980). Linkage Analysis in Man. In H. Harris & K. Hirschhorn (eds.) *Advances in Human Genetics*, vol. 10, p. 209. Plenum, · New York.

Davies, L., Wolska, B., Milbich, C., Multhaup, E., Martins, R., Simms, E., Beyreuther, K. G. & Masters, C. L. (1988). A4 amyloid protein depositions and the diagnosis of Alzheimer's disease: prevalence in aged brains determined by immunocytochemistry compared with conventional neuropathological techniques. *Neurology*, **38**, 1688–93.

Davies, P. (1986). Genetics of Alzheimer's disease: a review and a discussion of the implications. *Neurobiology of Aging*, **7**, 459–66.

Duyckaerts, C., Delaère, P., Hauw, J.-J., Abbamondi-Pinto, A. L., Sorbi, S., Allen, I., Brion, J. P., Flament-Durand, J., Duchen, L., Kauss, J., Schlote, W., Lowe, J., Probst, A., Ravid, R., Swaab, D. F., Renkawek, K. & Tomlinson, B. (1990). Rating of the lesions in senile dementia of the Alzheimer type: concordance between laboratories. *Journal of the Neurological Sciences*, **97**, 295–323.

Gibb, W. R. G., Mountjoy, C. Q., Mann, D. M. A. & Lees, A. J. (1989). A pathological study of the association between Lewy body disease and Alzheimer's disease. *Journal of Neurology, Neurosurgery and Psychiatry*, **52**, 701–8.

Goate, A. M., Owen, M. J., James, L. A., Mullan, M. J., Rossor, M. N., Haynes, A. R., Farrall, M., Lai, L. Y. C., Roques, P., Williamson, R. & Hardy, J. A. (1989). Predisposing locus for Alzheimer's disease on chromosome 21. *Lancet*, **i**, 352–5.

Goate, A., Chartier-Harlain, M.-C., Mullan, M., Brown, J., Crawford, F., Fidani, L., Giuffra, L., Haynes, A., Irving, N., James, L., Mant, R., Newton, P., Rooke, K., Roques, P., Talbot, C., Pericak-Vance, M., Roses, A., Williamson, R., Rossor, M., Owen, M. & Hardy, J. (1991). Segregation of a missense mutation in the amyloid precursor protein gene with familial Alzheimer's disease. *Nature*, **349**, 704–7.

Goldgaber, D., Lerman, M. I., McBride, O. W., Saffiotti, U. & Gajdusek, D. C. (1987). Characterization and chromosomal localization of a cDNA encoding brain amyloid of Alzheimer's disease. *Science*, **235**, 877–80.

Haass, C., Koo, E. H., Mellon, A., Hung, A. Y., & Selkoe, D. J. (1992a).

Targeting of cell surface beta-amyloid precursor protein to lysosomes – alternative processing into amyloid-bearing fragments. *Nature*, **357**, 500–3.

Haass, C., Koo, E. H., Mellon, A., Hung, A. Y., & Selkoe, D. J. (1992b). A second constitutive pathway for the beta-amyloid precursor protein – targeting of cell surface molecules to lysosomes. *Journal of Neuropathology and Experimental Neurology*, **51**, 358.

Jeffreys, A. J. (1979). DNA sequence variants in the $^G\gamma$-, $^A\gamma$-, δ- and β-globin genes of man. *Cell*, **18**, 1–10.

Kang, J., Lemaire, H.-G., Unterbeck, A., Salbaum, M., Masters, C. L., Grzeschik, K.-H., Multhaup, G., Beyreuther, K. & Muller-Hill, B. (1987). The precursor of Alzheimer's disease amyloid A4 protein. *Nature*, **325**, 733–6.

Khatchaturian, Z. A. (1985). Diagnosis of Alzheimer's disease. *Archives of Neurology*, **42**, 1097–105.

Kosaka, K. (1990). Diffuse Lewy body disease in Japan. *Journal of Neurology*, **237**, 197–204.

Laurie, D. A., Palmer, R. W. & Hultin, M. A. (1982). Chiasma derived genetic lengths and recombination fractions: chromosomes 2 and 9. *Annals of Human Genetics*, **46**, 233–44.

Lejcune, J., Gautier, M. & Turpin, R. (1959). Etudes des chromosomes somatiques de neuf enfants mongoliens. *Comptes Rendue Académie de Science*, **248**, 1721–2.

Levy, E., Carman, M. D., Fernandez-Madrid, I. J., Power, M. D., Lieberburg, I., van Duinen, S. G., Bots, B. T. A., Luyendijk, W. & Frangione, B. (1990). Mutation of the Alzheimer's disease amyloid gene in hereditary cerebral hemorrhage with amyloidosis of Dutch type. *Science*, **248**, 1124–6.

Lindenbaum, R. H., Clarke, G., Patel, C., Moncrieff, M. & Hughes, J. T. (1979). Muscular dystrophy in an X;1 translocation female suggests that Duchenne locus is on X chromosome short arm. *Medical Genetics*, **16**, 389–92.

Mann, D. M. A., Yates, P. O., Marcyniuk, B. & Ravindra, C. R. (1987). Loss of nerve cells from cortical and subcortical areas in Down's syndrome patients at middle age: quantitative comparisons with younger Down's patients and patients with Alzheimer's disease. *Journal of the Neurological Sciences*, **80**, 79–89.

Mann, D. M. A., Prinja, D., Davies, C. A., Ihara, Y., Delacourte, A., Defossez, A., Mayer, R. J. & Landon, M. (1989). Immunocytochemical profile of neurofibrillary tangles in Down's syndrome patients of different ages. *Journal of the Neurological Sciences*, **92**, 247–60.

McKusick, V. A. & Ruddle, F. (1977). The status of the gene map of human chromosomes. *Science*, **196**, 390–405.

Murray, J. M., Davies, K. E., Harper, P. S., Meredith, L., Muller, C. R., Goodfellow, P. N. & Williamson, R. (1982). Linkage relationship with a cloned cDNA sequence on the short arm of the X chromosome to Duchenne muscular dystrophy. *Nature*, **300**, 69–71.

Murrell, J., Farlow, M., Ghetti, B. & Benson, M. (1991). A mutation in the amyloid precursor protein associated with hereditary Alzheimer's disease. *Science*, **254**, 97–9.

Nakamura, Y., Leppert, M., O'Connell, P., Wolff, R., Holm, T., Culver, M., Martin, C., Fujimoto, E., Hoff, M., Kumlin, E. & White, R. (1987). Variable number tandem repeat markers for human gene mapping. *Science*, **235**, 1616–22.

Naruse, S., Igarashi, S., Aoki, K., Kaneko, K., Iihara, K., Miyatake, T., Kobayashi, H., Inuzuka, T., Shimizu, T., Kojima, T. & Tsuji, S. (1991). Missense mutation Val–Ile in exon 17 of amyloid precursor protein gene in Japanese familial Alzheimer's disease. *Lancet*, **337**, 978–9.

Navaratnam, D. S., Priddle, J. D., McDonald, B., Esiri, M. M., Robinson, J. R. & Smith, A. D. (1991). Anomalous molecular form of acetylcholinesterase in cerebrospinal fluid in histologically diagnosed Alzheimer's disease. *Lancet*, **337**, 447–50.

Oliver, C. & Holland, A. J. (1986). Down's syndrome and Alzheimer's disease: a review. *Psychological Medicine*, **16**, 307–22.

Ott, J. (1985). Variability of the recombination fraction. In S. H. Boyer, G. M. Green, R. T. Johnson, P. R. McHugh, E. A. Murphy, A. H. Owens, J. L. Spivak & B. H. Starfield (eds.) *Analysis of Human Genetic Linkage*, pp. 97–119. The John Hopkins University Press, Baltimore.

Pericak-Vance, M. A., Yamaoka, L. H., Haynes, C. S., Speer, M. C., Haines, J. L., Gaskell, P. C., Hung, W.-Y., Clark, C. M., Heyman, A. L., Trofatter, J. A., Eisenmenger, J. P., Gilbert, J. R., Lee, J. E., Alberts, M. J., Dawson, D. V., Bartlett, R. J., Earl, N. L., Siddique, T., Vance, J. M., Conneally, P. M. & Roses, A. D. (1988). Genetic linkage in Alzheimer's disease families. *Experimental Neurology*, **102**, 271–9.

Perry, R. H., Irving, D., Blessed, G., Fairbairn, A. & Perry, E. K. (1990a). Senile dementia of Lewy body type. A clinically and neuropathologically distinct form of Lewy body dementia in the elderly. *Journal of the Neurological Sciences*, **95**, 119–39.

Perry, R. H., Irving, D. & Tomlinson, B. E. (1990b). Lewy body prevalence in the ageing brain: relationship to neuropsychiatric disorders, Alzheimer-type pathology and catecholaminergic nuclei. *Journal of the Neurological Sciences*, **100**, 223–33.

Price, D. L., Borchelt, D. R., Walker, L. C. & Sisodia, S. S. (1992). Toxicity of synthetic Aβ peptides and modeling of Alzheimer's disease. *Neurobiology of Aging*, **13**, 623–5.

Race, R. R. & Sanger, R. (1975). *Blood Groups in Man*, 6th edition, pp. 594–618. Blackwell Scientific Publications, Oxford.

Rao, D. C., Keats, G. J. G., Morton, N. E., Yee, S. & Lew, R. (1978). Variability of human linkage data. *American Journal of Human Genetics*, **30**, 516–29.

Reeves, R. H., Robakis, N. K., Oster-Granite, M.-L., Wisniewski, H. M., Coyle, J. T. & Gearhart, J. D. (1987). Genetic linkage in the mouse of genes involved in Down syndrome and Alzheimer's disease in man. *Molecular Brain Research*, **2**, 215–21.

Richards, S.-J., Waters, J. J., Beyreuther, K., Masters, C. L., Wischik, C. M., Sparkman, D. R., White III, C. L., Abraham, C. R. & Dunnett, S. B. (1991).

Transplants of mouse Trisomy 16 hippocampus provide a model of Alzheimer's disease neuropathology. *EMBO Journal*, **10**, 297–303.

Robakis, N. K., Wisniewski, H. M., Jenkins, E. C., Devine-Gage, E. A., Houck, G. E., Yao, X.-L., Ramakrishna, N., Wolf, G., Silverman, W. P. & Brown, W. E. (1987). Chromosome 21q21 sublocalization of gene encoding β-amyloid peptide in cerebral blood vessels and neuritic (senile) plaques of people with Alzheimer's disease and Down syndrome. *Lancet*, i, 384–5.

Roses, A. D. (1989). A conservative viewpoint on linkage in Alzheimer's disease. *Neurobiology of Aging*, **10**, 427–9.

Rumble, B., Retallack, R., Hilbich, C., Simms, G., Multhaup, G., Martins, R., Hockey, A., Montgomery, P., Beyreuther, K. & Masters, C. L. (1989). Amyloid A4 protein and its precursor in Down's syndrome and Alzheimer's disease. *New England Journal of Medicine*, **320**, 1446–52.

Schellenberg, G. D., Bird, T. D., Wijsman, E. M., Moore, D. K., Boehnke, M., Bryant, E. M., Lampe, T. H., Nochlin, D., Sumi, S. M., Deeb, S. S., Beyreuther, K. & Martin, G. M. (1989). Absence of linkage of chromosome 21q21 markers to familial Alzheimer's disease. *Science*, **241**, 1507–10.

Schellenberg, G. D., Bird, T. D., Wijsman, E. M., Orr, H. T., Anderson, L., Nemens, E., White, J. A., Bonnycastle, L., Weber, J. L., Alonso, M. E., Potter, H., Heston, L. L. & Martin, G. M. (1992). Genetic linkage evidence for a familial Alzheimer's disease locus on chromosome 14. *Science*, **258**, 668–71.

St George Hyslop, P. H., Tanzi, R. E., Polinsky, R. J., Haines, J. L., Nee, L., Watkins, P. C., Myers, R. H., Feldman, R. G., Pollen, D., Drachman, D., Growden, J., Bruni, A., Foncin, J.-F., Salmon, D., Frommelt, P., Amaducci, L., Sorbi, S., Piacentini, S., Stewart, G. D., Hobbs, W. J., Conneally, P. M. & Gusella, J. F. (1987). The genetic defect causing familial Alzheimer's disease maps on chromosome 21. *Science*, **253**, 885–90.

St George Hyslop, P. H., Myers, R. H., Haines, J. L., Farrer, L. A., Tanzi, R. E., Abe, K., James, M. F., Conneally, P. M., Polinsky, R. J. & Gusella, J. F. (1989). Familial Alzheimer's disease: progress and problems. *Neurobiology of Aging*, **10**, 417–25.

St George Hyslop, P. H., Haines, J. L., Farrer, L. A., Polinsky, R., van Broeckhoven, C. and the FAD collaborative study (1990). Genetic linkage studies suggest that Alzheimer's disease is not a single homogeneous disorder. *Nature*, **347**, 194–7.

Tanzi, R. E., Gusella, J. F., Watkins, P. C., Bruns, G. A. P., St George Hyslop, P. H., van Keuren, M. L., Patterson, D., Pagen, S., Kurnit, D. M. & Neve, R. L. (1987). Amyloid β protein gene: cDNA, mRNA distribution and genetic linkage near the Alzheimer locus. *Science*, **235**, 880–4.

van Broeckhoven, C., Genthe, A. M., Vandenberghe, A., Horsthemka, B., Backhovens, H., Raeymaekers, P., van Hul, W., Wehnert, A., Gheuens, J., Cras, P., Bruyland, M., Martin, J. J., Salbaum, M., Multhaup, G., Masters, C. L., Beyreuther, K., Gurling, H. M. D., Mullan, M., Holland, A., Barton, A., Irving, N., Williamson, R., Richards, S.-J. & Hardy, J. A. (1987). Failure of familial Alzheimer's disease to segregate with the A4-amyloid gene in several European families. *Nature*, **329**, 153–5.

van Broeckhoven, C., van Hul, W., van Camp, G., Wehnert, A., Stinissen, P., Raeymaekers, P., de Winter, G., Gheuens, J., Martin, J. J. & Vandenberghe, A. (1988). The familial Alzheimer's disease gene is located close to the centromere of chromosome 21. *American Journal of Human Genetics*, **43**, A205.

van Broeckhoven, C., Backhovens, H., van Hul, W., van Camp, G., Stinissen, P., Wehnert, A., Raeymaekers, P., de Winter, G., Bruyland, M., Gheuens, J., Martin, J. J., & Vandenberghe, A. (1990a). Genetic linkage analysis in early-onset Alzheimer's dementia. In Bunney, Hippius, Laakman & Schmauss (eds.) *Neuropsychopharmacology*, pp. 86–91. Springer-Verlag, Berlin.

van Broeckhoven, C., Haan, J., Bakker, E., Hardy, J. A., van Hul, W., Wehnert, A., Vegter-van der Vlis, M. & Roos, R. A. C. (1990b). Amyloid β protein precursor gene and hereditary cerebral haemorrhage with amyloidosis (Dutch). *Science*, **248**, 1120–2.

van Duijn, C. M., Hendriks, L., Cruts, M., Hardy, J., Hofman, A. & van Broeckhoven, C. (1991). Amyloid precursor protein gene mutation in early-onset Alzheimer's disease. *Lancet*, **337**, 978.

Wyman, A. R. & White, R. (1980). A highly polymorphic locus in human DNA. *Proceedings of the National Academy of Sciences, USA*, **77**, 6754–8.

Yanker, B. A. & Mesulam, M. D. (1991). β-Amyloid and the pathogenesis of Alzheimer's disease. *New England Journal of Medicine*, **325**, 1849–57.

Yates, J. R. W. & Connor, J. M. (1986). Genetic linkage. *British Journal of Hospital Medicine*, **36**, 133–6.

Yoshioka, K., Miki, T., Katsuya, T., Ogihara, T. & Sakaki, Y. (1991). The Val–Ile substitution in amyloid precursor protein is associated with familial Alzheimer's disease regardless of ethnic groups. *Biochemical and Biophysical Research Communications*, **178**, 1141–6.

Zatz, M., Vianna-Morgante, A. M., Campos, P. & Diament, A. J. (1981). Translocation (X;6) in a female with Duchenne muscular dystrophy: implications for the localisation of the DMD locus. *Journal of Medical Genetics*, **18**, 442–7.

PART VII

Health care and social policy issues

Health-care policy and planning for dementia: an international perspective

BRIAN COOPER

Worldwide, the numbers of persons aged over 65 years are growing currently at an annual rate of 2.4%, more rapidly than the global population as a whole. This rate of growth will lead already by the year 2000 to a total of some 410 million elderly, of whom an estimated 59% will be living in the less developed countries, and will continue well into the twenty-first century (US Department of Commerce, Bureau of the Census, 1987). In the more developed regions of the world, it is, above all, the disproportionate increase in numbers of the very old that portends for the decades ahead a continuing massive growth in the public health problems of age-related disability and dependency. Thus, demographic projections for the period 1980–2020 have pointed to a relative increase of some 65% in the populations of these regions aged over 65 years, but well over 100% among those aged over 80 years (Siegel & Hoover, 1982). These demographic trends imply, in particular, a steeply rising frequency of dementia, whose age-specific prevalence has been shown to fit an exponential curve over the age range above 60 years (Jorm et al., 1987). While all forms of mental disorder associated with old age must be expected to present greater demands in future on the medical and social services, there can be no doubt that dementing disorders will pose the greatest challenge.

This chapter is concerned primarily with questions of care provision for old people with clinically diagnosable dementing disorders, although it also pays some attention to the public-health significance of so-called 'mild dementia', a topic now of increasing concern (see the section below and also Chapter 6).

In this context, the traditional epidemiological concept of a 'case' of illness usually refers to the severe and moderately severe degrees of dementia. The best available basis for estimating the extent of

Dementia and Normal Aging, eds. F. A. Huppert, C. Brayne & D. W. O'Connor.
© Cambridge University Press 1994.

needs, and hence for service planning, is provided by data on the frequency and distribution of such 'cases' in elderly populations, together with information on the affected persons' physical health status, family situation and social circumstances. Milder forms of cognitive deficit are here of interest chiefly as predictors of disease onset, and as diagnostic pointers in early case-detection. This approach is, however, fundamentally a pragmatic one, which does not necessarily imply a preference for one theoretical model of morbidity over another. It is important to emphasize that the notion of a 'case', while highly convenient in public-health epidemiology, depends ultimately on social judgements and, for research purposes, must be made operational by means of descriptive criteria, whichever theoretical model the investigators favour. The most useful tools of measurement will be those which permit the findings to be expressed in terms either of categories or of dimensions, because, as Cooper & Schwarz (1982) have argued with respect to the field of psychogeriatric illness more generally, where such an approach proves to be feasible, much of the heat will be taken out of the 'either–or' controversy.

Not a great deal is known about special service provision for old people with dementia in different countries and global regions, since the existing health information systems are not yet developed well enough for this purpose. The following brief review is restricted to those areas of the world, notably western Europe, North America and Australia, for which enough information about health care of the elderly is available to permit meaningful comparisons to be made and some broad conclusions to be drawn. In large measure, one has to rely upon official policy pronouncements, the published findings of ad hoc research projects and commissions of inquiry, and descriptive reports by individual observers and interest groups. The statistical and economic data available at national level usually pertain to much wider categories, such as psychiatric hospital services, long-stay care accommodation, services for the disabled and the dependent elderly, or community nursing and social services as a whole. While broad inferences can often be drawn from such information, it is obvious that large differences in both type and quality of provision for dementia can lie concealed behind the published data.

National expenditures on health care provide a case in point. The proportion of total medical expenditure accounted for by persons aged over 65 years is rising rapidly in all European countries, with a mean increase of from 37% in 1985 to an estimated 58% by 2015. There is, however, extensive variation among the countries concerned, both in

Table 22.1. *Health care and social expenditures of European Community countries, 1981–82, as a proportion of total gross domestic product*

Country	Health care (1981) (%)	Social budget (1982) (%)
Belgium	6.4	30.2
Denmark	6.9	29.3
France	9.3	27.2
Federal Republic of Germany	8.2	29.5
Ireland	8.2	22.0[a]
Italy	7.0	24.7
Luxembourg	9.5[a]	27.1
Netherlands	9.1	31.7
United Kingdom	5.9	23.5

[a]Data for 1980.
From Mangen (1985).

the baseline figures – from 18% to 44% in 1985 – and in the rates of increase – from 42% to 105% over the 30-year period (ILO, 1991). Moreover, the quality of services provided may not be reflected accurately in these statistics. Of the countries listed in Table 22.1, Denmark has one of the best developed service networks, despite a relatively low expenditure on health care. British psychogeriatric services enjoy a high reputation, although total health-care costs in the UK are well below the mean and the proportion devoted to the elderly is average only.

Again, while rates of institutional care for the elderly will obviously depend upon national levels of provision, the variation among affluent industrial nations appears to be as large as the differences between these and many less developed countries; for example, 11–12% of old people are in long-stay care in the Netherlands, but only 5–6% in France and Belgium. Very little of this variation can be explained by differences in age structure (OECD, 1991). The factors that govern the nature and standard of care provision in each country are complex, the situation being influenced by the structure of its population, the historical development and financial basis of its medical and social welfare services, its economic prosperity and, not least, the philosophy which informs its policy of care for disabled and handicapped citizens.

Dimensions of the public-health problem

International communication in medicine presupposes the use of gen- erally accepted diagnostic definitions and systems of classification. In the past, comparative studies of dementia have been hampered by uncertainty about the nature of the disorder and its relationship both to other clinical conditions and to normal aging (see Chapter 3). Modern definitions, such as that by the Royal College of Physicians (1981), stress that dementia is essentially a clinical syndrome, characterized by global impairments affecting memory and other higher cortical functions, performance of learned skills and control of emotional reac- tions, which can be caused by a number of different brain pathologies. This view has proved to be of great help in promoting scientific com- munication and has been incorporated into more recent definitions and standard classifications (see Chapter 5 and Chapter 6). Research workers in the different world regions can now be reasonably confident that they are dealing with a common diagnostic concept, although difficulties are still encountered with respect both to differential diag- nosis and to subdividing dementia according to its degree of clinical severity or the stage of its progression.

Predicting future levels of need and demand for services

Studies of the prevalence and distribution of dementing disorders in elderly patients are reviewed in this volume by Brayne (Chapter 9), and will not be discussed further here. The epidemiological data pro- vide a baseline for prediction of the future numbers and distribution of dementia cases in populations for use in forward planning, which must try to keep ahead of changes in the levels of need and demand for services. A number of workers have computed projected popu- lation figures against age-specific prevalence ratios for dementia, derived from one or more field studies. Thus, Kramer (1980) forecast a worldwide increase from nine to over 15 million in the number of dementia sufferers during the period 1975–2000. While this was a useful exercise in drawing attention to the global dimensions of the problem, more recent estimates based on pooled international data suggest that the prevalence ratios he employed may have been too high (Jorm et al., 1987; Hofman et al., 1991).

To make national service-planning as accurate as possible, attention must be paid to the country's population structure and demographic trends. Although data from area surveys in different European countries, and indeed in developed industrial societies more generally, point to a relative uniformity of age-specific prevalence ratios over the latter one-third of the life span, demographic projections for the different countries indicate that the continued aging of their populations will result in widely differing increases in case numbers over the next decades, even assuming that the age-specific prevalence ratios remain uniform. Jorm et al. (1988), who examined this question on the basis of pooled data from 22 field studies in different countries, found that the age-specific prevalence estimates from their pooled data conformed to a baseline model of the form:

$P_i = \exp(S_i - 13.50 + 0.137X)$

where:

P$_i$ is the prevalence ratio of dementia for persons aged X in study i

S$_i$ is a variable term, specific to study i but independent of age

X is age in years.

Although prevalence ratios differ between individual studies, their increase with age takes a similar exponential form in each, while the proportionate increase over a given base-year is invariant over values of exp (S$_i$). Hence, in predicting percentage increase in each study population, the formula can be reduced to:

$P_i = \exp(-13.50 + 0.137X)$

Applying this statistical model to UN population projections for 29 countries, Jorm et al. (1988) found that, in each, an overall increase, both in the numbers of the elderly and in dementia prevalence, could be predicted for the period 1980–2025, but that the increases showed no single consistent pattern. Projections for selected countries, shown in Figure 22.1, emphasize the range of variation.

At one extreme are the trends for Ireland, where, until about 2020, the rate of increase for the population as a whole will be greater than that for the elderly; at the other extreme is the pattern for Japan, where, by 2025, the total population will have increased by only 13% over that in 1980, but the number of the elderly will have increased by 128% and that of dementia sufferers by 215%, so that a dramatic increase in the demand for special services must be expected. Other countries with high projected increases in dementia cases include Australia, Bulgaria, Canada, Finland, Greece, New Zealand, Poland and Portugal. The large differences in national projections underline the need for care in making statistical predictions and the errors that can arise if forecasts for one country are extrapolated to others.

Economic costs of dementia

The most careful, detailed examinations of the economic consequences of late-life dementia have been undertaken in the USA. Three studies in the 1980s attempted to estimate the overall costs to the nation of caring for persons with dementia, taking into account the costs of diagnosis, treatment, nursing-home and community care, loss in terms of earned income and other indirect costs (Battelle Memorial Institute, 1984; Hu et al., 1986; Hay & Ernst, 1987). The estimates were based in each case on the expected number of new cases annually, derived from epidemiological field-studies in the USA and elsewhere, which were thought to provide reliable prevalence and incidence data. In fact, the projected numbers of new cases differed considerably between studies, but nevertheless the estimated total costs were of roughly the same order in each analysis: Hu et al. (1986) reached a figure of 38 billion dollars for 1983; the Battelle Memorial Institute (1984) estimated between 24 and 48 billion dollars for 1985; while Hay & Ernst (1987) computed from 28 to 31 billion dollars for dementia

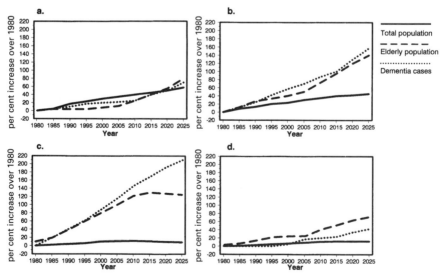

Figure 22.1. Projected increases in dementia cases, elderly population and total population for: (a) Ireland; (b) Australia; (c) Japan; (d) France. (Adapted from Jorm et al. (1988) with the permission of Munksgaard International Publishers Ltd, Copenhagen, Denmark.)

of the Alzheimer's type alone in 1983. These computations, which must be viewed against the background of a high GNP and an exceptionally costly health-care system, cannot be extrapolated to other countries, even in the developed industrial world. They are, none-the-less, of general value in emphasizing the importance of dementia as a burden on national economies, and the potential gains to be won from scientific advance in its prevention and treatment.

In many countries today, the main burden of costs for care of the demented elderly is borne, not by health insurance cover, but by social-security funds which are subject to means testing. Thus, an analysis of the total visible costs of mental-illness care for persons aged over 60 years in one area of Germany (Bundesministerium, 1986) revealed that 60% came from social-welfare funds, because geriatric-home care accounted for some two-thirds of the total budget and was not payable by health insurance, long-stay residential care not being part of medical treatment. In this study, the costs of geriatric-home care were 10 times as high as the total expenditure on ambulatory and domiciliary care for the elderly mentally ill. Such findings point to a need for redistributive action, not only to stop many old people from being pauperized by their ill-health, but also to ensure higher priority in future for community-based forms of care.

The public-health significance of mild dementia

Estimates of the amount of disability in elderly populations which is attributable to dementia, as well as the economic consequences of this disease category, will tend to underrate the true magnitude of the problem if they are based solely on the frequency of clinically manifest cases, ignoring the milder degrees of cognitive impairment. This point becomes at once apparent if a dimensional model is adopted (Brayne & Calloway, 1988), for the latter assumes that no point of rarity is to be expected on a continuum ranging from normal aging to severe, disabling dementia. It is, however, also compatible with a categorical disease model, since one consequence of the insidious onset and slow mental deterioration which characterize most dementing processes must be the presence of large numbers of mild cases in any cross-section of the elderly population.

Trying to quantify the contribution of mild forms of dementia to the total public-health burden is difficult none-the-less, for a number of reasons. Estimates of their prevalence in field surveys have varied widely, and appear in general to be much less reliable than those for dementia of clinical severity (Henderson & Huppert, 1984). This is perhaps unsurprising, in view of the unclear definition of mild dementia and the extent to which old people's performances on cognitive testing may be influenced by such non-specific factors as physical ill-health, sensory handicap, affective disturbance or poor literacy (see Chapter 6). While such consequences of severe dementia as gross memory loss, disorientation and confusion are readily apparent, mild dementia is associated with less conspicuous forms of abnormality, whose true cause may not be so easy to identify. Standardized screening tests show low efficiency in picking out cases of mild dementia, so that many persons are classified incorrectly and small differences of method may result in large discrepancies in the findings (Mowry & Burvill, 1988).

For all these reasons, little is known as yet about the public-health consequences of mild dementia, and one must rely on the tentative findings of a handful of community-based research projects which have paid attention to this question. Two recent studies, one in the UK and one in Germany, are relevant here because both were based on unselected general-practice populations and both made use of the 'CAMDEX' criteria (Roth et al., 1986; see Chapter 4) to assess the severity of individual cases. This procedure incorporates systematic guidelines which enable clinically trained researchers to allocate elderly persons on examination to one or other of five stages: severely, moderately, mildly or minimally demented, or cognitively unimpaired.

The British study (O'Connor et al., 1991) used CAMDEX to examine a sample of 481 Cambridge (UK) residents who were aged over 75 years and then examined a subsample of these (who were classified as being cognitively normal, minimally demented or mildly demented) on the Blessed–Roth dementia scale (Blessed et al., 1968). The latter scale is based on informants' responses to questions about memory, orientation and personal care, and can be regarded as being a crude measure of disability. While only 9.3% of the cognitively normal patients received a high disability score, this proportion increased to 27.5% among the minimally demented and 73.6% among those with mild dementia. The data are suggestive less of a threshold effect than of a continuous increase in disability risk over the whole range of cognitive loss. However, these findings may have been confounded to some extent because, actually, the Blessed–Roth scale measures a mixture of dementia-related impairments and less specific forms of disability.

The aims and method of the German research project (Cooper et al., 1992a, b) differed in certain respects. The study was based on a documentation of over 3000 consulting patients aged over 65 years, and the sample selected for more detailed investigation was stratified according to the general practitioners' assessments of their patients' mental functioning, those thought to be demented or impaired cognitively being systematically oversampled. In addition, assessments of disability, while based partly on informant interviews, also drew on direct interviewing of patients and observations made during home visits, and were rated on a series of scales, hence the associations between degree of cognitive impairment and disability in everyday life could be analysed in some detail. Table 22.2 presents the frequencies with which various indicators of disability and dependency were found in each of the CAMDEX severity grades.

Striking features of this table are the steepness with which most indicators increase in frequency across the severity grades and the extent to which elderly patients classified as being mildly demented were already handicapped in their everyday routines: 40% were unable to leave the house unaccompanied; 85% could not use public transport without help, and one-third had been admitted to long-term residential care. It appears, in short, that the stage of mild dementia, at any rate as defined by CAMDEX guidelines, is already associated with a pronounced loss of autonomy and capacity for normal living.

Of course one can object that, as mental and physical ill-health are known to co-exist in very many old people, and particularly among those who consult in medical practice, the disabilities represented in Table 22.2 might be determined less by cognitive disorder than by concomitant physical impairments. In fact, the research data provided only limited support for this argument. When the study sample was further subdivided, using operational criteria, into persons with, and those without, one or more severe physical impairments, the frequency of disability differed much less between these groups than it did between the cognitively normal and the demented. A severe degree of disability and dependency seems indeed to be found rather infrequently among elderly general-practice patients, in the absence of a dementing disorder or related cerebral pathology. Of a total of 79 severely disabled individuals in this sample, only eight (10.1%) were free from cognitive disorder, 21 (26.6%) suffered from dementing illness alone and 50 (63.3%) were both cognitively and physically impaired. Although cognitive disorders were less crucial in determining the milder degrees of disability, it is noteworthy that 42%

Table 22.2. *Disability and dependency on others among general-practice patients aged over 65 years, according to degree of cognitive impairment (n = 407)*

Indicators of disability and dependency	Degree of cognitive impairment (CAMDEX criteria)				
	No cognitive impairment (n = 223) (%)	Minimal dementia (n = 67) (%)	Mild dementia (n = 42) (%)	Severe or moderately severe dementia (n = 75) (%)	
Unable to leave apartment unaccompanied	2.7	19.4	40.5	64.0	
Use of public transport only if accompanied	13.5	55.2	85.7	100.0	
Cannot dress or wash without help	1.8	10.4	28.6	80.0	
Frequent urinary incontinence	1.3	10.4	11.9	58.7	
Frequent faecal incontinence	0.0	0.0	2.4	38.7	
Nursing care and supervision required	0.9	9.0	16.7	85.3	
Help and supervision for at least four hours daily	9.0	25.4	78.6	92.0	
Resident in long-stay geriatric home	1.8	9.0	33.3	46.7	

From Cooper et al. (1992a).

of the elderly patients in this category were also characterized by some degree of dementia. Furthermore, extrapolation of the sample findings to the background population of elderly general-practice patients suggested that, while 67% of all those dependent on others for care are suffering from dementia of clinical severity, an additional 13% manifest milder degrees of cognitive impairment which contribute to their infirmity and disablement. These findings underline the practical importance of the concept of 'mild dementia' and the need for its more systematic investigation.

Provision and co-ordination of special services for dementia

Issues of service provision

The new awareness of dementia as a medico-social problem has given rise in many countries to vigorous, and at times heated, discussion of the issues that arise in national health policy and planning. In fact, the most urgent problems are not specific to dementia, but relate to a more general increase in need for care of the disabled and dependent elderly. Nevertheless, it is without doubt the increase in numbers of the demented, the group making the heaviest demands on families and nursing services, that has contributed most to the developing crisis in care and has fuelled the ongoing public debate.

Because of their usually intractable and progressive character, late-life dementing disorders pose a number of difficult questions of health policy, which arise in most acute form wherever the tasks and responsibilities of different service agencies are demarcated rigidly. The inclusion of prolonged nursing and supportive care under health insurance cover; the advantages and drawbacks of geriatric nursing homes as compared to hospital facilities; the desirability of segregating demented old people from other residents within these establishments; the organization of extramural and domiciliary forms of care; the appropriate ways to help affected families and the part that should be played in diagnosis and case management by the general practitioner and his co-workers: each of these problems can be resolved most successfully where service structures and cost-bearing modalities are flexible enough to foster professional co-operation and an effective continuity of care.

Central to all the issues is the need for an integrated psychogeriatric service, with in-patient, day-care, out-patient and consultative functions. In order to respond adequately to the needs of the elderly and their families, such a service requires to be based on a defined population and to accept responsibility for the medical needs that arise within it. Arie (1989), reviewing the growth of old-age psychiatry in the UK, has emphasized that the services are based on health districts with an average of about 250 000 inhabitants, each with its own team for the elderly mentally ill. This size of population, which in western European countries today will include as many as 40 000 persons aged over 65 years, represents a practicable basis for the provision of a range of in-patient, extramural and complementary services (Cooper, 1991; Melzer et al., 1992), and hence for the organization of psychogeriatric teams.

Various 'norms' have been proposed over the years, as targets for an adequate standard of specialist psychogeriatric care, based on this size of population, but inevitably these have been heavily influenced by existing national scales of provision (Cooper, 1991). The figures set out in Table 22.3 are derived from recommendations for the UK, contained in the report of a joint working body (Royal College of Physicians and Royal College of Psychiatrists, 1989; Melzer et al., 1992), and refer explicitly to the British situation. It is axiomatic, however, that, whatever national targets are announced, the specialist team will have to work in close co-operation with nursing, remedial and social-work staff, with the local general practitioners and with medical geriatricians, if a satisfactory standard of care is to be achieved. Arie (1986) has also stressed the importance of such an integrated team system, based on area populations, for realizing in practice the basic principles of secondary and tertiary prevention, which in general have been neglected unjustly in the care and management of dementia.

Early detection and diagnosis

Opportunistic screening during the course of medical consultation may prove the most practicable approach to early case-detection of dementia, whether it relies upon a standardized test, recognition of cognitive disorder by the medical practitioner and his team at their contacts with elderly patients, or a combination of both approaches. A number of brief tests, such as the Mini-Mental State Examination (Iliffe et al., 1990) have been found to be effective for picking up undeclared cases in medical practice, although most of the cases identi-

Table 22.3. *Key resources needed to provide an adequate old-age psychiatric service to an area population including 40000 persons aged over 65 years*

In-patient and residential care	
Functional mental illness	24 beds
Short-stay care for organic mental illness (assessment and relief)	40 beds
Long-stay care	80–120 beds
Day-care places	
Functional mental illness	20–30 places daily
Dementia	80–100 places daily
Additional staffing (sessional workload – whole-time equivalents)	
Consultant psychiatrists	2
Psychiatrists under consultant grade	3–4
Clinical psychologists	1–2
Community psychiatric nurses	6–8
Occupational therapists	4
Physiotherapists	1–2
Social workers	2
Secretarial support	3–4

Based on the report of the Royal College of Physicians and Royal College of Psychiatrists (1989).

fied in this way appear to be at least moderately severe. The detection of 'mild dementia' presents greater difficulty, and tends to yield a high proportion of misclassified cases. While earlier studies found that many cases of dementia remain 'invisible' to general practitioners (Bergmann, 1982), more recent evidence suggests an improvement in their diagnostic sensitivity (O'Connor et al., 1988; Philp & Young, 1988; Cooper & Bickel, 1990), and thus offers some hope that early detection of cognitive decline in the elderly, making use of simple, reliable techniques, will become increasingly feasible in general practice. Similar methods could also be applied by community nurses providing home care for the elderly, who in their daily rounds make contact with many cases both of clinical and of mild dementia (Schäufele & Cooper, 1991).

The past decade has seen a rapid growth of new facilities for the diagnosis and management of cognitive disorders (Bayer et al., 1987; van der Cammen et al., 1987). Since the first Memory Clinic was set up in London (van der Cammen et al., 1987), others have been opened in many countries, including Switzerland, France, Belgium, Germany, Canada and the USA (Stahelin et al., 1989; Larrabee et al., 1993) and usually employ a team made up of psychiatrist, physician and psychologist, whose tasks are to assess evidence of memory deficits, to identify possible causes, including underlying depression, and to give counselling both to the patients and to their families. Diagnosis and treatment of potentially reversible conditions, including depression, behavioural disorders and confusional states associated with somatic illness, are important aims of the Memory Clinics. Patients may be referred by local practitioners, but, with the growth of public awareness, increasing numbers are now self-referred. A general problem of service facilities of this kind, intended to cater for the need of specified high-risk groups of the population, is that their clientele may in the event be drawn from sections of the public not characterized by the type of risk in question, but presenting other, less specific forms of need. Thus, Memory Clinics might be expected to attract large numbers of elderly persons who, on investigation, manifest no objective evidence of organic mental impairment, but in many instances prove to be depressed or hypochondriacal. In fact, the early reports suggest that this problem is less conspicuous than might have been feared.

Medical investigation, treatment and management

Communication between medical scientists in most regions of the world is today so rapid and efficient that one would not expect to find any major differences of opinion among experts, with respect to the choice of diagnostic investigations and treatment methods for late-life dementia. Indeed, international reviews of clinical trials, whether of cholinergic drugs, so-called cognition enhancers or other substances, have for the most part reported compatible findings. A scientific group convened by WHO (1986) reached agreement that there is as yet no effective therapy for primary degenerative dementia, and that management in the individual case devolves on a series of symptomatic and supportive measures.

Despite this measure of consensus, differences in emphasis are to be found between countries, and relate in part to the underlying health-service structures. Thus, in contradistinction to the WHO group, a German expert committee report published in the same year concluded that three nootropic substances (co-dergocrin mesilate, piracetam and pyritinol), although not specifics, are clinically efficacious in dementia (Kanowski, 1989), and indeed these and a variety of other substances are today being prescribed extensively for dementing disorders, in the medical practice of many countries.

Similar influences can be detected in differing attitudes towards diagnostic assessment, and to medical management more generally. In parts of Europe, diagnostic evaluation is still regarded as being a task for the hospital-based specialist, and, in consequence, a comprehensive set of laboratory tests and special investigations, including cranial computerized tomography (CT) and electroencephalograms (EEG), tend to be regarded as prescriptive or 'routine' in suspected cases of dementia, regardless of the age of onset. One must, however, suspect that the cases referred to neuropsychiatric centres for diagnosis in these countries form a highly unrepresentative group. In the USA, where office practitioners in neurology and psychiatry play a more prominent role, the American Medical Association (1986) has counselled a selective approach, careful diagnostic assessment being indicated if, for example, papilloedema, dysphasia or focal neurological signs are detected, or if no adequate explanation can be found for the mental deterioration. It is not made clear, however, whether or not old age alone should be considered to be an adequate explanation.

In the UK, the existence of a National Health Service, and, in the past two decades, that of a flourishing subspecialty of old-age psychiatry, has helped to foster medical co-operation in diagnostic assessment. Arie (1986) has questioned how much good would actually be achieved by detailed clinical investigation of all old people with a typical history and clinical picture of primary degenerative dementia, and has stressed the importance of an initial assessment based on a domiciliary visit, in which hospital specialist and family doctor meet by arrangement at the patient's home, discuss the problem with family care-givers, make their clinical assessment and try to draw up a scenario for case management. A strategy of this kind may be of great value in avoiding or postponing the need for institutional admission.

Long-stay hospital and residential care

The decline in hospital in-patient care

During the first half of the present century, the numbers of elderly persons occupying psychiatric hospital beds rose throughout the Western world. In the 30-year period from 1950 onwards, however, there was a large-scale shift in the 'locus of care' for the elderly mentally ill, as a result of changes in health-care structures and public attitudes. The shift set in earliest, and was most pronounced, in the USA, where the state mental hospital population began to fall in 1955, after more than 100 years of continuous increase. By 1973 the number of psychiatric in-patient episodes had fallen from 5.1 to 3.1 per 1000 in the population (Kramer, 1977). This trend could be accounted for chiefly by a decrease in the numbers of elderly patients. Whereas psychiatric first-admission rates for young adults continued to rise, those for persons aged over 65 years declined by 70%.

This striking development did not result from the introduction of new, more effective methods of treatment and rehabilitation. Rather than helping older persons, commented Kahn (1975, pp. 25–6), the 'great mental health revolution' had resulted only in their dropping out of the psychiatric care system. To the question of what happened to the elderly mentally ill in the USA during that period, an answer is supplied by the data on geriatric nursing homes, following on introduction of the cost-shifting programmes 'Medicare' and 'Medicaid'. The total number of nursing home residents increased from 554 000 in 1963 to 1 098 500, or almost double, only 10 years later. 'The nursing homes', in Kahn's words: 'have replaced the state and county hospitals as the custodial warehouses' (Kahn, 1975, p. 25–6).

Should this be seen as a characteristically American phenomenon? Probably not, but because of inadequate monitoring of health-care trends, the question cannot be answered with confidence. The data on psychiatric bed trends in western European countries, summarized in Table 22.4, suggest a very mixed picture. Countries such as Belgium and West Germany, which following the Second World War faced an acute bed shortage, were concerned to build up their hospital in-patient capacities; whereas in England and Wales, as in Ireland, which already had high bed ratios, psychiatric hospital capacity began to run down from the 1950s onwards.

Data from 22 European and North American countries for the period 1978–80, presented by Pirella (1987), demonstrate that, by

Table 22.4. *Psychiatric hospital beds in European countries: changes in bed numbers and bed ratios per 1000 inhabitants, 1950–80*

Country	Period covered	Change in total bed number (%)	Bed ratio at end of period
Belgium	1951–79	+23.8	2.6
Denmark	1951–79	−12.5	2.1
France	1952–77	+13.4	2.6
Federal Republic of Germany	1953–79	+24.6	1.9
Ireland	1951–79	−29.3	4.1
Italy	1954–79	−8.8	1.5
Netherlands	1950–79	+6.9	1.9
United Kingdom:			
England & Wales	1952–79	−43.5	1.9
Scotland	1952–79	−19.2	3.3
Northern Ireland	1952–79	+19.9	4.3

From Mangen (1985).

then, the overall trend in western European countries, as in the USA, was towards a decline in bed ratios, amounting to around 12% in Norway and Sweden, 18% in Denmark and nearly 40% in Italy (where, however, the introduction, in 1978, of a new law on health reform, the famous Law 180, resulted in a redesignation of many of the existing hospital beds). Apart from Canada, only the eastern European socialist bloc was characterized by a continued increase in psychiatric bed capacity during these years. One cannot assume, however, that the same trends occurred in relation to bed-occupancy by the elderly. In West Germany, for example, although psychiatric admission rates for the elderly continued to rise, the bed-occupancy per 1000 persons aged over 65 years declined over the decade from 1970, by proportions which varied from 20% to 40% in the different states. Jaeger (1987), who analysed these data, noted similar trends in the UK and Denmark, and concluded that a general shift from clinical to non-clinical forms of long-stay care for the elderly was under way in western Europe, although less pronounced than in the USA.

Geriatric nursing-home care

In recent years, the issue of long-stay care-provision for the elderly has become a subject of concern chiefly because of the growth of demand for geriatric-home places. Although the numbers of the demented elderly in long-stay residential care are nowhere systematically monitored, indirect evidence suggests a wide range of variation between countries. Grundy & Arie (1984), who collected data on the numbers and proportions of old people living in 'non-private households', for 10 developed countries during the 1970s, calculated a standardized population ratio (SNPHR) for each. For some countries they were also able to compute specific ratios for the numbers in long-stay medical or social-welfare institutions (SIR).

Among the European countries included in Table 22.5, the proportion in care varied from 1.9% in Spain to 10.5% in the Netherlands, or more than five-fold. The corresponding age-specific rates, which could be calculated for some of the countries, showed similar slopes, the overall differences between them being distributed over the whole age-range above 65 years. That this pattern of variation is relatively stable is indicated by a more recent survey of nine European Community (EC) nations, carried out as part of 'Age Care Research Europe', which has yielded a similar pattern of distribution, although the proportions in care are increasing (Jamieson, 1990). It should be noted, however, that all these frequency estimates are based on census survey data, and hence are subject to what Kastenbaum & Candy (1973) called the '4 per cent fallacy'. In fact, as they demonstrated for an American, and Bickel (1989) for a German population, the individual citizen's probability of ending up in a geriatric home is from three to four times as high as the proportion of the elderly population found to be in care at any given point in time.

As a result of the aging of populations, combined with the latter-day tendency to prefer residential to long-stay hospital care, more and more of those afflicted by dementia are now congregating in geriatric and old people's homes. Wherever the situation has been surveyed, increases in the numbers and proportions of demented persons in these establishments have been found: a trend which, to some extent, reflects a shift in the locus of care from the public to the private sector. In the UK, for example, the prevailing political ideology has resulted in a massive increase in the private sector and a corresponding decline in local authority and health service provision of long-stay care for the disabled and dependent elderly: the burden of costs being borne

Table 22.5. *Proportion of elderly population in non-private households[a]
in 10 countries, and standardized non-private household residence
(SNPHR)[b] ratios*

Country	Year	Persons in non-private households[a] per 100 aged 65+	SNPHR[b]
Northern Europe			
England & Wales	1971	5.30	100.00
Finland	1975	9.04	195.05
Scotland	1971	6.71	132.12
Western Europe			
Belgium	1970	4.78	95.25
W. Germany	1970	3.69	77.01
Netherlands	1971	10.48	216.57
Switzerland	1970	6.98	139.15
Southern Europe			
Spain	1970	1.90	37.75
Other			
USA	1970	5.50	100.93
Singapore	1970	3.98	89.72

[a]'Non-private households' subsumes all forms of long-stay care, including
hospital in-patient units, local authority geriatric and old people's homes,
and private nursing homes.
[b]SNPHR ratio is calculated by standardizing for age and sex against the
1971 elderly population of England and Wales, and taking the rate for
that population as 100.
From Grundy & Arie (1984).

increasingly by families (Wattis, 1992). Since the homes were intended
originally to accommodate either relatively independent, active old
people, or the physically infirm who require general nursing care, few
of them are suitable either in structure or in staffing for their new
task. Hence, demand is growing for the provision of new, more
specialized units for the elderly mentally ill or, more specifically, for
those with severe dementia.

Psychogeriatric nursing homes in the public sector are already an
established feature in some European countries, notably the Nether-

lands and Scandinavia, where one finds in combination a high proportion of elderly inhabitants and a well-developed system of social
welfare (Kane & Kane, 1976). While providing a pleasant, homely
environment, these specialized units have in effect taken over many
of the functions of geriatric hospital wards, as indicated by staffing
requirements which include full-time medical officers, physiotherapists
and occupational therapists, in addition to trained nurses (Moss, 1983).
In other countries, however, this policy has not found official favour,
because of the relatively high capital and maintenance costs that are
involved. A more usual arrangement is the incorporation of nursing-
care sections within old people's homes or hostels (Pritchard, 1989).
In the USA, skilled nursing facilities (SNF) are distinguished, with
respect to fee charges and subsidies, from the euphemistically termed
health-related facilities (HRF), often found within the same large complex. Care of demented residents then devolves mainly on the former
type of unit.

Doubts have been expressed about the wisdom of a policy of segregated care for the demented. It has been argued that the use of trained
nursing staff to supervise mobile, physically active old people suffering
from dementia is unjustified on economic grounds. Certainly, experience suggests that it is unrealistic to plan special units for demented
and confused old people without regard to the fact that a majority of
such persons also require heavy physical nursing care (Stilwell et al.,
1984). The growing evidence for a continuum of cognitive impairment,
from normal aging to severe dementia, also argues against a policy of
systematic segregation. Rabins (1986, p. 121), in a balanced commentary, has pointed out that the concept of specialized Alzheimer's disease units, which has captured the attention of those concerned to
improve the quality of care, 'has also been identified as a marketing
tool by the nursing-home industry'.

A number of alternatives to conventional nursing-home care have
been developed and tested in different parts of the world, although
their significance for the management of dementia is not always clear.
In Germany, Gössling (1986) has pioneered the development of geriatric day-centres which are linked closely to nursing-home care. In the
UK, the large-scale growth of sheltered housing for the elderly has
served to promote the setting up, in some places, of 'very sheltered'
forms of accommodation with trained nursing supervision (Tinker,
1987). In France, a type of communal living unit known as the *cantou*
has been used to provide long-stay care for old persons suffering from
dementia. A recently reported evaluative study of 10 such units found

that the residents were less dependent, more mobile and less handicapped by language impairments than a matched control group of long-stay hospital patients (Ritchie et al., 1992). However, the groups were not randomized, so that some of the differences may have been a consequence of selective admission. Systematic comparisons of outcome and relative costs have been carried out, in the USA, on geriatric nursing homes, day hospitals and so-called 'senior center programs' (Sherwood et al., 1986). As part of another research project, elderly hospital in-patients were assigned randomly to nursing-home placement or foster care with local families, and their outcomes compared (Oktay & Volland, 1987).

In Australia, special hostels for mobile dementia sufferers have proved to be more popular than special nursing homes, and have been encouraged as part of government policy (Rosewarne et al., 1991). 'Lodges' have been set up in community housing in the State of Victoria, so that dementia sufferers can live in family groups under the direction of a supervisor (Marshall & Eaton, 1980), and the Commonwealth Government has offered 'dementia grants' to enable the hostels to develop better facilities for caring for demented old people. A parallel development has been the setting up of units for the confused and disturbed elderly ('CADE' units), designed to accommodate small groups of dementia sufferers in a home-like atmosphere. Affected old people have been found to improve in behaviour following transfer from psychiatric hospital wards to these units, suggesting that the new environment is more appropriate for their needs (Fleming et al., 1989). The publication of a 'National Action Plan' for dementia services (Australian Department of Health, Housing and Community Services, 1992), with an initial budget allocation of 31 million dollars, will promote the implementation of these and other recent developments in care provision on a national scale.

Day-care and home-care programmes

Day-care and community services together can provide a degree of support that may enable many elderly dements to remain in their own homes for months or even years longer than would otherwise be possible. Some of these programmes concentrate on persons who are already on the waiting lists for admission, but most provide support for old persons referred by a variety of medical agencies, including many with evidence of multiple morbidity. Provision of both day-care

Table 22.6. *Proportion (%) of population aged 65 years and over who are receiving specific forms of care and support: selected European Community countries*

Country	Residential care[a] (%)	Home nursing[b] (%)	Home help only (%)
Denmark	6	17	12
Netherlands	12	12	4
UK	5	9	5
France	5	7	0.6
Federal Republic of Germany	4	3 (max.)[c]	10 (max.)[c]
Italy	1.5	—	—
Greece	<0.5	<0.5	<0.5

[a]Excludes hospitals, and also sheltered housing.
[b]Includes persons also receiving home help.
[c]During one year: point prevalence considerably lower.
— No information.
From Jamieson (1990).

and domiciliary support varies greatly among countries, in ways that are not related obviously either to the general economic standard or to the provision of long-stay beds. Table 22.6, which presents crude data for seven European Community countries, gives some indication of the disparities.

The burden on families caused by dementia is everywhere increasing as populations age (OECD, 1988). On average, the 'old-age support ratio' (ratio of persons aged 15–64 years to those aged over 65) will decrease in OECD countries from 5.7 in 1980 to 3.7 in 2025, amounting to a 35% fall over this period. In some countries, the decline will be considerably steeper: corresponding, for example, to 58% per cent in Japan, 52% in Canada and 49% per cent in Finland. These projections indicate that a growing crisis in care for the demented must be expected.

Increasing recognition of the crucial part played by family caregivers in maintaining community 'lines of defence' has led in many countries to a new focusing of research on their problems, material and emotional. In a review of the problem field, Morris et al. (1988) distinguished a number of major determinants of stress, including the demented individual's behavioural disturbance, distress due to the caregiver's emotional involvement, the interference with his or her own occupation, family life and leisure activities, and the degree of support received from other members of the family (see Chapter 13). Surveys in the UK (Levin et al., 1989), Australia (Wells et al., 1990) and elsewhere have found consistently: that caregivers are predominantly female; that a high proportion are themselves elderly; and that rates of psychiatric disturbance among them are disturbingly high. In a study carried out by the US Congress Office of Technology Assessment (1985), the types of provision named most often as being essential or important by the caregivers of dementia sufferers were: a paid companion to take over supervision and care for a few hours weekly, and to stay overnight on occasion; assistance in getting financial help; and assistance in locating people or organizations providing patient care. This theme is also relevant to the provision of brief in-patient care for the demented, which offers family caregivers the chance of a respite (Burdz et al., 1988; Lawton et al., 1989).

A number of intervention schemes, designed to help and to support the family caregivers of elderly dements, have been reported. Brodaty & Gresham (1989) have developed an innovative training programme in Sydney, organized in groups of two to four pairs of caregivers and dementia patients, who are admitted to hospital together for 10 days for the purpose. Following this training period, the group members are brought together regularly by conference telephone calls, and are encouraged to form their own mutual support network. To evaluate their experimental service, the authors assigned caregivers randomly to the full programme, or to an alternative training for dementia sufferers only, or to a waiting-list control group. The full programme led to a reduction in caregivers' subjective stress, which was most pronounced one year after completion of training and not seen in either of the other two groups. The programme was also associated with a decline in demand for residential care, so that after 30 months the number of cases admitted from the experimental group was only half that from the control group.

The role of primary health-care services

Milder forms of cognitive impairment may, as already noted, be medically significant either as prodromal signs of dementing illness or as contributors in their own right to the burden of disability and dependency in old age. While there is already a sizeable body of research focused on the concepts of 'mild dementia', 'minimal dementia', 'benign senescent forgetfulness' and 'age-associated memory impairment', and their relationships both to normal aging and to clinical dementia (Dawe et al., 1992), little attention has been paid so far to the implications for health-service research and planning. The most appropriate framework for such research would seem to be that provided by primary health-care (Cooper, 1992), since it is axiomatic that most of the affected persons must continue to rely less upon hospital-based specialist agencies than on the help of general practitioners, community nurses and social workers. A start has been made by a few recent studies of case recognition in general practice, whose findings suggest an increasing scope for the early detection of dementia in this setting (Cooper et al. 1992b) and a high level of compliance on the part of elderly patients and their families, when the approach is made by, or with the support of, their own doctors (O'Connor et al., 1993). Whether systematic screening of the highest age-groups, using standardized cognitive tests as part of a broader screening battery, will prove more effective than an opportunistic strategy, which exploits the normal practice routine of patient consultation and home visits, remains to be seen.

Early detection and diagnosis by general practitioners affords the promise of improved standards of case management in the community, but an awareness of such possibilities has yet to be reflected either in the research literature or in national health policy and planning documents. How the general medical services of different countries will cope in future with the rising flood of dementia cases is thus still a matter for conjecture. Guidelines provided by a few practitioners with special interest and experience in the subject (Almind, 1985; Graham, 1991) suggest that the scope for intervention, once a decline in cognitive capacity has been recognized, can be subsumed under the following headings:

(1) Decisions with regard to appropriate diagnostic investigations and the need for specialist referral at this point
(2) Prescription of symptomatic treatment (e.g. nocturnal tranquillizer), together with a review of the patient's medication and the elimination of any possible iatrogenic factors. Prescribing of more 'specific' drugs for dementia (cholinomimetics, nootropics, etc.) is not included here, since many experienced practitioners are sceptical of their value or prefer to leave this decision to the specialist

(3) Measures to diagnose physical co-morbidity, to improve the general health and nutritional status, and to prevent or reduce confusional episodes

(4) Explanation, counselling and moral support, directed both to the patient and to family members, although inevitably with a gradual change in relative emphasis as the illness progresses

(5) Mobilization of domiciliary and community care services as necessary, including advice and help with respect to social welfare benefits and caregivers' allowances

(6) Collaboration with mutual-help groups, voluntary agencies and neighbourhood schemes

(7) Help in arranging 'respite care' to give temporary relief to the family, and, in due course, suitable long-stay care

There is nothing in this short catalogue which can be held to lie outside the sphere of competence of general medical practice, or indeed beyond the range of professional activities of many family doctors today. It does, however, highlight the importance for this field of care of two features which are present only to a limited extent in contemporary practice, even in well-developed national health services. First, regular or frequent home visiting by the doctors is often a basic requirement in assuring an acceptable standard of care for the mentally impaired elderly. Secondly, a close co-operation with community nurses will also be essential in many cases. Experience suggests that this can be assured most readily when locally based nurses are linked to the individual practice by formal attachment schemes. More generally, the quality of care for such patients will tend to be improved by the growth of multi-disciplinary primary care teams.

Future prospects: research and services

Policy objectives with respect to dementia fall into two broad groups: those intended to diminish the magnitude and gravity of the problem for future generations, and those concerned mainly with amelioration for the present generation of affected persons and their families, and therefore of immediate practical relevance. Whereas the long-term objectives predicate a search for ways to reduce the incidence of dementing disorders in elderly populations by means of biomedical and epidemiological research, attainment of the short-term goals calls for health-services and evaluative research, but also depends heavily upon the political will and reforming spirit required to change public priorities and to bring about improvement in existing care structures.

Over the past 10 to 15 years, there has been an impressive growth of research into dementia: most notably in the USA, where the creation of the National Institute on Aging, as part of the National Institutes of Health, has had a powerful catalytic effect. Federal support for biomedical research on dementia rose from four to 65 million dollars annually over the decade 1976–86. Federal spending on health-services research related to dementia has remained at a much more modest level; in 1986, it was estimated at about 1.3 million dollars, or only 0.03% of the 4.4 billion dollar Federal outlay for long-term care of dementia patients (US Congress, Office of Technology Assessment, 1986).

Dementia research is also expanding in other developed countries, although expenditure remains very low compared to that in other fields of medicine. Modest funds from the Commission of the European Community have been deployed to conduct a meta-analysis of epidemiological data from different European countries (Hofman et al., 1991; Rocca et al., 1991), and, in a recent collaboration with the US National Institute on Aging, a meta-analysis of 11 case–control studies in different regions of the world has been undertaken to uncover possible risk factors of dementia of the Alzheimer type. The World Health Organization has come to realize the emerging importance of dementia as a public-health problem of developing countries, and its Mental Health Division is co-ordinating an epidemiological research project (WHODEMMS) which is currently in progress, with participating centres in Africa (Nigeria), Asia (Israel, India, Singapore and Korea), North America (Canada), Latin America (Brazil and Uruguay) and Europe (France and Spain) (WHO, 1990).

This growth of research activity and collaboration encourages a guarded optimism about the prospects for future scientific progress. With regard to the planning and organization of services, however, the outlook is much less encouraging. Here, the most urgent single problem is the growing crisis in nursing-care provision. Nursing is the backbone of long-term care, but in the geriatric field it commands low prestige, prospects and earning power. In the USA, a shortfall of 75 000 nurses in long-stay care has been estimated (US Congress, Office of Technology Assessment, 1986). Nursing aides, who provide 80% to 90% of all hours of direct contact spent with geriatric patients, are in general poorly paid, have low educational levels, and are not encouraged by career prospects to remain in post. A report to the

World Health Organization (Skeet, 1988) emphasizes that the concept of nursing as a hospital-based service still prevails in most member states and that the sharp dividing line between hospital and community has a detrimental effect on nursing care for the elderly. A new type of structure is required which will enable nurses to work flexibly in hospital or community according to the requirements of case assignment.

A closely related issue is the administrative division often drawn between medical treatment, as a response to acute or remittent illness, and the care necessary for cases of chronic impairment and disability. In many countries, systems of health insurance were introduced originally to ensure stability of the work force, and were regulated by definitions of illness that assumed the possibility of recovery and return to productive employment. Although socio-economic changes and the aging of populations have resulted everywhere in some modifications to this basic structure, its framework is still strong enough to impose constraining limits upon the further development both of long-stay care and of community support for the demented elderly. One solution now being canvassed widely in European countries is the introduction of 'ring-fenced' disability insurance, as a cover for the costs of prolonged care in old age. Such schemes could yield important advantages, but they cannot resolve the fundamental problem, which Andersen (1990) has stated bluntly:

> . . . the provision of health and social services is a part of the human rights which everybody should enjoy in his capacity of being a citizen, not only as part of the labour force. The housewives, the invalids, the jobless, the chronically ill, should not have services which are secondary to those of the strong and wealthy.

Hence, he went on to say, the responsibility given to the Danish local authorities to provide adequate services, including community nursing and home-help, sheltered housing and geriatric-home placement for those requiring more intensive care. Posed in these terms, provision for the demented elderly can be seen to take its place as an integral part of that much-maligned concept, the 'welfare state'.

References

Almind, G. (1985). The general practitioner and the dementia patient. *Danish Medical Bulletin*, **32**, (supplement 1), 65–72.

American Medical Association (Council of Scientific Affairs) (1986). Dementia. *Journal of the American Medical Association*, **256**, 2234–8.

Andersen, B. R. (1990). 'Social security and care of the elderly in the Nordic countries.' (Unpublished MS) Copenhagen.

Arie, T. (1986). Management of dementia: a review. In M. Roth & L. L. Iversen (eds.) *Alzheimer's Disease and Related Disorders. British Medical Bulletin*, **42**, 91–6.

Arie, T. (1989). Twenty years of geriatric psychiatry in Britain. In D. H. Sipsma & L. M. Punt (eds.) *The Future of Psychogeriatrics*, pp. 153–61. Nieuw Toutenburg, Noordbergum, Netherlands.

Australian Department of Health, Housing and Community Services (1992). *Putting the Pieces Together. A National Action Plan for Dementia Care. Mid-Term Review of the Aged Care Reform Strategy, Stage 2: 1991–92.* Australian Government Publishing Service, Canberra.

Battelle Memorial Institute (1984). *The Economics of Dementia.* Report prepared for the Office of Technology Assessment, US Congress.

Bayer, A. J., Pathy, M. S. J. & Twining, C. (1987). The Memory Clinic. A new approach to the detection of early dementia. *Drugs*, **33**, (supplement 2), 84–9.

Bergmann, K. (1982). A community psychiatric approach to the care of the elderly. Are there opportunities for prevention? In G. Magnussen, J. Nielsen & J. Buch (eds.) *Epidemiology and Prevention of Mental Illness in Old Age*, pp. 87–92. EGV, Hellerup, Denmark.

Bickel, H. (1989). Wahrscheinlichkeit und Dauer einer stationären Pflege im Alter (Probability and duration of care for the elderly in nursing homes). *Öffentliches Gesundheitswesen*, **51**, 667–73.

Blessed, G., Tomlinson, B. E. & Roth, M. (1968). The association between quantitative measures of dementia and of senile change in the cerebral grey matter of elderly subjects. *British Journal of Psychiatry*, **114**, 797–811.

Brayne, C. & Calloway, P. (1988). Normal ageing, impaired cognitive function, and senile dementia of the Alzheimer's type: a continuum? *Lancet*, **i**, 1265–6.

Brodaty, H. & Gresham, M. (1989). Effects of a training programme to reduce stress in carers of patients with dementia. *British Medical Journal*, **299**, 1375–9.

Bundesministerium (Bundesministerium für Jugend, Familie und Gesundheit (Federal Ministry of Health)) (1986). *Modellprogramm Psychiatrie: Regionales Psychiatriebudget.* Schriftreihe des BMJFG Nr. 181. Kohlhammer, Stuttgart.

Burdz, M. P., Eaton, W. O. & Bond, J. B. (1988). Effects of respite care on dementia and non-dementia patients and their care-givers. *Psychology and Ageing*, **3**, 38–42.

Cooper, B. (1991). Principles of service provision in old-age psychiatry. In R. Jacoby, & C. Oppenheimer (eds.) *Psychiatry in the Elderly*, pp. 274–300. Oxford University Press, Oxford.

Cooper, B. (1992). Late-life mental disorders and primary health care: a review of research. In B. Cooper & R. Eastwood (eds.) *Primary Health Care and Psychiatric Epidemiology*, pp. 213–33. Tavistock/Routledge, London.

Cooper, B. & Schwarz, R. (1982). Psychiatric case-identification in an elderly urban population. *Social Psychiatry*, **17**, 43–52.

Cooper, B. & Bickel, H. (1990). Early detection of dementia in the primary care setting. In D. Goldberg & D. Tantam (eds.) *The Public Health Impact of Mental Disorder*, pp. 166–75. Hogrefe und Huber, Göttingen.

Cooper, B., Bickel, H. & Schäufele, M. (1992a). Demenz und kognitive Beeinträchtigung bei älteren Patienten in der ärztlichen Allgemeinpraxis. (Dementia and cognitive impairment among elderly patients in general practice.) *Nervenarzt*, **63**, 551–60.

Cooper, B., Bickel, H. & Schäufele, M. (1992b). The ability of general practitioners to detect dementia and cognitive impairment in their elderly patients: a study in Mannheim. *International Journal of Geriatric Psychiatry*, **7**, 591–8.

Dawe, B., Procter, A. & Philpot, M. (1992). Concepts of mild memory impairment in the elderly and their relationship to dementia – a review. *International Journal of Geriatric Psychiatry*, **7**, 473–9.

Fleming, R., Bowles, J. & Mellor, S. (1989). Peppertree Lodge: some observations on the first CADE unit. *Australian Journal on Ageing*, **8**, 29–32.

Gössling, S. (1986). Tagespflegeheime – Alternative zur Heimversorgung? (Day-care homes – an alternative to long-stay care?) In S. Articus & S. Kardus (eds.) *Altenhilfe im Umbruch*, pp. 133–43. DVF, Frankfurt.

Graham, H. J. (1991). General practice and the elderly mentally ill. In R. Jacoby, & C. Oppenheimer, (eds.) *Psychiatry in the Elderly*, pp. 488–512. Oxford University Press, Oxford.

Grundy, E. & Arie, T. (1984). Institutionalization and the elderly: international comparisons. *Age and Ageing*, **13**, 129–37.

Hay, J. W. & Ernst, R. L. (1987). The economic costs of Alzheimer's disease. *American Journal of Public Health*, **77**, 1169–75.

Henderson, A. S. & Huppert, F. A. (1984). The problem of mild dementia. *Psychological Medicine*, **14**, 5–11.

Hofman, A., Rocca, W., Brayne, C., Breteler, M. B. B., Clarke, M., Cooper, B., Copeland, J. R. M., Dartigues, J. F., Droux, A. da Silva, Hagnell, O., Heeren, T. J., Engedal, K. Jonker, C., Lindsey, J., Lobo, A., Mann, A. H., Mölsa, P. K., Morgan, K., O'Connor, D. W., Sulkava, R., Kay, D. W. K. & Amaducci, L. (1991). The prevalence of dementia in Europe: a collaborative study of 1980–1990 findings. *International Journal of Epidemiology*, **20**, 736–48.

Hu, T. W., Huang, L. F. & Cartwright, W. S. (1986). Evaluation of the costs of caring for the senile demented elderly: a pilot study. *Gerontologist*, **26**, 158–63.

Iliffe, S., Booroff, A., Gallivan, S., Goldenberg, E., Morgan, P. & Harries, A. (1990). Screening for cognitive impairment in the elderly, using the Mini Mental State Examination. *British Journal of General Practice*, **40**, 277–9.

ILO (International Labour Organization) (1991). *From Pyramid to Pillar: Population Change and Social Security in Europe*. ILO, London.

Jaeger, J. (1987). Trends in der stationären gerontopsychiatrischen Versorgung in der Bundesrepublik Deutschland (Trends in psychogeriatric in-patient care in the FRG). *Zeitschrift für Gerontologie*, **20**, 187–94.

Jamieson, A. (1990). Care of old people in the European Community. In L. Hantrais, S. Mangen & M. O'Brien (eds.) *Caring and the Welfare State: Cross-national Research Papers*. Aston University, Birmingham, UK.

Jorm, A. F., Korten, E. & Henderson, A. S. (1987). The prevalence of dementia: a quantitative integration of the literature. *Acta Psychiatrica Scandinavica*, **76**, 465–79.

Jorm, A. F., Korten, A. E. & Jacomb, P. A. (1988). Projected increases in the number of dementia cases for 29 developed countries. Application of a new method for making projections. *Acta Psychiatrica Scandinavica*, **78**, 493–500.

Kahn, R. L. (1975). The mental health system and the future aged. *Gerontologist*, **15**, (supplement), 24–31.

Kane, R. L. & Kane, R. A. (1976). *Long-Term Care in Six Countries*. Dept. of Health, Education and Welfare, Washington, DC.

Kanowski, S. (1989). Somatotherapie. In K. P. Kisker, H. Lauter, J.-E. Meyer, C. Müller & E. Strömgren (eds.) *Psychiatrie der Gegenwart* (3. Auflage) Bd. 8: *Alterpsychiatrie*, pp. 271–312. Springer, Berlin; Heidelberg.

Kastenbaum, R. & Candy, S. E. (1973). The 4 per cent fallacy: a methodological and empirical critique of extended-care facility population statistics. *International Journal of Ageing and Human Development*, **4**, 15–21.

Kramer, M. (1977). *Psychiatric services and the changing institutional scene, 1950–1985*. DEW Publ. No. (ADM): 77–433. US Government Printing Office, Washington, DC.

Kramer, M. (1980). The rising pandemic of mental disorders and associated chronic diseases, associated chronic diseases and disabilities. In E. Strömgren, A. Dupont & J. A. Nielsen (eds.) *Epidemiological Research as Basis for the Organization of Extramural Psychiatry*, pp. 382–96. Munksgaard, Copenhagen.

Larrabee, G. J., Pathy, M. S. J., Bayer, A. J. & Cook, T. H. (1993). Memory Clinics: state of development and future prospects. In M. Bergener & S. I. Finkel (eds.) *Scientific Psychogeriatrics*. Springer, Berlin, in press.

Lawton, M. P., Brody, E. M. & Saperstein, A. R. (1989). A controlled study of respite service for caregivers of Alzheimer's patients. *Gerontologist*, **29**, 8–16.

Levin, E., Sinclair, T. & Gorbach, P. (1989). *Families, Services and Confusion in Old Age*. Avebury, Aldershot, UK.

Mangen, S. P. (1985). *Mental Health Care in the European Community*. Croom Helm, London.

Marshall, E. & Eaton, D. (1980). 'Forgetting but not forgotten: residential care of mentally frail elderly people'. Division of Community Services of the Uniting Church, Melbourne.

Melzer, D., Hopkins, S., Pencheon, D., Brayne, C. & Williams, R. (1992). 'Epidemiologically based assessment of services for people with dementia'. Unpublished report: Dept. of Public Health Medicine and University Dept. of Community Medicine, Cambridge, UK.

Morris, R. G., Morris, L. W. & Britton, P. G. (1988). Factors affecting the emotional wellbeing of the caregivers of dementia sufferers. *British Journal of Psychiatry*, **153**, 147–56.

Moss, B. (1983). *Dementia – Who Cares?* Moorfields Community for Adult Care, Melbourne, Australia.

Mowry, B. J. & Burvill, P. W. (1988). A study of mild dementia in the community using a wide range of diagnostic criteria. *British Journal of Psychiatry*, **153**, 328–34.

O'Connor, D. W., Pollitt, P. A., Hyde, J. B., Brook, C. P. B., Reiss, B. B. & Roth, M. (1988). Do general practitioners miss dementia in elderly patients? *British Medical Journal*, **297**, 1107–10.

O'Connor, D. W., Pollitt, P. A., Hyde, J. B., Miller, N. D. & Fellowes, J. L. (1991). Clinical issues relating to the diagnosis of mild dementia in a British community survey. *Archives of Neurology*, **48**, 530–4.

O'Connor, D. W., Fertig, A., Grande, M. J., Hyde, J. B., Roland, M. O., Silverman, J. D. & Wraight, S. K. (1993). Dementia in general practice: the practical consequences of a more positive approach to diagnosis. *British Journal of General Practice*, **43**, 185–8.

OECD (Organization for Economic Co-operation and Development) (1988). *Ageing Populations: the Social Policy Implications*. OECD, Paris.

OECD (Organization for Economic Co-operation and Development (1991). 'The care of the frail elderly: the issues'. (Unpublished report.) OECD, Paris.

Oktay, J. S. & Volland, P. J. (1987). Foster home care for the frail elderly as an alternative to nursing home care: an experimental evaluation. *American Journal of Public Health*, **77**, 1505–10.

Philp, I. & Young, J. (1988). An audit of a primary care team's knowledge of the existence of symptomatic demented elderly. *Health Bulletin* (Edinburgh), **46**, 93–7.

Pirella, A. (1987). Institutional psychiatry between transformation and rationalization: the case of Italy. In C. Breemer ter Stege & M. Gittelman (eds.) *Trends in Mental Health Care in Western Europe in the Past 25 Years. International Journal of Mental Health*, **16**, 118–41.

Pritchard, R. (1989). '*A Better Way*'. Report to the Winston Churchill Memorial Trust of Australia. Project to study developments in services for persons with dementia. Moorfields Community for Adult Care, Victoria, Australia.

Rabins, P. V. (1986). Establishing Alzheimer's disease units in nursing homes: pros and cons. *Hospital and Community Psychiatry*, **37**, 120–1.

Ritchie, K., Colvez, A., Ankri, J., Lédesert, B., Gardent, H. & Fontaine, A. (1992). The evaluation of long-term care for the dementing elderly. A comparative study of hospital and collective non-medical care in France. *International Journal of Geriatric Psychiatry*, **7**, 549–57.

Rocca, W. A., Hofman, A., Brayne, C., Breteler, M. B. B., Clarke, M., Copeland, J. R. M., Dartigues, J.-F., Engedal, K., Hagnell, O., Heeren, T. J., Jonker, C., Lindesay, J., Lobo, A., Mann, A. H., Mölsa, P. K., Morgan, K., O'Connor, D. W., Droux, A. da Silva, Sulkava, R., Kay, D. W. K. & Amaducci, L. (1991). The prevalence of vascular dementia in Europe: facts and fragments from 1980–1990 studies. *Annals of Neurology*, **30**, 817–24.

Rosewarne, R., Carter, M. & Bruce, A. (1991). 'Hostel Dementia Care: survey of programs and participants (Victoria)'. Report to Commonwealth

Department of Community Services and Health. Aged Care Research Groups, Lincoln School of Health Sciences, La Trobe University, Australia.

Roth, M., Tym, E., Mountjoy, Q., Huppert, F. A., Hendrie, H., Verma, S. & Goddard, R. (1986). CAMDEX: a standardized instrument for the diagnosis of mental disorder in the elderly. *British Journal of Psychiatry*, **149**, 698–709.

Royal College of Physicians (Committee on Geriatrics) (1981). Organic mental impairment in the elderly: implications for research, education, and the provision of services. *Journal of the Royal College of Physicians of London*, **15**, 3–29.

Royal College of Physicians and Royal College of Psychiatrists (1989). *Care of old people with mental illness: specialist services and medical training. A joint report*. London.

Schäufele, M. & Cooper, B. (1991). Dementia among the elderly patients of a community nursing service: a study in Mannheim. In G. Brenner & I. Weber (eds.) *Health Services Research and Primary Health Care*, pp. 162–5. Deutscher Ärzte-Verlag, Cologne.

Sherwood, S., Morris, T. N. & Ruchlin, H. S. (1986). Alternative paths to long-term care: nursing home, geriatric day hospital, senior centre, and domiciliary care options. *American Journal of Public Health*, **76**, 38–44.

Siegel, J. S. & Hoover, S. L. (1982). Demographic aspects of the elderly to the year 2000 and beyond. *World Health Statistics Quarterly*, **35**, 133–202.

Skeet, M. (ed.) (1988). 'The age of aging: implications for nursing'. (Unpublished report. IRP/HEE 114 2 6). World Health Organization, Geneva.

Stahelin, H. B., Ermini-Funfschilling, D., Grunder, B., Krebs-Roubiak, E., Monsch, A. & Spiegel, R. (1989). The Memory Clinic. *Therapeutisches Umschau*, **46**, 72–7.

Stilwell, J. A., Hassall, C. & Rose, S. (1984). Changing demands made by senile dementia on the National Health Service. *Journal of Epidemiology and Community Health*, **38**, 131–3.

Tinker, A. (1987). A review of the contribution of housing to policies for the frail elderly. *International Journal of Geriatric Psychiatry*, **2**, 3–17.

US Congress, Office of Technology Assessment (1985). *Technology and Aging in America*. (OTA-BA-264.) US Government Printing Office, Washington, DC.

US Congress, Office of Technology Assessment (1986). *Losing a Million Minds: Confronting the Tragedy of Alzheimer's Disease and Other Dementias*. (OTA-BA-323.) Government Printing Office, Washington, DC.

US Department of Commerce, Bureau of the Census (1987). *An Aging World* (September 1987). US Government Printing Office, Washington, DC.

van der Cammen, T. J. M., Simpson, J. M., Fraser, R. M., Preker, A. S. & Exton-Smith, A. N. (1987). The Memory Clinic. A new approach to the detection of dementia. *British Journal of Psychiatry*, **150**, 359–64.

Wattis, J. P. (1992). Needs for continuing care of demented old people: a model for estimating needs. *Psychiatric Bulletin*, **16**, 465–7.

Wells, Y. D., Jorm, A. F., Jordan, F. & Lefroy, R. (1990). Effects on caregivers of special day care programmes for dementia sufferers. *Australian and New Zealand Journal of Psychiatry*, **24**, 82–90.

WHO (World Health Organization) (1986). *Dementia in Later Life: Research and Action*. Technical Report Series 730. WHO, Geneva.
WHO (World Health Organization) (1990). WHODEMMS: Multicentre study of cognitive impairment and dementia. (Unpublished report. MNH/MND/90.16.) WHO, Geneva.

23

Public health implications of a continuum model of dementia

KAY-TEE KHAW

The debate about whether dementia does, or does not, represent the extreme of a continuum whether of pathology or of clinical function is not unique to dementia, but has analogies throughout medicine and sociology. The standard medical model is that diseases are biologically coherent disorders distinct from health; hence, health and disease are separate entities (or distributed bimodally). Illness represents specific derangements from some biological ideal. The continuum model, in contrast, suggests that health and disease are on a continuous distribution, albeit of various qualitative factors. The distinction between persons with disease and persons without disease is largely quantitative, and hence, fairly arbitrary. Whether we discuss social, psychological or biological conditions, the first (categorical) model views these as more or less dichotomous: a person does, or does not, have dementia, depression, dyslexia, atherosclerotic arterial disease, osteoporosis, glaucoma, cancer, etc. The continuum model views those with these conditions as being at one extreme end of the distribution in the population which may range, to take one example, from those with completely clear arteries, through varying degrees of arterial plaques resulting in vascular insufficiency, to complete arteriosclerotic occlusions resulting in tissue infarctions.

The evidence for either of these models in dementia has been discussed at length elsewhere in this volume. Dementia per se is a clinically defined syndrome. Some researchers argue that dementia is a distinct pathological entity with specific characteristics: Hirano bodies, granulovacuolar degeneration, vascular and parenchymal amyloid deposits. Plaques and tangles are pathological hallmarks of dementia of the Alzheimer's type. Thus, these characteristics are said to be distributed bimodally in the population. On the other hand, it has

Dementia and Normal Aging, eds. F. A. Huppert, C. Brayne & D. W. O'Connor.
© Cambridge University Press 1994.

been suggested that all these characteristics are found to a lesser extent in normal aging (though not in normal young and middle-aged people) and so they are part of a continuum of normal age-related changes in the brain; thus, it is argued that the apparent bimodal density distribution is a function of study design, in which persons at extreme ends of a normal distribution are compared. The term 'normal aging' is, I believe, a misnomer, since it begs the whole question or what does, or does not, constitute 'normal' aging, and the continuum debate really focuses on whether dementia is, or is not, qualitatively (as well as quantitatively) a distinct entity.

Which then, is the most appropriate model for dementia? The very difficulty in coming towards a consensus definition for dementia indicates that it not a clearcut homogeneous condition and, indeed, most researchers would agree that dementia as a clinical syndrome encompasses a variety of conditions. Most researchers would also agree that it is possible to identify definitely people who do or who do not have dementia. However, in between the two extremes, there is a nebulous area and even when specific criteria are employed, whether cognitive, neuropathological or neurochemical, it is clear that there is no absolute division between disease and non-disease. Plaque and tangle densities are correlated with each other and with degree of cognitive impairment. However, the relationship is neither specific nor perfect; some persons will have histological features without cognitive impairment while others will have severe cognitive impairment without (at post-mortem) the pathological features.

These models are not necessarily in conflict; their difference is rather one of focus, or emphasis. Arguments for both models have already been well rehearsed in the Platt–Pickering debate in the 1950s over the nature of hypertension: Platt insisted that essential hypertension was a distinct disease, while Pickering argued that hypertension was but the extreme of a distribution of blood pressure in the general population (Hamilton et al., 1954; Pickering, 1968). This debate has evolved over the years, the implications having been most fully developed and discussed by Geoffrey Rose in a series of landmark articles (Rose 1981; 1985; 1990). Examples from hypertension and cardiovascular disease may perhaps provide useful analogies for the arguments concerning dementia

The clinical conditions of stroke, myocardial infarction and malignant hypertension are well defined. Numerous population studies have shown that high blood pressure is a major risk factor for these clinical conditions. Blood pressure is distributed continuously, and more or less normally, in the population. Risk of cardiovascular disease – that is, stroke or heart attack, increases with increasing level of blood pressure across the whole normal distribution, such that the optimal blood pressure in terms of prognosis is, in fact, at the low end of the distribution. However, some strokes will happen in those with low blood pressure, and many persons with high blood pressure will not inevitably have a stroke. There is no threshold effect: various definitions of hypertension are set at some fairly arbitrary cutpoint criteria. Hence, it is possible to have blood pressure below the cutpoint but still to have increased risk of cardiovascular disease compared to those at the bottom of the distribution. To have average, or 'statistically normal' blood pressure is not the same as having optimal blood pressure. It is also clear that the prevalence of hypertension, as defined by blood pressure above a given cutpoint, is related to where the mean of the population distribution lies. Mean blood pressures tend to rise with increasing age, such that the whole population distribution shifts to the right with increasing age; hence, the prevalence of hypertensives also rises with increasing age.

However, studies in different communities indicate that the phenomenon of mean blood pressures rising with age is not a necessary concomitant of aging, since numerous communities exist in which mean blood pressures are low, and do not rise with age. That is, what constitutes 'normal' aging in western communities, at least, as far as blood pressure is concerned, is not at all what constitutes 'normal' aging in these low blood pressure communities. 'Normal' indicates merely 'usual' or average, and the average differs. In these communities, the prevalence of hypertensives at any age is low. Migration studies have indicated that, when communities with low blood pressures move to different environments, the whole blood pressure distribution shifts upwards, such that the prevalence of hypertensives increase (Poulter et al. 1990). Thus, differences between communities are largely due to environmental influences, and are probably dietary.

These observations are not unique to blood pressure alone but can be generalized to other physiological variables such as serum cholesterol, and weight, such that the prevalence of 'persons with hypercholesterolaemia' or 'obesity' is related to the population mean directly. For example, the Intersalt study, which examined blood pressure, weight and other variables including alcohol and sodium intake in 52 different communities in 28 different countries, found that the close correlation between prevalence of 'high risk' and the mean of the population applied not only to physiological variables such as blood pressure and weight but also to behavioural variables such as alcohol and sodium intake (Rose, 1990). That is, the prevalence of heavy drinkers, defined arbitrarily as being those drinking more than 300 ml alcohol a week, in each community was related directly to the mean alcohol intake in that community. Similarly, the prevalence of those with high sodium intakes (over 250 mmol/day) was also related to the mean sodium intake in the community. The concept that the amount of deviance, or disease, present in a community is a reflection of societal norms or means is not new; and was first noted when Durkheim (1897) observed that the rates of suicide varied greatly between different communities and postulated that these were related inversely to the degree of social cohesion in these communities.

Thus, the continuum model for dementia, drawn from analogies with cardiovascular disease, may not be as far fetched as it first appears. The Intersalt study showed its application not just to physiological risk factors but also to behavioural variables; more recently, there is also evidence that it may apply to neurological or psychological syndromes. Dyslexia is widely believed to be a biologically based disorder distinct from other, less specific reading problems; however, a recent study suggested that dyslexia may represent the lower tail of a normal distribution of reading ability. Shaywitz (1992, p. 149) concluded that 'dyslexia is not an all-or-none phenomenon, but, like hypertension and obesity, occurs in varying degrees of severity'.

Rose (1990) has suggested, therefore, that the distribution of health-related characteristics is continuous in a population: 'cases' or 'deviants' are but the tail end, or extreme, of the distribution. The prevalence of 'cases' or 'deviance' is related closely to the population mean. Figure 23.1 illustrates this, using cognitive function as an example; the prevalence of dementia in this case, using an arbitrary absolute cutpoint for diagnosis, varies depending on where the population distribution lies. This model could be applied equally by using other criteria, for example, pathological features such as the plaque or tangle density score; the higher the score, the greater the likelihood of dementia; the prevalence of dementia here would depend on the distribution and mean plaque score for the population. Based on observations for cardiovascular disease, Rose (1981) postulated that there were two major strategies for prevention in a population. The first, or high risk strategy, aims to identify those defined as being sick, or at high risk (e.g. hypertensives, or alcoholics) and to treat them to prevent further adverse consequences such as stroke. The second, or population strategy would be to shift the whole population distribution in a favourable direction, resulting in a reduction in the prevalence of the high risk group. These approaches are illustrated in Figure 23.2. Rose (1981) indicated that a small shift in population mean might have a profound effect on population prevalence and incidence.

How then might the analogies from cardiovascular disease apply to the disease/continuum models for dementia? Neither represents some absolute truth; rather, the value of a model depends on the use to which it is put. The approach of the dichotomous or categorical model would be to compare only well-established cases with 'normals', both groups of which would conform to strict criteria. This approach, which excludes those borderline persons who are not unambiguously cases and controls, thus maximizes possible differences between dementia and non-dementia and is helpful for research in terms of understanding the possible mechanisms of dementia. This model aims to establish why a specific individual has a condition, and explains disease in terms

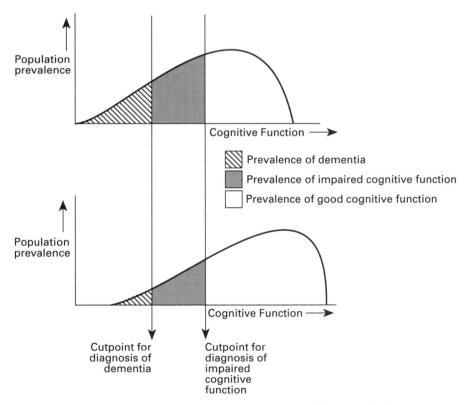

Figure 23.1. Model to illustrate that the prevalence of those with dementia is related to the population distribution of risk factor score, e.g. cognitive function.

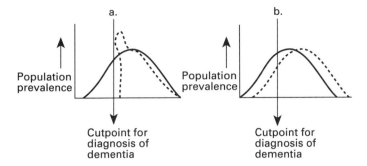

Figure 23.2. Strategies for prevention: (a) high risk (dichotomous approach) – the population is screened, and those below the cutpoint definition are treated; (b) population strategy (continuum approach) – an attempt to shift the distribution of the whole population in a favourable direction. (Solid lines indicate the baseline population prevalence distribution of cognitive function; dotted lines indicate the population prevalence distribution of cognitive function which is the target for the strategy.)

of derangements from ideal. If we are interested in optimal treatment for individuals, it is clearly essential to identify the specific aberrations that might occur, and how to remedy them. Should effective management be established in trials, it is also an appropriate approach to identify individuals for treatment who conform to well-established criteria, and who might be most likely to benefit, therefore.

However, the factors determining which specific individual in any given community gets a condition are not necessarily the same as those which determine incidence of a condition in the community. As Rose (1985) has pointed out, while it is clearly accepted that the cigarette smoking habit is an important cause of lung cancer, not everyone who smokes develops lung cancer. If a given exposure such as cigarette smoking is uniformly high in a community, no differences in cigarette smoking habit would be identified between individuals who develop lung cancer and those who do not; differences between cases and non-cases would reflect differences in susceptibility due to genetic or other reasons. However, a community where everyone smoked 20 cigarettes daily would have considerably higher lung cancer incidence than a community where nobody smoked.

The continuum model suggests that individuals with a condition such as dementia are but the tail end of a continuous distribution. While accepting that individuals at the one end of the distribution are different from those at the other end, this model would suggest that, in terms of research and prevention, we should try to identify what determines the population distribution of disease, and hence the prevalence or incidence of the condition. Action would be aimed at shifting the whole population distribution favourably.

Is there any evidence that the continuum model can be applied to dementia? Brayne & Calloway (1988, 1990) reported that cognitive function was distributed continuously in a population study and that the distribution of cognitive function scores shifted downwards with increasing age, such that mean scores decreased and prevalence of cognitive impairment increased. However, other factors such as educational level and socioeconomic status were also related independently of age to the distribution of scores; the whole distribution was shifted favourably to the right with higher education and socioeconomic level. Similarly a recent French study has also reported that rates of cognitive impairment, standardized for age and sex, varied according to previous educational level and principal occupation from 2% to 50% (Dartigues et al., 1992). The nature of this relationship is still debatable and persons with better educational levels may simply be better able to complete psychometric testing. Nevertheless, the possibility that exogenous factors (such as intellectual occupation or higher education) might delay or minimize decline has interesting implications. Theoretically, if the relationship is causal, even a small improvement in overall educational levels might be related to a halving of prevalence rates for poor cognitive function later in life.

However, a continuum model need not be confined to cognitive function, but may have other applications. Clinical manifestations of dementia are related to the quantity of features such as senile plaques, in which aluminosilicate deposits have been identified. While rare in the young, these appear with increasing frequency with increasing age. However, it has been suggested that environmental agents such as aluminium intake may be risk factors for the prevalence of such plaques, and consequent clinical disease (Martyn, et al., 1989; Graves et al., 1990a, b) or conversely, other agents such as antioxidants could modulate their development (Evans et al., 1992). Changing the environmental exposure in a population might thus influence the frequency of development of such features and, possibly, the consequent clinical manifestations. If research can identify factors which are causally related to shifting the distribution of cognitive function, or plaque formation in the population, a small favourable shift in population mean may result in a considerable reduction in the prevalence of the high risk group, as shown with cardiovascular disease.

The continuum model also has implications for services. As Shaywitz (1992) has pointed out for dyslexia, the notion that any disease is a discrete, definable entity is the basis of health policy that provides services only for those who satisfy what are seen as being specific, absolute criteria. However, accepting that disease is but one extreme of a continuum should not deny that individuals at one end require specialized diagnosis and interventions. 'Although limitations on resources may necessitate the imposition of cutoff points for the provision of services, physicians must recognize that such cutoffs may have no biologic validity. Instead, [those] who do not meet these arbitrarily imposed criteria may still require and profit from special help' (Shaywitz et al., 1992, p. 149).

References

Brayne, C. & Calloway, P. (1988). Normal ageing, impaired cognitive function, and senile dementia of the Alzheimer's type: a continuum? *Lancet*, **2**, 1265–7.

Brayne, C. & Calloway, P. (1990). The association of education and socio-economic status with Mini-Mental State examination and the clinical diagnosis of dementia in elderly people. *Age and Ageing*, **19**, 91–6.

Dartigues, J. F., Gagnon, M., Letenneur, L., Barberger-Gateau, P., Commenges, D., Evaldre, M. & Salamon, R. (1992). Principal lifetime occupation and cognitive impairment in French elderly cohort (Paquid). *American Journal of Epidemiology*, **135**, 981–8.

Durkheim, E. (1897). *Le Suicide: Etude de Sociologie*. Alcan, Paris.

Evans, P. H., Peterhans, E., Burge, T. & Klinowski, J. (1992). Aluminosilicate-induced free radical generation by murine brain glial cells in vitro: potential significance in the aetiopathogenesis of Alzheimer's dementia. *Dementia*, **3**, 1–6.

Graves, A. B., White, E., Koepsell, T. D., Reifler, B. V., van Belle, G. & Larson, E. B. (1990a). The association between aluminium-containing products and Alzheimer's disease. *Journal of Clinical Epidemiology*, **43**, 35–44.

Graves, A. B., White, E., Koepsell, T. D., Reifler, B. V., van Belle, G., Larson, E. B. & Raskind, M. (1990b). A case–control study of Alzheimer's disease. *Annals of Neurology*, **28**, 140–8.

Hamilton, M., Pickering, G. W., Roberts, J. A. F. & Sowry, G. S. C. (1954). The aetiology of essential hypertension: (1) the arterial pressure in the general population. *Clinical Science*, **13**, 11–35.

Martyn, C. N., Osmond, C., Edwardson, J. S., Barker, D. J. P., Harris, E. C. & Lacey, R. F. (1989). Geographical relation between Alzheimer's disease and aluminium in drinking water. *Lancet*, **i**, 59–62.

Pickering, G. W. (1968). *High Blood Pressure*, 2nd edition. Churchill, London.

Poulter, N. R., Khaw, K. T., Hopwood, B. E. C., Mugambi, M., Peart, W. S., Rose, G. & Sever, P. S. (1990). The Kenyan Luo migration study: observations on the initiation of a rise in blood pressure. *British Medical Journal*, **300**, 967–72.

Rose, G. (1981). Strategy of prevention. *British Medical Journal*, **282**, 1847–51.

Rose, G. (1985). Sick individuals and sick populations. *International Journal of Epidemiology*, **14**, 32–8.

Rose, G. (1990). The population mean predicts the number of deviant individuals. *British Medical Journal*, **301**, 1031–4.

Shaywitz, S., Escobar, M. D., Shaywitz, B. A., Fletcher, J. M. & Makuch, R. (1992). Evidence that dyslexia may represent the lower tail of a normal distribution of reading ability. *New England Journal of Medicine*, **326**, 145–50.

Index

abiotrophy
  Gowers' concept, 42–4
  and senile dementia of Alzheimer
      type, 48
abnormal behaviour, explanations for,
      261–2
acetylcholinesterase in dementia,
      438–40, (Table 19.1) 440–7
  in aging, 449
activity disturbances and normal aging,
      284
age-associated memory impairment
      (AAMI), concept, 87, 321–2
age changes, carers' attitudes and
      understanding, 257–71
  see also caring for people with
      dementia
age, chronological
  association with AD, 210–11
  risk factor in dementia, 239
age differences in memory, 308–11
  cross-sectional studies, 315–18
  longitudinal studies, 318–21
age-specific death rate, 230–1
age-specific incidence of dementia,
      190–2
age-specific prevalence of dementia, 4
AGECAT, 110, 111
aggressive behaviour and normal aging,
      284
aging
  -associated cognitive decline, concept,
      321–2
  cerebral, pathological changes,
      nineteenth century opinions,
      17–18
  definition, 230–1
  and dementia, relationship between,
      historical factors, 19–21
  and disease, 237–8
  disposable soma theory, 233–4
  evolution, 232

genetic factors, 234–5
mechanisms, 235–6
  and risk factors, 230–43
natural selection theory, 232–3
as programmed process, 232
selection at group level, 232
why it occurs, 231–4
aluminium salts
  neurofibrillary tangles, and AD, first
      described, 47
  role in AD, 210, 217
Alzheimer, first describes the disease,
      32–3
Alzheimer-type dementia, publications
      1964–90, 48
Alzheimer's disease (AD)
  aetiopathogenesis, research, 41–56
  as aging process continuum theory,
      57–8
    see also continuum model of
      dementia
  aging process or disease, 52
  as brain aging, 51–2
  brain weight and volume changes,
      387–98
  combined with multi-infarct dementia
      (MID), clinical change and
      progress, 62–3
  continuous measures, 244–53
  criteria for, 168–9, 180
  differential diagnosis in the
      community, 192–3
  early onset forms, 68–9
  family history of dementia, 213–14
  genetic studies, 511
  rating scale, behavioural pathology,
      276
  reception of the 'new' disease, 33–4
  relationship to senile dementia, 33,
      44–5, 46–7
  risk factors, 210–19
  Roth's early contributions, 45–7

Alzheimer's disease (AD) – *cont'd.*
  summary of genetic, clinical and
    research aspects, 503–10
  terminology, and research, 44–5
  see also dementia; and specific
    headings throughout
Alzheimer's and Related Disorders
    Association (ADRDA), 120; *see
    also* NINCDS—ADRDA
'amentia', first use of term, 22
amyloid deposits, 552
  brain, in normal aging and AD,
    426–7
amyloid precursor protein
  in AD, 69, 70
  β/A4 binding to tau, 506–7
  β/A4 deposits and aging pigments,
    482–3
  β/A4 deposits and neurofibrillary
    pathology, 483
  biochemical and clinical significance,
    470–2
  changes in processing, in aging and
    AD, 480–2
  genetics, and AD, 484, 504–6
anomia, *see* word finding
apoplectic dementia, early descriptions,
    31–2
apraxia, in dementia, 121
arterial pressure and continuous
    distribution, 64
arteriosclerotic dementia, concept, early
    twentieth century, 31
assessment schedules, mild dementia,
    110–12
astereognosis in DAT, 120, 121

backward visual masking tasks
  in AD, 369–70
  in normal elderly, 375
BEHAVE-AD, behavioural pathology
    rating scale, 276
behaviour
  changes
    explanation, images of dementia,
      262, 263–4
    and normal aging, 281–5
  definition, 272–3
  in dementia and normal aging, 271–90
  methods for assessing, 273–7
    direct observation, 274, *see also*
      expectations of age related to
      mental status

information from carers, 275–7
  objective measurement of specific
    behaviour, 274–7, (Table 14.1)
    278–9
behavioural measures in cognitive
    impairment and dementia, 176–8
benign forgetfulness of old age, 93–4,
    385
  see also memory function in dementia
    and normal aging
Binswanger's disease, neuropathological
    features, 457
Blessed dementia scale for cognitive
    impairment, 176, 526–9
brain
  in AD, 408, (Table 18.5) 410–15
  cells, changes in numbers and size,
    399–408
    in AD, 408
    in normal aging, 399–408, (Tables
      18.3, 18.4) 400–8
  cerebral pathology, 71–2
  changes
    and aging, historical accounts, 30–1
    systematic examination, 385–436
  changes in weight and volume, 386–98
    AD, 387–98
    normal aging, 386–7, (Table 18.1)
      388–93
  constituent changes, 409–27
    in AD, 409–15
    aging and dementia: amyloid
      deposits, 426–7; granulovacuolar
      degeneration, 417, 426; Hirano
      bodies, 417, 426
    development of plaques and tangles:
      in AD, 415–17; in aging, 416–17
    normal aging, 409
  derived neurotrophic factor, and aging
    and dementia, 439, 461
  microscopic changes, 398–409
    in dementia, 408, (Table 18.5)
      410–14
  nerve cell numbers and size in
    normal aging, 399–408, (Tables
      18.3, 18.4) 400–7
  'softening', historical accounts, 30

Calmeil, views on dementia, 24–5
CAMCOG, for cognitive impairment,
    175
CAMDEX (Cambridge Examination for
    Mental Disorders of the Elderly)

for cognitive impairment, 176
criteria for dementia, AD and
    multi-infarct dementia, (Table
    9.1) 168–9
criteria for mild dementia, 96, 97, 99,
    109, 110–11, 526–9
interview and criteria, 259–60
caring for people with dementia, 257–71
changes in perception, 264
discrepancies between lay and
    professional views, 267–9
expectations of age related to mental
    status, 260–6
explanations for seeing changes as
    being normal, 262
explanations for abnormal behaviour,
    261–2
Hughes Hall Project for Later Life,
    258–60
meaning of terms to different people,
    257
perceptions of dementia, 257–8, 260–1
providing information for assessments,
    275
provision and coordination of special
    services, 529–33
redefinition of the problem, 265–7
resistance to acknowledgment, 257–8
CDR (Clinical Dementia Rating scale),
    109
CERAD, efficacy of memory measures,
    303–6
cerebellar ataxia in DAT, 120, 121
choline acetyltransferase in brain,
    438–40, (Table 19.1) 441–7
in aging, 449–56
cholinergic changes
aging, 448–56
    AD, and Lewy body disease
        compared, 451, 457–60, (Table
        19.2) 452–3
    in dementia, 457–62
    in dementia and aging, 437–69
        methods of investigation, 438–48;
        parameters, 438–40, (Table 19.1)
        441–7
cholinergic depletion
in presenile and senile AD, first
    described, 47–8
research progress, 49
chromosome 21, in AD, 70, 498–503
Clinical Dementia Rating scale (CDR),
    109

cognitive decline and vascular risk
    factors in AD, 222
cognitive impairment and function, 58
behavioural measures, 176–8
classification, (Figure 15.7) 323
cognitive scales for population studies,
    174–5
components of case definition, 168–70
continuous measures, 244–53
    adjustment for education, 248–50
    advantages, 252
    description of method, 245–6
    illustration of method, 246–50
    limitations, 250–2
and continuum studies in dementia,
    555–6
in elderly people, is it benign? 93–4
epidemiology, 167–207
field studies, 174–92
mortality and population studies,
    173–4
response rates for surveys, 173
sample definition for population
    studies, 171–3
sources for population studies,
    173–4
types of diagnosis in population
    studies, 170–1
validity for the diagnosis, 171
see also language in dementia and
    normal aging; memory function in
    dementia and normal aging;
    visuospatial dysfunction
cognitive paradigm view, 15
community assessments of dementia,
    107–8
computerized tomography and
    dementia, 134–9
atrophy, 138
clinical applications, 135
clinical results, 139
effect of aging, 136–8
relationship to PET, 154–5
technical aspects, 134–5
Consortium to Establish a Registry for
    Alzheimer's Disease, see CERAD
continuity and discontinuity of
    neurobiological brain changes in
    AD, 66–7
continuity view, early twentieth century,
    21, 41–5
continuous distribution and arterial
    pressure, 64

continuum model of dementia
  AD as aging process, 57–8
  early twentieth century, 21
  for measuring dementia in community
    surveys, 244–53
  neuropathological features, 460–2
  normal aging and dementia, 277–85
    abnormalities in eating and weight,
      283
    other types of abnormal behaviour,
      284
    personality changes and dementia,
      280–2
    personality changes and normal
      aging, 280
    sleep disturbance and EEG
      recordings, 282
  public health implications, 552–60
    analogies from other diseases,
      553–6
    application, 558–9
    deciding on appropriate model,
      552–5
    neuropathological factors, 552–3
    using cognitive impairment and
      function, 555–6
  summary, 3–7, 10–11
  and incompatibility with threshold
    phenomena, 60
conversation, 346
  see also discourse
Cortex, entorhinal, cholinergic studies,
    437–69
  see also cholinergic changes;
    cholinergic depletion
cortical atrophy and dementia, 138
Cotard's syndrome, 29
Creutzfeldt–Jakob disease
  identifiable cause, 52
  neuropathological features, 457

Darwin, Erasmus, views on aging, 17
day-care programmes in dementia,
    539–41
decision tree, for diagnosing dementing
    diseases, 245
dementia
  age-specific, 190–2
  and aging
    history, 15–40; see also history of
      dementia and aging
    relationship between, historical
      factors, 19–21

of Alzheimer type
  continuum hypothesis, evidence,
    4–7
  description, 92
  disease process, evidence, 4–7
  severity, criteria and prognoses,
    96–7
  summary, 10–11
beginnings of signs of dementia, 92–3
behavioural measures, 176–8
CAMDEX, DMS-III-R, and
    NINCDS–ADRDA criteria,
    168–9
caring for people, 257–71
  see also caring for people with
    dementia
category or dimension, diagnostic
    criteria, 85
causes and criteria, 97–8
clinical/epidemiological, differing
    aspects, 197–8
cognitive scales for population studies,
    174–5
components of case definition, 168–70
continuous measures, 244–53
differential diagnosis, see diagnosis
early detection and diagnosis, 530–2
early terminology, 21, 22
early twentieth century fragmentation
    of different forms, 27
in the elderly, Roth's contribution,
    45–7
epidemiology, 167–207
field studies, 174–92
genetic affinities of different types,
    twentieth century opinions, 46–7
history of research, 41–6
  see also history of research
incidence, 190–2
levels of severity, assessment, 179
mild, see mild dementia
mortality and population studies,
    173–4
and normal aging
  relationship: as continuum
    hypothesis, 3–7; evidence
    favouring, 5–7; as disease
    process, evidence favouring, 7–10
and normal aging of the brain, 57–76
population studies and the continuum,
    195–6
prevalence studies, 180–90
  Europe, (Table 9.4) 184–5

other countries, (Table 9.6) 188–9
United Kingdom, (Table 9.3) 182–3
USA, (Table 9.5) 186–7
provision and co-ordination of special
    services, 529–33
recognition, 101–2
response rates for surveys, 173
role of post-mortem studies, 196–7
sample definition for population
    studies, 171–3
severe, disability and dependence on
    others, 527–9
sources for population studies, 173–4
terminology, 45–7
see also Alzheimer's disease;
    continuum model of dementia;
    senile dementia; and specific
    headings throughout
dementia praecox becomes
    schizophrenia, 28–9
demographic trends, elderly people, 519
dendrites and loss of dendritic spines
    in AD, 415
    in old age, 409
diagnosis
    criteria for memory impairment in
        dementia, 291–2
    criteria for research, 81–2
    decision tree, 245
    demented and non-demented subjects
        cerebral pathology, 71–2
        distinction between, in very old age,
            62–3, 65
    differential
        in the community, 192–4
        of dementia, 85–7
        in very old age, in demented and
            non-demented subjects, 179–80
    early, 542
    and health care policy, 532–4
    imaging, see imaging and dementia
    mild dementia, 105–6, 110–12
        criteria, 108–9
    neurological signs, 119–22
        reflection of accelerated or
            abnormal aging, 123–4
        results of three studies, 119–21
        subclinical, 123–4
        subgroups, 124–6
        summary, 10–11
        in uncontrolled studies, 121–2
        usefulness in diagnosis, 122–3
    in population studies, 170–1

problems in Alzheimer's disease,
    pathological and genetic aspects,
    503–10
standardized criteria, 79–90
validity, 171
see also risk factors
Diagnostic and Statistical Manual of
    Mental Disorders, third edition,
    revised, see DSM-III-R
diffuse Lewy body disease (DLBD), see
    Lewy body variant of Alzheimer's
    disease, abnormal neurological
    signs
disability and dependency, 528
discontinuity view, early twentieth
    century, 21
discourse, 353
    in dementia, 349–52
    macrostructure, 346–7
        in dementia, 350–2
        in normal aging, 347
    in normal aging, 347–9
    turn taking, 346
    use of pronouns, 347–50
discrepancies between lay and
    professional views of mental
    illness, 267–9
discrimination between dementia and
    normal aging, availability of tests,
    303–6
disease process hypothesis, summary,
    5–7, 10–11
disposable soma theory, 234–5, 238
DNA markers to local FAD, 497–503;
    see also familial Alzheimer's
    disease (FAD)
Down's syndrome, 63
    association with AD, 211–13
    family history, and AD, 216
    and neuropathology of AD, 498, 503
drug abuse, 133
drug use in mild dementia, 103
DSM-III-R
    criteria for dementia, 92–3
        AD and multi-infarct dementia,
            (Table 9.1) 168–9
    criteria for memory impairment, 291–2
    criteria for mild dementia, 109
    and DSM-IV, criteria for dementia, 82
    and ICD-10 compared, (Table 5.1) 83
    instruments for diagnosing dementia,
        84–5
    validity of criteria, 82–4

early detection and diagnosis of
    dementia, 542–3
eating, abnormalities, and the
    continuum hypothesis, 283
economic costs of dementia, 525–6
education
    cognitive score adjustment, 248
    level, and AD, 218
electroencephalogram recordings and
    sleep disturbance, and the
    continuum hypothesis, 282
environmental risk factors and AD, 50
epidemiology, 167–207
    cognitive scales for population studies,
        174–5
    community assessments, 107–8
    diagnostic criteria, 168–70
    field studies, 174–92
    incidence, 190–2
    mild dementia, 106–12
    mortality, 168, 173–4
    population statistics, 170–1
    post-mortem studies, 196–7
    prevalence studies, 180–90, 111–12
    response rates, 173
    risk factors, see risk factors
    sample definition, 171–3
    validity for diagnosis, 171
Esquirol, views on dementia, 23–4
EURODEM meta-analysis
    of AD, 192–3
    of vascular dementia, 194
European Community countries, health
    care and social expenditures,
    520–1
European Concerted Action on
    Dementias (EURODEM),
    prevalence studies, 181
expectations of age related to mental
    status, 260–6
    interpretations of mental illness by
        carers, 257–8, 263–7
    lay and professional discrepancies,
        267–9
expenditure, national, on health care,
    520–1
extensor plantar responses in dementia,
    121
extrapyramidal features in DAT, 120,
    121

familial Alzheimer's disease (FAD)
    chromosome defect, 493–7

example families, 495–7
    hunting the gene, 497–503
families' perceptions and dementia,
    102–3
family history of dementia, association
    with AD, 213–14
fluency tests, 315, 319
focal lobar atrophies, see Pick's disease
food intake, continuum hypothesis and
    normal aging, 283
forgetfulness, senescent, 385
    is it benign? 93–4
    see also memory function in dementia
        and normal aging
fragile X syndrome, 63
French views on dementia, nineteenth
    century, 23–8
frequency distributions, normal, and
    threshold effects, 59–61
frontal lobes
    atrophy, 154–5
    dementia, 150, 151, 154, 155
    HMPAO studies, 150–1
    oxygen and glucose reduction, 154
frontal release phenomena in DAT, 119,
    120, 121, 122
frontal release signs, descriptions, 127
future levels of need and demand for
    services, predicting, 522–4

gait
    in dementia, 121
    disturbance in DAT, 120, 121
general paralysis of the insane, 27–8
general practice perspective of mild
    dementia, 98–103
general practitioners, guidelines for
    intervention, 542–3
genetics
    dementias, twentieth century
        opinions, 46–7
    factors in aging, 234–5
    linkage
        in Alzheimer's disease, 492–516;
        APP gene studies, 504–6; Val–Ile
        mutation, 504–6; early/late onset,
        505; hunting the gene, 497–503;
        understanding AD, 503–11
    introduction and historical features,
        492–7
    recombination studies, 493–7
research progress, 49–50
Georget, views on dementia, 24

Geriatric Mental State (GMS)
  examination for continuous
  measuring, 246
Geriatric Mental State (GMS) schedule,
  110, 111
geriatric nursing-home care in dementia,
  534–5, 536–9
Gerstmann–Straussler disease
  APP mutations, 505
  neuropathological features, 457
glabellar tap
  in DAT, 120, 121
  description, 127
global–local stimuli
  in AD, 370–4
  in normal elderly, 375
glucose, cerebral metabolic rate, 154
glutamate N-methyl-D-aspartate
  (MK801) binding, normal aging
  and AD, (Figure 19.1), 450,
  450–1
GMS (Geriatric Mental State), 110, 111
Gowers' 'abiotrophy', 42–4
granulovacuolar degeneration, 552
  in Alzheimer-type changes, 57
  brain, aging and dementia, 417, 426
graphaesthesia in DAT, 120, 121
grasp responses
  in DAT, 120, 121
  in dementia, 121
  description, 127
growth rate of numbers of persons over
  65 years, 519
guilt after death, 268
Guislain, views on dementia, 25

Hallervorden–Spatz disease,
  neuropathological features, 457
hallucinations in Lewy body disease, 459
head trauma, association with AD,
  215–16, 221, 222
health care in dementia
  day-care and home-care programmes,
  539–41
  decline in hospital in-patient care,
  534–5
  early detection and diagnosis, 530–2
  future prospects, research and
  services, 543–5
  geriatric nursing home care, 534–535,
  536–9
  internationally, 519–51
  issues of service provision, 529–30

long-stay hospital and residential care,
  534
medical investigation, treatment and
  management, 532–3
nursing home residents, 534–5
provision and co-ordination of special
  services, 529–33
role of primary health-care services,
  541–43
and social expenditures of European
  Community countries, 1981–82,
  as proportion of total gross
  domestic product, 520–1
see also public health implications of a
  continuum model of dementia;
  public health problem
Health and Lifestyle Survey, 316
analysis for age differences in
  memory, 317
hippocampus, cholinergic studies, see
  cholinergic changes; cholinergic
  depletion
Hirano bodies, 552
brain, development in aging and
  dementia, 417–26
history of dementia and aging, 15–40
  before 1800, 21–2
  during 1800–1899, 23
  1800 to present day, 15–21
  fragmentation of concepts, 27
  French views, 23–6
  general paralysis of the insane, 27–8
  naming and accepting AD, 33–4
  specific terminology and diseases,
  28–33
history of research, 41–56
  1920–1955, 44–5
  early twentieth century, 41–5
  Gowers' 'abiotrophy', 42–4
HIV infection and dementia diagnosis,
  86–7
HMPAO imaging, 132–3, 147–51
hoarding and normal aging, 284
Hobart community study of dementia,
  246
home-care programmes in dementia,
  539–41
homocystinuria, 63
hospital care, 534–6
Hounsfield units (HU) and dementia,
  138–9
Hughes Hall Project for Later Life,
  258–60

Huntington's disease
    identifiable cause, 52
    neuropathological features, 457
hyperactive tendon reflexes in dementia,
    121

ICD-10
    chapter on mental and behavioural
        disorders, 79–87
    classification of the dementias, (Table
        5.2) 86
    criteria for dementia, 92–3
    criteria for memory impairment,
        291–2
    criteria of mild dementia, 109
    Diagnostic Criteria for Research, 81–2
    and DSM-III-R compared, (Table 5.1)
        83
    instruments for diagnosing dementia,
        84–5
    validity of criteria, 82–4
images of dementia by carers, 257–8,
    260–3, 264–7
imaging and dementia, 130–63
    case mix/spectrum, 131
    methods of data analysis, 132–4
    sensitivity, specificity, predictive
        values and disease, 133
    study design, 130–2
    see also specific techniques
incidence of dementia, 190–2
incontinence and normal aging, 284
institutional care for the elderly, rates,
        European Community countries,
        521
International Classification of
        Diseases-10, see ICD-10
international criteria and differential
        diagnosis, 79–90
international personality disorder
        evaluation, 81

12 kDA protein fragment, monoclonal
        antibody recognition, 472–3
Kety–Schmidt technique, 153

lack of understanding, see expectations
        of age related to mental status
language in dementia and normal aging,
        331–65
    changes across the lifespan, 331
    definition, 331
    directions for future research, 357–8
    misdiagnosis, 354–5
    reference and discourse structure,
        345–52, 353
    response time studies, 355
    syntax, 339–45
    word finding, 332–8
    see also fluency tests: name-finding
        difficulties; naming latency;
        vocabulary
lay and professional views of mental
        illness, 267–9
    implications of discrepancies, 268–9
Lesch–Nyhan syndrome, 63
leukoariosis, 137, 145, 222
Lewy body disease, 504
    AD and aging compared, for
        cholinergic changes in the brain,
        451, 457–60, (Table 19.2) 452–3
    neuropathological features, 457–60,
        461
Lewy body disorders, and AD
        compared, 507–8
Lewy body variant of Alzheimer's
        disease, abnormal neurological
        signs, 124–5
lexical decision tasks, 333
lipofuscin accumulation, changes in
        brain
    in AD, 409–15
    in normal aging, 409
lobar atrophies, see Pick's disease
long-stay hospital in dementia, 534

macrophages and senile atrophy, early
        opinions, 20–1
magnetic resonance imaging and
        dementia, 140–7
    clinical imaging, 142–5
    clinical results, 142
    general factors, 140
    magnetic resonance spectroscopy,
        145–7
    measurement of T_1 and T_2, 141–2
    relationship to PET, 154–5
Marc, views on dementia, 25–6
medical investigation, treatment and
        management, in dementia, 532–3
Memory Clinics, 532
memory function in dementia and
        normal aging, 291–330, 323–4,
        (Table 15.5) 324
    cross-sectional studies, 316–17
    diagnostic criteria, 291–2

discrimination between dementia and
    normal aging, 303–6
episodic memory, direct vs. indirect
    measures, 298–9
framework for analysing memory,
    292–4
longitudinal studies, 318–21
can memory impairment predict
    dementia? 306–7
memory performance in elderly
    population samples, 314–21
rates of forgetting, 299–300
remote versus recent memory, 300–1
selection of subjects, 295
semantic memory, 301–2, 311–14
similarities and differences in memory
    performance, 295–8
similarity between dementia- and
    age-related impairments, 307–8
younger/older adults, 308–11
mental disorders, ICD-10, 79–87
microtubule associated protein tau, see
    tau protein
mild cognitive disorder, ICD-10 criteria,
    87
mild dementia
    assessment schedules, 110–12
    clinical perspective, 91–117
    community assessments, 107–8
    community-minded perspective, 91
    diagnosis, 105–6, 108–9
    disability and dependence on others,
        527–9
    epidemiological perspective, 106–12
    families' perceptions, 102–3
    general practice perspective, 98–103
    general practitioner, psychiatric, and
        epidemiological viewpoints, 91–2
    German research project, 527
    importance of preventive strategies,
        103
    late referral to GP, 103
    management of tasks, 98–101
    practical consequences, 98–100
    progression, 95–8
    pseudo-dementia, 104–5
    psychiatric perspective, 103–5
    as public health problem, 525–9
    recognition, 101–2
Mini-Mental State Examination
    (MMSE), 175, 259, 305
    for cognitive impairment, 175, 177,
        181
for continuous measuring, 247
in mild dementia, 105, 109, 110
molecular changes
    analysis of structural changes in AD
        and in brains of normal aged,
        67–8
    neurodegenerative, 470–91
        characterization of neurofibrillary
            pathology of AD, 472
        distinguishing normal aging from
            AD, 470–91
        normal function and distribution of
            tau protein, 473–5
molecular genetics, research progress,
    49–50
monoclonal antibodies in AD diagnosis,
    472–3, 475–7
Morel, views on dementia, 26
mouse chromosome 16, involvement in
    AD, 503
multi-infarct dementia (MID), 60, 145
    CAMDEX, DMS-III-R, and
        NINCDS–ADRDA criteria,
        168–9
    threshold effects, 61
muscarinic receptor
    in AD and Lewy body disease, 459
    changes with aging, 450–1
muscle tone in DAT, 121
myoclonus in DAT, 121

name-finding difficulties, 311–14
naming latency, 333
national expenditures on health care,
    520–1
National Institute of Neurological and
    Communication Disorders and
    Stroke (NINCDS), 120
nerve cells
    numbers and size, brain changes,
        399–408
    in AD, 408
    in normal aging, 399–408, (Tables
        18.3, 18.4) 400–7
    and PHF in AD, 478
nerve growth factor receptor in brain
    cholinergic system studies,
    438–440, (Table 19.1) 441–7
    in aging, 449
neural aging and Alzheimer's dementia,
    50–2
neurodegenerative changes to distinguish
    normal aging from AD, 470–91

neurofibrillary tangles, 552
  absence, and AD diagnosis, 477
  AD-type changes, 57
    molecular analysis, 67–8
  and β/A4 deposits, 483–4
  development in brain
    in AD, 415–7
    in aging, 415–7
  immunoelectronmicroscopy, 472,
    (Figure 20.2) 473
  later twentieth century research, 45–7
  and pathological process of AD, 59
  PHF accumulation in AD, 477
  recognised by Alzheimer, 43
neurological aspects of dementia and
    normal aging, 118–29
  and accelerated or abnormal aging,
    123–4
  effect on diagnosis, 122–3
  identification of subgroups of DAT
    patients, 124–6
  increased neurological signs in DAT,
    119–22
neurons, brain, reserve capacity,
    208–210
neuropathology
  in dementia and normal aging,
    385–436
  development during the nineteenth
    century, 20
nicotine binding, age-related decline,
    normal aging and AD, 450–1
NINCDS–ADRDA criteria for
    dementia, AD and multi-infarct
    dementia, 3–4, (Table 9.1) 120,
    121, 168–9
non-demented and demented subjects
  cerebral pathology, 71–2
  distinction between, in very old age,
    62–3, 65
normal aging
  acceptable cutpoint, 195–6
  discrimination between normal aging
    and dementia, 303–6
  distinction from AD patients, 65–6
    molecular analysis, 67–8
  threshold model, 208–10
nucleolar volume
  reduction in brain
    in AD, 415
    in normal aging, 409
numbers of persons over 65 years,
    growth rate, 519

nursing care for the elderly, 544–5
nursing home care, geriatric, in
    dementia, 534–5, 536–9
nursing homes, alternatives, 539–40

olfaction, impaired in DAT, 120, 121
onset of symptoms, reserve capacity of
    brain, 208–10
organic apoplexy, early descriptions,
    31–2
oxygen, cerebral metabolic rate, 153–4

P-31 spectroscopy, 146
paired helical filament (PHF)
  accumulation
    in destruction of nerve cells in AD,
      478
    failure to correlate with β-amyloid
      deposits, 482
    as feature of AD not of aging,
      478–80
    in grey matter, and
      neuropathological lesions in AD,
      correlation between, 477
  as basis for immunochemical assay for
    AD, 475
  PHF-tau protein assays, 475–8
  in immunoelectronmicroscopy of
    neurofibrillary tangles, 472,
    (Figure 20.2) 473
palmomental reflex, description, 127
paratonia (gagenhalten), description, 127
parenchymal amyloid deposits, 552
  brain, in normal aging and AD, 427
parietal sensory signs in DAT, 120, 121
Parkinson's disease, neuropathological
    features, 461
pathological and normal aging in
    cerebrum, 71–2
  comparison with AD, 71–2
perception, changes at two-year
    follow-up, 264
perceptions of dementia, 257–8, 260–1
perfusion defects, 150–2
personality
  assessment, 277, (Table 14.1) 278–9
  changes
    and dementia, and the continuum
      hypothesis, 280–2
    and normal aging, and the
      continuum hypothesis, 280
  definition, 273
  in dementia and normal aging, 271–90

phenylketonuria, 63
Pick's disease
    abnormal neurological signs, 125–6
    identifiable cause, 52
    neuropathological features, 457
Pinel, and terminology for cognitive
        impairment, 22
plaques, 552
    and AD diagnosis, 470
    development in brain
        in AD, 415–17
        in aging, 415–17
    later twentieth century research, 45–7
    PHF accumulation in AD, 477
    recognised by Alzheimer, 43
    senile
        in Alzheimer-type changes, 57
        described by Simchowicz, 43
population studies, 167–207
    see also diagnosis: epidemiology
positron emission tomography and
        dementia, 153–5
    brain metabolism and age, 153–4
    clinical studies, 154
    relationship to CT and MRI, 154–5
'prehensile' release signs in dementia,
        121
premature senility, relationship to
        presenile AD, 43
presenile dementia, relationship to senile
        dementia, 43
present behavioural examination,
        interview, 275
prevalence, 111–12, 180–90
prevalence of dementia, 111–12, 180–90
primary health-care services, role in
        dementia, 541–43
prolonging life, concept, historical
        factors, 19–20
pronouns, use in discourse, 347–8
    in dementia, 349–50
    in normal aging, 347
proton spectroscopy, 146–7
pseudo-dementia
    characteristics, 104–5
    definition, 104
    and vesanic dementia, terminology
        during nineteenth century, 29–30
psychiatric hospital beds in European
        countries, numbers and ratios,
        1950–80, 534–5
psychiatric perspective of mild dementia,
        103–5

psychiatric referral in mild dementia,
        103–4
psychiatric service for old age, key
        resources, 532
psychogeriatric nursing homes in
        European countries, 537–8
public health implications of a
        continuum model of dementia,
        552–60
    analogies from other diseases, 553–6
    application, 558–9
    deciding on appropriate model, 552–5
    neuropathological factors, 552–3
    using cognitive impairment and
        function, 555–7
public health problem
    dimensions, 522–9
    economic cost of dementia, 524–5
    predicting future levels of need and
        demand for services, 522–4
    significance of mild dementia, 525–9
    see also health care in dementia

rating scales for behaviour, 274–7
reaction time performance
    in AD, 373–4
    in normal elderly, 375
reference and discourse structure in
        dementia and normal aging,
        345–52, 353
regression analysis to predict cognitive
        performance, 247–8
remote versus recent memory in
        dementia and normal aging,
        300–1
research, ICD-10 criteria, 81–2
research into dementia
    care for patients, 542, 543–5
    European Community, 544
    USA, 544
reserve capacity of brain, 208–10
residential care in dementia, 534
response time studies in normal aging
        and dementia, 355
restriction fragment length
        polymorphisms (RFLPs), to
        detect FAD, 497, 498
risk factors
    for AD, 210–19
        do certain exposures lower or raise
            age of onset? 220–1
        identification, dependence on
            statistical power, 219–20

risk factors – *cont'd.*
for AD – *cont'd.*
interaction between, and increasing
risk of AD, 221–2
and aging mechanisms, 230–43
for dementia, 208–29
aetiological aspects, 239–40
rooting, description, 127

schedule for clinical assessment in
neuropsychiatry, 81
schizophrenia, previously known as
dementia praecox, 28–9
screaming and normal aging, 284
segregated care for the demented,
policies, 538–9
semantic memory in dementia and
normal aging, 301–2,
311–14
senescence and evolution of aging,
232–3
senescent changes, timing, 236–7
senile dementia
and AD, naming, in 1910, 33
of Alzheimer type, publications
1964–90, 48
early twentieth century, relationships
and terminology, 42–5
genetic affinities, twentieth century
opinions, 46–7
of Lewy body type, *see* Lewy body
variant of Alzheimer's disease,
abnormal neurological signs
relationship to AD, 44–5
terminology, 44–5
see also dementia
senium praecox concept, 479
services for the elderly, future prospects,
543–5
sex incidence, 190
shouting and normal aging, 284
single photon emission tomography and
dementia, 147–52
clinical studies, 149–52
technical aspects, 147–9
sleep disturbance and EEG recordings,
and the continuum hypothesis,
282
smoking, role in AD, 217–18, 221
snout (or pout) reflex (response)
in DAT, 120, 121
in dementia, 121
description, 127

social and health care expenditures of
European Community countries,
1981–82, as proportion of total
gross domestic product, 520–1
social planning, *see* health care in
dementia
socioeconomic status and AD, 218
special services for dementia, 529–33
issues of service provision, 529
spectrin, changes in brain in AD, 415
storage of information, adults of
different ages, 311
strokes, and dementia, early
descriptions, 32
suck responses in dementia, 121
sucking, description, 127
synaptophysin, changes in brain
in AD, 415
in normal aging, 409
syntax in AD, 342–5
attention deficits, 343
involvement of memory, 343–4
linguistic vs. non-linguistic processing
demands, 343–4
syntax complexity test, 342
syntax and normal aging, 339–342
sentence comprehension and memory,
340–1

tangles, *see* neurofibrillary tangles
tau protein
binding to β/A4 amyloid, 506–7
changes in normal and pathological
aging, 478–80
distribution and normal function,
473–5
measure of changes in AD, 475–8
and PHF protein assays, 475–8
present in AD, 68, 475–7
technetium-99m HMPAO imaging, 132,
147–51
temporal lobe atrophy, 133
temporal perfusion defects, 152
threshold model for dementia, 208–10
threshold phenomena
in AD, 59–61
in common diseases, 63–6
incompatible with simple continuum
theories, 60
in other mental disorders, 61–3
thyroid disease as risk factor in AD, 216
'tip-of-the-tongue' memory difficulties,
313

tremor in DAT, 120, 121
trophic factors in the nervous system,
    and aging research, 461

Val–Ile mutation of APP gene, 504
vascular amyloid deposits, 552
    brain, in normal aging and AD, 427
vascular dementia, differential diagnosis
    in the community, 193–5
vascular risk factors and cognitive
    decline, in AD, 222
vesamicol binding, alterations, 458
vesanic dementias
    described in 1852, 25
    and pseudo-dementia, terminology
        during nineteenth century, 29–30
views of dementia by carers, 258–9,
    260–3, 264–7
visual–perceptual problems in AD,
    336–7
visuospatial dysfunction in Alzheimer's
    disease, past studies, 368–74
    backward visual masking tasks,
        369–70
    component processes, 369
    global–local stimuli, 370–4
    reaction time performance, 373–4
    temporal–parietal lobe involvement,
        368–9
visuospatial dysfunction in dementia and
    normal aging, 366–81
    general background, 366–7
    implications of past research findings
        on continuum versus categorical
        models, 376–7

visuospatial dysfunction in the normal
    elderly, past studies, 374–6
    backward visual masking tasks, 375
    cross-sectional studies, 375–6
    global–local stimuli, 375
vocabulary
    at 1 year, 332
    adult, 332
    see also word finding

wandering and normal aging, 284
Wechsler memory scale, exclusion
    criteria, 315
weight, abnormalities, and the
    continuum hypothesis, 283
Werner's syndrome, characteristics,
    58
WHODEMMS research project into
    dementia, 544
word finding, 332–8, 353–4
    in AD, 335–8
        lexical retrieval problems, 335
        'place fillers', 335
        semantically related words, 335
    background, 332
    in dementia
        lexical knowledge problems, 335
        visual–perceptual problems, 336–7
    in normal aging, 333–5
        retrieval deficits, 333–4
        semantic priming effects, 334
        storage of words, 333
        structure of lexical knowledge,
            333–4
word fluency tests in the elderly, 315